The Molecular Biology of Cancer

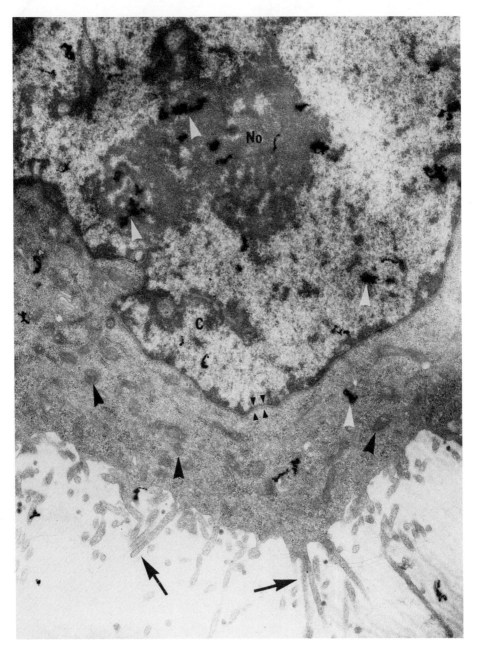

A margin of a nucleus and cytoplasm of a Novikoff hepatoma ascites cell. There are many lengthy microvilli (arrows) of the plasma membrane on the cytoplasmic surface. The two layers of the nuclear envelope are distinct (small pointer) as are the cytoplasmic mitochondria (large pointers). There are canaliculi (C) between the inner layer of the nuclear envelope and the nucleoplasm. This cell was exposed previously to labeled uridine for 60 minutes, and there are a number of grains (white pointers) in the nucleolus (No) and the nucleoplasm, as well as the cytoplasm (Courtesy of Drs. T. Unuma, K. Smetana, and Y. Daskal).

THE MOLECULAR BIOLOGY OF CANCER

Edited by

HARRIS BUSCH

DEPARTMENT OF PHARMACOLOGY
BAYLOR COLLEGE OF MEDICINE
TEXAS MEDICAL CENTER
HOUSTON, TEXAS

ACADEMIC PRESS   New York and London   1974
A Subsidiary of Harcourt Brace Jovanovich, Publishers

ACADEMIC PRESS, INC.
111 Fifth Avenue, New York, New York 10003

United Kingdom Edition published by
ACADEMIC PRESS, INC. (LONDON) LTD.
24/28 Oval Road, London NW1

LIBRARY OF CONGRESS CATALOG CARD NUMBER: 73-7442

PRINTED IN THE UNITED STATES OF AMERICA

DEDICATION

This book is dedicated to the millions of our fellow human beings who have died from cancer. It is our fervent hope that some day human endeavor will end the untold suffering produced by this disease.

Contents

PART I GENERAL ASPECTS OF MOLECULAR BIOLOGY OF CANCER

Chapter I Introduction

Harris Busch

Chapter II The Nucleus of the Cancer Cell

Harris Busch and Karel Smetana

Chapter III   **Chromosomes in the Causation and Progression of
Cancer and Leukemia**

Avery A. Sandberg and Masaharu Sakurai

Chapter IV   **DNA: Replication, Modification, and Repair**

Thomas W. Sneider

Chapter V   **Messenger RNA and Other High Molecular Weight RNA**

Harris Busch

Chapter VI   **Low Molecular Weight Nuclear RNA**

Tae Suk Ro-Choi and Harris Busch

Chapter XI   Oncogenic Viruses

Matilda Benyesh-Melnick and Janet S. Butel

PART III SPECIAL ASPECTS OF THE CANCER PHENOTYPE

Chapter XII   Molecular Correlation Concept

George Weber

Chapter XIII   Phenotypic Variability as a Manifestation of Translational Control

Henry C. Pitot, Thomas K. Shires, Geoffrey Moyer, and Carleton T. Garrett

Chapter XIV   Plasmacytomas

Michael Potter

List of Contributors

Numbers in parentheses indicate the pages on which the authors' contributions begin.

MATILDA BENYESH-MELNICK (403), Department of Virology and Epidemiology, Baylor College of Medicine, Houston, Texas

EDWARD BRESNICK (277), Department of Cell and Molecular Biology, Medical College of Georgia, Augusta, Georgia

HARRIS BUSCH (1, 41, 187, 241, 309), Department of Pharmacology, Baylor College of Medicine, Texas Medical Center, Houston, Texas

JANET S. BUTEL (403), Department of Virology and Epidemiology, Baylor College of Medicine, Houston, Texas

CARLETON T. GARRETT (523), Department of Oncology and Pathology, McArdle Laboratory, University of Wisconsin Medical School, Madison, Wisconsin

A. CLARK GRIFFIN (355), The University of Texas at Houston, M. D. Anderson Hospital and Tumor Institute, Texas Medical Center, Houston, Texas

ELIZABETH C. MILLER (377), McArdle Laboratory for Cancer Research, University of Wisconsin Medical Center, Madison, Wisconsin

JAMES A. MILLER (377), McArdle Laboratory for Cancer Research, University of Wisconsin Medical Center, Madison, Wisconsin

GEOFFREY MOYER* (523), Departments of Oncology and Pathology, McArdle Laboratory, University of Wisconsin Medical School, Madison, Wisconsin

MARK O. J. OLSON (309), Department of Pharmacology, Baylor College of Medicine, Houston, Texas

HENRY C. PITOT (523), Department of Oncology and Pathology, McArdle Laboratory, University of Wisconsin Medical School, Madison, Wisconsin

MICHAEL POTTER (535), Laboratory of Cell Biology, National Cancer Institute, National Institutes of Health, Bethesda, Maryland

* Present address: Department of Pathology, School of Medicine, University of California, Los Angeles, California.

TAE SUK RO-CHOI (241), Department of Pharmacology, Baylor College of Medicine, Texas Medical Center, Houston, Texas

MASAHARU SAKURAI (81), Department of Medicine C, Roswell Park Memorial Institute, Buffalo, New York

AVERY A. SANDBERG (81), Department of Medicine C, Roswell Park Memorial Institute, Buffalo, New York

THOMAS K. SHIRES* (523), Departments of Oncology and Pathology, McArdle Laboratory, University of Wisconsin Medical School, Madison, Wisconsin

KAREL SMETANA (41), Department of Pharmacology, Baylor College of Medicine, Texas Medical Center, Houston, Texas

THOMAS W. SNEIDER (107), Department of Pharmacology, Baylor College of Medicine, Houston, Texas

WESLEY C. STARBUCK (309), Department of Pharmacology, Baylor College of Medicine, Houston, Texas

GEORGE WEBER (487), Department of Pharmacology, Indiana University School of Medicine, Indianapolis, Indiana

* Present address: Toxicology Center, Departments of Pharmacology and Pathology, Medical School, University of Iowa, Iowa City, Iowa.

Preface

In the ten years since "An Introduction to the Biochemistry of the Cancer Cell" was published an enormous amount of progress has been made in the cancer field. The events that were underway at that time which provided a basis for the understanding of gene function and the various roles of DNA, RNA, gene control proteins, and other important elements of cellular function have partially reached fruition. A huge literature has developed which is difficult for the graduate student, fellow, and many workers in the field to fully comprehend, and, accordingly, it seemed appropriate at this time to once again attempt to prepare a treatise that would at least cover the broad areas of this field. The goal of this volume is to acquaint the student of oncology with the state of progress in the molecular biology of cancer and to provide literature references which hopefully will give a more detailed review of special topics.

The cancer cell is characterized by its ability to escape from homeostatic controls. It can metastasize, invade, and grow independently of host controls whereas other cells must contribute to the welfare of the host. It is still uncertain whether the special features of cancer cells are simply aberrant manifestations of normal gene readouts or whether new information is brought into the cell that produces unusual functions. This volume presents the current status of information regarding these aspects of molecular biology of cancer in Part I, a number of aspects of chemical and viral carcinogenesis in Part II, and some special features of the variable phenotypes of cancer cells in Part III.

In a sense the cancer problem is very similar to an iceberg in that only a peak of information on its complexity is visible. It is clear from the literature that enormous progress is required at the molecular level in cancer in important areas such as the chemistry of DNA and messenger RNA; it is unfortunately slow because of the serious difficulties in making technological advances in these fields. On the other hand, there is gratifying progress in the field of protein synthesis, including structural and functional information on contributory molecules and, recently, in the field of gene control by nuclear proteins. Unfortunately, it has not yet been possible to specifically single out either critical elements involved in cell growth or more importantly the special features of the cancer process.

In the fields of carcinogenesis, basic and meaningful advances have occurred in our understanding of metabolism of chemical carcinogens and in the multiple types of oncogenic viruses. Progress in these fields has been impressive at the experimental level, but extension or application of this information to the human problem has been slow and very difficult as indicated in Chapters X and XI.

As noted in "An Introduction to the Biochemistry of the Cancer Cell," cancer cells repress many phenotypic functions of their cells of orgin and derepress other phenotypic features. As pointed out in Chapter XII some of these alterations of phenotype reflect quantitative reductions of gene activity. Conversely, others reflect a production of new gene products such as species of molecules found only in embryos rather than in adult cells. Some of these events are apparently random and others may be of great importance to growth and survival of cancer cells. However, there is still no clear single phenotype that is characteristic of cancer cells.

Many of the older generation of research workers in the cancer field were greatly stimulated by Jesse Greenstein's "The Biochemistry of Cancer" and some of the earlier works that dealt primarily with carbohydrate metabolism. The enormous progress in molecular biology has reoriented cancer research by providing new methods, new concepts, and new information. Many of these important methods in cancer research are reviewed in the current series of ten volumes which deal specifically with the uses and evaluation of methods in this field (*Methods in Cancer Research*, H. Busch, ed.)

In connection with the literature covered, it should be noted that the amount of research in the cancer field as well as in allied disciplines is great. There are now multiple encyclopedias and other volumes on specific aspects of the problem. This volume is not intended to substitute for such works, but rather to balance a broad and general review with sufficient detail for comprehension of more specific literature. The authors are apologetic for the omission of many important contributory works, but the goals of this volume could simply not have been achieved by the broadest possible coverage. For more extensive and detailed reviews the readers are urged to consult either the primary literature or such distinguished series as *Advances in Cancer Research* (S. Weinhouse and G. Klein, eds.).

Although cancer is under attack in a wide variety of areas, the need is still pressing for intensive and unremitting dedication to the task for new ideas and for the development of interest in young and keen minds. The discrepancy between the urgency of the problem that confronts both patient and clinician and the slow but steady pace of progress is all too apparent to those of us who have seen loved ones slowly dying from this disease. Yet, we all recognize that patient effort, enormous stamina, and endurance as well as all of the other attributes of dedication are the only approaches to the solution of the problem.

The present state of knowledge of cancer is the result of idealism, devotion, and effort of many distinguished and dedicated scientists. Their accomplishments provide the basis of the hope that we and our successors can continue to develop new knowledge and methods to the point that cancer can be conquered.

Harris Busch

Acknowledgments

I am extremely thankful to each of the authors of the various chapters of this work for their diligence and promptness in preparing their chapters. It is clear that as each of the contributory fields to cancer research evolves the expertise of investigators in special fields is particularly critical for both comprehension and interpretation of various types of specific information. Accordingly, it seems clear that in future works of this type more rather than fewer specialized chapters will be required.

I am extremely appreciative for critical reading of the manuscripts and helpful suggestions by Dr. Ferenc Gyorkey, Professor of Pathology and Pharmacology, Baylor College of Medicine; Dr. Frank E. Smith, Associate Professor, Department of Pharmacology, Baylor College of Medicine; Dr. Yong C. Choi, Research Associate Professor, Department of Pharmacology, Baylor College of Medicine; Dr. Ross N. Nazar, Assistant Professor, Department of Pharmacology, Baylor College of Medicine, Dr. Stanley W. Crooke, Instructor, Department of Pharmacology, Baylor College of Medicine; Dr. Thomas O. Sitz, Instructor, Department of Pharmacology, Baylor College of Medicine, Mr. Charles W. Taylor, Instructor, Department of Pharmacology, Baylor College of Medicine; and Dr. Lynn C. Yeoman, Instructor, Department of Pharmacology, Baylor College of Medicine.

We wish to acknowledge the aid of the Public Health Service for support of much of the basic research reported; in particular, the Cancer Research Center Grant CA-10893, the Welch Foundation, the National Science Foundation, as well as the American Cancer Society for institutional and other support.

We wish to express our appreciation to the following for permission to reproduce figures: Dr. T. C. Hsu for Figures, 1.12 and 1.17; Dr. Avery Sandberg for Figure 1.13, Dr. David Hungerford for Figure 1.14; Dr. Arthur Cole for Figure 1.15; Professor G. Attardi for Figure 1.16; Dr. George G. Rose for Figure 2.2; Dr. Ferenc Gyorkey for samples for Figures 2.3, 2.11A, 2.18B, and 2.19; Dr. Robert Love for Figure 2.8, Dr. Edgar C. Henshaw for Figure 5.1a and b; Dr. Howard Savage for Figures 5.3a and b; Dr. Roger Chalkley for Figures 8.2 and 8.9; Dr. Vincent G. Allfrey for Figure 8.13; Dr. Pierre Chambon for Figure 8.14 and Dr. Andre Vorbrodt for Figure 8.15.

CHAPTER I

Introduction

HARRIS BUSCH

I. The Importance of Cancer as a Disease

Approximately 350,000 persons will die in the United States in 1974 from cancer or complications developing in the course of the disease. The number of new cases developed each year is estimated to be approximately twice the number. The long duration of the disease and its chronically debilitating effects produce a serious economic burden to the patients and to the community. Because cancer chiefly affects the older population, it produces a serious loss of valuable persons who have important knowledge and training. Aside from the fact that neoplastic disease is associated with death and debility, a major concern of both the laity and the medical profession is the intractable pain which may develop in the later stages of the disease. The nature of the disease and its prevalence have spurred the development of the National Cancer Act which provides for large research institutes for the study of cancer and allocation of funds to medical schools and universities for the study of fundamental aspects of the disease. Moreover, vast expenditures have been made by private agencies, pharmaceutical industries, and the government in an effort to find curative drugs, palliative drugs, and new measures for combating the disease. While advances have been made in therapy, they have not yet markedly affected the morbidity and the mortality of the disease. Accordingly, it has become increasingly clear that fundamental knowledge about the nature of the cancer cell and its distinguishing properties must be obtained before approaches can be made to therapy on truly rational grounds.

II. The Biological Nature of the Cancer Cell

The fundamental problem in cancer is the cancer cell (27) which exhibits the property of division that is not subject to the usual homeostatic control mechanisms of the host. Since the daughter cells from these divisions exhibit similar properties, the cancer problem is generally believed to be a genetic problem involving biochemical disorders or aberrations of normal molecular biology.

Neoplastic lesions, or tumors, consist of many cells which have an altered phenotype that results in differences in both histological and biological properties from other cells. For example, cancer cells have darker staining nuclei, more chromatin, and more mitoses than cells of the tissues of origin (Figs. 1.1–1.3). In addition, cancerous lesions exhibit the pathological properties of invasion of normal tissues and entry into cellular masses such as muscle cells. Metastasis is the escape of cancer cells from the original locus of the tumor and passage via the blood or lymphatic tissues to another tissue or organ where the cells lodge and produce secondary tumor masses, which may be much larger than those of the tissue of origin and may be lethal.

The tumor masses are generally composed of many millions of cells (10^7 to 10^9 cells) and the degree of damage to the host is dependent both on the rate of cell division and the anatomic locus of the tumors. Although tumors are divided into malignant (cancerous) and nonmalignant (benign) tumors, based upon considerations of their lethality, a benign tumor may have a very "malignant location," and a malignant tumor may be so located or so slowly growing that at least initially the damage it produces is very small.

Regardless of whether they are slowly or rapidly growing, malignant tumors ultimately kill the patient. This end result may develop through local effects such as erosion or penetration of blood vessels, hemorrhage, infection, displacement, restricted oxygenation, or mass effects, e.g., colonic obstruction and loss of liver function.

A. Morphological and Ultrastructural Properties

Many efforts have been made to give a specific definition of the cancer cell. Table 1.1A and 1.1B indicate the light and electron microscopic characteristics that have been found for neoplastic cells (123). The more malignant the tumor and the more rapid the growth rate the more of these changes are found (27, 123, 162, 167). For example, Fig. 1.1 demonstrates nucleolar aberrations and dense cytoplasmic basophilia. Figures 1.2–1.4 show the irregular form of nuclei of cancer or leukemic cells. Figures 1.3 and 1.4 show densities of chromatin structures in leukemic lymphoblasts. Figures 1.5 and 1.6 show irregularities of mitochondria including defective ultrastructures and swelling. Figure 1.7 shows filamentous structures in the cytoplasm of a leukemic monoblast and a dilated perinuclear space which may be related to nuclear abnormalities. Figure 1.8 shows similar filamentous structures in the cytoplasm of a hepatoma. Figures 1.9 and 1.10 show cytoplasmic variations in a human plasmacytoma and immature leukemic lymphocytes. In Fig. 1.9 the Golgi apparatus appears to be hypertrophic but in Fig. 1.10 it is small (hypotrophic). These ultrastructural variations, particularly with respect to the cytoplasmic structures, reflect differences in the degree of differentiation and dedifferentiation of cancer cells. These variations produce the greater or lesser phenotypic expressions of the cells of origin of these tumors (17, 33, 41, 123). In some cases, such as melanomas, insulinomas, and plasmacytomas, the tumors may produce sufficient signs and symptoms to permit early diagnosis of the disease.

B. The Nucleolus

One development of the 1930's that captured the attention of oncologists and later of molecular biologists was the report first from the Mayo clinic (101–103)

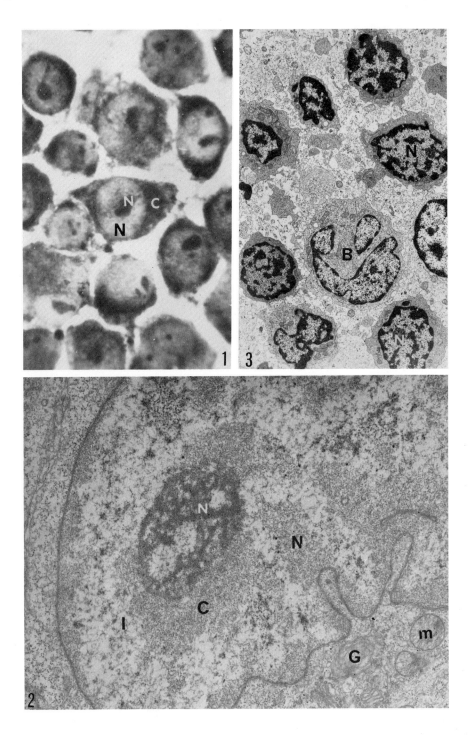

and later from Sweden (36) that the morphology of nucleoli was aberrant in cancer cells (Fig. 1.11). Large numbers of studies have been made on the morphology of neoplastic cells ever since the students of Virchow suggested that the "only constant feature of neoplasia was nucleolar aberration" in morphology and in function (33). Large, irregularly shaped nucleoli few in number but with increased density are found in tumors (33). Both of the main features of nucleolar morphology are abnormal: (a) the nucleolar shape is pleomorphic; while characteristic of rapidly growing tumors, this pleomorphism has been found to a limited extent in other rapidly growing tissues; and (b) the size is large, which is also found in a number of nontumor tissues as well as tumors. These morphological distortions are of interest, but it was apparent that the cancer problem must be approached with more incisive systems than with the tools of gross morphology. These early studies pointed to an important direction for cancer research which only recently has been approached at a molecular level (33) as discussed in Chapter V.

C. Unusual Properties of Cancer Cells

Unlike most mammalian cells, cancer cells are immortal in tissue culture. The HeLa cell, named after Helen Lane, the woman who bore and nurtured it, demonstrates the remarkable special properties of the cancer cell. Although the original host has been dead for over two decades, the HeLa cell continues to grow in tissue culture and has served as a useful experimental tool not only for studies on neoplastic disease, but also for studies on viruses. Another special feature of these cells is the occasional but characteristic multiple mitosis. Mitosis of cells generally implies division of the cells into two equal daughter cells. Even the germ cells which are capable of division into cells which are genetically unequal, carry out their "reduction division" in an orderly way with two "daughter" cells from each division (132). One pathognomonic histological characteristic which clearly differentiates tumor cells from other cells is the occurrence of multiple mitotic spindles which results in multiple divisions of the cancer

---

Fig. 1.1. Walker tumor cells of a rat as seen by light microscopy after staining with toluidine blue for the demonstration of RNA-containing structures. Note the intense staining of the cytoplasm (C) and nucleoli (white N) indicating a high content of RNA in these structures which is characteristic for rapidly proliferating malignant cells. Black N, nucleus. ×1400.

Fig. 1.2. Electron micrograph of a Walker tumor cell fixed in osmium tetroxide and postfixed in formaldehyde. After such fixation, RNA-containing structures such as the nucleolus (white N), dark granules in interchromatinic areas (I), and cytoplasmic ribosomes are very dense. The chromatin (C) is preserved but less dense (33). Black N, nucleus; G, Golgi apparatus; m, mitochondrion. ×11,000.

Fig. 1.3. Low magnification electron micrograph of a lymphocytic leukemic infiltrate in human bone marrow. Lymphoblast (B) represents one of the immature proliferating cells of this disease. A nucleolus (white N) is visible in another cell. Other cells are more mature and are characterized by their smaller size as well as by more condensed chromatin in their nuclei (black N). ×3600.

TABLE 1.1   ELECTRON MICROSCOPIC CHARACTERISTICS OF CANCER CELLS[a]

A. The Nucleus

1. The nucleus in interphase often has a more irregular form than normal and its size may be considerably increased. Every neoplasm, however, has its own pattern of nuclear behavior, and it is impossible to determine direct relationships between neoplastic transformation of a cell and hypertrophy of its nucleus.

2. Heterochromatin anomalies in the resting nucleus are very marked in tumors but have not shown specific features as yet.

3. Cancer cells often show an increased nuclear deoxyribonucleic acid content, but this increase varies in different tumors and even within the same tumor, along with changes of the nuclear volume and chromosome number.

4. The nucleolus is as a rule hypertrophic. There is no constant ultrastructural difference as compared with normal nucleoli.

5. The nuclear membrane frequently shows deep invaginations; its ultrastructure does not seem to be changed as compared with that of the normal nucleus.

6. The chromosomes show the most marked irregularities as to number and shape. Cancer cells are often heteroploid and the chromosomes may show considerable structural changes. There has never been any demonstration, so far, that these anomalies are a cause rather than a consequence of malignant transformation.

7. Mitotic anomalies are very frequent; but all such irregularities can be experimentally reproduced in noncancerous tissues.

8. Changes in the duration of mitosis are considerable. The metaphase seems to be relatively longer than in homologous normal tissues; the mitotic frequency is not increased in cancer tissue as compared with embryonic tissue in full growth.

9. Amitosis, in the classic sense of the word, does not seem to play a role in the multiplication of cancer cells.

B. The Cytoplasm

1. The number of mitochondria varies considerably from tumor to tumor. All the intermediate states between extreme richness and almost complete absence of chondriosomes are found; often, however, tumor cells tend to show fewer, smaller, and denser mitochondria. Phenomena of degeneration are also found, such as defective ultrastructure and swelling.

2. Cytoplasmic basophilia is as a rule more marked, but may also be absent. On the ultrastructural level, this basophilia corresponds to an increase of RNP granules, freely dispersed in the cytoplasm, and rarely to an increase of endoplasmic reticulum. The latter, on the contrary, tends to disappear in the cancer cell.

3. The Golgi apparatus can be very hypertrophic in certain tumors and may be hypotrophic in others. Its ultrastructure does not differ from that of the Golgi zone in normal cells.

4. The ultrastructure of the centriole in cancer cells does not seem to be abnormal. The position of this organelle and of the Golgi apparatus determines the polarity of the cells, which may be reversed or completely lost in dedifferentiated cancer tissue.

5. The cytoplasm of cancer cells may contain numerous inclusions of variable origin, resulting from degenerative processes, from partly preserved functional activity, from the phagocytic properties of certain cancers, or from the presence of virus particles in filterable tumors.

6. The ground substance shows no electron microscopic alterations.

7. The ultrastructure of the cell membrane of cancer cells also seems to be identical to that of normal cells.

8. So far it has been impossible to distinguish between normal and cancer cells on the basis of differences in staining dependent on any specific cytochemical reaction.

9. In filterable tumors, the electron microscope has made it possible to demonstrate virus particles contained in the nucleus or the cytoplasm. Highly polymorphous inclusions reveal a complex development of oncogenic viruses.

---

[a] From Oberling and Bernhard (123).

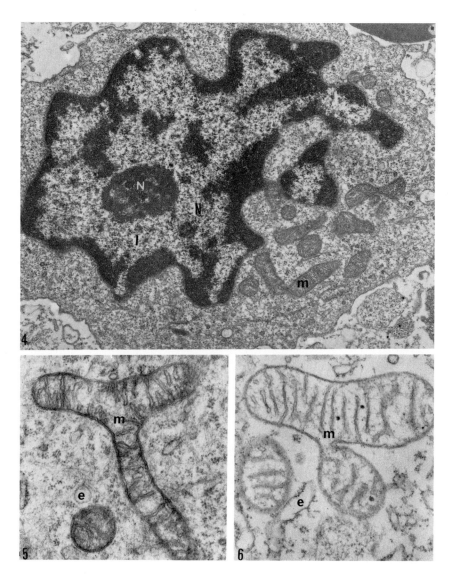

Fig. 1.4. Electron micrograph of a leukemic lymphoblast after fixation in glutaraldehyde and postfixation in osmium tetroxide. This procedure produces a very high density of nuclear chromatin structures. Nucleus, black N; nucleolus, white N. Interchromatinic areas (I) contain a large number of dense interchromatinic granules. The cytoplasm is rich in ribosomes (small dense granules) and poor in other structures (147a). Mitochondrion, m. ×31,200.

Fig. 1.5. Electron micrograph of an irregular T-shaped mitochondrion (m) in the cytoplasm of a Walker tumor cell. Smooth endoplasmic reticulum, e. Note that some ribosomes are in polysomal clusters. Fixation in oxmium tetroxide (147a–d). ×25,000.

Fig. 1.6. Electron micrograph of a T-shaped mitochondrion (m) in a human plasmacytoma cell after fixation in "alkaline" osmium tetroxide. Endoplasmic reticulum, e. ×24,000.

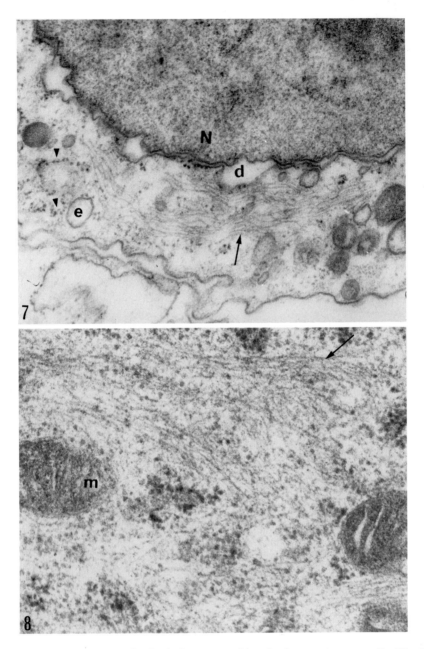

Fig. 1.7. Electron micrograph of a leukemic monoblast fixed in osmium tetroxide. The "peri-nuclear space" between two sublayers of the nuclear membrane is occasionally dilated form-ing cisternae (d). The cytoplasm contains bundles of fine filaments (arrow) and polysomes (points) as well as smooth endoplasmic reticulum (e) (33). N, Nucleus. ×50,000.

Fig. 1.8. Electron micrograph of the cytoplasm of an experimental cancer cell (Novikoff hepatoma) which is rich in fine filaments occasionally organized in bundles (arrow). Mito-chondrion, m. ×56,000.

cell. This process may result (p. 44) in formation of three, four, five, or as many as twelve daughter cells. Other biological properties of cancer cells are loss of mutual adhesiveness which is related to loss of "contact inhibition" which is a cessation of cell movement or cell growth when their plasma membranes are in contact; electron microscopic studies have shown surface changes in cancer cells which may be related to loss of contact inhibition (3, 109).

A startling characteristic of tumor cells is resistance to conditions which would produce serious damage to other cells. For example, cells of the brain or heart die within minutes when exposed to an environment lacking in oxygen or containing cyanide. On the other hand, tumor cells have remained viable and transplantable as long as three days in an environment containing cyanide and totally lacking in oxygen (163). Thus, the biological characteristics of cancer cells would seem to indicate that they are specialized for growth and survival under adverse conditions.

D. Cancer as a Genetic Disease

Historically, not long after the development of the fundamental theory of Schleiden (139) and Schwann (140), which stated that all living matter is composed of cells, the equally important statement was made by Virchow that "*omnis cellula a cellula,*" i.e., all cells come from preexisting cells (160). The development of this knowledge soon carried over into the field of oncology. Thiersch (158) reported that "*omnis cellula a cellula ejusdem generis,*" i.e., all cells come from cells of a genetically similar type. The connotation is that once a cell becomes neoplastic, the trait is transferred to all of the daughter cells. The intermediate events leading from the normal to the neoplastic state are the subjects of later chapters (cf. Chapters X, XI).

This genetic transmission of the cancer trait from mother to daughter cell is one of the cardinal features of the neoplastic process and it is readily affirmed in the simplest of laboratory experiments such as the injection of cells of transplantable tumors into normal animals. New tumors develop almost uniformly in the new host. Such transplantation experiments are routine in laboratories devoted to the study of neoplastic diseases and special techniques have been developed to simplify the process.

E. Origin of Cancer in Single Cells

The genetic transmission of the neoplastic character from mother to daughter cells has been supported by studies on transmission of neoplasia with single cells. A by-product of these studies is the demonstration that a single neoplastic cell suffices to produce cancer. With the aid of cell counting techniques and progressive dilution of media containing known numbers of cells, it was found that mouse leukemia (47) and the Yoshida sarcoma (62, 73) could be transmitted to susceptible animals with highly diluted preparations containing single

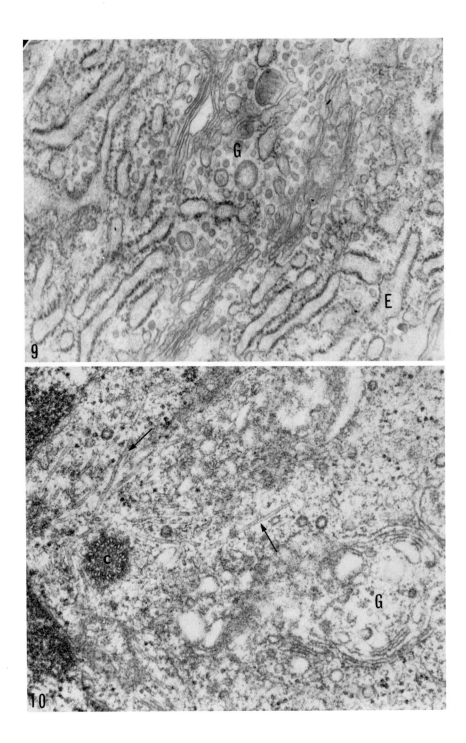

cells. The development of these neoplasms and their lethal effects were not significantly different from the results obtained with larger inocula. Since the "cancer trait" is genetically transmitted, it simply remains to define normal genetic transmission and the abnormalities of genetic transmission present in cancer cells (27, 153).

F. Concepts of the Genetic Origin of Cancer

The clinically significant aspects of these observations are (a) cancer cells do not revert to normal cells and (b) on subsequent division cancer cells give rise to cancer cells. This latter result has led to the general concept that cancer is a molecular biological disease, i.e., one involving abnormal genetics and further that the process is continued as a kind of a "mutation." At the present time there are four major concepts relating to the genetics of origin of cancer cells:

(1) All cells contain cancer genes, i.e., genes which when derepressed cause cancer. In noncancer cells these genes are repressed (27).

(2) Either at an early stage or following some type of viral or other infection, lysogeny (complete or partial) occurs as a result of which "cancer genes" or "growth genes" that are normally portions of viral genomes become incorporated into the cancer cell genome and are expressed, regardless of whether other viral genes are functional (150, 155; see Chapter XI).

(3) Cancer results from one or more "somatic mutations" (19).

(4) Cancer results from epigenetic (nongene) changes in cells (Table 1.2).

One of the difficulties in accepting the concept that cancer is a somatic mutation is the relative low frequency of such mutations* and the high frequency of cancer in man. In man, virtually every cell type is potentially neoplastic and cancers have been reported of almost every organ and every kind of cell. Some tumors increase in frequency with age to the point where almost the total population is affected, i.e., precancerous states of the prostate or frank prostatic cancer have been found in autopsies in 80% of patients above age 75. Moreover, tumors of endocrine origin and tumors of the gastrointestinal tract occur in such high frequency in the human population that mutational events would seem to be only a remote possibility for their causation.

At one time it was thought that disorders of the chromosomes were responsible for the development of neoplastic disease. However, it is now demonstrated that completely eukaryotypic cells (cells with a completely normal diploid

---

* Recently, Knudson (85, 85a) has suggested that some retinoblastomas and Wilms tumors in man may be the result of specific mutations.

Fig. 1.9. The well-developed Golgi apparatus (G) and rough endoplasmic reticulum (E) in a plasmocyte from human plasmacytoma (multiple myeloma) indicate that some malignant cells can retain secretory functions that are phenotypically characteristic for the cell type from which they originally developed. Fixation was in osmium tetroxide. ×32,000.

Fig. 1.10. Electron micrograph of a centriole (c), microtubules (arrows), and a relatively small Golgi apparatus (G) in an immature leukemic lymphocyte. Fixation with glutaraldehyde, postfixation in osmium tetroxide. ×57,000.

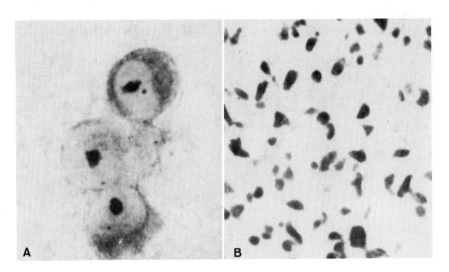

Fig. 1.11. A—Novikoff hepatoma ascites cells. B—isolated nucleoli of Novikoff hepatoma cells showing marked nucleolar pleomorphism.

TABLE 1.2

MAJOR THEORIES OF NEOPLASIA

Concept	Explanation
1. Viral genome insertion (150, 155)	Whole viral DNA or DNA produced by RNA-dependent DNA polymerase becomes inserted into cell genome and causes oncogenic effects
2. Activation of latent cancer DNA (27)	Cancer DNA may be present in all cells but is normally repressed; various extracellular and intracellular stimuli result in expression of this DNA
3. Deletion hypothesis (129)	Various cytoplasmic reaction series may exert specific controls on cell division; carcinogens may cause loss of these control reactions
4. Membron concept (128)	Messenger RNA is normally fixed to specific membrane sites in the cytoplasm; this membrane is abnormal in cancer cells
5. Somatic mutation theory (19)	Either chromosomal changes or point mutations cause alteration in cellular function
6. Abnormal cell respiration (163)	Cancer may arise as a result of cellular anoxia which results in excessive glycolysis
7. Defects in immune survey (50)	Carcinogenic substances alter the immune cell response to tumors and a failure to eliminate tumor cells
8. The cell rest theory (40, 124)	Precancerous cells or "rest" cells are present in many tissues; they are activated to cancer cells by oncogenic stimuli

chromosome complement) can be neoplastic. Presumably in such cells few if any changes have occurred in the DNA although point mutations cannot be excluded (121, 122).

One of the major problems with respect to the viral theory for human cancer is that only the Burkitt lymphoma which is very rare and has a defined epidemiological pattern has been shown to be a possible virus-induced tumor. Recently some evidence has been adduced that in small populations of Parsi women, a highly inbred sect in India, one form of breast cancer may be virus-induced. For the overwhelming mass of human tumors, however, it seems clear that the possibility of a viral etiology is remote in the absence of positive evidence and the negative epidemiological evidence (see Chapter XI).

G. Paramutation

If cancer is not a mutational event, some perpetuating mechanism must exist to produce its abnormal neoplastic phenotype or its insensitivity to growth regulation. An interesting parallel to an ongoing nonmutational phenotypic change is the "paramutation" described by Brink in speckled or mottled corn (22). In essence, Brink's initial experiment was carried out by altering temperature and other environmental conditions during growth of yellow or white corn (22). These were induced to produce a speckled product which then persisted over many generations. This speckled phenotype returned to normal when environmental conditions were again changed. Thus, during the many generations when the speckled corn was produced no changes occurred in the genome either during the "speckling" or on reformation of the normal phenotype. Presumably, the paramutational effect occurs through an operator gene responsible for the formation of the speckled product which was derepressed during the period of "speckling."

The fundamental concept of "paramutation" is that a gene product is produced that is sufficiently high in concentration in daughter cells that after mitosis its derepressor effect persists. In cancer cells, one mechanism by which such a derepressor effect may occur is related to the nucleolus which is both large and irregular in shape in actively dividing cancer cells. The rDNA genes, which produce the preribosomal products of nucleoli, presumably act through an operator mechanism which modulates their function (7). In some cells, such as resting liver cells, the nucleolus is small and composed substantially of fibrillar regions. In resting mature lymphocytes where the rDNA genes are largely repressed, the nucleolus is a small ring-shaped structure in which biosynthetic activity proceeds slowly, if at all. Even in such cells the rDNA is potentially functional because phytohemagglutinin markedly stimulates nucleolar activity as measured by RNA synthesis and ultrastructural appearance of granular and fibrillar elements in these hypoactive nucleoli (33).

In actively growing cancer cells, the nucleolus is large, pleomorphic, and extremely active as indicated by analysis of turnover of the nucleolar components (33). This extreme activity of nucleoli is one of the "pathognomonic" features of neoplastic cells and may result from a continued derepression of nucleolar rDNA genes. The fundamental mechanism by which this derepression occurs is not fully defined, but recent studies have shown that the newly synthesized RNA of neoplastic nucleoli may differ from that of nontumor cells. If nonneoplastic 28 S rRNA has binding sites that combine with derepressors of the nucleolar operator genes, a sufficient number of ribosomes would cause these derepressors to be reduced in concentration to the point where they are unavailable to nucleolar genes or no longer derepress them to produce maximal rRNA synthesis. Under such circumstances the nucleolus would be reduced in functional activity. If, on the other hand, in cancer cells a modified type of RNA is produced that has a reduced binding to derepressors, it would seem possible that these derepressors would no longer be reduced in concentration and, accordingly, nucleolar function would continue at maximal rates.

III. What and Where Are the Genes?

The broadest working definition of the gene is that it is a factor concerned with hereditary transmission of characteristics of the parent to the offspring, whether the parent be an individual cell such as an ameba or a multicellular organism. The molecular biology of the gene has now been extensively studied in terms of structure and function (164). In bacteria and some phages, and to a lesser extent in eukaryotic cells, gene loci have been established with great specificity at various sites on the chromosomes. Evidence for a genetic role of the cytoplasm has come from rather extensive evidence that "plasma-genes" (which may be viruses) may also function as hereditary determinants and the demonstration of mitochondrial DNA. Since there are different nucleic acids and proteins outside the nucleus than in the nucleus, it would appear that such genetic transmission may be different from that usually occurring at mitosis. Although our present knowledge is such that most genetic transmission is considered to be chromosomal, there is still much uncertainty as to the role of the cytoplasm in mammalian cells.

How Many Genetically Important Factors Are There in Normal Cells?

It is of some interest to inquire into the number of genetic factors which may be present in the nuclei of cells. It is certain that there is an enormous number of such factors, since even relatively simple characteristics are genetically transmitted. It has been pointed out that although there are, at present, over 3 billion persons inhabiting the earth, none of these look completely alike with the exception of identical twins. Another example of the enormous variations which are genetically permitted even in small characteristics is the contour of the fingerprint, which is such a specifically definitive mark that individual persons may be identified by this means. Indeed, one need not look farther than one's nose to find a structure which is genetically molded. As one views the population, there is frequently a remarkable similarity in the size, shape, and cartilaginous characteristics of the nose in siblings or in the various generations of a single family. Simpler features such as hair color, iris color, and skin color are also determined by the genetic apparatus.

Although it is not completely clear how many genes really exist and are functional in cells, some estimates have been made from the fact that eukaryotic nuclei contain about 10 pg (10^{-11} g) of DNA and the molecular weight of the DNA of cells is approximately 10^7. This molecular weight has been derived by studies on DNA isolated from a variety of mammalian cells. However, it now seems likely that whole chromosomes are single DNA molecules and accordingly, such molecular weights could be far too low. Since 10^7 gm of DNA or 1 mole would contain 6×10^{23} DNA molecules, there are about 600,000 DNA molecules in a given mammalian cell. Moreover, it may be calculated that a single DNA molecule with a molecular weight of 10^7 would contain approximately 30,000 nucleotides which would be sufficient information to code for 10,000 amino acids. Since proteins of molecular weight 50,000 contain approximately 400 amino acids, each of these molecules of 10^7 molecular weight would have enough information to code for approximately 25 protein molecules. Accordingly, there would be a total possible readout of $25 \times 600,000$ or approximately 15,000,000 proteins if the total DNA is read. Calculated another way: 10 pg = 10^{-11} g; since 325 g = 1 mole of nucleotide, 10 pg contain (6×10^{23}) $\times 10^{-11}/325$ or 1.85×10^{10} nucleotides; thus, the genome can code for 15×10^6 proteins. Assuming that only one strand of the DNA is actually read, then it seems most likely that information for 7×10^6 proteins could be the most coded for by the genome.

Many factors serve to modify the possible value of these numbers for estimating total gene numbers because proteins are quite heterogeneous in size. Some peptides have molecular weights ranging from 2000 to 3000 and some globulins have molecular weights in the millions. In addition, there is much evidence now that a large number of DNA segments are "reiterated," i.e., much of the DNA may exist in multiple copies for special functions and also, much of the DNA may be part of regulatory mechanisms that are related to gene:gene control. Although it is not possible to specify the number of genes involved in the overall transmission of characters, the number is probably in the millions.

The numbers and types of genes in a given species may be referred to as the genetic load which provides the biochemical apparatus for development of these complex characteristics of the species. Each somatic cell must initially have the same "genetic load" as the zygote since in the process of normal mitosis each cell should theoretically bear the same characters as the maternal cell. The remarkable studies on the blastula of the frog (20, 21) support this concept. These experiments were designed to explore the "totipotentiality" of cells at various levels of development of the fertilized frog egg. Nuclei were transplanted from cells of embryos in various stages of division into unfertilized eggs, and from these complete frogs developed. This result was obtained with the cells at various levels of development, i.e., at the 4-, 8-, and 16-cell stages. After

the gastrula stage, this totipotentiality was apparently lost, although some technical problems were involved in these experiments (82). Later experiments with
the intestine of the tadpole showed that nuclear totipotentiality was persistent
even in fully differentiated tissues. Advantage was taken of the fact that in
the tadpole, the intestine is not functional although it is fully differentiated.
Nuclei derived from these cells indeed demonstrated the same type of toti-
potency as that found in the cells of early stages of development (56).

However, the nuclei from the tumors they studied lacked this abiltiy. No
perfectly normal frog developed following the implantation of tumor nuclei
into enucleated eggs (82). In the occasional tadpole that formed, there was
usually some serious associated abnormality. Many of the earlier developmental
forms were remarkably abnormal. In some respects, it is quite surprising that
cell division and embryonic maturation proceeded as far as they did.

Since neoplastic transformation is one expression of such types of genetic
potential, it seems likely that the underlying genetic factors responsible for the
neoplastic phenotype must exist in many cells (27).

IV. How Many Genetic Changes Does It Take to Convert a Normal Cell to a Cancer Cell?

Regardless of whether neoplasia is the result of mutations in which new gene
characters are produced (which seems very unlikely) or introduced into cells
or existing repressed genes are released, it is apparent that the number of
changes involved are probably very small compared to the total genetic load.
In Knudson's studies one or two mutations were reported in retinoblastoma
or Wilms tumor (85, 85a). Thus, it is not surprising that in man and in most other
species, primary tumors are frequently not phenotypically differentiable from
the cells of origin. As Greenstein pointed out (52), a primary osteosarcoma
frequently makes bony structures similar to those made by the adjacent osteo-
blastic cells. In studies of the enzymes of tumors, a number of workers (93,
163, 168, 169) have commented on the identity of a series of enzymes isolated
from tumors as compared with those isolated from other tissues. Indeed, the
ability of tumors to produce hormones identical to those produced by adjacent
nontumor tissue is frequently the means for their clinical identification.

V. Random Repression of Normal Cell Phenotypes in Cancer Cells

The evolution of the cancer phenotype is in part associated with varying
degrees of suppression of the normal cell phenotype in cells in which the cancer
genes become activated. The gene sets functional for specialized readouts in
the tissue of origin are apparently more or less randomly shut off as the neoplastic process evolves. Fascinating clinical examples of this type of random repres-

sion are seen in neoplasms of the β-cells of the pancreas (insulinomas), neoplasms of the pigment cells of the skin (melanomas), and neoplasms of the plasma cells (plasmacytomas). Each of these neoplasms has a wide variety of phenotypes in any series of patients. For example, insulinomas may produce excessive amounts of insulin per cell, no insulin per cell, or any variation between these extremes. As a result, the patient may exhibit hyperinsulinism and hypoglycemia of a very serious degree, a moderate hyperinsulinism, or no hyperinsulinism. In cases of malignant melanomas, the neoplasms may be blue-black or black in color which is the normal color of melanocytes, or the neoplasms may be colorless, i.e., they may be amelanotic melanomas. Any variation between these extremes may result.

Another example is the plasmacytomas (Chapter XIV) formed from cells that normally produce γ-globulins. These tumors may produce a spectrum of proteins ranging from Bence-Jones proteins which are small segments (κ chains) of immune globulins to abnormal or normal immune globulins. Variations also occur between these extremes. As exemplified by these cases of human neoplasia, the cancer phenotype may exhibit a variety of levels reflecting the special characteristics of the cells at a given level of repression.

VI. Experimental Tumors

It is extremely difficult to carry out biochemical experiments with human neoplasms for a number of reasons. Among the most serious problems are the difficulty of reproducing experimental samples which frequently are obtained after complex surgery, the variety of phenotypes in any given patient, infection in human neoplasms which are in external or internal cavities, changes produced by antitumor therapy, and the presence of cells other than cancer cells. Moreover, in almost all human neoplasms there are large amounts of fibrous tissue, lymphocytes, and granulation tissue which are exceedingly difficult to separate from cancer cells.

For these reasons and in order to insure a continuing supply of tumor material for studies that necessarily will take many years, studies began almost 80 years ago on tumor transplantation and the evolution of strains of cancer cells that could be obtained in very high homogeneity. At present, many lines of neoplastic cells are available in laboratories and institutions specializing in cancer research. These vary from tumors that are transplanted from animal to animal to cells that are cultured over a period of years for "cloning" of special strains.

The process of development of neoplastic cells is a continuing one because all the strains obtained thus far have one or more problems from an experimental point of view. Among the series of malignant tumors, the "Morris hepatomas" (116) have been selected in such a way that they could vary in phenotype from cells that are very slow growing "liverlike" (minimal deviation hepatomas) to rapidly growing cells whose origin could not be defined unless one knew their source. These tumors vary with respect to their production of albumin, bile, glycogen, special enzymes of the liver, and other metabolic characteristics. Their variation is marked and orderly, and biochemical analyses have provided a "molecular correlation concept" that seeks to interrelate their growth rates and the various enzymatic activities and other biochemical parameters that have been assayed (Chapter XII). In brief, the fastest growing tumors have higher rates of glycolysis (production of lactic acid from glucose), more rapid rates of synthesis of nucleic acids and nuclear proteins, and less of the phenotypically important liver functions such as bile production, synthesis of glycogen, albumin synthesis, and special enzymes that characterize liver function. Correlations between growth rate, glycolytic rates, and loss of the usual liver functions have been developed (Chapter XII; 167).

VII. Number of Operating "Cancer Genes"

The exact number of genetic differences between tumors and other tissues can be probably set as $1(+?)$. Studies on chemical carcinogenesis (cf. Chapter V) have made it clear that the carcinogenic process involves two and possibly three steps (15, 16, 84). The first of these is the so-called "initiating step" in which a cell or a group of cells sustains some type of stimulus by contact with a carcinogen. This step can be demonstrated by application of a carcinogen such as 20-methylcholanthrene or some similar agent to the skin of an animal. While this stimulus alone may be sufficient to set off the development of the neoplasms, generally it is not and there is need for another step. This second step has been labeled the "promoting step," or the "precipitating step"; the development of the neoplastic lesion is hastened or induced. Experimentally, the procedure in this step may simply be weekly treatment with croton oil, an irritant, or a site previously treated with a carcinogen such as 20-methylcholanthrene. In some undefined ways, the irritant causes the tissue to develop the full neoplastic reaction to the carcinogen. Another example which has been receiving a great deal of recent attention is the development of lung cancer in man. There are a great many carcinogens in the atmosphere such as benzpyrene, a hydrocarbon carcinogen, or split products of diesel oils or commercial gasoline products (86, 87). Such molecules are capable of providing the "initiating" stimulus for the development of cancer of the lung, this being the first site at which such particles would lodge. The demonstration (171, 172) of the presence of carcinogens in the inhalate of cigarette smoke provided evidence for the ready availability of a carcinogen which might account for the development of neoplasms of the lung. Moreover, it is inherent in the characteristic pharmacological activities of the components of cigarette smoke that there would be a very marked irritating or "promoting" effect of cigarette smoke. There are some people who cannot remain in a room filled with smoke because of the remarkable irritating power of these combustion products and others who fear inhalation of cigarette products for their possible carcinogenic effects. It is thus conceivable that the cigarette smoker is the victim of this habit in two ways from the point of view of carcinogenesis: (a) the cigarette itself may provide carcinogens which may potentiate the activities of the normally present carcinogens in the atmosphere and (b) the irritants which are inhaled induce the necessary "promoting" effect which causes the proliferation of the neoplastic cells.

Although one genetic change must be involved in oncogenesis, it is by no means certain that more are not involved. An upper limit on the number of genes affected cannot be presently stated but it is not likely that the number is large compared to the total number of genes in these cells. It is clear that the ultimate sorting out of the particular genes which are specifically responsible for the neoplastic process will make the finding of the "needle in the haystack" look to be about as difficult as piloting a bobsled down a snowy hill in midwinter.

VIII. The Chromosomes

A. Morphology

The rapid growth of knowledge regarding chromosome structure and the relationship of chromosomal abnormalities to specific diseases has been the result of improvements in methods for the histological examination and identification of chromosomes. Most present-day studies are carried out with variations of the "squash" technique for flattening and spreading the chromosomes (64, 66–68, 159), "hypotonic" media for swelling the nucleus, phase microscopy for improved resolution, and cytostatic and other agents (159) which increase the number of cells in metaphase (Fig. 1.12). By careful study of selected cells, the chromosome patterns for individuals or species can be completely determined and the pictorial representation of the chromosomes in the order of decreasing size and complexity is referred to as the "idiogram" or "karyotype" (Fig. 1.13). This method is readily applied to cells in tissue culture. With relatively few variations it has been applied to human cells, including leukocytes from peripheral blood kept in culture (115) and marrow cells obtained directly from patients (83).

A number of terms are used to define the chromosomal structure. Chromatids are the individual halves of the double chromosomal structure and the kinetochore or the primary constriction is the site of attachment of the chromosome to the spindle. The term chromonema refers to the chromosomal strand which is visible in the light microscope. Since similar substructures have been visualized recently in mammalian chromosomes, it has been more or less assumed that mammalian chromosomes also contain the chromomeres and the interchromomeric regions. Recent light microscopic studies using quinacrine staining for fluorescence or the Giemsa stain have supported this concept of chromosomal structure for mammalian cells (6, 35, 42a, 65a).

With the aid of the improved techniques, normal idiograms have been established for man (65, 98), other animal species (14, 65), insects, and plants (98, 100). The characteristic finding is that there is a high degree of constancy

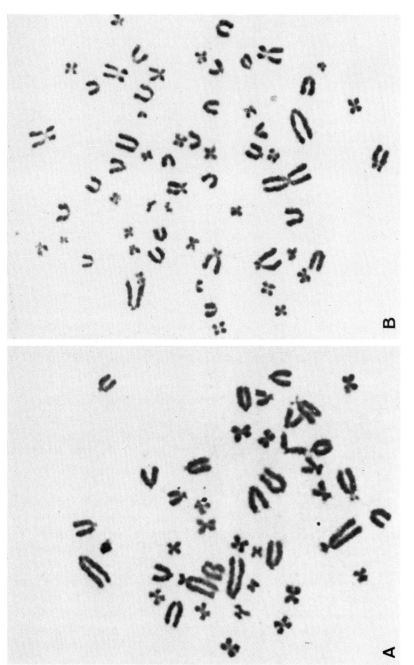

Fig. 1.12. Chromosomes of metaphases of (A) a normal embryonic cell of the rat and (B) a Walker tumor cell. The normal cell has 42 chromosomes and the modal number for the Walker tumor is 60–65 chromosomes per cell. Abnormal chromosomes are also found in the Walker tumor. (Courtesy of Dr. T. C. Hsu, M.D. Anderson Hospital, Houston.)

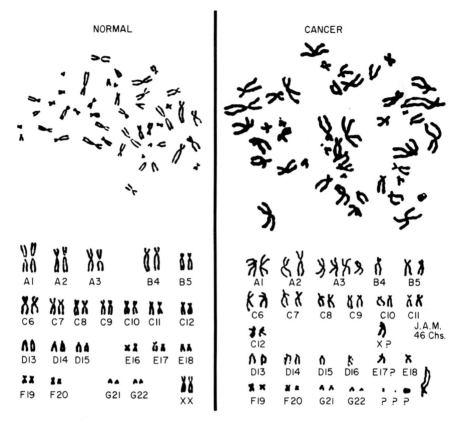

Fig. 1.13. Metaphases and karyotypes of normal (left) and colon cancer cells (right). In the colon cancer there are 4 additional chromosomes, an uncertain X chromosome (X?) and other unknown chromosomes (E17?0) and others shown as ?. There is also an elongated chromosome adjacent to the small abnormal chromosomes. One small chromosome is a double-ringed chromosome. (Courtesy of Dr. Avery Sandberg, Roswell Park Memorial Institute.)

in normal tissues (18, 53, 98, 111). Variations from the usual idiograms are associated with pathological states such as mongolism, Turner's syndrome, Klinefelter's syndrome (53), and other clinical syndromes (58b).

B. Chromosomes of Cancer Cells

Although only one is specific, abnormalities in chromosomes of cancer cells have been studied intensively during the last decade (118–122, Chapter III). Many tumors have abnormal numbers and types of chromosomes (118, 120, 122). It is uncertain whether these chromosomal aberrations are a cause of neoplasia or result from the activity of the tumor cells in subsequent deranged cell divisions. Some Morris hepatomas (the 9618A and 9633 hepatomas) have normal diploid karyotypes (122).

The wide variations in the phenotypes of neoplastic cells are associated with remarkable aberrations in the chromosome complement and types in tumor cells (Figs. 1.12–1.14). Chromosome numbers ranging from hypodiploid to greater than octaploid have been found. Although the numbers of chromosomes may be increased or decreased, the most characteristic feature of chromosomes of neoplastic cells is their aberration in number from precise multiples of the diploid state (118, 131, 151, 152). In normal human cells, 46 chromosomes represent the diploid state characteristic of somatic cells. In normal cells, variations in chromosome number may occur such that there are tetraploid cells containing 92 chromosomes or octaploid cells that contain 184 chromosomes. These variations are characteristic of normal cells. In many tumors, however, the chromosome number is aneuploid, i.e., not greater or less than the normal in multiples of 46. They are either hyper- or hypodiploid, hyper- or hypotetraploid, and hyper- or hypooctaploid. Thus, as few as 37 chromosomes have been found in leukemic cells and, in rare instances, as many as several thousand chromosomes have been found in individual cancer cells.

In addition to changes in numbers of chromosomes, some tumors are characterized by changes in specific chromosomes. A wide variety of aberrations has been found, including the presence of ring chromosomes, very large and complex chromosomes (Fig. 1.13), small chromosomes such as the Philadelphia chromosome (Fig. 1.14) that is pathognomonic for chronic myelogenous leukemia (119, 120), disorganized separation of anaphase chromosomes, chromatid bridges, and criss-cross bridges. Breaks, failure of complete unions, and other types of changes have been noted. Some abnormal chromosomes that are J-shaped or V-shaped have been related to such important properties as invasiveness, infiltration, and peritoneal transplantability. Losses of some chromosomes do not markedly limit the viability of the tumor cells. Apparently the losses are of segments of the genome that are unrelated to growth and cell division.

Although the problem of neoplasia was once viewed as a problem of "chromosome balance" (54, 97), the gene or "chromosome balance" has not been compared in tumors and other tissues. In tissue culture, the medium has definite effects on chromosomal structure and function (97) in cells from embryonic skin, normal spleen, brain, liver, and kidney cells. Even trypsinization of cells can lead to malignant changes and thus surface changes are capable of producing numerical and even structural chromosomal changes (99, 147). Trypsinization may alter some immune mechanisms that suppress malignant cells *in vivo* (127) or *in vitro* (138). Thus far no specific chromosomal changes have been found that are generally characteristic of neoplasia (115, 119, 122; see Chapter III).

C. Ultrafine Structure of Chromosomes

The gap between the studies of the microscopic structure of the chromosomes by staining techniques and the biochemical information on the deoxyribonucleoproteins is bridged in part by studies on the chromosomes by means of electron microscopy (Fig. 1.15) (133). Chromosomes contain many "chromofibrils" or

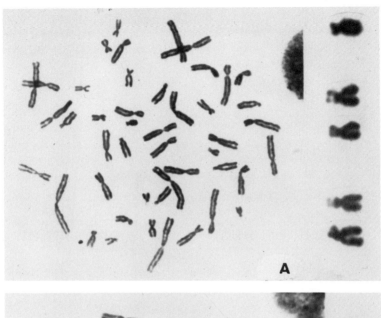

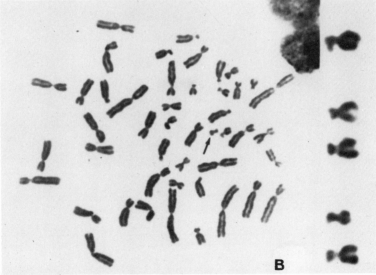

Fig. 1.14. Human chromosomes at metaphase from a normal white blood cell (upper) and a leukemic cell (lower) from cultured blood of a male patient with chronic granulocytic leukemic (CGL). The chromosome complement of the leukemic cell is characterized by the Philadelphia (Ph¹) chromosome (arrow), which is a chromosome deficient for approximately 40% of its normal amount of DNA. The small acrocentric chromosomes of these two cells are compared in the right margin. In (A) there are four normal autosomes and, uppermost, the Y chromosome. In (B) there are, in ascending order, a normal autosome, the Ph¹, two more normal autosomes, and the Y. This chromosome abnormality is found in blood cells of the vast majority of patients with CGL. Various chromosome abnormalities are found in other malignancies, but, other than the Ph¹, no constant type has been found to be characteristic of a specific kind of malignancy. (Courtesy of Dr. David Hungerford, Institute for Cancer Research.)

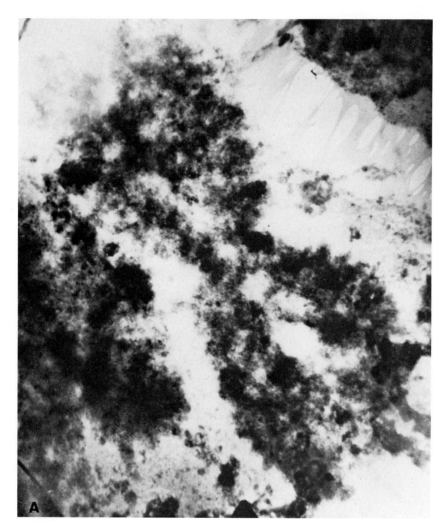

Fig. 1.15. (A) Electron micrograph of a metaphase chromosome.

"elementary chromosome fibrils" 150–220 Å in width and approximately 500–3000 Å and greater in length (133). Mammalian chromosomes seen under the light microscope apparently consist of eight or more strands of these subunits (Fig. 1.15) while the large salivary chromosomes of *Drosophila* apparently have up to 1000 times this number of strands.

The bands and interbands (chromomeres and interchromomeres, respectively) of the chromosomes result from varied degrees of cooling of the strands in localized segments of chromosomes. Although the chromomeres and heterochromatin are richer in nucleic acid than the euchromatin of the interchromomeric regions (interbands), the DNA fibers are continuous through the chromosomes. The functional significance of this coiling is not definitely known except in some specific examples of insect cell functions.

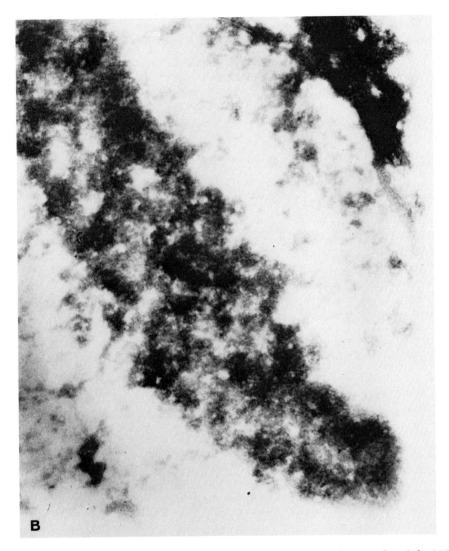

Fig. 1.15. (B) Telomere of a metaphase chromosome. (Courtesy of Dr. Arthur Cole, M.D. Anderson Hospital and Tumor Institute.)

D. Isolated Chromosomes

For isolation of intact metaphase chromosomes, methods usually have involved the use of mild homogenization of the nuclei or cellular preparations in metaphase in media containing divalent ions. Differential centrifugation in sucrose gradients (Fig. 1.16) has provided some concentration of some chromosomes such as those containing either secondary constrictions of nucleolar organizer regions (NOR's) in specific groups (Fig. 1.17). Analysis of the various chromosome bands for specific compositions has not revealed marked differences in

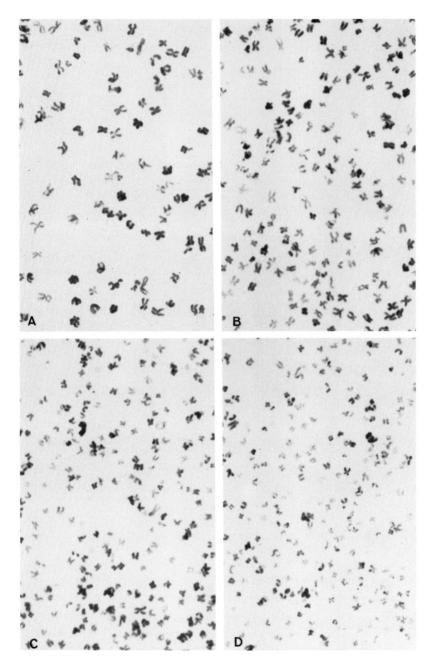

Fig. 1.16. Isolated and fractionated HeLa metaphase chromosomes. A small amount of a suspension in FM (fractionation medium) containing 30% glycerol of each pooled chromosome class from chromosome preparation I (see 69, 70) was spread on a clean glass slide and allowed to dry for 60 minutes. The half-wet chromosomes were then fixed in acetic acid-ethanol (3:2 v/v) for 10 minutes and stained in 1% orcein in lactic acid-acetic acid (1:1 v/v). Bright field ×800 (70). The different panels represent fractions of chromosomes taken from different regions of the sucrose density gradients. (Courtesy of Professor G. Attardi, California Institute of Technology.)

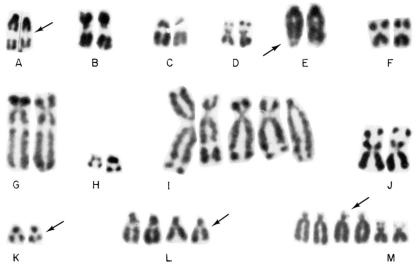

Fig. 1.17. Chromosomes of a number of species with secondary constrictions. The arrows represent the positions of the constrictions. Top row from left to right: A. *Spilogale putorius* (spotted skunk); B. *Mephitis mephitis* (striped skunk); C. *Mustela putorius* (ferret); D. *Felis catus* (domestic cat); E. *Cervus canadensis* (elk); F. *Sus scorfa* (domestic pig). Second row: G. *Carollia perspicillata* (fruit bat); H. *Pipistrellus subflavus* (Eastern pipistrelle); I. *Tamiasciurus hudsonicus* (red squirrel); J. *Chinchilla laniger* (chinchilla). Third row: K. *Tupaia glis* (tree shrew); L. *Alouatta caraya* (black howler); M. *Homo sapiens* (man). (Courtesy of Prof. T. C. Hsu, M.D. Anderson Hospital, Houston, Texas.)

their composition, i.e., they all contain about 30% DNA, 30% histones, 30% acidic proteins, and approximately 5–10% RNA (28, 34, 69, 70, 108). Thus, the condensed chromosomes and "chromatin" fraction isolated from interphase cells have similar compositions suggesting that the central DNA-histone core is surrounded by the layer of acidic ribonucleoproteins (33, 147a).

The development of these isolation methods should ultimately permit the isolation of the "nucleolar chromosomes" that contain rDNA, the templates for synthesis of 18 S and 28 S rRNA in the NOR's (nucleolus organizer regions). The 18 S and 28 S ribosomal RNA of HeLa cells hybridized best with the smaller chromosomes (70). On the other hand, the mRNA (presumably the template RNA for biosynthesis of the cytoplasmic proteins) hybridized with all of the chromosomes (70). The nucleolar chromosomes frequently contain secondary constrictions (Fig. 1.17).

E. Nucleoli, Puffs, and Balbiani Rings of Insects

The best examples of the functions of chromomeres and interchromomeric regions are found in the polytene chromosomes of the *Drosophila* and other flies, midges, and insects. The individual chromomeres become activated at different times by different hormonal influence and by other physiological factors. In *Chironomus tentans,* chromosomes II and III have NOR's, i.e., nucleolus organizing regions, that were located with relative ease (11–13, 125, 126). An "accessory nucleolus" may develop on chromosome IV, generally at the end of the chromosome.

Although the components of the Balbiani rings and puffs are not clearly defined, they do not serve for the formation of ribosomal precursors which is one of the main functions of the nucleoli (33, 43) which are present in these cells throughout their functional stages. The formation of Balbiani rings and puffs is associated with the development of specific secretory granules (12, 13), molting (39), hormone synthesis, particularly the juvenile hormone and ecdysone, a hormone that induces molting (38, 39, 92), and specific stages of cell function (95).

The chromosomal puffs are found at specific loci and contain both RNA and protein as is the case with the nucleoli. Swift (154) has found that they also contain DNA and histone. Intriguing studies have been made on the Balbiani rings of the salivary glands of the *Chironomus*. In *Chironomus thummi*, there are marked changes in morphological appearance during the last instar, a prepupal stage. These changes are associated with increases and decreases in the sizes of specific chromosomal puffs. Kroeger (92) utilized transplantation to produce puffing changes quite similar to those produced with purfied ecdysone or juvenile hormone.

Interestingly, $ZnCl_2$, $CdCl_2$, chloroform, butanol, and urethane all had effects similar to those of ecdysone. The effects of juvenile hormone could be duplicated by the wounding of the cells, X-radiation, or oxygen poisoning. The effects of these substances may not occur directly on the genes but rather on some cytoplasmic input elements that later produced altered gene readouts. This concept is similar to the one postulated for nucleolar synthesis of ribonucleoproteins (33).

Beerman (12) related the production of specific secretory granules in the salivary glands to a specific chromosomal locus. In the *Chironomus*, there are only four cells which are active in the production of the normal salivary secretions. These cells contain the biochemical apparatus for production of the secretory granules referred to as SZ granules. Some mutants lack the ability to produce the SZ granules, either because the cells are inactive or absent; the salivary secretions of this type of fly differ from that of the normal flies. The production of the secretory granules is dependent on the activity of one specific Balbiani ring on chromosome IV; if this specific puff is absent, these cells are not functional. Thus, it seems possible that each Balbiani ring or perhaps several of these rings acting together may produce specific biochemical activities in cells and thus may represent the intermediaries through which the chromosomes express genetic information. (See also Chapter V.)

IX. Evidence for the Role of DNA as Genetically Active Material

The development of the information with regard to DNA was initiated by the landmark studies of Griffith (55). He injected into mice a number of types of pneumococcal cultures, some attenuated and unencapsulated (rough) and some virulent and encapsulated (smooth). Injection of rough cultures of Type II forms did not induce pneumonia or pneumococcal peritonitis in mice, i.e., the culture was avirulent. Injection of heat-killed Type III pneumococci also did not induce either pneumonia or pneumococcal peritonitis. Injection of the viable Type III pneumococci produced an extensive peritonitis which was rapidly and uniformly fatal. The crux of Griffith's experiment was the simultaneous injection of a mixture of the heat-killed Type III pneumococci with the avirulent rough Type II strain. The one strain was not potent in producing disease and the other was "dead." The mixture of the two produced encapsulated Type III pneumococci, the lethal form which was easily cultured from the pneumococcal peritonitis that resulted.

The experiments of Griffith were readily confirmed. Alloway (4, 5) purified the component of the dead Type III pneumococci which possessed the "transforming activity," i.e., the ability to "transform" Type II to Type III pneumococci. Avery et al. (8) decisively established that the transforming factor was deoxyribonucleic acid (DNA). They utilized a strain of pneumococcus that did not revert to the smooth strain and also was responsive to the transforming factor. The Type III cells were treated with saline containing deoxycholate as a detergent. The deoxyribonucleoprotein precipitated with alcohol was dissolved in normal saline solution. The protein was precipitated out of the saline solution with chloroform.

The DNA obtained from this solution was stable from $-70°$ to $65°C$, was diphenylamine positive (42), had a ratio of nitrogen to phosphorus of 1.69, was resistant to hydrolysis by trypsin or ribonucleases, and was very sensitive to deoxyribonuclease.

On ultracentrifugation, the sedimentation of the transforming activity was simultaneous with the sedimentation boundary. Electrophoresis also provided evidence for purity and indicated that the mobility was consistent with that of nucleic acids. The absorption of light was minimal at 2350 Å and maximal at 2600 Å, which is also characteristic of nucleic acids. The purest material obtained was active in inducing transformation in quantities as low as 1.25 pg $(1.25 \times 10^{-12}$ gm$)$/ml.

Is the Transforming Factor a Genetic Entity?

By its mode of preparation the DNA obtained from the pneumococcus Type III was clearly a very large segment, if not all, of the DNA in the cells of these bacteria. Accordingly, it would seem that the total material might embody a large number of the genetic characteristics of the cells of origin. Since the molecule is very large, i.e., 5000–10,000 Å in diameter (63, 144, 174, 175), it is clear that entry into the cells of Type II pneumococcus must involve complex permeability factors or must occur when the cell wall is weak or opened (78, 178).

At present there are 40 known examples of DNA-produced transformation defined either by the surface antigens or bacterial sensitivity to antibiotics (1, 57, 58, 63, 79, 80, 94, 117, 134, 148, 175). Interestingly, one "transforming" factor was resistant to DNase (178).

A "positive mutation," i.e., a thymineless bacterial mutant, could be induced to form thymine following the uptake of DNA from bacteriophage T2 (10). Presumably, the phage contains the "template" synthesis of the enzyme. Both "transduction" and "lysogeny"* in which the genome of the phage is partially integrated into the host genome have been amply defined in biochemical terms in various phage systems (48, 74–78, 96, 178). The host cell not only makes what is required by its own nucleic acids but also what is demanded by the integrated or lysogenized viral nucleic acids.

X. Other Evidence for the Role of DNA in Hereditary Transmission

A. UV-Induced Mutation

Another kind of evidence for the role of DNA in hereditary transmission is the finding that the greatest sensitivity of mutability to light in various species is in the ultraviolet (UV) at which absorption is greatest by nucleic acids (44, 61, 81, 170). At other wavelengths there was less mutation. Although the peak of mutations (176) was 2650 Å, not much less mutation was found at 2800 Å. This result suggests that mutability may also be affected by UV light absorption of proteins.

B. DNA in Virus Infection

With regard to virus infection, both RNA and DNA are agents for genetic change. Hershey (59, 60) labeled T2 bacteriophage to demonstrate virus attachment to the cell membrane and injection of DNA of the phage through the cell wall (88–91). More than 97% of the phage protein remained on the cell surface in the form of a collapsed syringelike bag. It is apparent that DNA is the factor primarily responsible for the transmission of T2 phage characteristics (145, 146). Important oncogenic viruses such as the Rous virus (135–137) contain RNA and little DNA (see Chapter XI). Highly purified RNA has been isolated from enteroviruses and has also been shown to be active in the infectious process (149). In mutational events, it is generally considered that "reverse transcription" of the RNA of the virus to a host-integrated DNA is important (9, 155–157).

---

* Lysogeny is a characteristic of bacteria that permits them to destroy other bacteria by production of lysins. This property is phage mediated and integrated into the genome of the infected bacteria. Lysogenic strains of bacteria produce phage and have immunity to the homologous phage.

C. Bacterial Mating

Other evidence for the role of DNA in the transfer of genetic characteristics in bacteria emerged from "chromosome mapping" (74–78). Both the timing and the order of gene entry of ^{32}P-labeled DNA from one form of the bacteria to another were worked out by separating bacteria from one another by gentle blending. In similar studies the transfer of genetic characteristics was determined for bacteria virus (phage) infection to disrupt mating at a critical point. At this time, the transfer of genetic character and labeled DNA was compared. The sequence of transfer of the ^{32}P-labeled DNA correlated well with gene transfer in these bacterial matings.

XI. Less Direct Evidence for the Role of DNA in the Transfer or Retention of Hereditary Characteristics

The principal linear component of the chromosomes is the DNA (45, 112–114, 130, 144). The content of DNA in the "chromatin" is about 30% of the total dry weight; most of the rest is protein (28). About 30% of the weight of chromatin is histones, about 30–35% acidic protein, and about 5% RNA (28, 105). Thus, by weight, the proteins of the chromatin compose a much greater part of the mass than does the DNA.

A. Constancy of the Weight of DNA in Cells of a Species

In virtually all cells of the species or the individual, the content of DNA is constant, except for the haploid products of reduction division (18). However, the constancy of DNA content per nucleus (23–25, 42, 45) of the individual or the species does not eliminate individual variation in chromosomal DNA content. For example, the "minutes" found in mongoloids and other genetic diseases hardly change the DNA content of the cells.

B. Stability of DNA

It has been stated that if one were to seek a molecule which had an important role in genetic transmission, one of the properties of such a molecule would be its chemical stability. The metabolic stability of DNA was established by studies on metabolism of labeled adenine in rats, which indicated that the turnover of the nitrogenous bases of DNA was very slow (26, 46). Further evidence along the same line was obtained for both DNA and RNA in bacteria (143). This metabolic confirmation of the proposition of stability of DNA is rather satisfying but other nuclear products (28, 32) also turn over slowly (Chapters VI and VIII).

C. *Equal Division of DNA between the Daughter Cells*

In mitosis, the genetic transmitting substance is equally divided at the separation of the two daughter cells (110). However, this is a rather weak argument in favor of any substance as genetic material since almost all of the cellular components are equally divided at mitosis.

XII. Relevance of the Role of DNA as a Transmitting Substance to the Cancer Problem

Although much evidence establishes an important role for DNA in hereditary transmission (63, 144, 164–166), other nuclear or cytoplasmic components may be important. Nonetheless, it is clear that many aspects of the cancer problem will be resolved if differences can be established between the DNA and other hereditary factors of tumor cells and other cells (Chapter IV). The evidence available at present indicates that the DNA's have constancy in most cells in terms of weight, that the DNA's are probably quite stable metabolically, that the DNA's are present as an important part of the chromosomes, and that DNA's are important in viral infections and in the processes involved in "transformation," "transduction," and lysogeny. It is for these many reasons that there has been a great, if frustrating, emphasis on the role of DNA in both oncogenesis, or tumor-formation, and in cancer chemotherapy. In both of these areas, the information currently available falls short of the great expectations of the last two decades.

In oncogenesis, the role of DNA has been conceptually high-lighted in two major theories that have emerged in the last decade (Table 1.2). In a sense, both state that "cancer genes" (oncogenes) are responsible for the hereditary character of the neoplastic process and that this process is vertically transmitted by the simple events of DNA reproduction, chromosomal division, and continued, derepressed readout in the daughter cells. The concepts emerging from studies on "oncogenic viruses" (both DNA and RNA) have been summarized as indicating that either new DNA enters the cells and is lysogenized or integrated into host DNA (9, 51, 150, 155–157) or that the RNA of the virus is subjected to "reverse transcription" and that the DNA produced is integrated into the host genome (9, 155–157).

The other concept (27, 71) has suggested that the "cancer genes" are present in virtually all mammalian cells and that oncogenic stimuli, whether infectious, chemical, or physical, derepress these genes. Along with this derepression, other cellular functions may be simultaneously derepressed or repressed, depending upon the cells of origin of the tumors and other factors as yet undefined. Accordingly, it seemed possible that neoplastic cells would produce different products and both chemical and physical changes might be expected. In recent years, gene derepressions resulting from formation of some cancer cells has been highlighted. Some of these may be of diagnostic value, i.e., fetal proteins such as α-fetoglobulins and tissue-specific antigens such as gastrointestinal or colonic antigens (2, 49, 50, 72, 161, 177). At present, a great effort is in progress to establish immunological differences between tumors and other tissues with the goal of advancing immunotherapy of cancer. Although this search has not yet been of great practical value, it has offered sufficient promise that it is being widely investigated.

Another aspect of derepression of cancer genes in neoplastic transformation is the "oncogene hypothesis" (71). It is suggested that C-particles of RNA viruses form in tumor cells of various types of intracellular templates that are carried genetically as part of the mammalian cell genome. This may also be an expression of latent genes that emerge following exposure of cells to "oncogenic" or "carcinogenic" substances.

Chemotherapeutic attack has been made on DNA synthesis from many directions (27, 31, 164–166, 173). The problem of specific attack on "cancer DNA" or "cancer genes" regardless of whether it is genetically transmitted as part of the normal genome or is extrinsic DNA brought into cells from exogenous sources remains as an immense challenge to both molecular biologists and therapists alike. Thus far, none of the current drugs specifically attack DNA of cancer cells, i.e., all are generally toxic to any cell that is undergoing cell division. No method currently available distinguishes cancer DNA or even the DNA critical to growth or cell division from any other DNA templates in the cell. At present, sequence or structural information on nucleic acids is available only for RNA and only in a few cases such as transfer RNA, 5 S RNA, some small nuclear RNA's, and ribosomal RNA (32, 33). It would be miraculous indeed if there were sufficient information from any of these molecules to permit differentiation of cancer cells, other growing cells, and nontumor cells, particularly since such readouts of the genome are expressions of only several of the thousands of gene sets being read in any mammalian cells (see Chapters IV–VII). Since complementarity of the DNA to the RNA readouts is guaranteed by the Watson-Crick concept (165, 166), some information on DNA can be obtained from these studies. Unfortunately, none of the sequences of mammalian DNA have been determined because no method has been developed to define them.

Inasmuch as the endeavor with respect to DNA has seemed inordinately complex and, in truth, definition of "cancer DNA" per se has been almost completely lacking, it is not surprising that individuals working on the ,complex problems of molecular biology and genetics of cancer cells have turned their attention to events that mirror the activities of DNA. Thus, many studies have been undertaken in the more tractable fields of nuclear structures, chromosomes, nucleoli, chromatin, mitotic apparatus, and a variety of nuclear constituents that will be dealt with in subsequent chapters.

XIII. Problems in Isolation and Analysis of Nuclear Components

The key advances in cancer research and other areas of research are those involving the development of methods for dealing with special problems (29). Although many technical problems have been solved in the isolation of nuclei, nucleoli, chromosomes, and the mitotic apparatus (33, 34, 37, 104, 106, 107, 121), there are many supplementary problems that need further study (Table 1.3). In addition, there are critical problems involved in isolation of native, undegraded, and unaggregated nucleic acids, proteins, lipids, and membrane fractions from all portions of both normal and tumor cells. Other problems are involved in such studies including: (1) separation of the various types of nucleic acids into their individual molecular species, (2) analysis of the primary, secondary, and tertiary structures of these individual molecular species, and (3) determination of the functions of the individual molecules in tumors and other tissues. It is of very real importance to the cancer problem that the last decade has brought forward an increasing number of precise and definitive methods for the approach to all of these problems (29). The fact that little definitive information has yet been obtained to precisely differentiate cancer cells and other cells is simply a reflection of the vast scope of the problem rather than the inadequacy of the advances made thus far. In this connection, it cer-

TABLE 1.3

SUMMARY OF PROCEDURES FOR ISOLATION OF NUCLEAR COMPONENTS

A. *Following Initial Isolation of Nuclei*
   1. *Isolation of nucleoli:* Either by sonication of nuclei prepared in 0.0033–0.005 M $CaCl_2$ and 2.2 M sucrose or by compression and rapid decompression of nuclear preparations in the French pressure cell; purification by differential centrifugation
   2. *Isolation of chromosomes:* By gentle procedures employing cells in metaphase; aspiration and ejection from syringes followed by centrifugation in sucrose solutions 0.0005 M with respect to Mg^{2+} and Ca^{2+}
   3. *Isolation of nuclear ribonucleoproteins:* Extraction from nuclei of calf thymus by 0.15 M NaCl or 0.01 M Tris buffers containing 0.001 M $MgCl_2$ followed by differential centrifugation
   4. *Isolation of deoxyribonucleoproteins:* Either by extraction of nuclei with 2 M NaCl or with water followed by precipitation of the deoxyribonucleoproteins from solutions 0.10–0.20 M with respect to NaCl
   5. *Nucleolochromosomal apparatus:* A residual fraction obtained after successive extraction of nuclei with 0.15 M NaCl and 2 M NaCl; bears many similarities to the nuclear ribonucleoprotein network, but probably contains other components including the nuclear membrane

B. *Without Initial Isolation of Nuclei*
   1. *Nucleoli:* Obtained from tumors without extensive nuclear preparation inasmuch as it is not possible to remove cytoplasmic components in the presence of calcium ions at concentrations required to maintain the integrity of the nucleoli; techniques are the same as in A,1, above
   2. *Deoxyribonucleoproteins:* Obtained as a residue following prolonged treatment of nuclear preparations with isotonic saline solutions

tainly may be hoped that the passage of the National Cancer Act of 1971 will provide the financial means to rapidly advance the problem to the point of a precise chemical definition of the cancer problem.

XIV. Molecular Biology of Human Cancer

The objective of cancer research is the destruction of the neoplastic cells. While our present knowledge of molecular biology is rapidly increasing (29, 30, 52, 56a, 81a, 130, 142), relatively little is known about what differentiates the neoplastic cell from other cells. In the case of human neoplasms which are apparently considerably more complex than the animal models studied, fewer definitive studies have been made and much information on control tissues is required (58a). The hope that the study of human cancer would provide more definitive biochemical clues to the cancer problem in man has not been borne out thus far (141). The many attempts to characterize human tumors on the basis of their enzymatic, glycolytic, and other activities have not been fruitful by comparison with other types of studies. In part, this is because of the enormous complexities of the variations in the phenotypic readouts in human neoplasms which may vary markedly even in a single patient, let alone in a series of studies on one type of cancer. Although the increased use of human tumors in tissue culture and the improved cooperation of clinicians and pathologists handling cancer patients has brought about extensions of the studies on experimental neoplasms, at least to this point, the primary investigational tool in neoplastic disease continues to be tumors of rodents and other lower species. Because of their reproducibility and ready availability hopefully the initial clues to the solution of the cancer problem can emerge from such studies and be quickly evaluated for human tumors.

References

1. Abe, M., and Mizuno, D. (1959). *Biochim. Biophys. Acta* **32**, 464–469.
2. Abelev, G. I., Assecritova, I. V., Kraevsky, N. A., Perova, S. D., and Perevodchikova, N. I. (1967). *Int. J. Cancer* **2**, 551–558.
3. Abercrombie, M., and Ambrose, E. J. (1962). *Cancer Res.* **22**, 525–548.
4. Alloway, J. L. (1932). *J. Exp. Med.* **55**, 91–99.
5. Alloway, J. L. (1933). *J. Exp. Med.* **57**, 265–278.
6. Arrighi, F. E., Hsu, T. C., Saunders, P., and Saunders, G. F. (1970). *Chromosoma* **32**, 224–236.
7. Attardi, G., and Amaldi, F. (1970). *Ann. Rev. Biochem.* **39**, 183–226.
8. Avery, O. T., MacLeod, C. M., and McCarty, M. (1944). *J. Exp. Med.* **79**, 137–157.
9. Baltimore, D. (1970). *Nature (London)* **226**, 1209–1211.
10. Barner, H. D., and Cohen, S. S. (1954). *J. Bacteriol.* **68**, 80–88.
11. Bauer, H. (1935). *Z. Zellforsch. Mikroskop. Anat.* **23**, 280–313.
12. Beermann, W. (1961). *Chromosoma* **12**, 1–25.
13. Beermann, W. (1963). *Amer. Zoologist* **3**, 23–32.

14. Bender, M. A., and Mettler, L. E. (1958). *Science* **128**, 186–190.
15. Berenblum, I. (1941). *Cancer Res.* **1**, 807–814.
16. Berenblum, I. (1952). "Man Against Cancer." John Hopkins Press, Baltimore, Maryland.
17. Bernhard, W. (1963). *Progr. Exp. Tumor Res.* **3**, 1–34.
18. Boivin, A., Vendrely, R., and Vendrely, C. (1948). *C. R. Acad. Sci. Paris* **226**, 1061–1063.
19. Boveri, T. (1929). "The Origin of Malignant Tumors." Williams and Wilkins, Baltimore, Maryland.
20. Briggs, R., and King, T. J. (1952). *Proc. Nat. Acad. Sci. U.S.* **38**, 455–463.
21. Briggs, R., and King, T. J. (1959). *In* "The Cell" (J. Brachet and A. E. Mirsky, eds.), Vol. I, pp. 537–617. Academic Press, New York.
22. Brink, R. A. (1964). *In* "The Role of Chromosomes in Development" (M. Locke, ed.), pp. 183–230. Academic Press, New York.
23. Brody, S. (1953). *Acta Chem. Skand.* **7**, 495–501.
24. Brody, S. (1953). *Acta Chem. Skand.* **7**, 502–506.
25. Brody, S. (1958). *Nature (London)* **182**, 1386–1387.
26. Brown, G. B., Roll, P. M., Plentl, A. A., and Cavalieri, L. F. (1948). *J. Biol. Chem.* **172**, 469–484.
27. Busch, H. (1962). "An Introduction to the Biochemistry of the Cancer Cell." Academic Press, New York.
28. Busch, H. (1965). "Histones and Other Nuclear Proteins." Academic Press, New York.
29. Busch, H. (1967–1973). "Methods in Cancer Research," Vol. I–X. Academic Press, New York.
30. Busch, H. and Davis, J. R. (1961). *Ann. Rev. Med.* **12**, 165–184.
31. Busch, H. and Lane, M. (1967). "Chemotherapy." Yearbook Medical Publ., Chicago, Illinois.
32. Busch, H., Ro-Choi, T. S., Prestayko, A. W., Shibata, H., Crooke, S. T., El-Khatib, S. M., Choi, Y. C., and Mauritzen, C. M. (1971). *Persp. Biol. Med.* **15**, 117–139.
33. Busch, H., and Smetana, K. (1970). "The Nucleolus." Academic Press, New York.
34. Cantor, K. P., and Hearst, J. E. (1966). *Proc. Nat. Acad. Sci. U.S.* **55**, 642–649.
35. Caspersson, T. O., Farber, S., Foley, G. E., Kudynowski, J., Modest, E. J., Simonsson, E., Wagh, U., and Zech, L. (1968). *Exp. Cell Res.* **62**, 219–222.
36. Caspersson, T. O., and Santesson, L. (1942). *Acta Radiol. Suppl.* **46**, 1–105.
37. Chorazy, M., Bendich, A., Borenfreund, E., and Hutchison, D. J. (1963). *J. Cell Biol.* **19**, 59–69.
38. Clever, U. (1963). *Chromosoma* **14**, 651–675.
39. Clever, U. (1966). *Develop. Biol.* **14**, 421–438.
40. Cohnheim, J. (1889). "Lectures on General Pathology," Vol. II, p. 789. New Sydenham Soc., London.
41. Dalton, A. J. (1959). *Lab. Invest.* **8**, 510–537.
42. Dische, Z. (1930). *Mikrochemie* **8**, 4–32.
42a. Drets, M. E., and Shaw, M. W. (1971). *Proc. Nat. Acad. Sci. U.S.* **68**, 2073–2077.
43. Edström, J.-E., and Dan3holt, B. (1967). *J. Mol. Biol.* **28**, 331–343.
44. Emmons, C. W. and Hollaender, A. (1939). *Amer. J. Bot.* **26**, 467–475.
45. Feulgen, R. (1913). *Z. Physiol. Chem. Hoppe Seyler's* **84**, 309–328.
46. Furst, S. S., Roll, P. M. and Brown, G. B. (1950). *J. Biol. Chem.* **183**, 251–266.
47. Furth, J., and Kahn, M. C. (1937). *Amer. J. Cancer* **31**, 276–282.
48. Garen, A., and Zinder, N. D. (1955). *Virology* **1**, 347–376.
49. Gold, P. (1967). *Cancer* **20**, 1663–1667.
50. Green, H. N. (1954). *Brit. Med. J.* **2**, 1374–1380.
51. Green, M. (1970). *Ann. Rev. Biochem.* **39**, 701–756.
52. Greenstein, J. P. (1954). "Biochemistry of Cancer." Academic Press, New York.
53. Griboff, S. I. and Lawrence, R. (1961). *Amer. J. Med.* **30**, 544–563.
54. Griffen, A. B. (1958). *Ann. N.Y. Acad. Sci.* **71**, 1156–1162.
55. Griffith, F. (1928). *J. Hyg.* **27**, 113–159.
56. Gurdon, J. B. (1963). *Quart. Rev. Biol.* **38**, 54–78.

56a. Haddow, A. (1955). *Ann. Rev. Med.* **6**, 153–186.
57. Hall, R. H. and Gale, G. O. (1959). *Fed. Proc.* **18**, 950.
58. Hall, R. H. and Gale, G. O. (1959). *Soc. Exp. Biol. Med.* **1**, 487–491.
58a. Heidelberger, C. (1961). *Nature (London)* **189**, 627–628.
58b. Hecht, F., Wyandt, H. E., and Magenis, R. E. (1974). *In* "The Cell Nucleus" (H. Busch, ed.), Vol. II. Academic Press, New York.
59. Hershey, A. D. (1955). *Virology* **1**, 108–127.
60. Hershey, A. D., and Chase, M. (1952). *J. Gen. Physiol.* **36**, 39–56.
61. Hollaender, A. and Emmons, C. W. (1941). *Cold Spring Harbor Symp. Quant. Biol.* **9**, 179–186.
62. Hosokawa, K. (1950). *Gann* **41**, 236–237.
63. Hotchkiss, R. D. (1952). *In* "Phosphorus Metabolism" (W. D. McElroy and B. Glass, eds.), pp. 426–439. Johns Hopkins Press, Baltimore, Maryland.
64. Hsu, T. C. (1952). *J. Hered.* **43**, 167–172.
65. Hsu, T. C. (1967–1971). "An Atlas of Mammalian Chromosomes, " Vol. 1–5. Springer-Verlag, New York.
65a. Hsu, T. C., and Arrighi, F. E. (1971). *Chromosoma (Berl.)* **34**, 243–253.
66. Hsu, T. C. and Kellogg, D. S., Jr. (1960). *J. Nat. Cancer Inst.* **24**, 1067–1093.
67. Hsu, T. C., and Pomerat, C. M. (1953). *J. Hered.* **44**, 23–29.
68. Hsu, T. C., and Somers, C. E. (1961). *Proc. Nat. Acad. Sci. U.S.* **47**, 396–403.
69. Huberman, J. A., and Attardi, G. (1966). *J. Cell Biol.* **31**, 95–105.
70. Huberman, J. A. and Attardi, G. (1967). *J. Mol. Biol.* **29**, 487–505.
71. Huebner, R. J., and Todaro, G. J. (1969). *Proc. Nat. Acad. Sci. U.S.* **64**, 1087–1094.
72. Hull, E. W., Carbone, P. P., Gitlin, D., O'Gara, R. W., and Kelly, M. G. (1969). *J. Nat. Cancer Inst.* **42**, 1035–1044.
73. Ishibashi, K. (1950). *Gann* **41**, 1–14.
74. Jacob, F. (1955). *Virology* **1**, 207–220.
75. Jacob, F., and Monod, J. (1961). *J. Mol. Biol.* **3**, 318–356.
76. Jacob, F., and Wollman, E. L. (1955). *C. R. Acad. Sci. Paris* **240**, 2566–2568.
77. Jacob, F., and Wollman, E. L. (1956). *C. R. Acad. Sci. Paris* **242**, 303–306.
78. Jacob, F., and Wollman, E. L. (1961. "Sexuality and the Genetics of Bacteria." Academic Press, New York.
79. Jesaitis, M. A. (1961). *J. Gen. Physiol.* **44**, 585–603.
80. Kaiser, A. D., and Hogness, D. S. (1960). *J. Mol. Biol.* **2**, 392–415.
81. Kaplan, R. W. (1932). *Z. Naturforsch.* **71**, 221–304.
81a. Kensler, C. J. and Petermann, M. L. (1953). *Ann. Rev. Biochem.* **22**, 319–340.
82. King, T. J. (1966). *In* "Methods in Cell Physiology" (D. M. Prescott, ed.), Vol. II, pp. 1–36. Academic Press, New York.
83. Kinlough, M. A., Robson, H. N., and Hayman, D. L. (1961). *Nature (London)* **189**, 420.
84. Kline, B. E., and Rusch, H. P. (1944). *Cancer Res.* **4**, 762–767.
85. Knudson, A. G., Jr. (1971). *Proc. Nat. Acad. Sci. U.S.* **68**, 820–823.
85a. Knudson, A. G., Jr., and Strong, L. C. (1972). *J. Nat. Cancer Inst.* **48**, 313–324.
86. Kotin, P., and Falk, H. L. (1956). *Cancer* **9**, 910–922.
87. Kotin, P., Falk, H. L., and Thomas, M. (1956). *Cancer* **9**, 905–909.
88. Kozloff, L. M., and Lute, M. (1957). *J. Biol. Chem.* **228**, 529–536.
89. Kozloff, L. M., and Lute, M. (1957). *J. Biol. Chem.* **228**, 537–538.
90. Kozloff, L. M., and Lute, M. (1959). *J. Biol. Chem.* **234**, 539–546.
91. Kozloff, L. M., Lute, M., and Henderson, K. (1957). *J. Biol. Chem.* **228**, 511–529.
92. Kroeger, H. (1963). *J. Cell Comp. Physiol.* **62**(1), 45–59.
93. Kubowitz, F., and Ott, P. (1943). *Biochem. Z.* **314**, 94–117.
94. Lacks, S., and Hotchkiss, R. D. (1960). *Biochim. Biophys. Acta* **45**, 155–163.
95. Lara, F., and Hollander, F. (1966). IEG No. 7, Memo No. 766.
96. Lennox, E. S. (1955). *Virology* **1**, 190–206.
97. Levan, A. (1958). *Yearbook Cancer (Netherlands)* **8**, 110–126.

98. Levan, A. (1959). *In* "Genetics and Cancer," pp. 151–182. Univ. of Texas Press, Houston, Texas.
99. Levan, A., and Biesele, J. J. (1958). *Ann. N.Y. Acad. Sci.* **71**, 1022–1053.
100. Lunden, A. P. (1960). *Euphytica* **9**, 225–234.
101. MacCarty, W. C. (1936). *Amer. J. Cancer* **26**, 529–532.
102. MacCarty, W. C. (1937). *Amer. J. Cancer* **31**, 104–106.
103. MacCarty, W. C., and Haumeder, E. (1934). *Amer. J. Cancer* **20**, 403–407.
104. Maio, J. J., and Schildkraut, C. L. (1967). *J. Mol. Biol.* **24**, 29–39.
105. Mauritzen, C. M., Roy, A. B., and Stedman, E. (1952). *Proc. Roy. Soc.* **B140**, 18.
106. Mazia, D. (1955). *Symp. Soc. Exp. Biol. No. 9* 335–357.
107. Mazia, D. and Dan, K. (1952). *Proc. Nat. Acad. Sci. U.S.* **88**, 826–838.
108. Mendelsohn, J., Moore, D. E., and Salzman, N. P. (1968). *J. Mol. Biol.* **32**, 101–112.
109. Mercer, E. H., and Easty, G. C. (1961). *Cancer Res.* **21**, 52–56.
110. Meselson, M., and Stahl, F. W. (1958). *Proc. Nat. Acad. Sci. U.S.* **44**, 671–682.
111. Metz, C. W., and Armstrong, L. S. (1961). *Growth* **25**, 89–106.
112. Mirsky, A. E., and Pollister, A. W. (1942). *Proc. Nat. Acad. Sci. U.S.* **28**, 344–352.
113. Mirsky, A. E., and Ris, H. (1947–48). *J. Gen. Physiol.* **31**, 7–19.
114. Mirsky, A. E., and Ris, H. (1950–51). *J. Gen. Physiol.* **34**, 475–492.
115. Moorehead, P. S., Nowell, P. C., Mellman, W. J., Battips, D. M., and Hungerford, D. A. (1960). *Exp. Cell Res.* **20**, 613–616.
116. Morris, H. P., and Wagner, B. P. (1967). *In* "Methods in Cancer Research" (H. Busch, ed.), Vol. IV, pp. 125–152. Academic Press, New York.
117. Nester, E. W., and Lederberg, J. (1961). *Proc. Nat. Acad. Sci. U.S.* **47**, 52–55.
118. Nowell, P. C. (1965). *Progr. Exp. Tumor Res.* **7**, 83–103.
119. Nowell, P. C., and Hungerford, D. A. (1960). *Science* **132**, 1497.
120. Nowell, P. C., and Hungerford, D. A. (1961). *J. Nat. Cancer Inst.* **27**, 1013–1035.
121. Nowell, P. C., and Morris, H. P. (1969). *Cancer Res.* **29**, 969–970.
122. Nowell, P. C., Morris, H. P., and Potter, V. R. (1967). *Cancer Res.* **27**, 1565–1579.
123. Oberling, C., and Bernhard, W. (1961). *In* "The Cell: Biochemistry, Physiology, Morphology" (J. Brachet and A. E. Mirsky, eds.), Vol. V, pp. 405–496. Academic Press, New York.
124. Osgood, E. E. (1964). *Geriatrics* **19**, 208–221.
125. Pelling, C. (1959). *Nature (London)* **184**, 655.
126. Pelling, C., and Beermann, W. (1966). *Nat. Cancer Inst. Monograph* **23**, 393–410.
127. Penn, I. (1970). "Malignant Tumors in Organ Transplant Recipients." Springer-Verlag, New York.
128. Pitot, H. C. (1969). *Arch. Pathol.* **87**, 212–222.
129. Potter, V. R. (1957). *Univ. Mich. Med. Bull.* **23**, 400–412.
130. Rhoads, C. P. (1959). *Persp. Biol. Med.* **2**, 318–334.
131. Richards, B. M., and Atkin, N. B. (1959). *Brit. J. Cancer* **13**, 788–800.
132. Richards, B. M., and Bajer, A. (1961). *Exp. Cell Res.* **22**, 503–508.
133. Ris, H. (1957). *In* "The Chemical Basis of Heredity" (W. D. McElroy and B. Glass, eds.), pp. 23–62. Johns Hopkins Press, Baltimore, Maryland.
134. Roger, M., and Hotchkiss, R. D. (1961). *Proc. Nat. Acad. Sci. U.S.* **47**, 653–669.
135. Rous, P. (1910). *J. Exp. Med.* **12**, 696–710.
136. Rous, P. (1936). *Amer. J. Cancer* **28**, 233–272.
137. Rubin, H. (1955). *Virology* **1**, 455–473.
138. Saksela, E., Saxen, E., and Penttinen, K. (1960). *Exp. Cell Res.* **19**, 402–404.
139. Schleiden, M. J. (1938). Muller's Arch. Anat. Physiol. II; *Transl.:* Sydenham Soc., London, 1847.
140. Schwann, T. H. (1939) Berlin; *Transl.:* Sydenham Soc., London, 1847.
141. Shonk, C. E., and Boxer, G. E. (1967). *In* "Methods in Cancer Research," (H. Busch, ed.), Vol. II, pp. 579–661. Academic Press, New York.
142. Siebert, G. (1953). *Freiburger Symp. Med. Univ.* **2**, 82–86.
143. Siminovitch, L., and Graham, A. F. (1956). *J. Histochem.* **6**, 508–515.

144. Sinsheimer, R. L. (1957). *Science* **125**, 1123–1128.
145. Sinsheimer, R. L. (1959). *J. Mol. Biol.* **1**, 37–42.
146. Sinsheimer, R. L. (1959). *J. Mol. Biol.* **1**, 43–53.
147. Sisken, J. E. and Kinosita, R. (1961). *Exp. Cell Res.* **22**, 521–525.
147a. Smetana, K. (1970). *In* "Methods in Cancer Research" (H. Busch, ed.), Vol. V, pp. 455–478. Academic Press, New York.
147b. Smetana, K., and Busch, H. (1963). *Cancer Res.* **23**, 1600–1603.
147c. Smetana, K., and Hermansky, F. (1966). *Folia Haematol.* **86**, 36–46.
147d. Smetana, K., Unuma, T., and Busch, H. (1968). *Exp. Cell Res.* **51**, 105–122.
148. Spizizen, J. (1959). *Fed. Proc.* **18**, 957–965.
149. Sprunt, K., Redman, W. M., and Alexander, H. E. (1959). *Proc. Soc. Exp. Biol. Med.* **101**, 604–608.
150. Steplewski, Z., and Koprowski, H. (1970). *In* "Methods in Cancer Research" (H. Busch, ed.), Vol. V, pp. 156–191. Academic Press, New York.
151. Stich, H. F., and Emson, H. E. (1959). *Nature (London)* **184**, 290–291.
152. Stich, H. F., Florian, S. F., and Emson, H. E. (1960). *J. Nat. Cancer Inst.* **24**, 471–482.
153. Strong, L. C. (1958). *Ann. N. Y. Acad. Sci.* **71**, 807–1241.
154. Swift, H. (1964). *In* "The Nucleohistones" (J. Bonner and P. Ts'o, eds.), pp. 169–183. Holden Day, San Francisco, California.
155. Temin, H. M. (1965). *J. Nat. Cancer Inst.* **35**, 679–693.
156. Temin, H. M. (1966). *Cancer Res.* **26**, 212–216.
157. Temin, H. M., and Mizutani, S. (1970). *Nature (London)* **226**, 1211–1213.
158. Thiersch, C. (1865). "Der Epithelial Krebs." Engelmann, Leipzig.
159. Tjio, J. H., and Levan, A. (1956). *Hereditas* **42**, 1–6.
160. Virchow, R. (1855). *Arch. Pathol. Anat.* **8**, 1–39.
161. Von Kleist, S., and Burtin, P. (1969). *Cancer Res.* **29**, 1961–1964.
162. Wallach, D. F. H. (1969). *N. Eng. J. Med.* **280**, 761–767.
163. Warburg, O. (1926). "Uber den Stoffwechsel der Tumoren." Springer, Berlin.
164. Watson, J. D. (1965). "Molecular Biology of the Gene." Benjamin, New York.
165. Watson, J. D., and Crick, F. H. C. (1953). *Nature (London)* **171**, 737–738.
166. Watson, J. D., and Crick, F. H. C. (1953). *Nature (London)* **171**, 964–967.
167. Weber, G., and Lea, M. A. (1967). *In* "Methods in Cancer Research" (H. Busch, ed.), Vol. II, pp. 524–578. Academic Press, New York.
168. Weinhouse, S. (1951). *Cancer Res.* **11**, 585–591.
169. Weinhouse, S., Millington, R. H., and Wenner, C. E. (1951). *Cancer Res.* **11**, 845–850.
170. Witkin, E. M. (1958). *Proc. Int. Congr. Genet., 10th, Montreal* **I**, 280–299.
171. Wynder, E. L., Graham, E. A., and Croninger, A. B. (1953). *Cancer Res.* **13**, 855–864.
172. Wynder, E. L., and Hoffman, D. (1968). *In* "Methods in Cancer Research" (H. Busch, ed.), Vol. IV, pp. 3–52. Academic Press, New York.
173. Yarbro, J. W. (1970). *Geriatrics* **25**, 135–148.
174. Zamenhof, S. (1959). "The Chemistry of Heredity." Thomas, Springfield, Illinois.
175. Zamenhof, S., Alexander, H. E., and Leidy, G. (1953). *J. Exp. Med.* **98**, 373–397.
176. Zelle, M. R., Ogg, J. E., and Hollaender, A. (1958). *J. Bacteriol.* **75**, 190–198.
177. Zilber, L. A. (1958). *Advan. Cancer Res.* **5**, 291–329.
178. Zinder, N. D. and Lederberg, J. (1952). *J. Bacteriol.* **64**, 679–699.

CHAPTER II

The Nucleus of the Cancer Cell

HARRIS BUSCH AND KAREL SMETANA

I. Introduction

The discovery of the cell nucleus by Fontana (1781), Brown (1830), and Purkinje (1827) along with a remarkable accumulation of evidence led to the cell theory of Schleiden (1838), Schwann (1839), and Purkinje (1839). The growing research in cellular pathology (197) that followed these discoveries indicated that nuclear size was greater in cancer cells than other cells and led to diagnostic criteria for neoplasia. Lebert (93) was among the first who noted that the average size of the nucleus and nucleolus is greater in cancer cells than in nontumor cells. After others pointed out that the nucleus to cytoplasm ratio was greater in cancer cells than in other cells (83), such observations were much extended by MacCarty and others (71, 110–113) who showed that in tumor cells the nucleolar size was more consistently increased than the nuclear size. Similar findings were reported in experimental tumors (14, 36) confirming the results of studies on human cancer cells.

A. Nuclear Aberrations

From the point of view of the pathological anatomy of neoplastic cells, the changes in the nucleus are the most diagnostically useful markers of cancer. When stained with the hematoxylin and eosin stains or other stains in common clinical usage, the most characteristic features of cancer cells are the increased density of the chromatin, the presence of excessive numbers of mitotic figures, pleomorphism of the nucleoli (Fig. 2.1), and unusual numbers of spindles in the mitotic cells (Fig. 2.2). Along with other morphological manifestations of neoplasia, including penetration of the basement membranes of various tissues or invasiveness and penetration of regions that are normally separated from other types of cells, the diagnosis of cancer is generally made from nuclear abnormalities (25, 83, 93, 197).

The various causes of such aberrations have been well defined for some of these morphological phenomena. For example, the hyperchromicity of the nuclear chromatin is generally related to the increased rate of cell division of cancer cells and even more to the heteroploidy and hyperploidy of the chromosomes (see Chapter III). The increased number of mitotic figures seen throughout tumors is another manifestation of the increased rate of cell division in many types of tumors. However, some tumors do not exhibit either of these common characteristics of neoplastic change. In such cases, other diagnostic criteria are required.

Although there are few "pathognomonic" features of cancer cells from a morphological point of view, the presence of three or more mitotic spindles or division of the cells into three or more daughter cells is rare except in cancer cells. On rarer occasions there may be division of cancer cells into as many as twelve daughter cells (Fig. 2.2). However, such phenomena as multiplicity of the spindles are uncommon and more frequently the diagnosis of cancer at the light microscopic level is made by the abnormalities of the cytoarchitecture and the irregularities of nuclear as well as nucleolar size and shape that are grouped together as "pleomorphism" (28, 110–113).

Although nucleolar pleomorphism is found in many types of dividing cells in tissue culture or in cellular regeneration, the marked aberrations of nucleolar morphology in cancer cells were noted by cytologists more than 100 years ago (25, 83, 93). The studies of MacCarty and his associates (110–113) at the Mayo Clinic in the 1930's indicated that the diagnostic value of nucleolar pleomorphism for malignancy was statistically meaningful, and Caspersson and Santesson (28) further suggested that nucleolar aberrations in size and shape were "pathog-

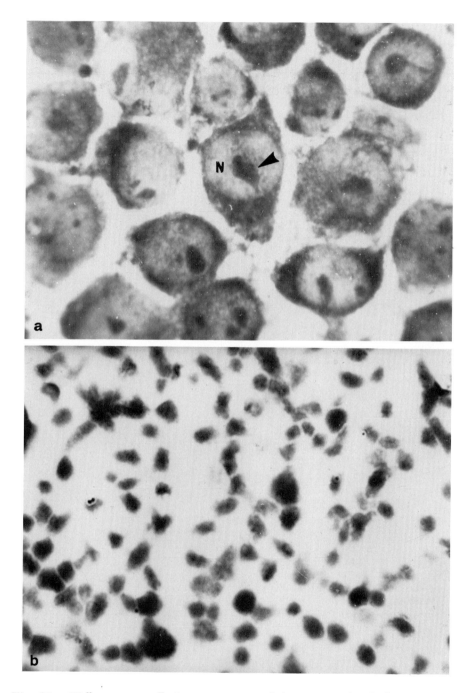

Fig. 2.1a. Walker tumor cells in a smear stained for RNA with toluidine blue (25). The nucleoli and cytoplasm are intensely stained and the chromatin of the nucleus (N) is not stained. The nucleoli are pleomorphic, i.e., they exhibit marked variations in shape and size as well as number. ×1600.

Fig. 2.1b. Isolated nucleoli from a Novikoff ascites hepatoma in a smear stained for RNA. These nucleoli also exhibit marked pleomorphism (T. S. Ro-Choi *et al.* in preparation). ×1400.

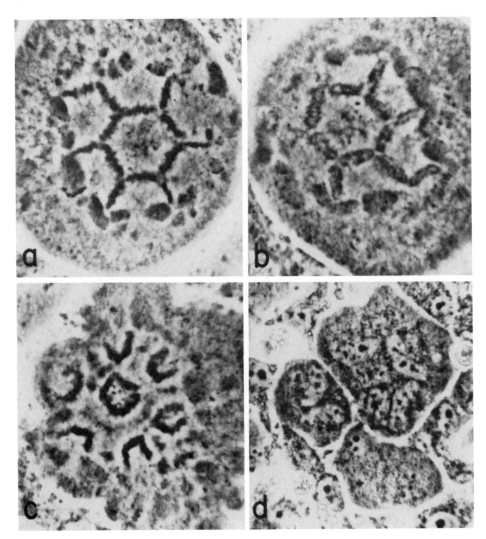

Fig. 2.2. Mitotic events producing multiple nuclei in a single nucleated giant KB cell. (a) unusual hexagonal mitotic figure, (b) and (c) metaphase and telophase, and (d) separated cell masses containing multiple nuclei. (Courtesy of Dr. George G. Rose, University of Texas Dental Branch, Houston, Texas.)

nomonic" for cancer. At present, a more precise statement would be that along with other criteria for malignancy, nucleolar pleomorphism provides an important aid to diagnosis of cancer (25, 139).

The nucleoli of rapidly growing experimental or human neoplasms exhibit the most marked pleomorphism of all of the types of neoplastic cells. In solid tumors, ascites tumor cells, and preparations of isolated nucleoli (Fig. 2.1, 2.3–2.6), there are enormous variations in the nucleolar sizes and shapes of tumor cells. In their microdissections of tumor nucleoli, Kopac and Mateyko (84, 85) noted that the shapes of many of these nucleoli were simply not readily

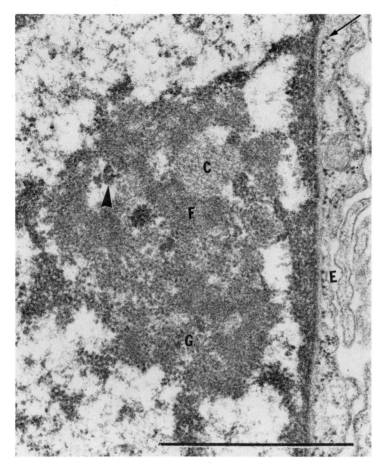

Fig. 2.3. A nucleolus in an epithelial cell of the human prostate gland; this nucleolus is composed of aggregated or coalescent nucleolonemas and contains a prominent fibrillar center (C), fibrillar elements (F), granular elements (G), intranucleolar chromatin (pointer), ribosomes attached to the external layer of the nuclear envelope (arrow), and endoplasmic reticulum (E). These samples and most of the others used for electron microscopy in this chapter were fixed in glutaraldehyde and osmium tetroxide. Samples of the human prostate were kindly provided by Dr. F. Györkey. ×52,000.

describable in usual terms. It is not known why the nucleoli of tumor cells undergo these "tortured" modifications in shape. It is unlikely that such changes simply result from increased synthesis of ribosomes since simple nucleolar hypertrophy, such as that observed in the nucleoli of livers of thioacetamide-treated rats (Fig. 2.7) is not accompanied by pleomorphism (25).

Even in a given tumor cell (Fig. 2.1), the nucleoli may differ markedly in size and shape. In a tumor mass, the extent of nucleolar variation depends on whether the cells are in the G_0 state, whether occasional cells are rapidly growing and dividing, or whether most tumor cells are growing and dividing. The fewer cells active in cell division, the fewer with enlarged and aberrant nucleoli. In some instances, the nucleoli may appear to be enlarged and essen-

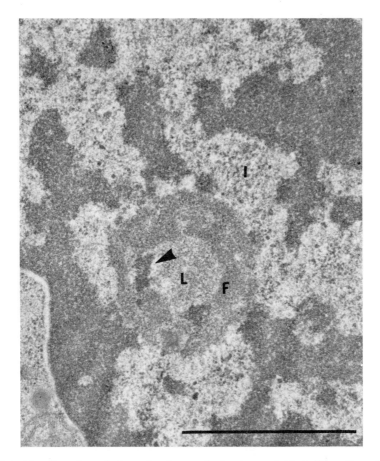

Fig. 2.4. Ring-shaped nucleolus of a human leukemic myeloblast. The ribonucleoprotein elements are in the nucleolar periphery forming a ringlike shell which surrounds a central light area (L). The fibrillar dense elements (F) are mostly present in the central light area. Condensed chromatin (pointer); interchromatin areas adjacent to the nucleolus (I) contain interchromatin granules (from 168a). ×46,000.

tially spherical and in others, the nucleoli may be small and several may be present. Thus, on a cell by cell basis, as is the case for most criteria of malignancy, nucleolar pleomorphism is not an adequate criterion of malignancy in a single cancer cell. However, its presence is very helpful for diagnosis especially in exfoliative cytology when considered with the morphology of other cellular components and previous therapy of the patient or treatment of experimental animals (52, 57, 136, 157, 158).

B. Nucleolar Size and Number

In general in human cancer cells, the nucleoli are enlarged and their mean diameters range from 0.5 to 3.0 μm. Their mean nucleolar areas range from 1.4

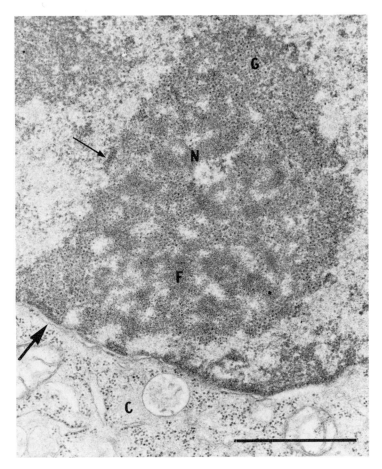

Fig. 2.5. A nucleolus of a Walker tumor cell at the nuclear membrane (large arrow). The nucleolus is composed of nucleolonemas (N), nucleolar fibrillar elements (F), granular elements (G), and nucleolus-associated chromatin (thin arrow). Cytoplasm (C) is also seen (from 25). ×33,000.

to 8.7 μm^2 (Table 2.1) and their nucleolar volumes from 10 to 25 μm^3 (30, 65, 67, 72, 118, 127, 132, 142, 156, 160, 177, 207). This increase in nucleolar mass is not strictly accompanied by a proportionate increase in the size of the nucleus and, accordingly, the size ratios of nucleolus:nucleus are greater than those for either normal cells or cells of benign tumors (59, 67, 71, 108, 110–113, 133). In general, a nucleolus:nucleus ratio of greater than 0.25 may be taken as one criterion of malignant growth with the provisos noted above with respect to other types of cells or cells adjacent to the tumors (21, 24, 27, 29, 55, 64, 120, 128, 149). For example, the mean nucleolar diameter was 1.49 μm in ovarian cystadenocarcinomas of the low malignancy grade I, 2.0 μm in the more malignant grade II, and 2.97 μm for the most malignant grade III. For an ovarian cystadenoma, a benign tumor, the corresponding diameter was 1.3 μm. Corresponding changes occur in the nucleolar areas (Table 2.1).

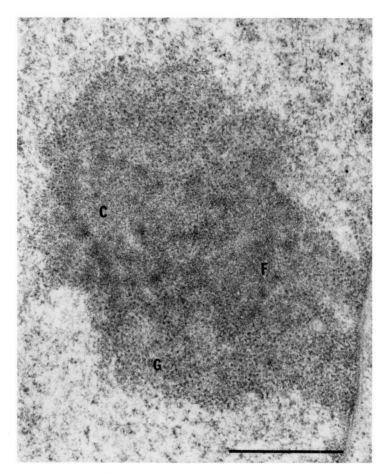

Fig. 2.6. A compact nucleolus of an Ehrlich ascites tumor lacking distinct nucleolonemas. It contains fibrillar elements (F), granular elements (G), and a fibrillar center (C). Fixation in osmium tetroxide and formaldehyde (from 192). ×31,000.

Under a variety of neoplastic and preneoplastic conditions there are marked changes in the sizes and shapes and occasionally in the numbers of the nucleoli in each cell. Although nucleolar enlargement has been found after application of noncarcinogenic substances on the skin of mice, there is a more pronounced nucleolar enlargement following application of carcinogens to the skin (34–36, 130, 131, 141); in the cells of methylcholanthrene-treated mouse skin, those cells that underwent malignant change had larger nucleoli than those that did not. Similarly, treatment with azo dyes, acetylaminofluorene, or ethionine produced enlargement of the nucleoli of liver cells and production of hepatomas (19, 31, 53, 63, 68, 79, 130, 179). As in carcinogen-treated cells, nucleolar enlargement has been observed in cells infected with oncogenic viruses and other viruses. However, these changes are more variable and less marked than those observed with chemical carcinogens (60–62, 117, 143, 148, 163).

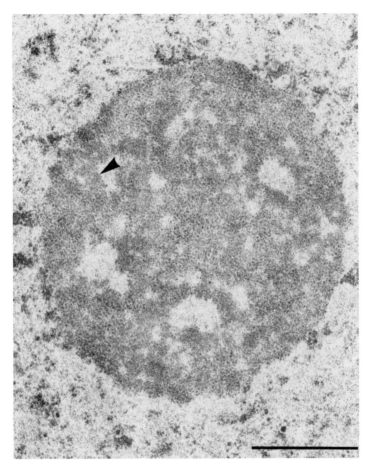

Fig. 2.7. Enlarged nucleolus of a thioacetamide-treated liver cell (8 days, 50 mg/kg daily). The nucleolus is composed of less distinct nucleolonemas and mainly contains granular elements. The amount of fibrillar elements (pointer) seems to be reduced. ×29,600.

Changes in nucleolar number seem to be very variable in neoplastic cells. For example, in hepatomas, whether human or experimentally produced in animals there was generally a decrease in the number of nucleoli per cell as compared to the normal liver. In normal liver, the mean number of nucleoli per cell is 2.7 and in hepatomas, the mean number is 1.3 nucleoli per cell. These data indicate that there are either special activities of specific nucleolar organizers or some sort of fusion of either nucleolar products or active sites. Frequently, many types of neoplastic cells have a single very large nucleolus and perhaps one or more small ones. In a few types of neoplastic cells, however, there may be a larger nucleolar number. For example, in some leukemic cells and in some cells of ovarian cystadenocarcinomas, there are marked increases in the numbers of nucleoli. If the change in nucleolar number is to be used as a criterion of malignancy, the number must be significantly increased or

TABLE 2.1
Mean Nucleolar Area in Various Human
Malignant Tumors Related to the
Histological Grading of the
Malignancy[a]

| | Grade of malignancy | | | |
Carcinoma	1	2	3	4
Thyroid	2.4	3.7	5.0	5.9
Breast	2.6	3.3	5.6	6.6
Liver	—	3.2	6.7	8.5
Stomach	—	3.2	3.8	4.9
Rectum	3.8	3.7	7.9	14.6
Ovary	2.1	4.7	4.6	—
Uterine cervix	—	5.3	9.7	6.0
Endometrium	2.6	3.4	4.5	8.3

[a] Values in μm^2; from Ferreira, 51.

decreased by comparison with control values for the specific tissue (25, 162). In virus-infected cells and virus-transformed cells, the changes of nucleolar size are less pronounced as compared with changes in the nucleolar shape, number, and appearance (4, 7, 11, 12, 38, 41–43, 46, 48, 49, 60–62, 69, 78, 86, 116, 121, 138, 145).

Although changes in nucleolar shape are related to the overall nucleolar pleomorphism of cancer cells, it has long been apparent that many types of cells contain irregularly shaped nucleoli (5, 22, 25, 40, 52, 75, 84, 85, 95, 97, 98, 103, 109, 142, 149, 177, 178, 207). In rapidly growing nontumor cells, such as those of regenerating liver, tissue culture cells, fibroblasts in young granulation tissue, proerythroblasts, and other cells in early prophase, nucleolar shapes may be as varied as those seen in tumor cells. Although in some instances it has been found that the tissue culture cells have undergone malignant transformation, this is probably not the whole explanation of these pleomorphic changes.

C. "Anisonucleolinosis"

"Anisonucleolinosis" is a term applied by Love and his associates (104, 105, 107) to changes in the morphology of some "light spaces" (Fig. 2.3) of nucleoli in tumor cells which may be "fibrillar centers" (105, 146). The nucleononemas of normal cells form the spongy matrix of the nucleolus and the spaces between these structures are less electron dense on electron microscopy.[1] Some of these spaces contain fibrillar structures which stain particularly well with toluidine blue and certain heavy metals (104–107). These structures, or somewhat larger

[1] The presence of metal ions in nuclei of tumors and other cells has been studied. In prostatic carcinomas, zinc ion was localized to nucleoli (66).

coalescences of these structures, become visible by light microscopy and are referred to as "nucleolini" (Fig. 2.8).

In nucleoli of normal cells, the number of nucleolini is approximately 10–25 and they are relatively constant in size and shape (104–107). "Isonucleolinosis" refers to the constancy of number, size, and shape of nucleolini. In neoplastic cells, the marked differences in the size and shape of the nucleolini is referred to as "anisonucleolinosis" (104, 105, 107).

There are changes in the sizes and shapes of these nucleolini in long term cultures (106, 107). After 26 generations, one previously "normal" cell line was transformed to a malignant cell line and under these conditions there was a change from "isonucleolinosis" to "anisonucleolinosis." The changes occurred simultaneously, suggesting that the control mechanisms involved in the "anisonucleolinosis" were relevant to the neoplastic change. A variety of pathological states also produce anisonucleolinosis, including treatment of cells with actinomycin D, 2-deoxy-5-fluorouridine, and the carcinogens, 2-nitroquinoline and thioacetamide. Infection of cells with herpes, polyoma, and SV40 viruses also produces such changes (25, 104–107, 122).

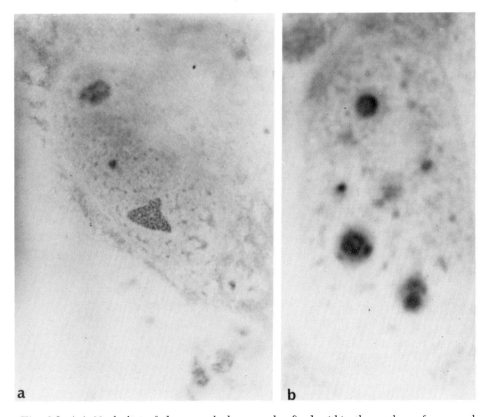

a   b

Fig. 2.8. (a) Nucleolini of dense nucleolar granules fixed within the nucleus of a normal cell (WI-38). All of the nucleolini are of approximately equal size. (b) Nucleolini of a tumor cell showing anisonucleoinosis; i.e., differences in the sizes of nucleolini. (Courtesy of Dr. Robert Love, Jefferson Medical College.)

II. Electron Microscopic Studies on Nucleoli of Cancer Cells

The characteristics of the nucleoli of human cancer cells seem to be related to growth rates of the cells (169a). In general, those cells with high growth rates have compact large nucleoli with less distinct nucleolonemas (Figs. 2.3–2.6) that contain many granular elements which are now believed to be precursors of cytoplasmic 60 S ribonucleoprotein (RNP) particles (Fig. 2.9). In tumor cells with lower growth rates, the nucleoli may be small and contain many light spaces or nucleolini (6, 10). Occasionally, the overall electron microscopic appearance of the nucleoli may be one of a skeinlike structure that occasionally resembles a large filament with concentric loops (25). In addition, there may be fibrillar cores surrounded by a ribonucleoprotein shell in such nucleoli (ring-shaped nucleoli) that show little evidence of rapid synthetic reactions involved in new RNA synthesis (25). The proliferative capacity of neoplastic cells with

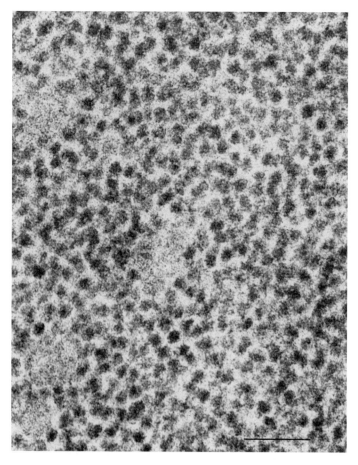

Fig. 2.9. Granular RNP elements isolated from nucleoli of thioacetamide-treated rat liver cells (from 87). ×180,000.

ring-shaped nucleoli seems to be decreased (140, 168a). The fibrillar elements have been noted to contain high molecular weight RNA precursors of the nucleolar RNP granules on the basis of electron microscopic autoradiography (12, 25). Another component of these fibrillar elements is apparently the low molecular weight U3 nucleolar RNA and possibly other low molecular weight RNA's (See Chapter VI) including 5 S, 5.5 S, and 8 S RNA (25).

Because they vary markedly in growth rates, the appearance of nucleoli of human tumors may differ markedly from those experimental tumors in which the growth rates are generally quite high. However, in the series of Morris rat hepatomas there was a similar variation in nucleolar electron microscopic appearance (25, 193). The nucleoli of the faster growing type contained large concentrations of the granular elements and those with lower growth rates had ultrastructural patterns similar to those of the normal liver. For some of the slowest growing of the tumors, the ultrastructural features were not significantly different from those of the normal liver (25, 193).

A. Nucleolar Dense Granules

Although there are a number of nucleolar components whose function remains to be determined (Figs. 2.3–2.6), e.g., the components of the fibrillar elements and the light spaces, some information has recently been accumulated about nucleolar granular elements. These granular elements of the nucleolus are of two types, one of which is essentially the same size as the 60 S ribosomal subunits (Fig. 2.9); the other is a structure that has a much larger size and greater electron density (Fig. 2.10). Many studies are now under way on the former because they are probably processing particles in which the nucleolar "assembly line" is functioning not only in properly sizing the RNA for delivery to the cytoplasm but also in stepwise addition of the most tightly bound ribosomal proteins and other protein elements of the ribosomes. These proteins are under intensive study with regard to their relationship to the cytoplasmic ribosomal proteins and their RNA-binding sites. Fortunately, excellent methods have been developed for the isolation of these RNP particles of the "dense granules" (Fig. 2.9) and the crucial problems at the present time are the insurance that these products are "native" and contain only undegraded elements.

Unfortunately there are few studies on the very "dense" granules of nucleoli (Fig. 2.10) (161, 163b, 194a, 196). These granules were best described in plant nucleoli where they are commonly found (76a, 180). However, they are also present in small numbers in normal liver nucleoli as well as under various experimental conditions (25) and in greater number in nucleoli of tumor cells. Their presence in these cells is probably a manifestation of the growth phenomena rather than a manifestation of the neoplastic characteristics of these cells since they are also present in cells of other rapidly growing tissues. For optimal demonstration of these granules the samples should be fixed in collidine-osmium tetroxide (25, 196). Hopefully it will not be too long until methods become available for their isolation and analysis.

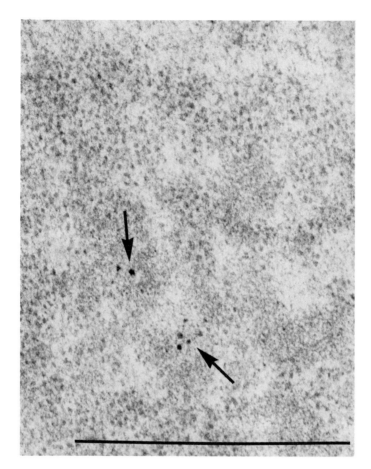

Fig. 2.10. Large dense particles (arrows) associated with fibrillar elements in a nucleolus of a Walker tumor cell. To demonstrate these particles, it is necessary to fix the sample in collidine buffered-osmium tetroxide (from 25). ×75,000.

B. Nucleolar Chromatin

Electron microscopic as well as light microscopic cytochemical studies (12, 25, 97, 98, 167, 168) indicate the presence of intranucleolar chromatin as well as perinucleolar chromatin (Fig. 2.11). The chromatin structures are present within the nucleolar body in a number of physical states including: (a) dispersed fine filaments about 20 Å in diameter (Fig. 2.12), (b) fibrils of various widths, or (c) chromatin structures organized in clusters of condensed chromatin (Fig. 2.11). At high magnifications these fibrils are also composed of coiled fine filaments 20 Å in width (Fig. 2.12). Quantitative planimetric measurements indicated that nucleoli of experimental hepatoma cells in rats contain more condensed intranucleolar chromatin than normal liver cells (194).

The perinucleolar chromatin is mostly composed of chromatin fibrils that form a discontinuous ring around the nucleolar body (Fig. 2.11). The proximal portion of the perinucleolar chromatin is an integral part of the nucleolus. It is connected with the intranucleolar chromatin by chromatin filaments or threads and has not been removed from the isolated nucleoli regardless of the isolation procedures used (Fig. 2.11B). In early light microscopic cytochemical studies, the nucleolus-associated chromatin was considered to be a part of the nucleolar apparatus. The proportion of the perinucleolar chromatin and intranucleolar chromatin may be different in nonproliferating normal liver and rapidly proliferating Novikoff hepatoma cells (194). For example, the areas of the perinucleolar chromatin appear to be relatively smaller in proliferating rat hepatoma cells than in normal rat liver cells. It is not clear why there are different relative proportions of perinucleolar and intranucleolar chromatin in normal and proliferating cells. These differences might reflect altered functional activities of the DNA of these cells. Much of DNA associated with the nucleolus does not code for rRNA but its function remains to be clarified.

III. Effects of Anticancer Agents on Nucleolar Ultrastructure

Among the anticancer agents, actinomycin D, daunomycin, and a number of clinically less useful agents produce dramatic alterations of nucleolar ultrastructure. They cause a marked reduction of synthetic reactions of the nucleolus in the fibrillar regions which are generally believed to be the site of synthesis of high molecular weight precursors of ribosomal RNA (25, 201). These RNA species are rapidly read off the nucleolar rDNA which is presumably monofilamentous in these regions (Fig. 2.12). In addition to the synthetic reactions which are apparently stopped abruptly by administration of such drugs (25, 77, 81, 151, 152, 208), there are transport reactions which are apparently unaffected. Such transport reactions cause a consolidation of the nucleolar granular elements at the edges or at one pole of the nucleolar body (Fig. 2.13) while the fibrillar elements are either left in the central mass of the nucleolar body or appear at the other pole.

The zonal separation of the nucleolar elements (Fig. 2.13) is referred to as "nucleolar segregation" by most electron microscopists (8, 12, 25, 144, 147, 165, 166, 173, 182–185, 189). Svoboda and his associates (144, 183–185) have introduced the term, "microsegregation" of the nucleolar elements, which indicates that there are masses of segregating nucleolar elements which are aggregated. Among the usual nucleolar components in such areas, not infrequently there are also central fibrillar masses, similar to those found in nucleoli of fetal tissues. Dense granules or larger masses of the same type that have been referred to as "microspherules" are often found in these areas.

A. Nucleolar "Microspherules"

In enlarged nucleoli of rapidly growing cells that are treated with inhibitors of nucleolar RNA synthesis, there are frequently noted relatively large dense

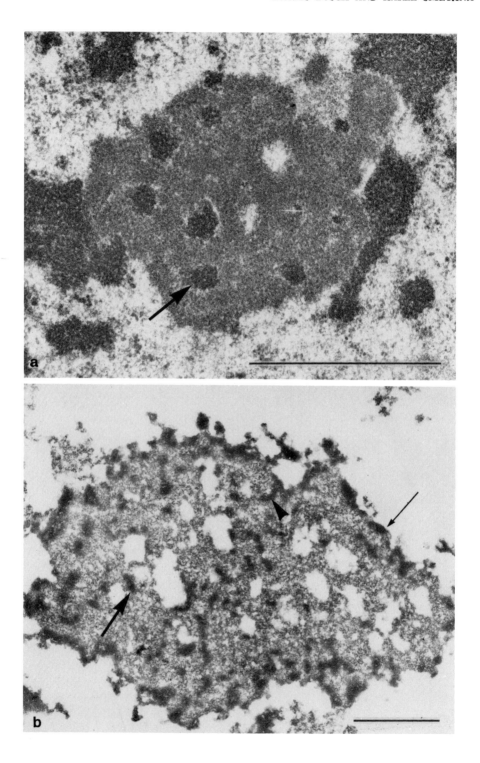

elements (Fig. 2.14) that have been referred to as "microspherules" (192). Large dense plaques have also been found in such nucleoli, but they seem to represent a type of intranucleolar segregation phenomenon in cells where the nucleolar size is too great to permit separation of the overall nucleolar mass into blocks as can be seen in Fig. 2.13. The macrosegregations of nucleoli may be sufficiently large that they are visible as "caps" in the light microscope (25); formation of microspherules is not visible by light microscopy.

B. Nucleolar Dark Substance

The schematic picture developed by Simard and Bernhard (166) (Fig. 2.15) shows that a dense substance appears under some circumstances during the course of macrosegregation. In nucleoli of cells treated with aflatoxin, appearance of this dark substance gave the nucleolus a "Mickey Mouse" appearance (25). The composition of the dark substance is not clearly defined but it may be similar to that of the microspherules. Much of the nucleolar substance contains RNA as shown by decreased density after RNase treatment of cells and tissues before fixation or even after some types of fixation. Similarly RNase treatment decreased the density of the segregated nucleolar elements and also decreased the density of the nucleolar "microspherules." Treatment with pepsin alone had no effect and pepsin together with RNase had no greater effect than RNase alone. For these reasons, it may be assumed that the "dark masses" or microspherules are composed primarily of RNA but also other substances are present, possibly glycoproteins or mucoproteins.

C. Types of Mechanisms Involved in Nucleolar Segregation

There are marked variations in both the effects and the mechanisms involved in the various forms of segregation of nucleolar elements. All of the compounds in Table 2.2 inhibit RNA synthesis but there are notable differences in both the results and mechanisms. For example, both actinomycin D and aflatoxin B_1 inhibit RNA polymerase (25, 58, 77, 90, 165, 176). However, when the nucleotide composition of the newly synthesized RNA was determined, that produced in the aflatoxin B_1-treated nucleoli did not differ markedly from the control but that produced after actinomycin D treatment has a high content of AMP and UMP. Thus, actinomycin D treatment produces a preferential shutoff of rDNA readouts but aflatoxin B_1 is apparently less specific. Among the substances

---

Fig. 2.11a. Nucleolus of a neoplastic cell from a human hepatocellular carcinoma. The nucleolus contains large clusters of the condensed chromatin (arrow). The sample was kindly provided by Dr. F. Györkey. ×51,000.

Fig. 2.11b. Condensed chromatin structures in and on the surface of an isolated nucleolus from Novikoff hepatoma cells. Nucleolus-associated chromatin (thin arrow), intranucleolar condensed chromatin (thick arrow), septalike structures penetrating from the perinucleolar chromatin into the nucleolar body (pointer). Fixation in formaldehyde and trichloroacetic acid. (T. S. Ro-Choi et al., Exp. Cell Res.) ×22,500.

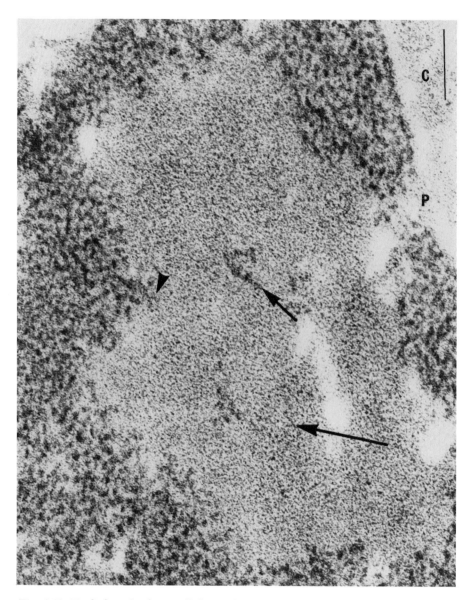

Fig. 2.12. Nucleolus of a liver cell digested with RNase after a short fixation in formaldehyde prior to embedding to facilitate demonstration of the intranucleolar chromatin. A chromatin fibril (small arrow) is composed of fine filaments. A solitary chromatin filament (large arrow) in the nucleolar body represents intranucleolar dispersed chromatin. Penetration of chromatin filaments from the perinucleolar chromatin into the nucleolar body is also seen (pointer). Cytoplasm (C), region of the nuclear pore (P). ×185,000.

that have been shown to have direct inhibitory effects on the RNA polymerase system are chromomycin A_3, lasiocarpine, nickel carbonyl, and 4-nitroquinoline-N-oxide (25, 134, 135, 147, 181).

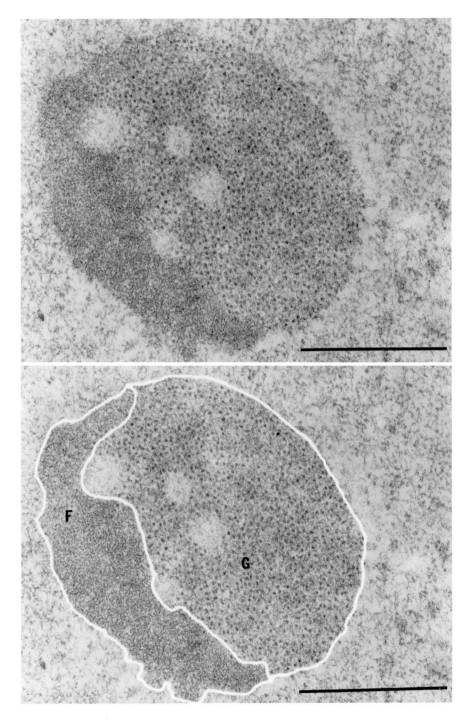

Fig. 2.13. Nucleolar segregation in a liver cell produced by actinomycin D. Separated areas containing fibrillar elements (F), granular elements (G). This sample was fixed in osmium tetroxide (from 173). ×40,000.

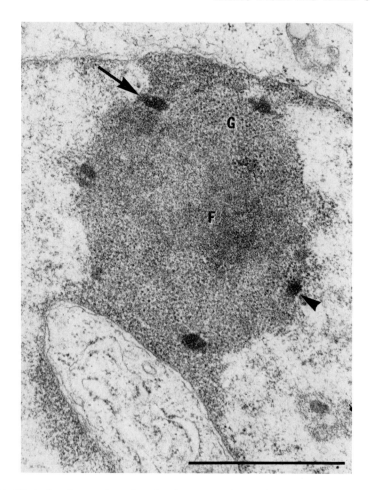

Fig. 2.14. Nucleolar dense microspherules (pointer and arrow) in an actinomycin D-treated nucleolus of an Ehrlich ascites tumor cell. Fibrillar elements (F), granular elements (G). Fixation in osmium tetroxide (from 192). ×42,000.

TABLE 2.2

ANTIBIOTICS CAUSING NUCLEOLAR
SEGREGATION AND INHIBITION
OF RNA SYNTHESIS[a]

Actinomycin D	Mitomycin D
Aflatoxin B₁	Nogalomycin
Anthramycin	Olivomycin
Chromomycin A₃	Puromycin
Cordecypin	Quinomycin A
Cycloheximide	Rifamycin
Daunomycin	Streptovaricin
Echinomycin	Triostin C
Mithramycin	Toyocamycin

[a] From Busch and Smetana, 25.

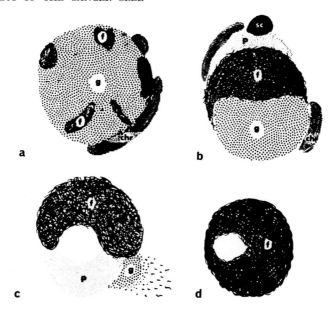

Fig. 2.15. Morphological sequence of nucleolar segregation. g, Granular elements; f, fibrillar elements; p, pars amorpha; sc, dense substance; chr, nucleolus-associated chromatin (166).

Some of the inhibitory agents were reported to intercalate into the DNA structure and thereby inactivate the rDNA; such substances include mitomycin C, proflavine, ethidium bromide, and actinomycin D (99, 150, 198). Some physical changes in the DNA produce marked inhibition of its function. Heat, X-radiation, and UV radiation produce specific scission, separation of strands, or base changes in DNA (125, 165, 198). Such changes in the nucleolar DNA-protein complexes markedly interfere with the biosynthetic reactions of the nucleolar synthetic system.

One interesting area of investigation is the migration of nucleolar elements out of the nucleolar substance after definitive granular elements have been laid down. It seems clear that dynamic events are involved in the production of the physical elements of the nucleolus that only now are beginning to be appreciated. Some energy-dependent reactions result in their migration to the nuclear membrane and then to the cytoplasm but it is clear that these are unaffected by the variety of agents that result in the inhibition of nucleolar synthetic reactions. In essence, the migration of the products to the nucleoplasm results in the "segregation" of the various types noted above. This aspect of nucleolar function is quite important in view of the interplay that seems to exist among hormonal chromosomal function, nucleolar gene readouts, and transport of special polysomes to the cytoplasm.

D. Stimulation of the Nucleolus

Most of the antibiotics, analogs, or other organic agents that affect the nucleolus are inhibitors of its biosynthetic activities. However, it is quite apparent that there are physiological activators of nucleolar function including hormones, feedback derepressors, and direct nucleolar activators (Table 2.3). Although it has been generally considered that many hormones act through feedback control systems, recently it was suggested that an initial primary effect of cortisone is directly on the nucleolus (206). The time sequence of biosynthetic reactions is first the synthesis of GC-rich nucleolar RNA followed by synthesis of messenger type AU-rich RNA. A similar type of result was found for synthesis of RNA in the prostate following the administration of androgens (100, 101). The generalization has been proposed that biosynthetic events following administration of hormones are initiated with nucleolar systhesis of GC-rich ribosomal RNA which is an obligate preparatory step for the readout and utilization of the specific cellular messengers that emerge into the cytoplasm as polysomes (188). Although proof of this concept is lacking to this point, the number of experiments supporting the idea is impressive.

Other types of nucleolar stimulatory substances are of interest from the point of view of carcinogenesis and the immunological systems. From the marked increase in the size of the nucleolus following the administration of thioacetamide to rats, it seemed possible that either thioacetamide had a direct effect on the nucleolus or functioned through a feedback system. Some evidence has been obtained in recent months for the former idea, i.e., incubation of nucleoli with thioacetamide may actually increase the activity of the nucleolar RNA polymerase system directly. However, there are marked effects of thioacetamide on the distribution of RNase and the content of ribosomal RNA in the cytoplasm which may produce the conditions necessary for the rapid synthesis of new ribosomal RNA as a compensatory process (32, 33).

In the cytoplasm of liver cells exposed to thioacetamide, the RNase content does not undergo such a marked increase but instead changes from a "latent" to an active RNase and also from particle-bound to free RNase. Apparently, the RNase that is well protected in the liver lysosomes or is membrane or structure bound undergoes a marked redistribution. Under these conditions, the lysosomal membranes are broken or the RNase inhibitors utilized first to block activity of the free RNase become insufficient for binding additional RNase

TABLE 2.3
NUCLEOLAR STIMULATORS

Stimulator	Mode of action	
	Direct	Feedback
Hormones		
Cortisone	++	?
Estrogens	++	?
Androgens	++	?
Activators		
Phytohemagglutinins	?	++
Thioacetamide	?	++

that becomes liberated. Within 24 hours after administration of thioacetamide, there is a 20% decrease in the content of cytoplasmic "microsomes" and by 9 days there is a 40% decrease. Presumably this decrease activates the "feedback" control system which then results in the enormous nucleolar activation. The nucleolar hypertrophy produced results in the appearance of enormous nucleoli. Their rates of synthesis of preribosomal RNA have been found to approximate twice the rates of regenerating liver and ten times the rates of normal liver, i.e., they produce approximately 30 femtograms of RNA per nucleolus per minute (25).

This rate of synthesis of 45 S nucleolar RNA is approximately the same as that found in rapidly growing tumor cells, i.e., approximately 45 fg of RNA per nucleolus per minute. There is no clear explanation for the morphological differences of the nucleoli of tumors as compared to those of the normal or even thioacetamide livers in which the nucleoli are almost all spherical, although there may be some relationship to either impending or completed cell division. Some relationships may be presumed between the synthetic activity of the nucleoli in both tumors and thioacetamide treated cells. The probability is that both represent cases of nucleolar release from repressors (37). If the administration of thioacetamide is discontinued, there is an increase in the amount of ribosomes in the liver cells and a decrease in nucleolar synthesis and nucleolar size. Thus, in these cells normal nucleolar control mechanisms are still functional.

E. PHA-Stimulated Lymphocytes

Following the administration of phytohemagglutinin (PHA) to normal animals or animals with acute leukemia or even lymphocyte preparations *in vitro*, there is a marked increase in the biosynthetic activity of the nucleoli, although it may be less or slower in leukemic lymphocytes (2, 25, 154a). This stimulatory effect is correlated with an increase in the overall protein synthetic activity of these cells along with an apparent restoration of cell division and ability to respond to immunological challenge. The change in the nucleoli is particularly marked since there is only a "ring-shaped (annular)" or "shell-like" nucleolus in the resting or mature lymphocyte which is an "idling" state (25). On administration of PHA, however, the massive increase in nucleolar size is associated with ultrastructural changes from a largely inactive structure with only a shell of ribonucleoprotein elements to a compact, "immature" nucleolus with large amounts of granular and fibrillar components (25, 189b).

Neither the rates of synthesis of RNA in the nucleoli of these PHA-stimulated cells nor the mechanisms of derepression of their nucleolar biosynthetic activities are known, so no clear-cut comparisons can be made with similar processes in tumor cells or thioacetamide-treated liver cells. However, it is clear that in the normal or resting lymphocytes there is a virtually complete repression of nucleolar biosynthetic reactions which are then derepressed in these stimulated cells. It is of great interest to determine the mechanisms of these derepressions as well as the nature of the normal repressors of nucleolar function in lymphocytes.

IV. Nuclear RNP Particles in Tumor Cells

Nuclei of neoplastic cells contain a variety of ribonucleoprotein (RNP) particles (11, 25). One type is found in the granular components of nucleoli (p. 53), which can be isolated in good yield from a variety of cells including normal and thioacetamide-treated liver cells (Fig. 2.10). These nucleolar RNP particles closely resemble the cytoplasmic ribosomal 60 S rRNP subunits both in size and shape (87, 89, 102, 163a, 199, 200). This finding is of interest in view of the postulated role of the nucleolus as a site of both biosynthesis and processing of the ribosomal precursors. It is not clear whether the nucleolar product is a mature RNP particle that is ready to serve as the fully formed ribosomal subunit or whether such particles serve some special function as "nascent" particles that are ready for further processing possibly in the nuclear RNP network (Fig. 2.16).

Another type of RNP particle is the "informosome" or a particle that is reputed to contain messenger RNA in a "packaged" form for delivery to the cytoplasm. Although there is little specific information on this subject, it seems certain that these particles do contain an AU-rich RNA that may be of the proper size to serve as messenger RNA's for specific cytoplasmic protein synthesis.

In addition to these particles, many of the nuclei of neoplastic cells contain a variety of other ribonucleoprotein (RNP) structures. The composition of these structures and their function in the cell nucleus is much less clear than that of the nucleolar ribonucleoprotein granules.

A. The Interchromatin Granules

Interchromatin areas of the nucleus contain a complex RNP network. Within this network only interchromatin granules (Fig. 2.16b, 2.17) have been morphologically characterized (124, 165, 171). The number of interchromatin granules is usually high in neoplastic cells. The size of these granules ranges between 100 and 300 Å. Cytochemical ultrastructural studies indicated that although interchromatin granules contain RNA they are resistant to RNase. This resistance of interchromatin granules to the RNase decreases after pretreatment with pronase in ultrathin sections (124) or it is completely lost when the suspended cells are predigested with pepsin prior to embedding for electron microscopy (171) indicating that the RNA in these particles is protected against RNase by proteins.

Although the biochemical composition and the function of interchromatin granules remain to be clarified, some of the interchromatin granules may be particles isolated from the nuclear sap. The biochemical analysis of such isolated particles suggested that they contain a rapidly labeled polydisperse DNA-like RNA with messenger properties (120a, 155). The isolated 40 S nuclear particles which are similar to the interchromatin granules in respect to their ultrastructure and cytochemistry contain rapidly labeled RNA (120a, 124, 124b, 155). However,

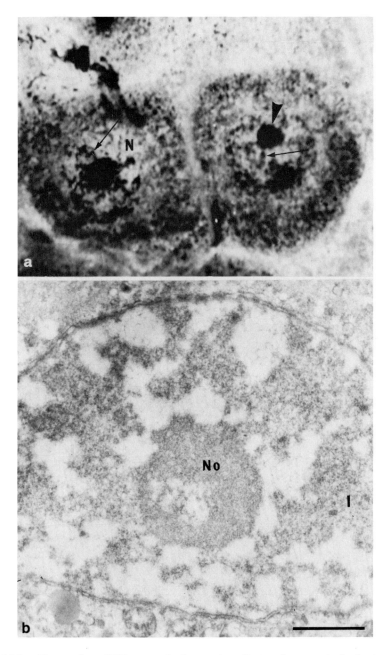

Fig. 2.16a. The nuclear RNP network (arrows) radiating from nucleoli (pointer) in a liver cell extracted with 0.14 *M* NaCl prior to smearing and staining with toludine blue for RNA; nucleus (N) (from 173a). ×2100.

Fig. 2.16b. The RNP network in a Walker tumor cell after treatment with 0.14 and 2 *M* NaCl prior to fixation in osmium tetroxide and embedding. The chromatin is extracted and the RNP network apparently corresponds to the various filaments and granules of the interchromatin areas (I) to which the nucleolus (No) seems to be attached (from 161a). ×22,000.

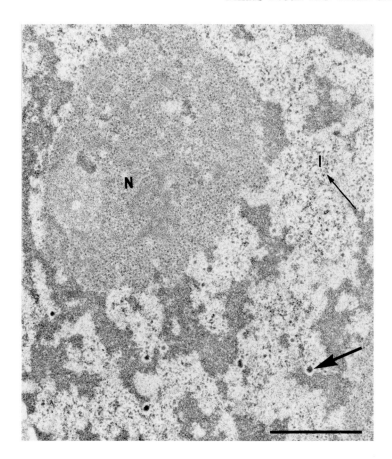

Fig. 2.17. Perichromatin granules (large arrow) surrounded by a distinct light halo in a human myeloblast. Numerous interchromatin granules in interchromatin areas (I), nucleolus (N), cluster of interchromatin granules (small arrow). ×24,000.

ultrastructural autoradiographic studies indicated that interchromatin granules contain slowly labeled RNA species (50a). Isolated polyribosomelike structures composed of monomeric "informofers" bound to the D-RNA strand have a similar ultrastructural appearance to the interchromatin granules *in situ* that are linked by dense filaments (155).

B. The Perichromatin Granules

These granules are frequently seen in nuclei of neoplastic and normal cells (Fig. 2.17). They are surrounded by a clear halo and are usually localized at the periphery of the condensed chromatin. Occasionally they can be found in interchromatin areas and within chromatin clusters. They can be rarely observed in interchromatin areas or within condensed chromatin. The size of perichromatin granules is relatively large ranging from 200 to 500 Å. Cytochemical studies indicate that the perichromatin granules are composed of fine filaments containing RNA and not DNA (195) since they are positively stained with the EDTA method which preferentially stains RNA-containing structures. They are also sensitive to digestion with pronase followed by RNase (195). These perichromatin granules increase in number when the nucleolar RNA synthesis is blocked but the synthesis of other rapidly labeled species of nuclear RNA is continuing (124a, 172). This result suggests that the formation of these granules might be related to extranucleolar RNA synthesis and nuclear transport of RNP particles (124a). It is possible that some of the perichromatin granules are rapidly labeled nuclear RNP particles such as informosomes (195).

C. The Perichromatin Fibrils and Coiled Bodies

Perichromatin fibrils were demonstrated by Bernhard's EDTA procedure (9, 124). They are present at the margins of condensed chromatin and their width ranges between 30 and 50 Å. Experiments in which nuclear RNA synthesis in liver cells is increased by cortisone or refeeding of starved animals produces an increase in the perichromatin fibrils suggested that these structures might represent the morphological expression of the rapidly labeled chromosomal or "DNA-like" RNA synthesis as found by corresponding biochemical studies (137). This suggestion is also supported by high resolution autoradiography which indicates the presence of silver grains over areas containing perichromatin fibrils when the cells were labeled with tritiated RNA precursors (50a, 195). The presence and morphology of RNP coiled bodies has been described (124) but their function in the cell nucleus is not known. Classic fixation and staining procedures did not readily permit their detection but they were easily seen after staining by the EDTA procedure of Bernhard (9). The size of the coiled bodies ranges from 0.3 to 0.5 nm in diameter. At higher magnifications, these bodies are composed of coiled RNP threads 400–600 Å in width (124).

D. Nuclear Bodies

Since the first descriptions of nuclear bodies (41, 202), their ultrastructural morphology and presence has been described for various cells (15, 18, 26, 44, 74, 80, 88, 91, 175, 186, 203). However, their function and their composition have not been satisfactorily clarified (15, 26, 45, 82, 88, 164, 203).

The ultrastructure of nuclear bodies is variable and several classifications of these bodies were proposed (15, 45, 126, 139). The simplest nuclear bodies are represented by relatively compact spherical fibrillar or filamentous structures with diameters of 0.3–0.5 nm (Fig. 2.18A). Some of the larger fibrillar nuclear bodies (0.5–0.8 nm in diameter) are composed of circularly oriented fibrils 50–100 Å wide (Fig. 2.18B). More complex nuclear bodies consist of a micro-fibrillar cortex surrounding a central core that contains dense structures of varying morphology and number. These include granules 200–250 Å in diameter,

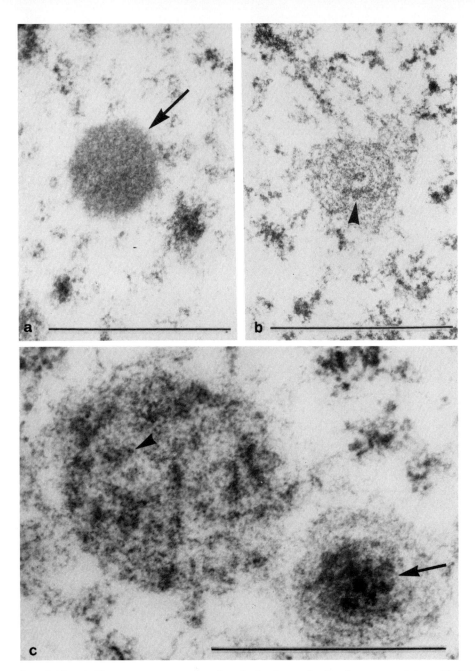

Fig. 2.18a. A filamentous compact nuclear body (arrow) of a human prostate epithelial cell (from 169). ×44,100.

Fig. 2.18b. Nuclear body (pointer) in a human prostate epithelial cell composed of a filamentous concentrically arranged cortex and a central core which contains a few structures of higher density than the cortical filaments. The sample was kindly provided by Dr. F. Györkey. ×45,000.

Fig. 2.18c. Complex nuclear bodies from the same specimen as in Fig. 15b. The larger body contains fibrillar and filamentous structures of varying density. Some of the dense fibers appear to be composed of dense twisted filaments. This body resembles the "coiled body" described by Monneron and Bernhard (124). The smaller nuclear body is composed of concentrically arranged filaments and a central core composed of dense particles (arrow). ×55,800.

TABLE 2.4
THE PRESENCE OF NUCLEAR BODIES IN
VARIOUS HUMAN TUMORS

Tumor	Ref.
Leukemias	18, 88, 170a
Hodgkin's disease	18, 88
Multiple myeloma	13, 170
Intracranial teratoma	88
Adenoma of the chorioid plexus	88
Ependymoma	15
Gliomas	15, 88, 154
Meningiomas	153
Mixed salivary tumors	82
Bronchial carcinomas	15
Cervical cancer	73
Mammary cancer	73
Wilms tumor	88
Melanoma	126
Keratoacanthoma	26

larger granules or globules, fibrils, or microtubularlike structures (1, 15, 80, 82, 126, 164, 203). Large nuclear bodies composed of fibrils and threadlike dense structures (Fig. 2.18C) may be the coiled bodies described recently (124).

Nuclear bodies are frequently found in neoplastic cells of malignant as well as benign human and animal tumors (Table 2.4). On the other hand, nuclear bodies have also been found in other diseases of human and animal as well as plant cells under normal and experimental conditions (1, 15, 26, 44, 45, 74, 88, 91, 96, 123, 139, 164, 172, 186, 191, 203). Thus, their presence is not characteristic for nuclei of neoplastic cells. Interestingly, nuclear bodies have been found in human meningiomas but not in normal meninges (153).

The origin of these nuclear bodies is still being evaluated. Simple filamentous compact nuclear bodies seem to originate from various filamentous or fibrillar nucleolar components including chromatin structures associated with the nucleolus (50, 169). The more complex nuclear bodies composed of the fibrillar cortex and granular or fibrillogranular cortex also appear to be of nucleolar origin (82). On the other hand, some studies on nuclear bodies suggested that these structures represent nuclear organelles developing from simple to more complex structures as the result of the cellular hyperactivity under various physiological experimental, and pathological situations (15, 44, 45, 50, 72a, 80, 82, 169–171). The formation of structures similar to nuclear bodies has been observed during inhibition of nucleolar synthesis with actinomycin D (44a, 70, 172).

E. The Nuclear Fibrillar Bundles or Rodlike Inclusions

Fibrillar bundles or rodlike inclusions are less frequently found than nuclear bodies, usually in nerve cells or gliomas (47, 115, 154, 187), and only occasionally in other cells (3, 74, 139). Rodlike inclusions are relatively large (0.5–10 nm in length, 0.5–2 nm in width) and sometimes some are surrounded by a filamentous shell which is similar to that of nuclear bodies (74).

The rodlike inclusions are composed of arrays of parallel fibers ranging in width from 60 to 100 Å. Their composition has not been clarified although they are resistant to digestion with ribonuclease and partially sensitive to the treatment with pronase or pepsin (159). The significance of rodlike inclusions in the nucleus is unknown. However, they were found in nerve cells, oocytes, and embryonic cells after treatment with actinomycin D (78a, 92, 115). The relationship of rodlike inclusions to the nucleolus or nuclear bodies is uncertain (115, 139, 187) but they are closely associated with these structures in some cells (47, 187).

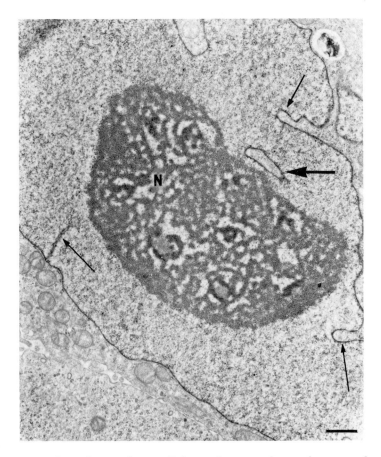

Fig. 2.19. A nucleus of a neoplastic cell from a human malignant hepatoma showing cytoplasmic invaginations into the nucleus (thin arrows). The cross section of the invagination is a nuclear pseudoinclusion (thick arrow). Nucleolus (N). Samples were kindly provided by Dr. F. Györkey. ×8250.

F. Cytoplasmic Invaginations into the Nucleus, Nuclear Pockets, Pseudoinclusions, and Inclusions

In electron micrographs irregularity of nuclear shape is a common feature of neoplastic cells (129). Some of these irregularities are due to the cytoplasmic invaginations of various sizes, content and morphology into the nucleus, or nuclear evaginations (56, 76, 94, 119, 129, 174, 190, 204, 205). Depending on their position in ultrathin sections, the cytoplasmic invaginations may appear to be nuclear inclusions (Figs. 2.19–2.21). However, they are surrounded by a double-layered nuclear envelope and represent pseudoinclusions or nuclear

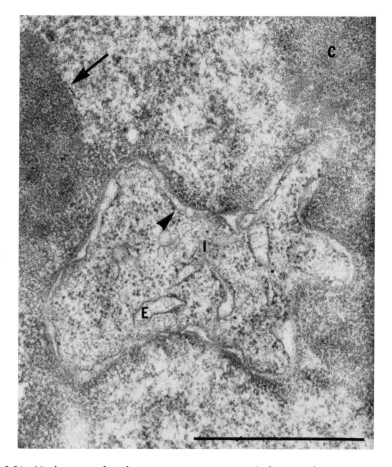

Fig. 2.20. Nuclear pseudoinclusion—a cross section of the cytoplasmic invagination (I) which is surrounded by the double-layered nuclear envelope (pointer) and contains characteristic cytoplasmic structures such as endoplasmic reticulum (E) and ribosomes. Nucleolus (arrow), chromocenter (C). Novikoff ascites hepatoma cell fixed in osmium tetroxide. ×46,000.

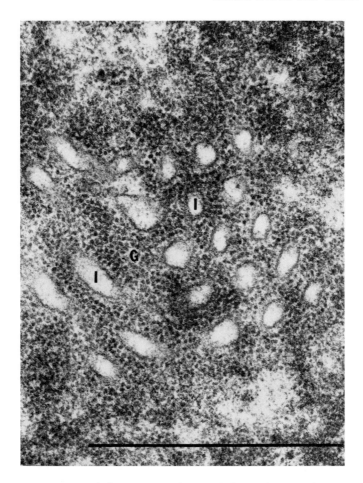

Fig. 2.21. Invaginations of the inner membrane of the nuclear envelope into the nucleus and nucleolus of a Novikoff hepatoma cell (in cross section). Such invaginations (I) may represent protrusions of the perinuclear space (limited by two layers of the nuclear envelope) into the nucleus and nucleolus adjacent to the nuclear envelope. They probably correspond to the modified nucleolar channel system found by Terzakis in endometrial secretory cells (189a). Granular nucleolar components surrounding the invaginations (G). ×69,000.

blebs (pockets) which usually contain characteristic cytoplasmic structures (Fig. 2.19). All of these structures increase the nuclear surface and their formation may be related to nucleocytoplasmic interactions (23, 94, 182, 204, 205) as has been suggested for the "nuclear pockets" (Fig. 2.22). The association of some of these structures with the nucleolus may facilitate the migration of ribosomal precursors to the cytoplasm. However, no evidence for passage of the nuclear or nucleolar material through nuclear pores has been noted in the regions of the nucleolar attachment to the nuclear membrane (50).

The nuclear inclusions that are surrounded by a single membrane are believed to be of cytoplasmic origin (17, 54, 56, 114, 169–171). Such inclusions seem

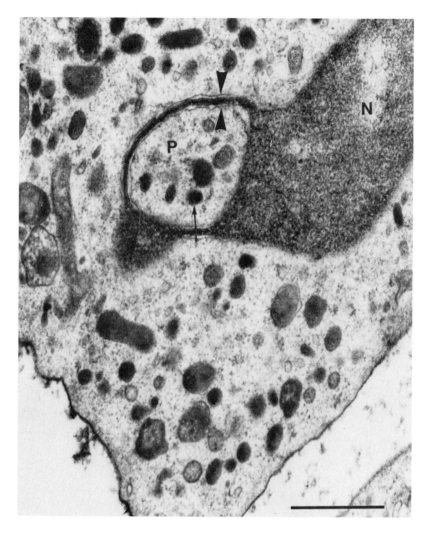

Fig. 2.22. A nuclear pocket (P) containing cytoplasm with granules (arrow) in a leukemic neutrophil. Nuclear membrane (pointers), nucleus (N). ×25,000.

to originate from various cytoplasmic invaginations. The original two-layered nuclear envelope is apparently transformed to a single-layered inclusion membrane. The sequence of changes occurring during such transformations is poorly understood at present. The content of inclusion bodies surrounded by a single membrane is very variable and often depends on the cell type. For example, in plasmocytes of some multiple myelomas, these inclusions contain dense protein globules that are also present in the endoplasmic reticulum (114). In a variety of cells single membrane-limited inclusions can contain lipid and protein droplets, glycogen particles, and/or some cytoplasmic organelles and their fragments (39). The nucleolar channel system found in endometrial cells (189a) probably represents a regularly organized invagination of the inner layer into the nucleolus of the nuclear membrane envelope (Fig. 2.21).

The nuclear inclusions without limiting membranes may originate from membrane-limited inclusions by disintegration of their membranes or by trapping of certain cytoplasmic structures into the nucleus during mitosis (16, 175). However, the inclusions originating by trapping of cytoplasmic organelles in the nucleus during mitosis are uncommon and have been observed only in leukemic cells or Rous intracranial sarcoma cells (16, 20). Fat, protein, and glycogen nuclear inclusions without limiting membranes are believed to originate by passage of these substances into the nucleus without visible changes in the morphology of the nuclear envelope (1).

V. Summary

Studies on the morphology of the nuclei and nucleoli of cancer cells have indicated that the sizes of the nucleoli are generally increased in rapidly growing tumor cells and that the nucleus to cytoplasm ratio is greater in tumor cells than in other cells. For the most part these changes are reflections of the increased synthetic activity of these nuclei and nucleoli as part of cell growth. It is not yet clear whether some special feature of cancer cells is reflected in these aberrations from normal cells. As yet, it is not known whether the discrepancy between nuclear and cytoplasmic size of tumor cells reflects a special feature of cancer or is a special feature of the rapid growth of these cells. It is also uncertain whether the marked pleomorphism of nucleoli of neoplastic cells is an expression of their rapid growth or is cancer related.

Alterations of the mitotic figures in cancer cells have been visualized and some of these may be pathogonomic for cancer cells. The relationship of the chromatin content of neoplastic cells to chromosome number requires statistical evaluation but for the present it appears that the chromatin reflects the hyperploidy of the neoplastic cells.

Many drugs produce marked changes in nucleolar ultrastructure. In particular, segregation of the granular and fibrillar elements of the nucleolus is produced by a variety of antibiotics and other agents that inhibit nucleolar RNA polymerase. On the other hand, nucleolar synthesis of ribosomal precursor products is stimulated by a variety of hormones and some other agents including phytohemagglutinin and thioacetamide. Since conversion of cells from hypofunctional, nongrowing states to rapid growth requires increased synthesis of ribosomes and polysomes, the stimulated cell exhibits a compensatory hypertrophy of nucleolar function. In cancer cells, nucleolar function is very active and the precise nature of the derepressors involved in the increased function of nucleoli of cancer cells is of great interest.

Although in the past, the nucleus was considered to be relatively amorphous, recently a wide variety of particulate elements have been found in the nucleoplasm. In addition to the granular and fibrillar elements of the nucleolus, the nucleoplasm contains perichromatinic and interchromatinic granular elements and many other types of dense granular and fibrillar structures.

Although no clear indication of their function has been developed yet, the broad array of morphological structures suggests they may subserve special functions. It is too early to specify whether any of these have a definitive relationship to neoplasia.

References

1. Altmann, H. W., and Pfeifer, U. (1969). *Virchows Arch. Abt. B. Zellpath.* **2**, 220–228.
2. Astaldi, G., and Lisiewicz, J. (1971). "Lymphocytes, Structure, Production, Functions." Idelson, Naples.
3. Bencosme, S. A., Allen, R. A., and Latta, H. (1963). *Amer. J. Pathol.* **42**, 1–21.
4. Bereczsky, E., Dmochowski, L., and Gray, C. E. (1961). *J. Nat. Cancer Inst.* **27**, 99–129.
5. Berman, C. (1951). "Primary Carcinoma of the Liver." Lewis, London.
6. Bernhard, W., (1958). *Exp. Cell Res. Suppl.* **6**, 17–50.
7. Bernhard, W. (1960). *Cancer Res.* **20**, 712–727.
8. Bernhard, W., (1963). *Progr. Exp. Tumor Res.* **3**, 1–34.
9. Bernhard, W. (1969). *J. Ultrastruct. Res.* **27**, 250–265.
10. Bernhard, W., Bauer, A., Gropp, A., Haguenau, F., and Oberling, C. (1955). *Exp. Cell Res.* **9**, 88–100.
11. Bernhard, W., and Granboulan, N. (1963). *Exp. Cell Res. Suppl.* **9**, 19–53.
12. Bernhard, W., and Granboulan, N. (1968). *In* "The Nucleus" (A. J. Dalton and F. Haguenau, eds.), pp. 81–149. Academic Press, New York.
13. Bessis, M., and Thiery, J. P. (1962). *N. R. F. Hemat.* **2**, 577–601.
14. Biesele, J. J., Poyner, H., and Painter, T. S. (1942). *Texas Univ. Publ.* #4243, 1–62.
15. Bouteille, M., Kalifat, S. R., and Delarne, J. J. (1967). *J. Ultrastruct. Res.* **19**, 474–486.
16. Brandes, D., Schofield, B., and Auton, E. (1965). *Science* **149**, 1373–1374.
17. Brittin, G. M., Tanaka, Y., and Brecher, G. (1963). *Blood* **21**, 335–357.
18. Brooks, R. E., and Siegel, B. V. (1967). *Blood* **29**, 269–275.
19. Brux, de, J., and Marchand, C. (1949). *Presse Med.* **49**, 704–705.
20. Bucciarelli, E. (1966). *J. Cell Biol.* **30**, 664–665.
21. Bucher, O., and Gattiker, R. (1954). *Z. Mikroskop.-Anat. Forsch.* **60**, 467–502.
22. Burke, M. D., and Melamed, M. R. (1968). *Acta Cytol.* **12**, 61–74.
23. Burns, E. R., Soloff, B. L., Hanna, C., and Buxton, D. (1971). *Cancer Res.* **31**, 159–165.
24. Busch, H., Byvoet, P., and Smetana, K. (1963). *Cancer Res.* **23**, 313–339.
25. Busch, H., and Smetana, K. (1970). "The Nucleolus." Academic Press, New York.
26. Caputo, R., and Bellone, A. G. (1966). *J. Invest. Dermatol.* **47**, 141–146.
27. Caspersson, T. O. (1950). "Cell Growth and Cell Function. A Cytochemical Study." Norton, New York.
28. Caspersson, T. O., and Santesson, L. (1942). *Acta Radiol. Suppl.* **46**, 1–105.
29. Caspersson, T. O., and Thorsson, K. G. (1953). *Klin. Wochschr.* **31**, 205–212.
30. Castren, H. (1926). *A. R. B. Patrol. Inst. U. Helsingforsch.* **4**, 240–318.
31. Catchpole, H. R., and Gersh, I. (1950). *Discuss. Faraday Soc.* **9**, 471–480.
32. Chakravorty, A. K., and Busch, H., (1967). *Biochem. Pharmacol.* **16**, 1711–1718.
33. Chakravorty, A. K., and Busch, H. (1967). *Cancer Res.* **27**, 789–792.
34. Cooper, N. C. (1956). *Bull. N. Y. Med. Soc.* **32**, 79–82.
35. Cowdry, E. V. (1956). *Ann. N. Y. Acad. Sci.* **63**, 1043–1053.
36. Cowdry, E. V., and Paletta, F. X. (1941). *J. Nat. Cancer Inst.* **1**, 745–759.
37. Crippa, M. (1970). *Nature (London)* **227**, 1138–1140.

38. Dave, C. J. and Law, L. W. (1959). *J. Nat. Cancer Inst.* **23**, 1157–1165.
39. David, M. (1964). "Submikroskopische ortho und pathomorphologie der leber." Ak. Verl. Berlin, MacMillian, New York.
40. Davis, J. M. G. (1963). *Phil. Trans. Roy. Microscop. Soc.* [B] **246**, 291–303.
41. DeThe, G., Riviére, M. R., and Bernhard, W. (1960). *Bull. Cancer* **47**, 569–584.
42. Dmochowski, L. (1960). *Cancer Res.* **20**, 977–1015.
43. Dourmashkin, R., and Bernhard, W. (1959). *J. Ultrastruct. Res.* **3**, 11–38.
44. Dumont, A., and Robert, A. (1971). *J. Ultrastruct. Res.* **36**, 483–492.
44a. Duprat, A. M., Beetschen, J. C., Zalta, J. P., and Duprat, P. (1965). *C. R. Acad. Sci. Paris* **261**, 5203–5206.
45. Dupuy-Coin, A. M., Lazar, P., Kalifat, S. R., and Bouteille, M. (1969). *J. Ultrastruct. Res.* **27**, 244–249.
46. Duryee, W. R. (1956). *Ann. N. Y. Acad. Sci.* **63**, 1280–1302.
47. Dutta, C. R., Siegesmund, K. A., and Fox, C. A. (1963). *J. Ultrastruct. Res.* **8**, 542–551.
48. Edwards, G. A. (1960). *Nat. Cancer Inst. Monograph* **4**, 313–321.
49. Edwards, G. A., Ruska, C., Ruska, H., and Skiff, J. V. (1959). *Cancer* **12**, 982–1002.
50. Erlandson, R. A., and deHarven, E. (1971). *J. Cell Sci.* **8**, 353–397.
50a. Fakan, S., and Bernhard, W. (1971). *Exp. Cell Res.* **67**, 129–141.
51. Ferreira, A. E. M. (1941). *J. Lab. Clin. Med.* **26**, 1612–1628.
52. Fidler, H. K. A. (1935). *Amer. J. Cancer* **25**, 772–779.
53. Flaks, B. (1968). *Eur. J. Cancer* **4**, 513–521.
54. Flaks, B. and Flaks, A. (1970). *Cancer Res.* **30**, 1437–1443.
55. Foot, N. C. (1937). *Amer. J. Pathol.* **13**, 1–11.
56. Frühling, L., Porte, A., and Kempf, J. (1960). *C. R. Acad. Sci. Paris* **251**, 794–796.
57. Gati, E., Inke, G., Bajtai, A., and Gyarfas, J. (1967). *Acta Morphol. Acad. Sci. Hung.* **7**, 343–350.
58. Gelboin, H. V., Wortham, J. S., Wilson, R. G., Friedman, M., and Wogan, G. N. (1966). *Science* **154**, 1205–1206.
59. Gonzalez, P., and Nardone, R. M. (1968). *Exp. Cell Res.* **50**, 599–615.
60. Granboulan, N., and Riviére, M. R. (1962). *J. Microsc.* **1**, 23–27.
61. Granboulan, N., Riviére, M. R., and Bernhard, W. (1960). *Bull. Cancer* **47**, 291–307.
62. Granboulan, N., Tournier, P., Wicker, R., and Bernhard, W. (1963). *J. Cell Biol.* **17**, 423–440.
63. Grishem, J. W. (1960). *Gastroenterology* **38**, 792–793.
64. Grundmann, E. (1964). "Allgemeine Cytologie." Thieme, Stuttgart.
65. Guttman, P. H. (1935). *Amer. J. Cancer* **25**, 802–806.
66. Györkey, F., Min, K. W., Huff, J. A., and Györkey, P. (1967). *Cancer Res.* **27**, 1348–1353.
67. Haam, E. von, and Alexander, H. G. (1936). *Amer. J. Clin. Pathol.* **6**, 394–414.
68. Hadjiolov, A. A. (1958). *Z. Krebsforsch.* **62**, 361–369.
69. Haguenau, F. (1960). *Nat. Cancer Inst. Monograph* **4**, 211–249.
70. Han, S. M. (1967). *Amer. J. Anat.* **120**, 161–183.
71. Haumeder, E. (1934). *Z. Krebsforsch.* **40**, 105–116.
72. Heilmayer, L., and Begemann, H. (1955). "Atlas der Klinischen Hämatologie und Cytologie." Springer, Berlin.
72a. Henry, K., and Petts, V. (1969). *J. Ultrastruct. Res.* **27**, 330–343.
73. Hinglais-Guilland, N., Moricard, R., and Bernhard, W. (1961). *Bull. Cancer* **48**, 283–316.
74. Horstmann, E. (1965). *Z. Zellforsch.* **65**, 770–776.
75. Hughes, H. E. and Dodds, T. S. (1968). "Handbook of Diagnostic Cytology." Williams and Wilkins, Baltimore, Maryland.
76. Huhn, D. (1967). *Nature (London)* **216**, 1240.
76a. Hyde, B. B., Shankarnarayan, K., and Birnstiel, M. L. (1965). *J. Ultrastruct. Res.* **12**, 652–667.
77. Jacob, S. T., Steele, W. J., and Busch, H. (1967). *Cancer Res.* **27**, 52–60.
78. Jensen, F., Koprowski, H., Pagano, H. S., Pontén, J. A., and Ravdin, R. G. (1964). *J. Nat. Cancer Inst.* **32**, 917–937.

78a. Jones, K. W. (1967). *J. Ultrastruct. Res.* 18, 71–84.
79. Karasaki, S. (1969). *J. Cell Biol.* 40, 322–335.
80. Karasek, J., Dubinin, J., Oehlert, W., and Konrad, B. (1970). *Neoplasma* 17, 389–397.
81. Kaziro, Y., and Kamiyama, M. (1967). *J. Biochem.* 62, 424–429.
82. Kierszenbaum, A. L. (1969). *Ultrastruct. Res.* 29, 459–469.
83. Koller, P. C. (1963). *Exp. Cell Res. Suppl.* 9, 3–14.
84. Kopac, M. J., and Mateyko, G. M. (1958). *Ann. N. Y. Acad. Sci.* 73, 237–282.
85. Kopac, M. J., and Mateyko, G. M. (1964). *Advan. Cancer Res.* 8, 121–190.
86. Koprowski, H., Pontén, J. A., Jensen, F., Ravdin, R. G., Morhead, P., and Saksela, E. (1962). *J. Cell Comp. Physiol.* 59, 281–292.
87. Koshiba, K., Chandra, T., Daskal, Y., and Busch, H. (1971). *Exp. Cell Res.* 68, 235–246.
88. Krishan, A., Uzman, B. G., and Hedley-Whyte, E. T. (1967). *J. Ultrastruct. Res.* 19, 563–572.
89. Kumar, A., and Warner, J. R. (1972). *J. Mol. Biol.* 63, 233–246.
90. LaFarge, C., Frayssinet, C., and Simard, R. (1966). *C. R. Acad. Sci. Paris* 263, 1011–1014.
91. Lafontaine, J. G. (1965). *J. Cell Biol.* 26, 1–17.
92. Lane, N. J. (1969). *J. Cell Biol.* 40, 286–291.
93. Lebert, H. (1851). "Traité Practique des Maladies: Cancreuses et des Affections Curables Confondues ave le Cancer." Bailliere, Paris.
94. Leduc, E., and Wilson, W. (1959). *J. Biophys. Biochem Cytol.* 6, 427–430.
95. Leighton, J., Kline, J., and Orr, H. C. (1956). *Science* 123, 502–503.
96. Lemaire, R. (1963). *Arch. Biol.* 3, 342–375.
97. Lettré, R., and Siebs, W. (1954). *Naturwissenschaften* 41, 458.
98. Lettré, R., and Siebs, W. (1954). *Z. Krebsforsch.* 60, 19–20.
99. Li, H. J., and Crothers, D. M. (1969). *J. Mol. Biol.* 39, 461–477.
100. Liao, S., Barton, R. W., and Lin, A. H. (1966). *Proc. Nat. Acad. Sci. U.S.* 55, 1593–1600.
101. Liao, S., and Lin, A. H. (1967). *Proc. Nat. Acad. Sci. U.S.* 57, 379–386.
102. Liau, M. C., and Perry, R. J. (1969). *J. Cell Biol.* 42, 272–282.
103. Long, M. E., and Taylor, H. C. (1955–56). *Ann. N.Y. Acad. Sci.* 63, 1093–1106.
104. Love, R. (1966). *Nat. Cancer Inst. Monograph* 23, 167–180.
105. Love, R., and Soriano, R. Z. (1971). *Cancer Res.* 31, 1030–1037.
106. Love, R., and Walsh, R. J. (1968). *Exp. Cell Res.* 53, 432–446.
107. Love, R., and Walsh, R. J. (1970). *Cancer Res.* 30, 990–997.
108. Ludford, R. J. (1954). *Brit. H. Cancer* 8, 112–131.
109. Luse, S. H., and Reagan, J. W. (1954). *Cancer* 7, 1167–1181.
110. MacCarty, W. C. (1928). *J. Lab. Clin. Med.* 13, 354–365.
111. MacCarty, W. C. (1936). *Amer. J. Cancer* 26, 529–532.
112. MacCarty, W. C. (1937). *Amer. J. Cancer* 31, 104–106.
113. MacCarty, W. C., and Haumeder, E. (1934). *Amer. J. Cancer* 20, 403–407.
114. Maldonado, J. E., Brown, A. L., Jr., Bayrd, E. D., and Pease, G. L. (1966). *Arch. Pathol.* 81, 484–500.
115. Masuwrovsky, E. B., Benitex, M. H., Kim, S. U., and Murray, M. R. (1970). *J. Cell Biol.* 44, 172–191.
116. Mayor, H. D. (1964). *J. Exp. Med.* 119, 433–441.
117. Mayor, H. D., Stinebaugh, S. E., Jamison, R. M., Jordan, L. E., and Melnick, J. (1962). *Exp. Mol. Pathol.* 1, 397–416.
118. McCormach, C. J. (1935). *Proc. Staff Meetings Mayo Clinic* 10, 24–29.
119. McDuffie, N. G. (1967). *Nature (London)* 214, 1341–1342.
120. McGrew, E. (1965). *Acta Cytol.* 9, 58–60.
120a. McParland, R., Crooke, S. T., and Busch, H. (1972). *Biochim. Biophys. Acta* 209, 78–89.
121. Melnick, J. L. (1962). *Science* 135, 1128–1130.
122. Mironescu, S., Encut, J., Mironescu, K., and Liciu, F. (1968). *J. Nat. Cancer Inst.* 40, 917–933.

123. Niyai, K., and Steiner, J. W. (1965). *Exp. Mol. Pathol.* **4**, 525–566.
124. Monneron, A., and Bernhard, W. (1969). *J. Ultrastruct. Res.* **27**, 266–288.
124a. Monneron, A., Lafarge, C., and Frayssinet, C. (1968). *C. R. Acad. Sci. Paris* **267**, 2053–2056.
124b. Monneron, A., and Moulé, Y. (1968). *Exp. Cell Res.* **51**, 531–554.
125. Montgomery, P. O'B., and Reynolds, R. C. (1964). *Lab. Invest.* **13**, 1243–1253.
126. Naseman, T., and Braun-Falco, O. (1968). *Klin Worschr.* **46**, 534–540.
127. Naidu, V. R. (1935). *Proc. Staff Meetings Mayo Clinic* **10**, 356–362.
128. Nieburgs, H. E., Parets, A. D., Perez, V., and Boudreau, C. (1965). *Arch. Pathol.* **80**, 262–272.
129. Oberling, C., and Bernhard, W. (1961). *In* "The Cell" (J. Brachet and A. E. Mirsky, eds.), Vol. 5, pp. 405–496. Academic Press, New York.
130. Opie, E. (1946). *J. Exp. Med.* **84**, 91–106.
131. Page, R. C. (1938). *A.M.A. Arch. Pathol.* **26**, 800–813.
132. Page, R. C., Carpenter, W., and MacCarty, W. C. (1937). *A.M.A. Arch. Pathol.* **24**, 1–7.
133. Page, R. C., Regan, J. F., and MacCarty, W. C. (1938). *Amer. J. Cancer* **32**, 383–394.
134. Paul, J. S., Reynolds, R. C., and Montgomery, P. O'B. (1967). *Nature (London)* **215**, 749–750.
135. Paul, J. S., Reynolds, R. C., and Montgomery, P. O'B. (1969). *Cancer Res.* **29**, 558–570.
136. Peters, K. (1963). *In* "Strahlenpathologie der Zelle" (E. Scherer and H. S. Stender eds.), pp. 32–46. Thieme, Stuttgart.
137. Petrov, P., and Bernhard, W. (1971). *J. Ultrastruct. Res.* **35**, 386–402.
138. Pontén, J. A., Jensen, F., and Koprowski, H. (1963). *J. Cell. Comp. Physiol.* **61**, 145–154.
139. Popoff, N., and Stewart, S. (1968). *J. Ultrastruct. Res.* **23**, 347–361.
140. Potmesil, M., and Goldfeder, A. (1971). *Cancer Res.* **31**, 789–797.
141. Pullinger, B. D. (1940). *J. Pathol. Bacteriol.* **50**, 463–471.
142. Quensel, U. (1928). *Acta Med. Scand.* **68**, 458–501.
143. Rabson, A. S., Kirschstein, R. L., and Legallais, F. Y. (1965). *J. Nat. Cancer Inst.* **35**, 981–991.
144. Racela, A., Grady, H., and Svoboda, D. (1967). *Cancer Res.* **27**, 1658–1671.
145. Rake, G., and Blank, H. (1950). *J. Invest. Dermatol.* **15**, 81–93.
146. Recher, L., Whitescurver, J., and Briggs, L. (1970). *J. Cell Biol.* **45**, 479–492.
147. Reddy, J., Harris, C., and Svoboda, D. (1968). *Nature (London)* **217**, 659–661.
148. Reissig, M., and Melnick, J. L. (1955). *J. Exp. Med.* **101**, 341–352.
149. Reitalu, R. (1957). *Acta Pathol. Microbiol. Scand.* **41**, 257–266.
150. Ringertz, N. R., and Bolund, L. (1969). *Biochim. Biophys. Acta* **174**, 147–154
151. Ro-Choi, T. S., and Busch, H. (1964). *Cancer Res.* **24**, 1630–1633.
152. Ro-Choi, T. S., and Busch, H. (1967). *Biochim. Biophys. Acta* **134**, 184–187.
153. Robertson, D. M. (1964). *Amer. J. Pathol.* **45**, 835–848.
154. Robertson, D. M., and MacLean, S. D. (1965). *Arch. Neurol.* **13**, 287–296.
154a. Rubin, A. D. (1968). *Nature (London)* **220**, 196–197.
155. Samarina, O. P., Lukanidin, E. M., Molnar, J., and Georgiev, G. P. (1968). *J. Mol. Biol.* **33**, 251–263.
156. Saxen, A. (1926). *Arb. Pathol. Inst. Univ. Helsingfors* **4**, 1–130.
157. Scherer, E., and Fiebelkorn, H. J. (1954). *Folia Haematol.* **72**, 143–148.
158. Scherer, E., Ringleb, D., and Ventske, L. E. (1953). *Strahlentherapie* **90**, 41–52.
159. Seite, R., Escaig, J., and Couineau, S. (1971). *J. Ultrastruct. Res.* **37**, 449–478.
160. Seybolt, J. F., Papnicolaou, G. N., and Cooper, W. A. (1951). *Cancer* **4**, 286–295.
161. Shankaranarayan, K., and Busch, H. (1965). *Exp. Cell Res.* **38**, 434–437.
161a. Shankaranarayan, K., Steele, W. J., Smetana, K., and Busch, H. (1967). *Exp. Cell Res.* **46**, 65–77.
162. Shea, J. R., Jr., and Leblond, C. P. (1966). *J. Morphol.* **119**, 425–434.
163. Shein, H. M., and Enders, J. F. (1962). *Proc. Nat. Acad. Sci. U.S.* **48**, 1164–1172.
163a. Shepherd, J., and Maden, B. E. H. (1972). *Nature (London)* **236**, 211–214.

163b. Shinozuka, H. (1970). *J. Ultrastruct. Res.* **32**, 430–442.
164. Simar, L. J. (1969). *Z. Zellforsch.* **99**, 235–251.
165. Simard, R. (1970). *Int. Rev. Cytol.* **28**, 169–212.
166. Simard, R., and Bernhard, W. (1966). *Int. J. Cancer* **1**, 463–479.
167. Smetana, K., and Busch, H. (1964). *Cancer Res.* **24**, 537–557.
168. Smetana, K., and Busch, H. (1966). *Cancer Res.* **26**, 331–337.
168a. Smetana, K., Gyorkey, F., Gyorkey, P., and Busch, H. (1969). *Exp. Cell Res.* **58**, 303–311.
169. Smetana, K., Györkey, F., Györkey, P., and Busch, H. (1971). *Exp. Cell Res.* **64**, 133–139.
169a. Smetana, K., Györkey, F., Györkey, P., and Busch, H. (1972). *Cancer Res.* **32**, 925–932.
170. Smetana, K., Hermansky, F., Kobliskova, H., and Pospisil, V. (1971). *Neoplasma* **18**, 3–13.
170a. Smetana, K., Hermansky, F., Janele, J., and Busch, H. (1968). *Folia Haematol.* **89**, 1–14.
171. Smetana, K., Lejnar, J., Vlastiborova, A., and Busch, H. (1971). *Exp. Cell Res.* **64**, 105–112.
172. Smetana, K., and Potmesil, M. (1968). *Z. Zellforsch.* **92**, 62–69.
173. Smetana, K., Shankaranarayan, K., and Busch, H. (1966). *Cancer Res.* **26**, 786–796.
173a. Smetana, K., Steele, W. J., and Busch, H. (1963). *Exp. Cell Res.* **31**, 198–202.
174. Smith, G. F., and O'Hara, P. T. (1968). *J. Ultrastruct. Res.* **21**, 415–423.
175. Sobel, H. J., Schwarz, R., and Margret, E. (1969). *Arch. Pathol.* **87**, 179–192.
176. Steele, W. J. (1966). In "The Cell Nucleus—Metabolism and Radiosensitivity" (H. M. Klouwen, ed.), pp. 203–220. Taylor and Francis, London.
177. Stenius, F., (1923). *Arb. Pathol. Inst. Univ. Helsingfors* **3**, 27–190.
178. Stenram, U. (1958). *Acta Path. Microbiol. Scand.* **44**, 239–246.
179. Stowell, R. E. (1949). *Cancer* **2**, 121–131.
180. Sun, C. N. (1961). *Exp. Cell Res.* **25**, 213–215.
181. Sunderman, F. W., and Esfahani, M. (1968). *Cancer Res.* **28**, 2565–2567.
182. Svoboda, D. (1964). *J. Nat. Cancer Inst.* **33**, 315–339.
183. Svoboda, D., Grady, H., and Higginson, J. (1966). *Amer. J. Pathol.* **49**, 1023–1051.
184. Svoboda, D., and Higginson, J. (1968). *Cancer Res.* **28**, 1703–1733.
185. Svoboda, D., Racela, A., and Higginson, J. (1967). *Biochem. Pharm.* **16**, 651–657.
186. Swanbeck, G., and Thyresson, N. (1969). *Acta Dermato Vernereol.* **44**, 105–106.
187. Tani, E., Ametani, T., Ishijima, Y., Higashi, N., and Fujihara, E. (1971). *Cancer Res.* **31**, 1210–1217.
188. Tata, J. R. (1968). *Nature (London)* **219**, 331–337.
189. Terao, K., Sakakibara, Y., Yamaraki, M., and Nigaki, K. (1971). *Exp. Cell Res.* **66**, 81–89.
189a. Terzakis, J. A. (1965). *J. Cell Biol.* **27**, 293–304.
189b. Tokuyasu, K., Maden, S. C., and Seldis, L. J. (1968). *J. Cell Biol.* **39**, 630–660.
190. Toro, I., and Olah, I. (1966). *Nature (London)* **212**, 315–317.
191. Ulrich, J., and Kidd, M. (1966). *Acta Neuropath. (Berlin)* **6**, 359–370.
192. Unuma, T., and Busch, H. (1967). *Cancer Res.* **27**, 1232–1242.
193. Unuma, T., Morris, H. P., and Busch, H. (1967). *Cancer Res.* **27**, 2121–2233.
194. Unuma, T., Smetana, K., and Busch, H. (1967). *Exp. Cell Res.* **48**, 665–671.
194a. Uzman, B. G., Foley, G. E., Farber, S., and Lazarus, H. (1966). *Cancer* **19**, 1725–1742.
195. Vasquez-Nin, G., and Bernhard, W. (1971). *J. Ultrastruct. Res.* **36**, 842–860.
196. Verbin, R. S., Goldblatt, P. J., Saez, L., and Farber, E. (1969). *Exp. Cell Res.* **56**, 167–169.
197. Virchow, R. (1863–1867). "Die Krankhaften Geschwulste." Hirschwald, Berlin.
198. Waring, M. J. (1968). *Nature (London)* **219**, 1320–1325.
199. Warner, J. R. (1966). *J. Mol. Biol.* **19**, 383–398.
200. Warner, J. R., and Soeiro, R. (1967). *New England J. Med.* **276**, 563–570, 613–617, 675–680.

201. Warner, J. R., and Soeiro, R. (1967). *Proc. Nat. Acad. Sci. U.S.* **58**, 1984–1990.
202. Weber, A., and Frommes, S. P. (1963). *Science* **141**, 912–913.
203. Weber, A., Whipp, S., Usenik, E., and Frommes, S. (1964). *J. Ultrastruct. Res.* **11**, 564–576.
204. Wessel, W. (1958). *Virchows Arch.* **331**, 314–328.
205. Yasuzumi, G., Tsubo, T., Okada, K., Terawaki, A., and Enomoto, Y. (1968). *J. Ultrastruct. Res.* **23**, 321–332.
206. Yu, F.-L., and Feigelson, P. (1971). *Proc. Nat. Acad. Sci. U.S.* **68**, 2177–2180.
207. Zadek, J. (1933). *Acta Med. Scand.* **80**, 78–92.
208. Zbarsky, S. H. (1964). *Can. J. Biochem.* **42**, 563–566.

CHAPTER III

Chromosomes in the Causation and Progression of Cancer and Leukemia

AVERY A. SANDBERG AND MASAHARU SAKURAI

I. Introduction

Even though general agreement seems to exist that the neoplastic process in mammalian cells is caused by alterations in the function of chromosomal chromatin (DNA), the possibility has not been ruled out that the cancerous state may also be caused and abetted by abnormalities resident outside the DNA and nucleus, i.e., in the histones and other proteins associated with the chromosomes, in the nucleolus, the elements present within the cytoplasm, or the cell membrane. Furthermore, agreement exists that minor molecular rearrangements within genes, certainly not detectable visually even with the most sophisticated microscopic techniques presently available, may lead to the development of cancer or leukemia. Hence, in discussing the role of chromosomal changes in the causation of cancer and leukemia in human subjects and animals, it must be realized that one is discussing only those cytogenetic abnormalities that are visibly recognizable and consisting primarily of numerical and morphological deviations of the chromosomes.

In the present chapter chromosomal changes in human neoplasia will be interpreted as they relate to the causation and progression of cancer and leukemia, though appropriate observations in animals will be presented to support (or not to support) and supplement the findings in human subjects. This chapter will contain only those references which appear to us to be germane. For more detailed cytogenetic findings in human cancer and leukemia, the reader may wish to consult several recent comprehensive reviews (19, 26, 33, 34).

This presentation will further develop concepts previously discussed regarding the role of chromosomal changes in cancer causation. The general thesis is that the development of cancer and leukemia in human subjects is usually not associated with or due to karyotypic abnormalities, though it is possible that some cases may develop such cytogenetic aberrations concomitant with or as result of the neoplastic state. Only a small number of relatively specific entities of human cancer and leukemia may be caused primarily by chromosomal changes (Fig. 3.1).

The consistency and morphological integrity of the chromosomal set in mammalian cells are guaranteed by the remarkable process of DNA replication and cellular mitosis. As a result of these events the amount of DNA per cell, as reflected in the relative stability of the chromosome number and morphology, is kept essentially identical in all somatic cells. Thus, when the chromosome number is determined in normal cells it is found to be constant ($2n = 46$ in the human, 40 in the mouse, 42 in the rat, etc.). Furthermore, the structure and relative length of the chromosomes are remarkably similar from cell to

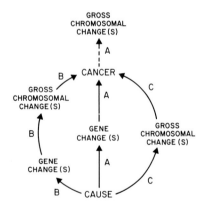

Fig. 3.1. Schematic presentation of 3 possible paths leading to cancer and chromosomal changes. In path A the direct causation of cancer is a change of function at the gene level with the chromosomal changes being secondary to the development of the cancerous state. This path probably operates in the preponderant number of cancers and most of the leukemias. The broken arrow leading from cancer to gross chromosomal changes in path A indicates that chromosomal changes may not necessarily accompany the neoplastic state. In path B the chromosomal changes are induced by genic malfunction with the karyotypic aberrations possibly being directly responsible for the cancerous condition. Additional chromosomal changes may or may not be induced by the already established cancerous state. Path B may be the one which is associated with human chronic myelocytic leukemia and its blastic phase. In path C the chromosomal changes are produced by agents which affect chromosomal structure directly without intervening genic involvement. The chromosomal abnormalities are then directly responsible for the induction of the cancerous state (33).

cell and from tissue to tissue, allowing rather facile classification of the chromosomes, at least in the human, into fairly specific groups. This has afforded the recognition of unique karyotypic abnormalities in various diseases and the deciphering of certain abnormal states on the basis of specific cytogenetic anomalies.

II. The Chromosomes in Normal Cells

Even though the diploid number of 46 (Fig. 3.2) is very constant and in some cells (under certain conditions) metaphases with the diploid number of chromosomes may constitute 100% of the cell population, some deviations exist and are worthy of note.

Examination of bone marrow cells by a direct technique, without subjecting them to *in vitro* culture conditions, reveals that about 10% of the cells are aneuploid (> or < than 46 chromosomes). Admittedly, it is probable that some of the hypodiploid cells result from random loss of chromosomes, possibly due to the mechanics of preparing the cytological material which requires swelling of the

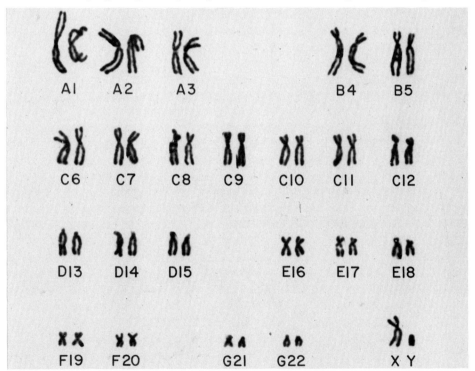

Fig. 3.2. Karyotype of a normal diploid human cell containing 46 chromosomes: 22 pairs of autosomes and one pair of sex chromosomes (gonosomes); in this case the sex chromosomes are those of a male, X and Y chromosomes. A normal female cell contains two X chromosomes. The chromosomes have been classified according to their length, location of the centromere (kinetochore) and the ratio of the short to long arms.

metaphase cells followed by procedures which could readily rupture the cell and lead to the loss of chromosomes. However, it has recently been shown that the Y chromosome may be absent in the marrow cells of males, particularly the elderly (65 years and older), leading to hypodiploidy with 45 chromosomes (30, 31). Cells with 47 or more chromosomes are probably generated by nondisjunction of daughter chromosomes at anaphase. Other tissues, in addition to marrow, have also been shown to contain cells with chromosome numbers deviating from the diploid. The role these aneuploid cells play in human cancer or leukemia is uncertain. Generally, though, normal tissues are characterized by over 90% of their cells being diploid.

III. The Chromosomes in Benign and Malignant Neoplasia

A. General Considerations

So-called benign tumors are diagnosed and classified on the basis of their histological appearance, failure to metastasize or invade adjoining tissues, relatively slow rate of growth, and lack of untoward metabolic or nutritional effects in the host. These criteria, however, do not exclude the possibility that parts of a benign tumor may undergo malignant transformation or that some of these tumors may not represent the least variant of malignant tumors.

The cytogenetic picture of benign tumors is almost always diploid, with the preponderant number of cells having normal karyotypes. Any consistent or unique deviation from the diploid picture is compatible with cancerous transformation of the benign tumor.

The amount of cytogenetic information available on benign tumors is rather meager. This is primarily due to the very low mitotic index of such tumors, with the result that few metaphases are present in the cytological preparations. If resort is made to *in vitro* culturing of the cells, the possibility always arises that the diploid cells found may not have originated from the tumor but from normal elements present in the tissue. Obviously, much more data are needed to establish the correct karyotypic profile of benign tumors of various origin and morphology.

Visibly recognizable chromosomal changes are not usually involved directly in the causation of neoplasia, though they may play an important role in the progression, metastatic spread, response to therapy, and other biologic aspects of cancer or leukemia. It is possible that rare cases of cancer or leukemia may be due to a direct involvement of a chromosomal change in the genesis of the neoplastic process, either in collaboration with another underlying cause or as a single factor in this process.

The section to follow is concerned primarily with those karyotypic changes which can be observed by visual microscopy, i.e., changes in the number or gross morphology of chromosomes (Fig. 3.3). Abnormalities at the gene level, which are submicroscopic, escape detection by the methods presently available.

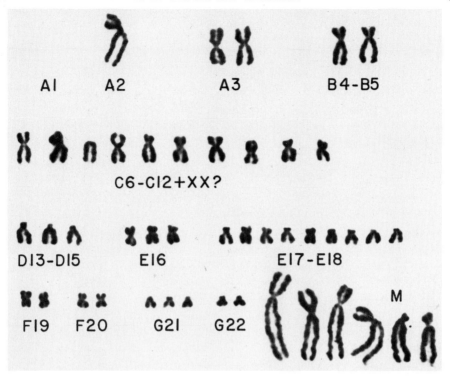

Fig. 3.3. Karyotype of a cancer cell from the peritoneal effusion of a patient with cancer of the ovary. Note the abnormal distribution of the chromosomes, with autosomes missing in groups A1, A2, C, and D and extra chromosomes being present in groups E and G. The 6 chromosomes (M) shown in the lower right-hand corner are abnormal "marker" chromosomes, possibly resulting from fusion of some of the missing chromosomes. Such "marker" chromosomes are not unusual in cancer or leukemia cells and almost invariably indicate the presence of a malignant neoplastic process.

However, recent developments in the preparation and staining of chromosomal material may afford new insight into the role of cytogenetic changes in cancer causation. These new methods of fluorescent staining and "banding" patterns reveal subchromosomal structure which, when studied in detail, may ultimately yield information which is specific and characteristic for certain cancers or leukemia, similar to the Ph[1] chromosome in chronic myelocytic leukemia (CML) in man (Section III,C,7,a).

B. The Chromosomes in Animal Tumors and Leukemia

Since the chromosomal changes in human neoplasia are difficult and often impossible to study throughout the genesis of the cancer or leukemia, animal studies are required to obtain cytogenetic information regarding this facet of carcino- and leukemogenesis. Spontaneous tumors and those induced by a number of different agents in animals are used to obtain data on the importance of karyotypic changes in the development and induction of cancer and leukemia in a variety of species.

Studies of chromosomes in various animal neoplasms have been performed to elucidate their role in carcinogenesis because the chromosomal changes are studied only after they have been well established in human cancer and leukemia. There is some possibility in animal studies that such changes can be found during the process of initiation and progression of these diseases. The effect of carcinogens on chromosomes can also be studied in the latter. In the following sections a comparison is attempted of the chromosomal changes in various neoplasms, mainly primary ones, induced by various agents.

1. Spontaneous Tumors and Leukemia

There have not been many reports of chromosomes studied on spontaneous tumors or leukemias of animals, particularly in recent years. This is probably due to the fact that such studies, similar to those in human cancer and leukemia, cannot contribute much to the understanding of the role of chromosomal changes in the causation of these states, since when these are studied they are fairly well established. Nevertheless, early observations indicated that mammary carcinoma and leukemia of mice were accompanied by a diploid or hyperdiploid chromosome constitution and that bovine lymphosarcoma was characterized by either diploidy or aneuploidy, the latter being either hypo- or hyperdiploid.

2. Tumors Due to Nutritional or Endocrine Imbalance

The findings presented in Table 3.1 indicate that the least malignant thyroid tumors were diploid, and hence, resembled in some respects normal thyroid tissue (1). The more undifferentiated the thyroid tissue became, the more complex were the chromosomal anomalies. However, convincing evidence was not found that the chromosomal changes contributed to the causation of the thyroid tumors. The karyotypic changes could just as well have been the result of the underlying neoplastic process, the metabolic changes, or the iodine deficiency.

Little is available on chromosomal findings in early thyroid tumors in the human. Frank cancers of the thyroid have been invariably found to be aneuploid,

TABLE 3.1

CHROMOSOMAL FINDINGS IN THYROID TUMORS OF RATS[a]

Type of tumor	Conditions of growth	Rate of growth	Chromosome findings
Dependent	Iodine deficiency and thyroidectomy	Slowly growing	Diploid (42)
Transitional	Growth faster in iodine deficiency and thyroidectomy	Slowly growing	Hypodiploid (41); missing #15
Autonomous	No dependence on iodine deficiency and thyroidectomy	Fast growing	Hyperdiploid (42–43); missing #15

[a] Al-Saadi and Beierwaltes, (1).

without any consistent karyotypic picture and with each cancer having its own unique chromosomal profile. No two tumors had identical chromosomal changes. Even though the cytogenetic findings in rats with thyroid tumors presented above (Table 3.1) were relatively more homogeneous than the findings in human cases, they were, nevertheless, variable within the groups studied. In addition, it is probable that the relative hereditary homogeneity of the rats used led to a somewhat more stable and characteristic karyotypic picture than obtained in human tumors, the latter possibly as a result of the extremely variable heredity of human subjects.

There is no absolute proof that nutritional or endocrine imbalance causes cancer of the thyroid in human subjects, although this is an area which is being intensely investigated in a number of places. It is possible that a number of human tumors may result from endocrine or metabolic imbalance, e.g., adrenal tumors possibly due to hypothalamic-pituitary imbalance, ovarian tumors due to pituitary malfunction, or cancer of the prostate due to hormonal factors. However no definitive proof exists that there is a relationship between the hormonal or metabolic upheaval and development of any cancer. Nevertheless, when cancers or benign tumors develop in these tissues, the chromosomal characteristics are not specific or unique and the malignant tumors tend to have a variable karyotypic picture. The benign tumors are invariably accompanied by chromosomal diploidy.

3. CHEMICAL CARCINOGENS

A host of chemicals has been shown to cause cancer and leukemia in a number of animals. Studies have also been performed on the role of chromosomal changes in the production of these tumors; the general opinion is that most, if not all, experimental tumors start out as diploid. Karyotypic changes become evident with either the biological progression of the tumor, transformation to a more malignant phase, or in the metastases of the tumor. Agreement also appears to exist that chromosomal abnormalities are not required for chemical carcinogens to induce tumor development or growth and that tumors with quite different karyotypes may exist at the same time in the same organ of an animal.

The mechanism for the production of a chromosomal change by chemicals, whether they are carcinogenic or not, is poorly understood. Heterochromatically altered regions in chromosomes, generated during carcinogen-induced malignant transformation, may be responsible for nondisjunction of chromosomes, leading to nonrandom rearrangement of a chromosomal complement with neoplastic, biochemical and cytological characteristics. An example of such a heterochromatic region is that of a C1 chromosome in DMBA-induced leukemia in rats (43). The importance of gaps and deletions in chromosomes induced by chemicals followed by changes in ploidy due to nondisjunction and/or duplication of chromosome sets have also been stressed (49).

Even though many chemicals play a role in the causation of human cancer and leukemia, only a few have been strongly implicated in these diseases. Benzene is probably a cause of acute leukemia in some subjects exposed to this chemical. Chromosomal changes, consisting primarily of gaps, breaks, deletions, translocations, and others, have been described in the cultured lymphocytes and marrow cells of subjects exposed to benzene, particularly during the severe anemic phase of the toxicity (46). When leukemia supersedes, the cytogenetic findings do not differ from those observed in other human acute leukemias (Section III,C,6). Many other chemicals have been shown to produce chromosomal changes of a nonspecific nature and whether these changes play any role in the development of neoplasia in human subjects is a moot point, since only a few chemicals have been imputed as carcinogenic.

Thus, a survey of the data (Table 3.2) and a review of the literature of experimentally induced tumors in animals, as well as the data pertaining to human subjects, appear to indicate that the genesis of the neoplastic state by these chemicals does not require any alteration of the chromosomal set from diploidy. It is possible that some chromosomal changes are involved in the causation of neoplasia in animals, but the overwhelming evidence appears to indicate that the development of such a state can occur just as readily in the presence of a diploid set of chromosomes, without any evident alterations.

4. Oncogenic Viruses

Many reports exist regarding the chromosomal changes in virus-induced tumors or leukemias in animals. Generally, no outstanding abnormalities have been observed in conditions induced by RNA viruses. These abnormalities are more striking in tumors or leukemia induced by DNA viruses.

a. RNA Viruses. *i. Friend Leukemia Virus.* Even though there are no significant alterations in the chromosome number or karyotypes in mice infected with Friend leukemia virus, apparently a significant correlation between the number of secondary chromosomal constrictions and progression of the disease was observed (9). As the weight of the spleen increased, the number of secondary constrictions per metaphase also increased. Furthermore, there was an inverse relationship between the increased weight of the spleen and the number of diploid cells with no secondary constrictions. Since the secondary constrictions were observed early in the disease and appeared to progressively increase throughout the course of the study, the authors felt that the changes had significant mutational importance in relation to the development of leukemia.

ii. Rous Sarcoma Virus (RSV). Several interesting studies have been performed on the chromosome constitution in mice infected with RSV. The chromosomes were examined in the primary tumors induced by the Schmidt-Ruppin strain of RSV in Chinese hamsters, such an analysis being performed on 42 tumors in 29 animals (18). Twenty-eight different karyotypes were found in 68 tumor stemlines and sidelines. About 40% of the stem- and sidelines and 52% of the stemlines had a normal karyotype. The most common karyotypic abnormality observed was the presence of extra two or three chromosomes. The proportion of normal cells in any given tumor correlated inversely with

TABLE 3.2

CHROMOSOMAL CHANGES IN TUMORS INDUCED BY CHEMICAL CARCINOGENS

Chemical	Animal	Neoplasia	Chromosome findings	Ref.
3-Methylcholanthrene	Mice	Subcutaneous sarcoma	Mostly diploid, some hyperdiploid	13
	Wistar rats	Leukemia	Diploid	25
	Golden hamsters	Primary tumors (subcutaneous)	Diploid, aneuploid, heteroploid	24
7,12-Dimethylbenz(a)anthracene	Mice	Thymic lymphoma	Hyperdiploid	41
	African mice	Sarcoma	Pseudodiploid, hypo- and hypertetraploid	14
	Rats	Leukemia	Trisomy of specific chromosomes (40% trisomy of C1, some of A6)	20
N-2-Fluorenylacetamide	Rats	Hepatic nodules	Diploid	5
		Hepatoma	Diploid, subtetraploid	
3'-Methyl-4-dimethylaminoazobenzene	Rats	Hepatoma	Diploid, hypo- and hyperdiploid	16
4-Nitroquinoline 1-oxide	Golden hamsters	Malignant transformation of embryo cells	Diploid, near tetraploid	49
Urethane	Mice	Thymic lymphosarcoma	Diploid, some cells with 41 chromosomes (hyperdiploid)	7

the age of such a tumor. The conclusion reached was that malignant transformation may be initiated without any visible chromosomal changes.

Earlier studies *in vitro* on the effect of RSV on cultured Chinese hamster fibroblasts indicated a higher incidence of chromosomal breakage than observed in control cells (17). Apparently, the spontaneous and virus induced breakages were distributed nonrandomly among the cells, the chromosomes, and chromosomal regions. Most of the breaks were localized in three specific regions of the chromosomes. Furthermore, a correlation was demonstrated between the pattern of chromosomal breakage and secondary constrictions. The most significant difference, however, was found between the patterns of distribution of spontaneous and virus-induced chromosomal alterations.

A more recent study dealt with the cytogenetic findings in 50 primary Rous sarcomas induced in the rat (22). About 80% of the sarcomas had a normal diploid stemline, although about half of these had some minor alterations of the chromosomal number in the cell population. These alterations most commonly consisted of hyperdiploidy with trisomy of one group or another being the predominant karyotypic anomaly. Pseudodiploidy appeared to occur as the second most common karyotypic aberration. The karyotypic changes during the development of heterodiploidy appeared to be of nonrandom nature. One extra telocentric or subtelocentric chromosome or both were found in 76% of all heteroploid cells and in about 70% of all variant cells. There appeared to be no relationship between the latent period of tumor development and the chromosomal findings. With increase in age of the tumor the number of diploid cells decreased and this was associated with a progressive histological anaplasia of the tumors.

Studies of the chromosomal constitution of 16 metastatic Rous sarcomas in rats revealed the close karyotypic relationship between the primary sarcomas and their metastases (23). The outstanding difference was an accelerated chromosomal progression in the secondary tumors, this progression being associated with a decrease in the histological maturity of the tumors. In 56% of the metastases heteroploid stemlines were found, as compared to 23% in primary tumors. Furthermore, about one-third of the primary sarcomas with normal diploid chromosomes constitutions had some cytogenetically abnormal cells, whereas about two-thirds of the metastatic tumors had such abnormal cells.

b. DNA Viruses. As indicated previously, the tumors induced by DNA viruses have chromosomal abnormalities more consistently than those induced by RNA viruses. Thus, it has been shown that the chromosomes of 8 primary tumors induced by adenovirus type 12 in Syrian hamsters were characterized by a karyotypically heterogeneous cell population, consisting of aneuploid, pseudodiploid, and polyploid cells (42). These changes were accompanied by marker chromosomes in some of the tumors and by a relatively high incidence of chromosomal and mitotic irregularities, including chromatid and isochromatid breaks, gaps, overcontracted chromosomes, and chromosome fragmentation. Each tumor contained many clones of cells with abnormal karyotypes, but a karyotypically predominant abnormal stemline was not present. They also speculated that the chromosomal instability was a reflection of the host genetic alteration associated with the viral-induced antigenic changes.

To date, there is no cogent definitive evidence that any human cancer or leukemia is caused by a virus. Hence, one cannot ascertain whether any of the karyotypic abnormalities observed in human neoplasia have been contributed to or are a result of viral effects. The chromosomal changes observed following infection with various viruses (some of which may in the future be shown to be oncogenic) have been observed primarily in cultured lymphocytes. These changes, which may persist for relatively long periods of time, have consisted primarily of gaps, breaks, fragmentation, and occasionally more serious alterations in chromosomal morphology. To our knowledge, no change in ploidy or the production of consistent marker chromosomes has been demonstrated to occur as a result of or concomitant with such a viral infection. The chromosomal changes just described have also been observed in early lesions, not necessarily cancerous ones, of the uterine cervix in human subjects and some workers have related these changes to the presence of virus in the tissue, with the possibility that such a virus may play a role in the oncogenic process leading to carcinoma of the cervix. No definite correlation, however, has been shown to exist between the presence of such a virus, the chromosomal changes in the cervical cells, and the subsequent development of neoplasia.

5. Contagious Tumors

An allegedly contagious reticulum cell sarcoma of the Syrian hamster has been studied following the subcutaneous implantation of such a tumor or after fragments of tumor were fed to animals, and in tumor-free animals who were caged with tumor-bearing ones (8). The stock tumor, maintained by serial subcutaneous passage in male hamsters, had a sharp modal number of 51, including a small marker chromosome. Tumors developing in animals of either sex or induced by several modes of implantation were shown to have karyotypes identical to those of the parent tumors (with only one exception). The chromosomal makeup of 17 cases of venereal tumors of dogs obtained in distantly separate localities and at different times in Japan have been investigated (21). All the tumors had stemlines with the chromosomal number of 59, instead of the normal number of 78, with one tumor having 58 chromosomes. The karyotypes of the various tumors were very similar and included a number of marker chromosomes. In these two examples, the transmission of intact tumor cells from animal to animal is more likely rather than the induction of the same chromosomal changes in a succession of primary tumors.

To our knowledge, no contagious tumors, particularly warts (verruca vulgaris), have been studied in human subjects. Such studies should be performed, since warts in all probability have a rather high mitotic index and should be a source of sufficient metaphase plates. To date, however, no human cancers or leukemias have been shown to be contagious.

6. Minimal Deviation Hepatomas

The most comprehensive study today was performed on 42 transplantable rat hepatomas, including the so-called "minimal deviation" hepatomas (29).

The tumors were divided into three groups according to the chromosomal findings: 9 were diploid, 17 had abnormal chromosome numbers with minimal deviation of the morphology of the chromosomes, and 16 had major changes in the
chromosome number and morphology. Transplanted tumors, studied in hosts
of the opposite sex from which they originated, allowed the investigators to
distinguish contaminating host cells from those of the original tumor. Metabolic
studies indicated that the "minimal deviation" tumors had enzymic alterations
which certainly were more than minimal and with considerable variation from
tumor to tumor. Interestingly, one of the hyperdiploid tumors (45 chromosomes)
was metabolically less "deviated" than any of those with the diploid number
of chromosomes. The conclusion was that a diploid chromosome complement
did not guarantee that a tumor was "minimally deviated" from normal hepatic
tissue either in its growth rate or metabolic profile. In addition, aneuploid tumors
did not necessarily have striking morphological or metabolic deviations. Thus
"regardless of how normal these cells appear by other criteria, the term 'minimally deviated,' compared with normal liver cells, would seem inappropriate,
at least from a cytogenetic standpoint" (29). A more recent study showed that
two of the diploid hepatomas previously reported had undergone transition to
an aneuploid state (28).

C. The Chromosomes in Human Tumors and Leukemia

1. CHROMOSOMES IN MENINGIOMAS

The closest human tumors to "minimal deviation" hepatomas are the meningiomas. These tumors have usually been considered to be benign in character
since they do not metastasize or invade adjacent tissues and, except for occasional sarcomatous transformation, they look "benign" histologically. When a
large number of these tumors was examined, it was found that a substantial
percentage of meningiomas was aneuploid with a fairly characteristic cytogenetic
anomaly being present in a significant number of these tumors (39). The latter
karyotypic abnormality consists of a missing G-group autosome, thus leading
to the presence of only 45 chromosomes in the cells of the meningiomas. The
loss of this chromosome appeared to be unrelated to the sex of the patients.
The other aneuploid meningiomas have a very variable chromosomal picture
and no consistency is found in the cytogenetic profiles among the various tumors.
The findings in meningioma confront the cytogenetist, pathologist, clinician,
and cancer biologist with a serious problem. What is the role of chromosomal
findings in the definition of cancer? Does the presence of an abnormal chromosome constitution indicate irrevocable evidence for neoplasia?
The types of changes found in meningioma indicate the presence of malignancy and point to a malignant transformation of the meningioma cells, however
early the change may be on the basis of other cytological and clinical data.
The results with meningiomas also indicate that there is no correlation between

the nature of the karyotypic changes and the degree of malignancy of a tumor. The meningiomas with chromosomal changes probably represent the least malignant human tumors, yet the cytogenetic aberrations may be extreme and similar to those observed in most anaplastic cancers. Thus, the presence of chromosomal changes similar to those found in meningiomas indicate the presence of malignancy.

2. CHROMOSOMES IN BURKITT'S LYMPHOMA

This tumor in the human may possibly be caused by a virus (Epstein-Barr virus), as demonstrated by means of immunological and/or electron microscopic techniques. Most of the Burkitt's lymphomas have been found to have a diploid chromosome constitution. For a while, a heterochromatic region involving one of the C-group chromosomes (chromosome #10) was thought to be characteristic for this disease. However, this abnormality has not been found consistently in Burkitt's lymphoma and probably does not have the significance originally attributed to it. Initially, it was thought that this cytogenetic change affecting the #10 autosome may be due to the presence of E-B virus, but recent observations indicate that the abnormality may be present in the absence of the virus and the presence of the virus does not necessarily lead to the heterochromatic region on the #10 chromosome (15).

When chromosomal changes are present in Burkitt's lymphoma they are protean in nature and, hence, no characteristic or unique cytogenetic picture has emerged for this disease. Bilateral Burkitt's tumors and their metastasis to the regional lymph nodes of the head and neck area were found to have different karyotypes: on one side both the facial tumor and its metastasis were diploid, whereas on the contralateral side the tumor and its metastatis were aneuploid (12). Unless one wishes to impute two different agents in the causation of this disease in the same patient, the conclusion must be reached that Burkitt's lymphoma does not require visibly recognizable changes in the chromosome set for its development.

3. CANCER OF THE UTERINE CERVIX

Lesions of the cervix probably afford the best and most direct means of studying neoplastic lesions during their various stages in human subjects. Thus, it is possible to study simple dysplasia, carcinoma *in situ*, and invasive cancer. The nature of the findings in cervix lesions varies with the methods used for analysis, i.e., examination of the tumor cells with or without previous *in vitro* culture, site from which specimens were obtained, diagnostic criteria in labeling the lesion, etc. Furthermore, in early lesions and in normal cervical tissue the number of metaphases may be very small due to the low incidence of dividing cells and, hence, the results may have to be based on rather sparse data. In addition, although there is every likelihood that, in dysplasia and carcinoma *in situ* and rarely in invasive carcinoma, diploid cells may truly be neoplastic and the shift to aneuploidy is only an indication of the biological change in these cells, the possibility cannot be excluded that some diploid cells are of normal origin.

The chromosomes in early lesions, i.e., dysplasia, have been shown to be preponderantly diploid, although some cytogenetically abnormal cells may be present in very low or high numbers (2). In carcinoma *in situ* the chromosomal findings are usually much more abnormal than in dysplasia and this would be compatible with the more malignant aspects of carcinoma *in situ* when compared to dysplasia. The chromosome number in the former is usually in the near-tetraploid range; multiple abnormalities are not uncommon. However, diploid cells are usually present in carcinoma *in situ*. The variation around the modal number of chromosomes, even in diploid cases, is more marked in carcinoma *in situ* than in dysplasia, and, in fact, several different modes may be present in the former. This applies even more to some of the invasive carcinomas of the cervix. Both dysplasia and carcinoma *in situ* progress to frank cervical cancer (usually invasive) in somewhat less than 50% of the cases. When that happens, the chromosome number usually changes from the near-tetraploid to the near-triploid range. Nevertheless, varying percentages of cells in the diploid and tetraploid ranges may be present in invasive cancer (47). Most of the invasive cancers of the cervix have a chromosomal number in the diploid range.

The finding of cells with an aneuploid karyotype in any cervical lesion indicates that the state is cancerous and not precancerous. In almost all cases, such cells would progress to become an invasive malignancy with all its dire consequences. Some cervical lesions with exfoliated cells with characteristics highly suggestive of malignancy and abnormal chromosomal constitutions are encountered which fail to develop into clinical cancer. There seems little doubt that the human is capable of spontaneously destroying cancer cells, possibly through an immunological mechanism, and cervical lesions are no exception. This may happen in some cases of aneuploid cervical lesions. Until proved otherwise, chromosomally abnormal cells (not of congenital or hereditary origin) in a tumor should be regarded as being cancerous.

4. Breast Cancer

An examination of various lesions of the breast has revealed a diploid picture in benign lesions. Lobular carcinoma *in situ* contained mostly diploid cells with a few aneuploid ones. When aneuploidy occurs in breast cancer it is most often in the triploid range, although diploid cancers tend to be just as readily metastasizing as aneuploid ones. Cytogenetic observations indicate that the progress of breast lesions from benign and localized into an invasive stage is not always associated with a gross change in the chromosome constitution (45). For some reason the presence of multiple abnormalities in the karyotype of breast cancers, e.g., fragments, rearrangements, multiradials, rings, and marker chromosomes, tends to be associated with a poorer prognosis of the tumor because of its apparent higher malignancy.

5. ADENOMA OF THE COLON

Benign adenomas of the colon are diploid, although pseudodiploid and hyperdiploid cells may be found frequently (4). However, it is known that atypical areas of cells may be found in some regions of the adenomas and are considered to be incipient cancer *in situ*, if not already malignant. In such adenomas the incidence of aneuploid cells is high and the morphological karyotypic changes resemble those found in established cancer of this organ. The preponderant number of adenomas of the colon is diploid when their histology is benign and no clinical evidence of malignancy is found. On the other hand, in patients with multiple adenomas of the colon in which some had undergone malignant changes, there is a high incidence of aneuploid cells in the adenomas not directly involved in the cancer transformation. The finding of aneuploid cells in adenomas is supporting evidence for malignant transformation in the benign adenoma, although such a process may occur in the absence of any evident cytogenetic alterations. Thus, a precancerous lesion may be malignant, particularly when chromosomal changes are established.

The gist of the findings presented is that early cancerous lesions are diploid and that aneuploidy is a common accompaniment of a malignant transformation and progression of a neoplastic process. Even though tumors of certain organs may have a unique chromosome constitution that favors or is associated with its invasiveness and metastasizing ability, such chromosomal modes differ from tissue to tissue (diploid range in cervical cancer, hypotetraploid in bladder cancer, hypodiploid in cancer of the colon, etc.).

6. ACUTE LEUKEMIA

Acute leukemia in human subjects is the best example of a neoplastic disease which may not be associated with deviations of the karyotype from diploidy. At least 50% of the cases with either acute myeloblastic or acute lymphoblastic leukemia do not have any recognizible cytogenetic changes in their leukemic cells. It is rare for a diploid acute leukemia to develop aneuploidy, even after several courses of remission and relapse and a number of different therapeutic regimens. However, the development of aneuploidy in a previously diploid acute leukemia has been reported.

No characteristic picture has been established for any form of acute leukemia and the cytogenetic changes vary from one case of acute leukemia to another. Observations (36) some years ago that acute lymphoblastic leukemia tends to be invariably pseudo- or hyperdiploid, whereas acute myeloblastic leukemia may have a chromosomal mode ranging from impressive hypodiploidy to hyperdiploidy (rarely above 55 chromosomes), have been supported by more recent observations (Fig. 3.4). Very high chromosomal numbers (above 80) occur more often in acute lymphoblastic leukemia than in acute myeloblastic leukemia and, in fact, very high chromosome counts are rather rare in the latter disease.

An interesting finding (Fig. 3.5), possibly bearing on the basic causation of acute leukemia, is the fuzzy and ill-defined appearance of the leukemic chro-

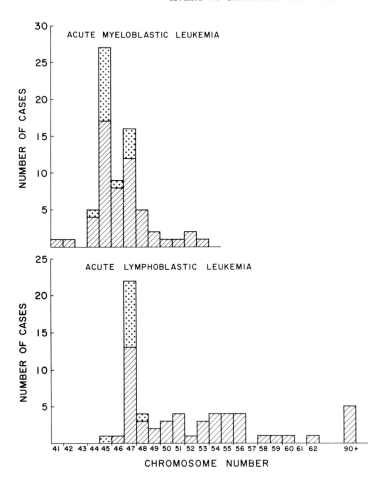

Fig. 3.4. Distribution of modal chromosome numbers in patients with acute myeloblastic or lymphoblastic leukemia. Note that acute lymphoblastic leukemia almost invariably tends to be hyperdiploid when chromosomal changes are present, whereas acute myeloblastic leukemia may be either hypo-, pseudo-, or hyperdiploid. The striped areas represent patients with preponderantly aneuploid cells and the stipled areas cases in which the aneuploid cells constituted a minor population in the marrow.

mosomes in most cases of acute leukemia, including the diploid ones (35). It has been difficult to establish the exact reason for this peculiarity of staining and/or morphology of the leukemic chromosomes and the deciphering of this unusual observation may provide important clues regarding the basic mechanism of human leukemogenesis.

Recent studies have correlated the survival of acute myeloblastic leukemia patients with the chromosomal picture (32). Patients who do not have any normal metaphases in their marrow (AA patients) at any stage of the disease have the shortest survival time and die much sooner following initiation of therapy than those subjects who have a mixed population of cells, i.e., diploid

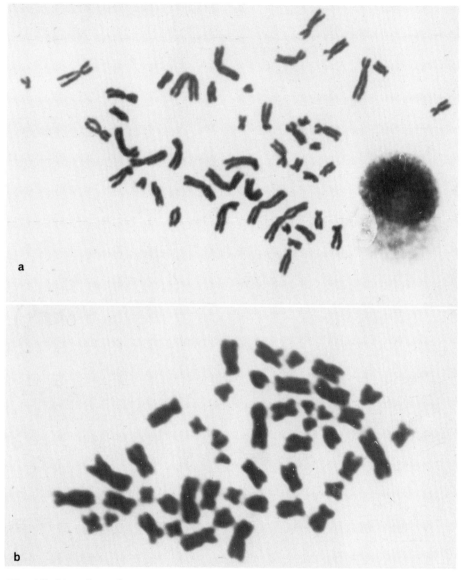

Fig. 3.5. Metaphases from a patient with acute lymphoblastic leukemia. Figure 3.5a shows a normal diploid cell with thin and well-defined chromatids, as compared to the ill-defined and fuzzy chromatids shown in Fig. 3.5b. The fuzzy and ill-defined appearance of the chromosomes in acute leukemia occurs in at least 50% of the cases and is an intriguing observation awaiting explanation.

and aneuploid cells, and those with only diploid marrows. AA patients apparently have no normal cells with which to repopulate the marrow following response of the leukemic cells to therapy and the short survival of these subjects may be related to this parameter. Erythroleukemia patients tend, more often than not, to fall into the AA group of acute myeloblastic leukemia. This study repre-

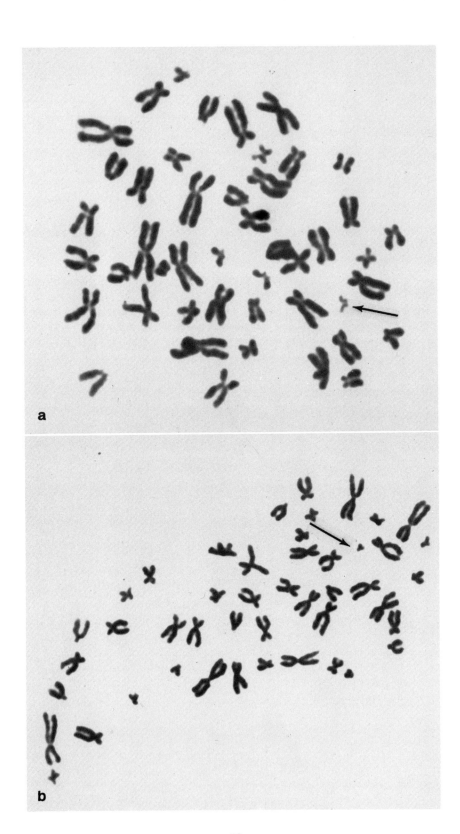

sents a possible application of cytogenetic findings in leukemia or cancer to certain therapeutic and/or clinical parameters and justifies the continuation of such studies in many human neoplastic conditions.

The aneuploid cells in acute leukemia may disappear completely, particularly in acute lymphoblastic leukemia, when the disease responds to therapy. When remission occurs, the leukemic cells reappear with the same karyotypic picture that characterized them prior to remission and this cycle may repeat itself several times. In fact, the appearance of occasional metaphases with an aneuploid chromosome constitution in an otherwise normal marrow may herald the relapse of the acute leukemia and this may prove to be a valuable therapeutic index in chemotherapy. Appearance of aneuploid cells in acute myeloblastic leukemia, in the presence of myeloblasts in the marrow, indicates that the leukemic cells are probably of different origin than the myeloblasts observed in the marrow during complete remission.

7. Chronic Leukemia

a. Chronic Myelocytic Leukemia. Chronic myelocytic leukemia (CML) is the only neoplastic condition in mammalian characterized by a specific and consistent karyotypic abnormality, the Ph^1 chromosome, (Fig. 3.6) (27). This cytogenetic abnormality is present in the leukemic cells of over 85% of the patients with chronic myelocytic leukemia. Apparently, the anomaly involves all the cells of the marrow, i.e., normoblastic, granulocytic, and megakaryocytic, and persists throughout the course of the disease, regardless of the response of the leukemia to therapy. The Ph^1 is an acquired chromosomal abnormality, as supported by the fact that it is found only in the affected members of identical twins.

When CML undergoes transformation to the blastic phase, the Ph^1 persists and may, in fact, duplicate or triplicate itself in some of the cells prior to or concomitant with the blastic changes. The cytogenetic changes which take place as a result of the blastic transformation vary from case to case, though hyperdiploidy is more common than hypodiploidy. A substantial number of CML cases, that go into the blastic phase, do not develop further karyotypic changes besides the Ph^1. It is possible for the chromosomal changes consequent to the blastic phase transformation to disappear upon response of the leukemia to therapy, but the Ph^1 persists in the cells of the marrow.

Patients with Ph^1-positive CML respond to therapy more readily and survive for a much longer period of time than Ph^1-negative patients with the same type of leukemia (10, 44). It is possible that Ph^1-negative CML may be a different entity than Ph^1-positive CML and more akin to acute leukemia, particularly myeloblastic leukemia, than to CML.

Fig. 3.6. Metaphases from 2 different patients with chronic myelocytic leukemia and containing the Philadelphia (Ph^1) chromosome (arrows). In Fig. 3.6a the shortening of the long arms of the Ph^1 chromosome, when compared to the other group G chromosomes, is particularly evident.

b. CHRONIC LYMPHOCYTIC LEUKEMIA (CLL). No characteristic cytogenetic picture has emerged for CLL. An abnormal G-group autosome, the Ch¹ chromosome, has been described in a family with a high incidence of CLL (11). But, so far, some of the affected members of the family have not developed CLL. The chromosomal change is found in all of the somatic cells examined, and thus, appears to constitute a hereditary karyotypic defect. Furthermore, the finding of a Ch¹ chromosome in CLL is an extremely rare (although interesting) finding in CLL, and in other instances of familial CLL no such cytogenetic abnormality has been found.

The chromosomal findings in human chronic leukemia, particularly the Ph¹, indicate that the karyotypic anomaly may play a direct role in the causation of CML. However, no cases with the Ph¹ without any cytological or clinical evidence of leukemia have been described to date, so that it is difficult to ascribe to the Ph¹ a specific role in the causation of CML. Until more is known about the mechanism by which the Ph¹ is generated, the fate of the missing DNA in the G22 autosome contributing to the Ph¹ and the correlation between the appearance of this abnormal chromosome and the genesis of CML, some caution should be exercised in ascribing to this abnormal chromosome a crucial and direct role in leukemia causation.*

8. OTHER HEMATOPOIETIC CONDITIONS

The chromosomal findings in other neoplastic conditions affecting the marrow, e.g., multiple myeloma and lymphosarcoma, do not differ from those of other cancers (Section III,C,9) and indicate that by the time these diseases become evident, either histologically or clinically, the cytogenetic aberrations are well established. Thus, it is difficult to ascertain the exact role the chromosomal changes play in the causation of these diseases because of the advanced stage in which they are examined. The emphasis on certain marker chromosomes as being typical of multiple myeloma or paraproteinemia has not withstood the test of time and further analysis. Besides, similar marker chromosomes can be observed in tumors of other tissues and not all cases of multiple myeloma or paraproteinemia have the marker chromosomes in their cells. Some of these cytogenetic abnormalities observed in the cells of patients with the above diseases, particularly cells following *in vitro* culture, may be a result of immunological effects due to derangement of this parameter in these patients. This effect may be mediated either through factors in the blood or by direct involvement of the cells in question.

9. THE CHROMOSOMES IN CANCER AND METASTASES

Human cancer may be many disease entities and it is not surprising that the chromosomal changes in cancerous tissues are very diverse, without any tumor having a characteristic chromosomal picture. Diploid human cancer is

---

* Recently it has been demonstrated by means of quinacrine fluorescence and Giemsa staining (30a) that the missing part of chromosome #22 is translocated onto the long arm of #9. Whether the amount translocated is equal to that missing from the Ph¹ has not been established with certainty. Others (including our laboratory) have confirmed this important finding, but whether it occurs in all cases of CML remains to be ascertained.

very rare; this is probably due to the fact that when such tumors become evident, they are already well established and advanced, including the cytogenetic abnormalities. The chromosome number in human cancer varies from very impressive hypodiploidy to very high counts. Furthermore, tumors of the same origin may have chromosome numbers which span a wide range (shown in Table 3.3). In fact, no two human cancers have been shown to have identical karyotypes.

Metastatic lesions show the same chromosome number variability as do primary tumors, though high ploidy tends to be more common in metastatic lesions than in primary tumors. Nevertheless, the karyotypic picture in metastatic lesions is usually a variation on the cytogenetic theme displayed by the primary tumor.

When cancer effusions containing aneuploid malignant cells respond to therapy, the cancer cells disappear (37). However, when the effusion recurs, the karyotypic picture has been found to be very similar to the original one or to vary from it only mildly, even when the recurrence is at a different site, e.g., the initial effusion may be peritoneal and the recurrent one pleural. This is similar to the reappearance of leukemic cells with very similar cytogenetic profiles in acute leukemia following remission.

These data indicate that the neoplastic cell selected has the karyotypic constitution that endows it with growth potential and biological advantages apparently not given to other karyotypes. The rarity of diploid cancers and metastases points to the possibility that (a) either the aneuploid karyotype allows the cancer cells definite survival and invasive potentials not supplied by a diploid

TABLE 3.3

DISTRIBUTION OF MODAL NUMBER OF CHROMOSOMES IN 91 CASES
OF HUMAN PRIMARY CANCERS AND IN 129 CANCEROUS
EFFUSIONS REPORTED IN THE LITERATURE[a]

Chromosome type	Range of modal chromosome no.	Primary cancers (%)	Effusions (%)
Diploid			
Hypo-	35–45	17	17
Pseudo-	46	9	14
Hyper-	47–57	35	17
Group total		61	48
Triploid			
Hypo-	58–68	12	16
Pseudo-	69	2	1
Hyper-	70–80	14	23
Group total		28	40
Tetraploid			
Hypo-	81–91	10	6
Pseudo-	92	1	0
Hyper-	93–133	0	6
Group total		11	12

[a] Sandberg and Hossfeld (34).

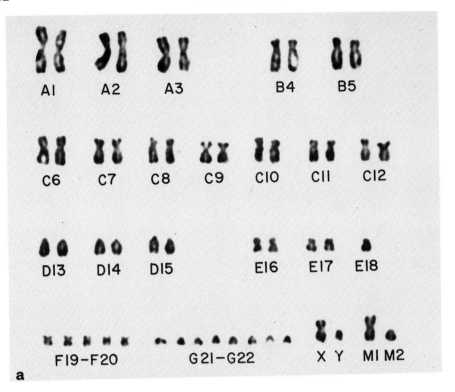

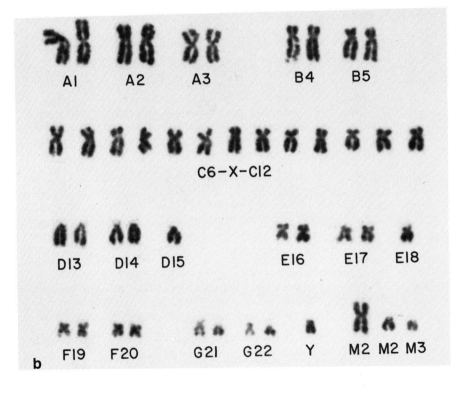

set of chromosomes or (b) that the cancerous state leads almost invariably to a change of the cytogenetic make-up of the cells.

The large array of chromosomal changes in human cancer and the seemingly endless variety of karyotypic pictures are probably secondary phenomena to the cancerous state and not its primary cause (Fig. 3.7). It is probable that the truly remarkable cytogenetic findings in human cancer are more a reflection of the variability of the human genome among different individuals and, thus, the chromosomal changes in cancer are but another phenotypic expression of the diversity of the genetic differences among human subjects and not the direct cause of the cancerous state.

10. MARKER CHROMOSOMES

Much has been made of marker chromosomes in cancer. These chromosomes differ morphologically from any of the chromosomes in the human set and are usually easily recognized in metaphase plates. Except for the Ph^1 chromosome (possibly also the Ch^1 chromosome), no marker chromosome has been shown to have a unique significance for any tumor in humans. Similar markers may occur in tumors of different tissue origin, either in hypo- or hyperdiploid cells; they are present in either a small or large percentage of the cells, and they bear no particular relationship to the cytological picture, malignancy, or response to therapy of the tumors.

The genesis of marker chromosomes is poorly understood, though most often they appear to originate from the fusion of one or more normal chromosomes. This has been demonstrated by means of autoradiographic techniques and the more recently developed methods of fluorescent staining and banding patterns (38, 48). It is possible that the latter methods may reveal that apparently normal chromosomes in cancer or leukemic cells may be abnormal chromosomes due to the fusion of certain chromosomes leading to the appearance of morphologically normal markers, e.g., fusion of a D-group autosome with a G-group one, leading to a C-grouplike autosome. It is certain that much of the genesis of marker chromosomes will be learned by the newly available techniques.

D. The Chromosomes in Conditions Predisposing to Neoplasia

1. CHROMOSOMES AND RADIATION

Ionizing radiation of whatever source shares with a number of other physical, chemical, and biological agents the ability to produce transient and possibly

---

Fig. 3.7. Karyotypes from paternal twins with congenital acute myeloblastic leukemia (AML). Since the cause of the leukemia must have been identical in these 2 subjects, the AML having developed *in utero*, the difference in the karyotypes (one containing only 45 and the other more than 50 chromosomes) is probably a reflection of the difference in the genetic makeup of the twins and points to the secondary nature of the chromosomal changes in acute leukemia.

permanent damage to the visible integrity of human chromosomes. The immediate effect of ionizing radiation is to produce damage to the chromosomes; this damage consists of deletions, translocations, acentric fragments, multicentric and ring chromosomes, and others, which are probably deleterious to further cellular division. Apparently, such changes may be latently present in human cells for as many as 20 years (3). Whether ionizing radiation is capable of producing permanent karyotypic changes visible microscopically which can be related directly to carcinogenesis is not certain. That they do produce changes in the human genome at a submicroscopic level is undoubted, as evidenced by the high incidence of cancer and leukemia in subjects exposed to one or another form of irradiation. The perplexing aspect is that not all subjects (as a matter of fact a rather small percentage of those exposed to radiation or oncogenic and/or chromosome damage-producing chemicals and viruses) develop neoplasia, and the same statement applies to those in whom chromosomal changes have been demonstrated. Besides, cancer and leukemia may develop in subjects exposed to radiation and in whose blood or other cells no changes in the chromosomes have been shown. Thus, the means by which ionizing radiation produces cancer or leukemia in human subjects is unknown and probably does not require modification of the visible chromosomal structure or number for the induction of neoplasia.

2. Congenital or Hereditary Chromosomal Conditions Predisposing to Neoplasia

A number of conditions in the human associated with a higher incidence of neoplasia and congenital chromosomal anomalies has been described. The high incidence of acute leukemia in Down's syndrome, a condition with G21 trisomy, is well established (40) though much remains unknown, e.g., only a small percentage of patients with Down's syndrome develops acute leukemia and there is a very low incidence of chronic myelocytic leukemia in this disease. In Fanconi's anemia and Bloom's syndrome (6) there is increased breakage of the chromosomes, particularly in cultured lymphocytes. Both conditions are associated with a high incidence of leukemia and cancer, though not all patients with the karyotypic abnormalities develop these complicating diseases. It is of interest that heterozygous members of families of patients with Fanconi's anemia, Bloom's syndrome, or ataxia telangiectasia may also have the chromosomal breakages in their cells.

As an extension of the chromosome breakage syndromes alluded to above, attempts have been made at establishing susceptibility of certain individuals to neoplasia by studying the malignant transformation in the cells of such individuals by certain oncogenic viruses or by determining the frequency of chromosomal changes in cells when these are exposed to X-ray. Both approaches have yielded interesting information. Cells from subjects with Fanconi's anemia, Down's syndrome, Klinefelter's syndrome (XXY), and Bloom's syndrome and XYY males show a much higher incidence of aberrations by either method. Cells from subjects with an XO chromosome constitution are resistant to X-ray-induced chromosomal damage, at least as much as the cells from normal subjects. Apparently, similar observations have been reported by others. Thus, it is conceivable that only cells from subjects with chromosome breakage syndromes or having extra autosomes or gonosomes are subject to a high incidence of malignant transformation and/or X-ray-induced damage. The relationship of these findings to the development of neoplasia remains to be elucidated.

References

1. Al-Saadi, A., and Beierwaltes, W. H. (1967). *Cancer Res.* **27**, 1831–1842.
2. Auersperg, N., Corey, M. J., and Worth, A. (1967). *Cancer Res.* **27**, 1394–1401.
3. Awa, A. A., and Bloom, A. D. (1967). *Jap. J. Human Genet.* **12**, 69–75.
4. Baker, M. C., and Atkin, N. B. (1970). *Proc. Roy. Soc. Med.* **63**, 9–10.
5. Becker, F. F., Fox, R. A., Klein, K. M., and Wolman, S. R. (1971). *J. Nat. Cancer Inst.* **46**, 1261–1269.
6. Bloom, G. E., Warner, S., Gerald, P. S., and Diamond, L. K. (1966). *New England J. Med.* **274**, 8–14.
7. Colnaghi, M. I., Porta, G. D., Parmiani, G., and Caprio, G. (1969). *Int. J. Cancer* **4**, 327–333.
8. Cooper, H. L., MacKay, C. M., and Banfield, W. G. (1964). *J. Nat. Cancer Inst.* **33**, 691–706.
9. Elliott, S. C., Helm, R. M., and Myszewski, M. E. (1972). *Cancer Res.* **32**, 776–780.
10. Ezdinli, E. Z., Sokal, J. E., Crosswhite, L. H., and Sandberg, A. A. (1970). *Ann. Intern. Med.* **72**, 175–182.
11. Fitzgerald, P. H., and Hamer, J. W. (1969). *Brit. Med. J.* **3**, 752–754.
12. Gripenberg, U., Levan, A., and Clifford, P. (1969). *Int. J. Cancer* **4**, 334–349.
13. Hellstrom, K. E. (1959). *J. Nat. Cancer Inst.* **23**, 1019–1034.
14. Huang, C. C., and Strong, L. C. (1963). *Cancer Res.* **23**, 1800–1807.
15. Huang, C. C., Minowada, J., Smith, R. T., and Osunkoya, B. O. (1970). *J. Nat. Cancer Inst.* **45**, 815–829.
16. Ikeuchi, T., and Honda, T. (1971). *Cytologia* **36**, 173–182.
17. Kato, R. (1967). *Hereditas* **58**, 221–247.
18. Kato, R. (1968). *Hereditas* **59**, 63–119.
19. Koller, P. C. (1972). "The Role of Chromosomes in Cancer Biology." Springer-Verlag, New York.
20. Kurita, Y., Sugiyama, T., and Nishizuka, Y. (1968). *Cancer Res.* **28**, 1738–1752.
21. Makino, S. (1963). *Ann. N.Y. Acad. Sci.* **108**, 1106–1122.
22. Mitelman, F. (1971). *Hereditas* **69**, 155–186.
23. Mitelman, F. (1972). *Hereditas* **70**, 1–14.
24. Nachtigal, M., Popescu, N. C., and Nachtigal, S. (1967). *J. Nat. Cancer Inst.* **38**, 697–721.
25. Nowell, P. C., Ferry, S., and Hungerford, D. A. (1963). *J. Nat. Cancer Inst.* **30**, 687–703.
26. Nowell, P. C. (1965). *Progr. Exp. Tumor Res.* **7**, 83–103.
27. Nowell, P. C., and Hungerford, D. A. (1960). *Science* **132**, 1497.
28. Nowell, P. C., and Morris, H. P. (1969). *Cancer Res.* **29**, 969–970.
29. Nowell, P. C., Morris, H. P., and Potter, V. R. (1967). *Cancer Res.* **27**, 1565–1579.
30. O'Riordan, M. L., Berry, E. W., and Tough, I. M. (1970). *Brit. J. Haematol.* **19**, 83–90.
30a. Rowley, J. D. (1973). *Nature (London)* **243**, 290–293.
31. Pierre, R. V., and Hoagland, H. C. (1972). *Cancer* **30**, 889–894.
32. Sakurai, M., and Sandberg, A. A. (1973). *Blood* **41**, 93–104.
33. Sandberg, A. A. (1966). *Cancer Res.* **26**, 2064–2081.

34. Sandberg, A. A., and Hossfeld, D. K. (1970). *Annu. Rev. Med.* **21**, 379–408.
35. Sandberg, A. A., Ishihara, T., Crosswhite, L. H., and Hauschka, T. S. (1962). *Cancer Res.* **22**, 748–756.
36. Sandberg, A. A., Ishihara, T., Kikuchi, Y., and Crosswhite, L. H. (1964). *Ann. N.Y. Acad. Sci.* **113**, 663–716.
37. Sandberg, A. A., Yamada, K., Kikuchi, Y., and Takagi, N. (1967). *Cancer* **20**, 1099–1116.
38. Scheres, J. M. (1972). *Humangenetik* **15**, 253–256.
39. Singer, H., and Zang, K. D. (1970). *Humangenetik* **9**, 172–184.
40. Stewart, A., Webb, J., and Hewitt, D. (1958). *Brit. Med. J.* **1**, 1495–1508.
41. Stich, H. F. (1960). *J. Nat. Cancer Inst.* **25**, 649–661.
42. Stich, H. F., and Yohn, D. S. (1965). *J. Nat. Cancer Inst.* **35**, 603–615.
43. Sugiyama, T. (1971). *J. Nat. Cancer Inst.* **47**, 1267–1275.
44. Tjio, J. H., Carbone, P. P., Whang, J., and Frei III, E. (1966). *J. Nat. Cancer Inst.* **36**, 567–584.
45. Toews, H. A., Katayama, K. P., Masukawa, T., and Lewison, E. F. (1968). *Cancer* **22**, 1296–1307.
46. Tough, I. M., Smith, P. G., Court Brown, W. M., and Harnden, D. G. (1970). *Eur. J. Cancer* **6**, 49–55.
47. Wakonig-Vaartaja, T. (1970). *In* "Gynecological Oncology" (R. K. Barber and E. A. Graber, eds.) pp. 80–88. Williams & Wilkins, Baltimore, Maryland.
48. Yamada, K., and Sandberg, A. A. (1966). *J. Nat. Cancer Inst.* **36**, 1057–1073.
49. Yosida, T. H., Kuroki, T., Masuji, H., and Sato, H. (1970). *Gann* **61**, 131–143.

CHAPTER IV

DNA: Replication, Modification, and Repair

THOMAS W. SNEIDER

I. Introduction*

The heritable alterations of host cells that result in their escape from control mechanisms that normally regulate cellular replication is the unifying trait underlying the diversity of cancer cell types (Chapter I). The two problems that have occupied experimental oncologists for the past several decades are (a) what are the molecular mechanisms governing normal cellular replication and (b) how do known oncogenic agents interact with these mechanisms to effect their disarrangement? Considering the dearth of data on the genetic loci in

---

* Abbreviations used: TdR, 2′-deoxythymidine; dTTP, 2′-deoxythymidine-5′-triphosphate; ATP, adenosine-5′-triphosphate; FUdR, 5-fluoro-2′-deoxyuridine; dNTP, the 5′-triphosphate of a 2′-deoxyribonucleoside; A, adenine; G, guanine; C, cytosine; T, thymine.

mammalian cells that control the various processes that make up cell division and the absence of an understanding of how disparate but coordinate eukaryotic cellular processes are integrated at the level of genetic control, it may be unrealistic at this time to make hypotheses on a mechanism for control of cell replication. Since the normal control mechanism(s) of cellular replication is unknown, there is little concrete information on how oncogenic agents presumably alter these controls to produce neoplastic cells.

One fact is strikingly apparent: the functional alteration is apparently inherited by the progeny of the original transformed cell. Although there are mechanisms of cytoplasmic inheritance and the process has been implicated in the establishment of neoplasia (360), most attention has focused on genomic alterations by oncogenic agents to explain the stability and, inferentially, the mechanism of neoplastic transformation (49).

The developments that led to the concept of DNA as the genetic material have been presented in Chapter I. This chapter will review the present state of knowledge of the enzymes responsible for DNA synthesis in simpler prokaryotic systems and in mammalian cells and what is known of *in vivo* replication of DNA. Along with the properties of some DNA-polymerizing enzymes, the complex problem of the structure and replication of DNA in higher organisms will be considered. Attention will be also given to two other areas—DNA modification by chemical carcinogens and DNA repair mechanisms—that are being studied in sufficient detail to enable the construction of hypotheses concerning the role of molecular alterations of DNA in neoplasia.

II. Historical Perspectives: The Structure of DNA

Much evidence supports the contention that DNA constitutes the genetic material of the cell (Chapter I). The progression from Miescher's initial isolation of "nucleinic acid" from salmon sperm to the demonstration of the role of DNA in specification of hereditary traits to the understanding of the structure of DNA (11, 31, 175, 190, 324, 435, 436, 471, 472, 491) required almost 80 years.

Extensive base compositional studies of RNA's and DNA's from many sources showed the molar equivalencies of 6-amino and 6-keto constituents of DNA, i.e., DNA-A = DNA-T and DNA-G = DNA-C (86–88). These data, combined with X-ray diffraction studies (147, 148), enabled Watson and Crick to construct their model of the structure of DNA (472) (Fig. 4.1). The DNA is composed of two separate chains each of which is composed of the four bases of DNA attached in glycosidic linkage to deoxyribose moieties which in turn are connected by 3′,5′-phosphodiester linkages. The two chains are wound about the same axis in a right-handed helix. The chains are antiparallel with the sequences of atoms in one chain running in the opposite direction from the sequences in the second chain. The DNA bases are arranged perpendicular to the long or fiber axis of the molecule. The chains are held together by base pairs formed between a purine base on one strand hydrogen-bonded to a pyrimidine base

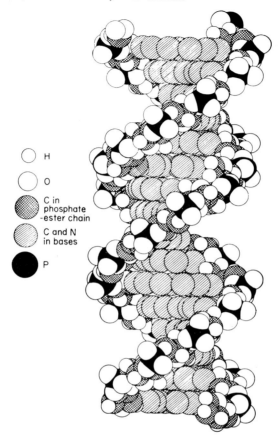

Fig. 4.1. A space-filling model of double helical DNA (from Busch, 73).

on the opposite strand. Under physiological conditions only specific pairs of bases can hydrogen-bond, i.e., adenine with thymine and guanine with cytosine. Although a purine must always be opposite a pyrimidine to account for the known dimensions of the molecule, the sequence of bases on a given strand is not restricted. Given a strand with a linear array of bases, however, the base sequence on the opposite strand is "automatically determined." Each chain acts as a template for the formation of a new complementary strand, yielding two new pairs of duplexes, each pair possessing the same linear base sequence information as the original duplex DNA molecule (473).

The essential correctness of this mode of duplication of duplex DNA was shown by the experiments of Meselson and Stahl (314). DNA extracted from *Escherichia coli* B at varying times after diluting the culture (which had been grown in $^{15}NH_4Cl$ as sole nitrogen source) with a tenfold excess of $^{14}NH_4Cl$ was centrifuged to equilibrium in cesium chloride density gradients. DNA from cells analyzed at the time of the shift from "heavy" to "light" nitrogen source and from cells analyzed after only one cell division in "light" medium showed a single peak of UV absorbance while DNA from cells sampled after two cell divisions in "light" medium showed two equal peaks of UV absorbance. The results (Fig. 4.2) constitute direct evidence for the "semiconservative" mode of DNA replication.

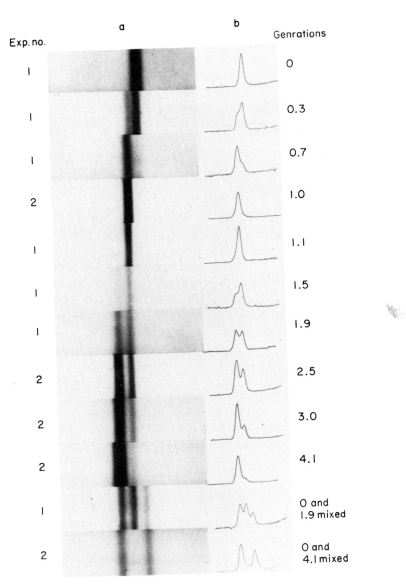

Fig. 4.2. Ultraviolet absorption photographs (a) and microdensitometric tracings (b) of DNA bands from cesium chloride density gradient centrifugation of lysates of bacteria sampled at various times after addition of an excess of ^{14}N substrates to a growing culture prelabeled with ^{15}N substrates. Density increases to the right. At generation 0, all DNA is heavy; at generation 1, all DNA bands at a lesser "hybrid" density; at generation 1.9, one-half the DNA bands at hybrid density (i.e., one strand of the duplex heavy and the other light) and one-half at a totally light density (from Meselson and Stahl, 314).

III. DNA Synthesis: Enzymic Aspects

A. Enzymes of DNA Synthesis in Simpler Organisms

1. DNA POLYMERASE I OF Escherichia coli

Originally, it was not certain whether a special enzyme would be required to polymerize the components into the DNA strands or if the DNA strand itself could serve as sort of an autocatalytic template (473, 474). Kornberg *et al.* (244) reported a very low level *in vitro* conversion of ^{14}C-labeled TdR into a product, the properties of which resembled DNA, with crude extracts of *E. coli*. Subsequently, they (245) prepared highly radioactive (1.5 × 10⁶ cpm/mole) ^{32}P-labeled dTTP to unequivocally demonstrate that a combination of two partially purified fractions from *E. coli* catalyzed the incorporation of [^{32}P]dTTP into DNA, that the reaction required the presence of all four deoxyribonucleoside triphosphates for maximal activity, and that the reaction depended very strongly upon the presence of "primer" DNA (see reviews in 168, 169, 234, 242, 243, 377).

DNA polymerase I from *E. coli* is a single polypeptide chain (of 109,000 daltons) which is folded in an unknown manner into a globular molecule 65 Å in diameter. The purified enzyme requires an oligonucleotide "primer" (either oligoribonucleotides or oligodeoxyribonucleotides; see following section) possessing a free 3'-hydroxyl group, a DNA template which must either contain internally located nicks (cleaved phosphodiester links) or else be duplex DNA, the 5'-end of which carries a single-stranded "tail," the presence of all four deoxyribonucleoside triphosphates and Mg²⁺ (although some controversy exists concerning the phosphorylation level of the nucleotide precursors *in vivo;* see Section IV, B, 1. DNA produced *in vitro* under these conditions is a faithful replica of the template as deduced from "nearest neighbor frequency" analysis (217).

There exist several distinct regions within the active site of the enzyme that are associated with the catalysis of polymerization (Fig. 4.3): A site for binding of the template DNA strand, a site for binding the elongating primer strand of DNA, a specific site for the 3'-hydroxyl terminus of the primer, and in very close proximity to this last named site a region for binding all four deoxyribonucleoside triphosphates. Figure 4.4 illustrates the polymerization step: Incoming deoxynucleoside triphosphate binds in close proximity to the primer 3'-hydroxyl terminus and in proper relationship to the template strand so that base-pairing can occur. The juxtaposition of the 3'-OH group and the triphosphate on the catalytic surface culminates in a nucleophilic attack by the 3'-OH on the 5'-phosphate (the α-phosphate) of the deoxynucleoside triphosphate resulting in elimination of pyrophosphate and formation of a new 3' to 5' phosphodiester bond. The template with its "hybridized" newly elongated primer (growing strand) presumably moves with respect to the enzyme such that the 3'-OH binding site and the triphosphate binding site is again free to accept the next nucleotide.

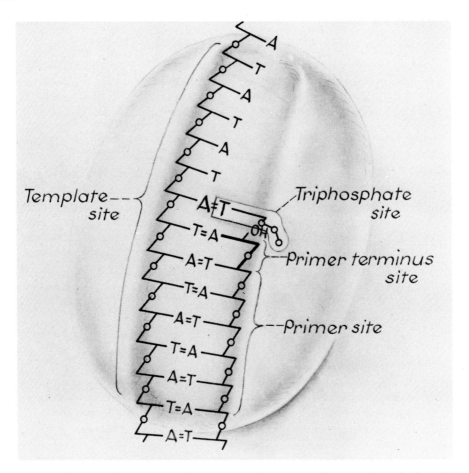

Fig. 4.3. Schematic illustration of the regions within DNA polymerase I involved in DNA polymerization (from Kornberg, 243).

The fidelity of synthesis probably resides in the fact that all "correct" base pairs have very similar dimensions and geometry which the active site of the enzyme might be able to "sense" quite accurately. A correctly made base pair might fit.on the enzyme and in so doing elicit subsequent steps in diester bond formation (243).

The ability of DNA polymerase I to exonucleolytically degrade DNA may also contribute to the precision and fidelity of DNA replication. DNA polymerizing activity and 3′ to 5′ exonucleolytic activity can be separated from 5′ to 3′ exonucleolytic activity of polymerase I by proteolytic cleavage of the enzyme (63, 237, 238, 399). The enzymic properties of the intact enzyme and the two proteolytic fragments are contrasted in Table 4.1. A possible biological role for the 5′ to 3′ exonucleolytic function is discussed in the section on DNA repair (Section VI).

The 3′ to 5′ exonuclease function acts only on single-stranded DNA or on helical duplex DNA with frayed ends, which suggests that this exonuclease

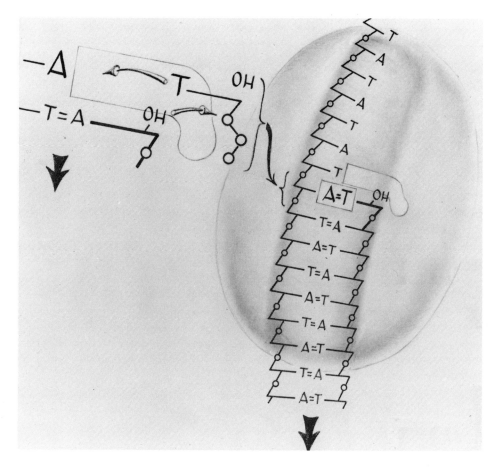

Fig. 4.4. Schematic illustration of the polymerization step catalyzed by DNA polymerase I. See text for explanation (from Kornberg, 243).

TABLE 4.1

DISTINCTION BETWEEN THE NUCLEASE ACTIVITIES OF DNA
POLYMERASE I FROM *E. coli*[a]

	3' to 5' Nuclease	5' to 3' Nuclease
Start of reaction	3' End (primer terminus)	5' End (OH, P, PPP)
Nucleotide products	100% Mononucleotides	80% Mononucleotides
		20% Di- and trinucleotides
Excision of oligomers	No	Yes
DNA structure	Frayed, single strand	Double strand
Influence of concomitant		
polymerization	Blocked	Enhanced 10-fold
Phage T4 polymerase	Possesses 3' to 5' nuclease	Does not have 5' to 3' nuclease

[a] From Kornberg (243)

function might serve to remove a primer terminus (3′) improperly based-paired to the template (243). Hence, artificial template primer duplexes containing matched or mismatched nucleotides at the 3′ terminus of the primer were incubated with the large fragment of polymerase I (62). The results unequivocally demonstrate that the very great fidelity of replication by polymerase I may be a consequence of both recognition of correct base-pair dimensions and geometry and a "proofreading" step occurring immediately after the primer terminus is elongated by one nucleotide (243).

2. *In vivo* MECHANICS OF DNA SYNTHESIS

Early *in vitro* studies on the enzymological aspects of DNA synthesis were paralleled by efforts to analyze DNA replication *in vivo* in "simple" prokaryotic systems. However, certain difficulties arose from the proposed DNA structure and its postulated semiconservative mode of replication. The X-ray diffraction data and model building led Watson and Crick (474) to postulate that the two strands of a DNA double helix must be plectonemically coiled, i.e., one single helix wound about and through the second helical strand. During semiconservative replication the parental DNA helices must be separated either by strand breakage, by "unscrewing" one helix past its complement (or by pulling in an axial direction the opposite ends of the two helices), or by actively unwinding the intertwined helices. The actual mechanism of strand separation remains unknown, but of the possibilities just mentioned, the concepts of strand breakage or an active unwinding of helices have been incorporated into many models of replication. Recently, a number of proteins have been partially purified from bacteriophage, bacterial, and eukaryotic systems which can direct and/or cause the melting out of the DNA double helix (3).

An even more fundamental difficulty became apparent from biochemical (76, 77) and genetic studies (338, 432) which showed that *in vivo* DNA replication begins at a fixed origin and proceeds sequentially and unidirectionally from that origin. Autoradiographic analyses (76, 77) provided direct confirmation of this conclusion. The self-portrait of an *E. coli* DNA molecule in the process of duplicating itself is shown in Fig. 4.5a. Study of DNA molecules extracted after varying periods of replication led Cairns (76) to conclude that the chromosome of at least two strains of *E. coli* exists as a circular length of double-stranded DNA 700–900 nm long, that the DNA duplicates by forming a **Y**-shaped fork the stem of which consists of both parental strands of DNA and the two limbs of which each consist of one strand of parental DNA and the complementary newly synthesized daughter strand, that there is probably only one replication fork per chromosome, and that the two new semiconservatively synthesized double helices are joined at their ends (i.e., distal to the replication fork and at the origin of replication). The distal union of the two new double helices was postulated to act as a swivel or rotation point which might be the site of the mechanism responsible for unwinding parental duplex DNA and rewinding the daughter duplexes (Fig. 4.5b).

The conclusion seemed inescapable that both strands of DNA in the duplex were synthesized simultaneously and sequentially from a fixed origin to a termi-

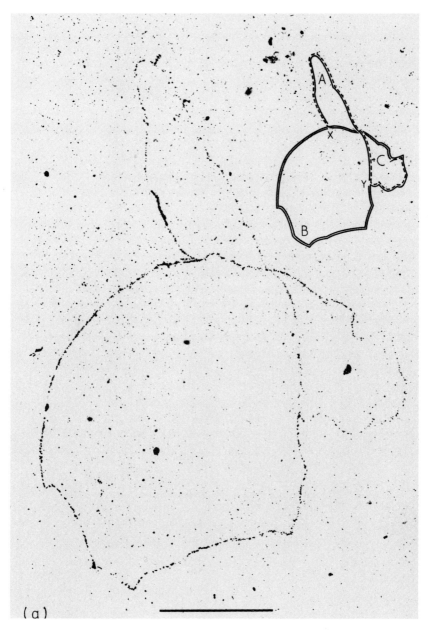

(a)

Fig. 4.5a. Autoradiograph of the chromosome of *E. coli* K12 Hfr labeled with [³H]TdR for two generations followed by DNA extraction and autoradiography. Scale represents 100 μm. Upper-right portion of figure is a diagrammatic representation of the autoradiograph with points X and Y denoting two forks, one of which may be the replication fork and the second of which might act as a swivel point. In this figure, segments XBY and XAY represent the newly duplicated double helices whereas segment YCX represents that portion of the parental DNA to be duplicated. Point X is the origin-termination point of duplication and Y the growing point. The dashed line represents an unlabeled DNA strand. The half-labeled segment (YC) and totally labeled segment (CX) is presumably obtained because the label was introduced prior to completion of the original duplex (from Cairns, 77).

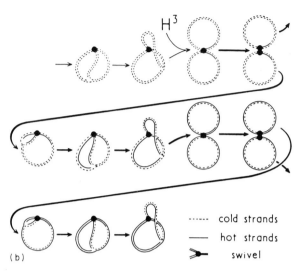

Fig. 4.5b. Cairns' interpretation of the replication of a circular chromosome based upon his autoradiographic studies. Each round of replication is assumed to begin at the same location and proceeds in the same direction as the previous round. The distal union of the two duplexes acts as a swivel upon which the DNA can wind and unwind in the process of replication (from Cairns, 77).

nus even though the two strands were of opposite polarity, i.e., one strand's deoxyribose phosphate backbone oriented with 5′ to 3′ phosphodiester linkages and the opposite strand's in the 3′ to 5′ direction. Synthesis in the 5′ to 3′ direction could occur as shown in Fig. 4.4 (Section III,A,1). Continual synthesis of the 3′ to 5′ strand of DNA at the same single growing point could theoretically occur by several mechanisms (see, e.g., 325), but the catalytic properties of *E. coli* polymerase I do not support such models (116, 377).

Recent experiments (343, 344) suggest, however, that sequential DNA replication need not necessarily be continuous, but that discontinuous chain growth could explain the simultaneous replication of antiparallel DNA strands. In this model (Fig. 4.6), DNA polymerase catalyzes the polymerization of monomers into a new strand of DNA in a 5′ to 3′ direction from the 3′ to 5′ parental strand and then switches to copy the 5′ to 3′ strand but in the reversed or 3′ to 5′ sense. The synthesis of short segments of both DNA strands but with a cyclical reversal of direction yields, macroscopically, unidirectional synthesis of antiparallel strands solely by 5′ to 3′ synthesis. The short pieces of newly synthesized strands could then be linked together to form a continuous daughter strand. Evidence supporting this model derives from pulse labeling studies with *E. coli;* after very short pulses of [³H]TdR, all newly synthesized DNA sedimented in sucrose gradients as very short fragments with sedimentation coefficients of 7 to 11 S corresponding to 1000–2000 nucleotide residues long. With longer "chase" times, the short labeled pieces were found to sediment more and more rapidly, presumably reflecting the covalent linkage of discontinuously synthesized pieces into a continuous DNA strand. The fact that all newly synthesized material was found in short pieces indicates that synthesis from both

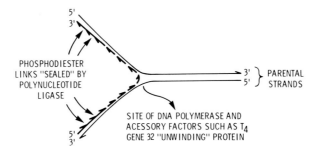

Fig. 4.6. A schematic representation of the model of discontinuous DNA synthesis suggested by the experiments of Okazaki and co-workers (Okazaki *et al.*, 343, 344). DNA polymerase I synthesizes new strands of DNA in the 5' to 3' direction using the 3' to 5' strand of the parental DNA as template. At short intervals the polymerase switches over to copy the 5' to 3' strand of parental DNA but in the reverse or 3' to 5' direction. By switching back and forth between the two strands, short segments of DNA are produced from both strands of the DNA being read in the 5' to 3' direction. The incomplete phosphodiester links are subsequently closed by the enzyme polynucleotide ligase. The overall macroscopic appearance is that of simultaneous synthesis of both the 5' to 3' and the 3' to 5' parental strands of DNA by an enzyme that can presumably synthesize DNA only in the 5' to 3' direction.

the 3' to 5' and the 5' to 3' parental strands occurred discontinuously. Digestion of newly synthesized DNA with specific nucleases proved that the direction of synthesis was 5' to 3'.

The joining of short pieces of newly synthesized DNA into continuous strands is thought to be catalyzed by an enzyme which catalyzes the formation of a phosphodiester linkage between adjacent nucleotides (one of which must bear a 3'-OH and the other a 5'-phosphoryl group) at single strand "gaps" in DNA chains. Such "polynucleotide ligases" have been noted in bacterial, phage, and mammalian systems by many investigators (162, 283, 477) and act by the formation of an enzyme-adenylic acid intermediate with the subsequent release of one mole of adenylic acid per phosphodiester link formed.

Many different variants of this scheme have been proposed to accommodate one or another facet of *in vivo* DNA replication in various experimental systems including the "rolling circle" model (163), the "knife and fork" scheme (178), the "prefork" model (186), and a pyrophosphate bridge model (330) among others. These models are discussed in detail elsewhere (168, 169, 234, 277).

3. PROBLEMS OF *E. coli* DNA POLYMERASE I

Although polymerase I is capable of *in vitro* synthesis of a biologically active ϕX174 DNA molecule (170, 171), a number of facts have cast doubt on its role in *in vivo* DNA replication. The ability of polymerase I to degrade double-stranded DNA in a 5' to 3' direction—the direction of DNA synthesis—is greatly stimulated by the presence of all four deoxynucleoside triphosphates (243). This property, desirable enough for an enzyme carrying out repair replication (see Section VII,A), is difficult to reconcile with semiconservative genome duplication. Polymerase I catalyzes synthesis of highly branched and aberrant DNA

(205); it cannot utilize native "unnicked" DNA as template, but can use with great facility nicked templates which might arise as a result of repair processes (243).

Polymerase I catalyzes DNA synthesis only in a 5′ to 3′ direction, whereas *in vivo* synthesis of both the 5′ to 3′ and the 3′ to 5′ strands must occur. As noted in the previous section, discontinuous 5′ to 3′ synthesis in concert with polynucleotide ligase made feasible the construction of models for simultaneous synthesis of antiparallel strands by an enzyme capable of synthesizing a strand only in one direction. Recent experiments (479, 480) suggest that TdR may not be the actual precursor of the DNA-thymine and that quite different results are obtained from short pulse studies if one employs labeled thymine. Furthermore, some polynucleotide ligase mutants, which presumably cannot easily join "Okazaki fragments," (Fig. 4.6) grow normally (168, 377). Polymerase I is unable by itself to initiate the synthesis of new strands of DNA (167).[*] Finally, a fairly large number of *E. coli* mutants thermosensitive for DNA replication were found to have normal levels of monomer precursors of DNA and of polymerase I under both permissive and nonpermissive temperatures (75, 177, 192). Thus, polymerase I in *E. coli* may not be involved in replicative DNA synthesis.

4. *E. coli* POLYMERASE I MUTANTS AND ADDITIONAL DNA POLYMERASES

A mutant of *E. coli* induced by N-methyl-N′-nitro-N-nitrosoguanidine contained 0.5% of the wild-type level of polymerase I (121) and was a nonsense mutation (amber) which, additionally, had no defect in genetic recombination (176). The mutant, termed *polA1*, grew normally in minimal and complete medium at 25° and 42°C but possessed a marked increase in sensitivity to ultraviolet light and to methylmethanesulfonate (121). The preponderance of evidence is that polymerase I, absent or defective in *polA1* mutants, is involved in DNA repair and/or recombinational systems (54, 220) (see Section VI,A).

Availability of *E. coli* mutants lacking polymerase I quite naturally led to a search in these mutants for an enzyme or enzymes that could account for the obvious ability of the mutant to replicate DNA. As a starting point, several groups of investigators examined more organized cell fractions of *polA1* mutants for polymerase activity since the possibility for an organized replication complex (212) had received some experimental support, e.g., a membrane-associated DNA polymerase (158). Both membrane fragment systems (240, 345, 414) and permeable cell systems (135, 329, 332, 460) were found to support semiconservative DNA synthesis at rates comparable to those observed *in vivo*, i.e., approximatey 10^5 nucleotides polymerized per cell per minute. The replicative DNA synthesis was dependent upon the presence of all four deoxyribonucleoside triphosphates,

---

[*] However, single-stranded M13 and φX174 DNA can be converted to their double-stranded replicative forms by polymerase I after a short piece of RNA is synthesized (presumably by DNA-dependent RNA polymerase which can initiate new strands) which RNA then acts as a "primer" for the DNA polymerase (64, 464). There is also a requirement of RNA synthesis *in vivo* in *E. coli* for initiation of DNA replication (265, 433). Thus, the inability of polymerase I to initiate synthesis of new strands of DNA *in vitro* may only reflect the artificiality of the test systems and may not define the role of the polymerase *in vivo*.

Mg^{2+}, and ATP and was inhibited by sulfhydryl reagents such as N-ethyl-maleamide. Both the membrane and permeable cell systems have indicated the existence of enzyme(s) in *polA1* mutants capable of carrying out replicative DNA synthesis. Several groups have subsequently purified DNA polymerases from both *polA1* mutants and from wild-type *E. coli* that are distinctly different from DNA polymerase I (161, 241, 246, 247, 333, 334, 482, 483).

DNA polymerase II has been purified to homogeneity. The enzyme requires a primer with a 3'-hydroxyl terminus, does not efficiently utilize native DNA, fully single-stranded DNA or nicked native DNA as template. It synthesizes in a 5' to 3' direction and possesses a 3' to 5' exonucleolytic activity but no 5' to 3' exonuclease action. It is inhibited by sulfhydryl reagents, does not require ATP for activity, has an estimated molecular weight of 120,000 daltons, and is not inhibited by antibody prepared against polymerase I. The actual function of DNA polymerase II as the *in vivo* replicative polymerase is uncertain. There are less than 17 molecules of polymerase II per bacterial cell and on the basis of its *in vitro* activity this amount of enzyme could catalyze the incorporation of only 800 nucleotides per cell per minute into DNA, thus nowhere near the *in vivo* rate of 3×10^5 nucleotides per cell per minute (482, 483). Neither purified polymerase I nor purified polymerase II demonstrates thermosensitivity when isolated from two mutant strains of *E. coli* thermosensitive in DNA synthesis (335). Thus some of the same properties that disinherited polymerase I from its role as the *in vivo* replicative enzyme are shared by polymerase II. The suggestion has been made (482, 483) that polymerase II also serves a DNA repair function.

Another enzyme, DNA polymerase III, has been found in several *E. coli* mutants, is separable from polymerase II by phosphocellulose chromatography, insensitive to antiserum prepared against polymerase I, one-fifth as stable to heat as polymerase II, three times more sensitive to N-ethylmaleamide than polymerase II, and inhibited by concentrations of ammonium sulfate that stimulated polymerase II activity (160, 247). Although detailed properties of this polymerase are not yet known, polymerase III from some *E. coli* strains carrying dnaE temperature-sensitive mutations for DNA synthesis exhibited thermosensitivity *in vitro*. It is not yet clear, however, if polymerase III is responsible for *in vivo* replication of DNA in *E. coli* or if it merely plays an accessory, albeit important, role.

The difficult tasks facing molecular biologists concerned with eukaryotic systems—and experimental oncologists who wish, additionally, to know how oncogenic agents perturb these systems to produce heritable neoplastic transformations—will become evident in the next section.

B. Enzymes of DNA Synthesis in Higher Organisms

In contrast to the extensive "molecular" characterization of microbial and phage DNA polymerases, not as much is known at that level about the enzyme(s) that catalyzes the synthesis of DNA in mammalian cells (Table 4.2).

TABLE 4.2

Animal tissue	Cellular localization	Sedimentation coefficient and/or molecular weight	Mg^{2+} optima (mM)	pH optima	Activity with 4 deoxynucleoside triphosphates as % of complete reaction		
					+3 dNTP	+2 dNTP	+1 dNTP
Rat liver	Nonhistone chromosomal protein	—	10	8.5–9.0	54	37	24
	Nuclear	—	10–15	9.0	—	35	—
	"Ribosomal"	—	10–15	9.0	—	35	—
	Smooth membranes	—	7–10	8.0	—	10	0
	Cytoplasmic	9 S	"Required"	6.8–7.4	"All 4 dNT's required"		
	Nuclear	3.4 S	"Required"	7.4–8.0	"All 4 dNTP's required"		
	Cytoplasmic	3.5 S 49,000 daltons	10	7.4–8.0	—	—	0
Mouse Ehrlich ascites	Unknown; probably both nuclear and cytoplasmic	4.8 S	7	7.4	1.2	1.9	2.5
Human KB cells	Cytoplasmic	2.4 S; 21,000 daltons	4	6.6	50	30	5
Human HeLa cells	Nuclear "I"[a]		15–25	9.0	—	—	4.5
	Nuclear "II"[a]		5–10	6.5–7.0	—	—	1.5
	Cytoplasmic[a]		5–10	6.5–7.0	—	—	9.5
Rabbit marrow	Nuclear and cytoplasmic	3.39 S; 40,000 to 50,000 daltons	5–20	8.6	5	2	1.
	Cytoplasmic	6–8 S	4–8	7.0	16	—	1

[a] Nuclear II elutes prior to nuclear I on Sephadex G-200; cytoplasmic cochromatographs with nuclear II.

Demonstration of a mammalian DNA polymerase (36, 37) utilized an aqueous supernatant fraction derived from centrifugation of a homogenate from "regenerating" rat liver. Incorporation of [³H]TdR into DNA *in vitro* was dependent upon added DNA and was stimulated by the presence of all four deoxyribonucleoside triphosphates. The level of cytosol polymerase activity correlated well with the *in vivo* incorporation of labeled orotic acid into nuclear DNA for the first 24 hours after partial hepatectomy thus implicating the measured *in vitro* enzyme activity in replicative DNA synthesis (38). Since these early reports, DNA polymerase activity in crude cellular fractions (e.g., cytosol versus nuclear supernatants) or in partial purifications from such fractions have been reported for many tissues from many species. These studies have included analysis of normal and "regenerating" rat and mouse liver (17–19, 24, 26, 68, 89, 90, 200, 201, 230, 305, 306, 348, 349, 356, 465, 468), calf thymus (32, 34, 35, 252, 500), rat thymus (466), beef and guinea pig adrenal glands (290, 308), Ehrlich ascites tumor cells (384, 385, 411, 412, 465), mouse L cells (164, 285), BHK 21 cells (228), sea urchin embryos (141, 287–289), Novikoff hepatoma cells (153, 154), human KB nasopharyngeal carcinoma cells (172–174), HeLa cells (13, 150, 184, 299, 395, 478), and rat liver mitochondria (219, 315). This

PROPERTIES OF SOME MAMMALIAN "DNA POLYMERASES"

Template preferences (%)			Nuclease activity	Terminal transferase activity	Increase in input DNA	Ref.
Native	Denatured	"Activated"				
++	+	+++	Present	Present	—	200, 201, 356, 467
22	7	100	Endonuclease	Not detected	—	17, 19
16	4	100	Endonuclease	Not detected	—	17, 19
3	2	100	Not detected	Not detected	—	17, 19
100	72	—	—	Not detected	—	89, 90
100	11	—	—	Not detected	—	89, 90
3	1	100	Not detected	Not detected	8-fold using poly-dAT	26
2	8	100	Exonuclease	Not detected	1-fold	384, 385
4	2	100	Exonuclease	Not detected	4.5-fold	174
12	0	100	—	Not detected	—	395, 478
4	<1	100	—	Not detected	—	395, 478
<1	<1	100	—	Not detected	—	395, 478
"Activated" DNA or initiated templates			Not detected	Not detected	1-fold	82–85
+	++	+++	"Present"	Not detected	1-fold	82–85

list of studies on DNA "polymerases" from eukaryotic cells could be expanded even further.

Mammalian cells apparently possess three more or less clearly defined enzymes or enzyme systems that catalyze the polymerization of deoxyribonucleoside triphosphates into DNA: a terminal deoxynucleotidyl transferase which does not require template direction (also called terminal transferase, "addase," nonreplicative polymerase), a relatively low molecular weight template-directed deoxynucleotidyl transferase presumably nuclear and cytoplasmic in cellular localization, and a relatively higher molecular weight template-directed deoxynucleotidyl transferase presumably restricted to the cytoplasm. Properties of the three enzymes are summarized in Table 4.3.

Terminal deoxynucleotidyl transferases will only briefly be noted here since very little is known of their significance, if any, with respect to DNA replication. Although terminal transferases from both calf thymus nuclei (166, 229, 250–252) and calf thymus cytoplasm (32, 33, 39, 81, 82, 226, 500) catalyze the consecutive addition of nucleoside triphosphates onto the 3'-OH terminus of single-stranded DNA, enzyme from the two sources differ in a number of fundamental properties.

As well characterized as calf thymus nuclear and cytoplasmic terminal trans-

TABLE 4.3
PROPERTIES OF ENZYME SYSTEMS THAT CATALYZE DEOXYRIBONUCLEOTIDE TRIPHOSPHATES

Enzyme System	Location	Properties
3.39 S Replicative polymerase	Nucleus	40,000–50,000 daltons Alkaline pH optimum 5–20 mM Mg^{2+} No detectable correlation with proliferation Tight complex with DNA Inhibited by antibody to 6–8 S polymerase
3.39 S Replicative polymerase	Cytoplasm	Similar if not identical to nuclear 3.39 S
6–8 S Replicative polymerase	Cytoplasm	100,000 daltons Neutral pH optimum 4–8 mM Mg^{2+} Positive correlation with proliferative state No complex with DNA Inhibited by antibody to 6–8 S
Terminal transferase (166)	Nucleus	Adds nucleoside triphosphate to denatured DNA primer Requires Mg^{2+}; Mn^{2+} cannot substitute Cannot use oligodeoxynucleotides as primers Adds only one NTP to 3′OH of primer (i.e., cannot polymerize ribose to ribose) but can add many dNTP's thereby forming chains
Terminal transferase (39, 226, 500)	Cytoplasm	Found only in thymus tissues of number of species $s_{20,w}$ of 3.65; about 35,000 daltons; two subunits of 8,000 and 26,500 daltons Adds monomeric ribo- or deoxyribonucleoside triphosphates to the 3′-OH terminus of single-stranded DNA or oligodeoxyribonucleotides pH optimum near 7.0; Mg^{2+} optimum of 2–8 mM; Mn^{2+} can substitute

ferases are, no known biological function can be ascribed to them. The cytoplasmic enzyme has no detectable nucleolytic or phosphorolytic activity and thus may not serve in a degradative role (80). It was suggested (227) that the terminal transferase might represent a subunit of a replicative deoxynucleotidyl transferase, but more recent work does not support that hypothesis. Ammonium sulfate fractionation followed by sucrose density gradient centrifugation to separate putative replicative deoxynucleotidyl transferase (about 100,000 daltons) from terminal transferase (about 32,000 daltons) was carried out on nuclei and cytoplasm from many different tissues from a variety of animal species (80). Terminal transferase activity was found in every species examined but only in thymic tissue. Measurements made on the same tissues that showed no detectable terminal transferase activity demonstrated levels of replicative DNA polymerase that varied with the presumed proliferative state of the tissue. These data constitute strong evidence against terminal transferase being a subunit of replicative DNA polymerase. Thus, the function of terminal transferase remains enigmatic but it might be related to some special function of thymic tissue (80).

1. REPLICATIVE DEOXYNUCLEOTIDYL TRANSFERASE(S)

Although there have been numerous reports of DNA polymerases in mammalian tissues, insufficient purification and characterization combined with preconceptions of the cellular localization and substrate preferences made the construction of an intelligible pattern from extant data extremely difficult. Classifications of DNA polymerases according to whether or not the enzymic activity is greater with native or denatured DNA may not be meaningful since template preferences vary with assay conditions (385) and with the degree of purification of enzyme presumably because of the extent to which cofractionated nucleases are removed (84). The strandedness of DNA *in vivo* at the site of interaction with replicative polymerase is not known, so classification of polymerase by *in vitro* substrate preference is very difficult.

Until recently a reasonable description of a mammalian replicative DNA polymerase was that of a protein, presumably monomeric, of 110,000 daltons requiring Mg^{2+}, all four deoxyribonucleoside triphosphates, and single-stranded DNA template for activity, possessing an alkaline metal-dependent nucleolytic activity, capable of catalyzing only one doubling of input DNA template with an optimal pH near neutrality, and generally located in the cytoplasm (234). However, a number of DNA polymerases (17, 200, 201, 305, 356) show consistent preference for "native" DNA at least in some stages of their purification. More extensive characterization of DNA polymerase(s) by several groups may force a recasting of the above description (Table 4.2). All of the enzymes studied are replicative transferases in that they require template direction. The templates were, as far as determinable with methods at hand, faithfully copied into complementary products. The results in Table 4.2 are at first sight notable for their multiple divergences from the description of DNA polymerase given above.

However, when Table 4.2 is studied in relation to recent work (80, 83–85) an intelligible pattern begins to emerge. In studying tissue and species distribution of terminal transferase, in addition to the usual 6–8 S 100,000-dalton replicative deoxynucleotidyl transferase, a low molecular weight deoxynucleotide-polymerizing activity which required template direction (hence replicative) was present in rabbit spleen and bone marrow (83). The enzyme had no terminal transferase activity and was present in both nucleus and cytoplasm. Nuclei from a wide variety of tissues from many species contained only the 3.39 S polymerase whereas the cytoplasm from these tissues had both the 3.39 S polymerase (with properties very similar to nuclear 3.39 S enzyme) and the "usual" 6–8 S DNA polymerase (84). A number of nuclear and membrane-associated DNA polymerases studied by others (17, 19, 26, 90, 200) have properties similar to the nuclear and cytoplasmic 3.39 S polymerase.

Incorporation of label in incomplete systems *in vitro* may be due to synthesis of numerous short regions of DNA from DNA template regions containing less than all four bases (Table 4.2). If numerous "nicks" in "activated" DNA are enlarged with exonuclease III, the same polymerase preparation will then show more stringent requirements for all four nucleotides (84).

The replicative polymerases can be classed as occurring in both nucleus and cytoplasm (3.39 S enzyme) or only in the cytoplasm (6–8 S enzyme). The higher molecular weight polymerases that some have found in nuclei (e.g., 465) may be contaminants since 6–8 S polymerase is absent in rabbit marrow nuclei treated with Triton X-100 which removes the outer nuclear membrane with its attached cytoplasmic "tags" (84). Such "tags" could conceivably include the DNA polymerase associated with smooth membranes of the endoplasmic reticulum (17, 19). The pattern that has emerged from all of these studies is shown in Table 4.3.

Despite this emergent pattern, many questions remain unanswered concerning the enzymic mechanisms of mammalian DNA replication. One of the more pressing questions is the relationship of 3.39 S enzyme to 6–8 S enzyme. A partially purified immunoglobulin from rabbits injected with purified calf thymus 6–8 S polymerase was tested for its effects on a number of types of partially purified deoxynucleotidyl transferases from various species (85). The results (Table 4.4) show that 6–8 S antibody inhibits 3.39 S enzyme as well as 6–8 S enzyme from many different species while not inhibiting calf thymus cytoplasmic terminal transferase, E. coli DNA polymerase I, or E. coli DNA polymerase II. An antibody depletion study implied that the partially purified immunoglobulin prepared against 6–8 S enzyme contained only one antibody even though it reacted

TABLE 4.4

IMMUNOLOGIC RELATIONSHIPS OF SOME MAMMALIAN "DNA POLYMERASES"[a]

Species	Enzyme	Antibody to	Inhibition[b] (%)	Antibody dilution for stated % inhibition
Calf	Thymus 6–8 S	Calf thymus 6–8 S	48	1/32
	Thymus 3.39 S	Calf thymus 6–8 S	45	1/8
	Thymus terminal transferase	Calf thymus 6–8 S	0	2/3
	Thymus 6–8 S	E. coli pol I	0	2/3
Rat	Regenerating liver 6–8 S	Calf thymus 6–8 S	37	1/64
	Regenerating liver 3.39 S	Calf thymus 6–8 S	72	1/32
	Liver mitochondria	Calf thymus 6–8 S	63	1/16
Mouse	L cells 6–8 S	Calf thymus 6–8 S	66	1/64
	L cells 6–8 S	Calf thymus 6–8 S	36	1/16
Human	PHA lymphocytes 3.39 S and 6.8 S	Calf thymus 6–8 S	86	1/3
	PHA lymphocytes 3.39 S	Calf thymus 6–8 S	70	1/8
Rabbit	Bone marrow 3.39 S	Calf thymus 6–8 S	59	1/16
E. coli	Pol I	Calf thymus 6–8 S	0	1/3
	Pol II	E. coli pol I	88	1/96
	Pol III	Calf thymus 6–8 S	0	2/3

[a] From Chang and Bollum (85).

[b] Related to enzyme activities of control samples of appropriate enzyme that had been incubated with purified α-globulin or serum from nonimmunized rabbits.

against both the 3.39 S and 6–8 S enzymes. Thus there are common antigenic determinants in the 3.39 S and 6–8 S polymerases and, most interestingly, these common antigenic determinants have apparently been reasonably well conserved in divergent species.

2. MEMBRANE ASSOCIATION OF REPLICATIVE DNA POLYMERASES

Thus, the two types of replicative DNA polymerase in mammalian cells are compartmentalized within the cell, the 3.39 S being distributed in both nucleus and cytoplasm, the 6–8 S enzyme presumably restricted to cytoplasm (22, 84, 230). Yet the 6–8 S polymerase located in the cytoplasm is the only DNA polymerase known at this time whose level correlates positively with the state of cell proliferation.

This fact is at first sight difficult to reconcile with the nuclear site of replication of DNA. Earlier studies (141, 150, 164, 285, 288, 289) considered in light of more recent results (17, 19, 83–85) may help to resolve this paradox. Levels of DNA polymerase activities were examined in supernatant and pellet fractions obtained by centrifugation of lysed mouse L-cells harvested at varying times after release from DNA synthesis blockade induced by 5-fluorodeoxyuridine (285) or by FUdR plus deoxyadenosine (164). Both sets of results were comparable—supernatant polymerase activity decreased 21% over a 3-hour period after release from S-phase blockade but polymerase activity in the pellet increased by 21% over the same period. After correcting for the difference in absolute activities between supernatant and pellet, the average absolute increase in pellet activity was 9% of the decrease in activity of the supernatant. Both studies suggest a translocation of polymerase from cytoplasm to nucleus during active DNA synthesis in L-cells. This interpretation could also apply to data on polymerase distribution in amethopterin-synchronized HeLa cells (150). A similar phenomenon has been studied in developing sea urchin embryos (141, 288, 289). During the first 16 hours of rapid cell division and DNA synthesis after fertilization of sea urchin eggs there was no change in whole embryo levels of DNA polymerase but there was an increasing recovery of activity in isolated nuclei with a concomitant loss of activity from cytoplasmic fractions. There was little protein turnover in early embryo development and no preferential synthesis of DNA polymerase. The change in localization of polymerase activity must therefore represent a physical migration of enzyme from cytoplasm to nucleus (288).

That something more than a simple "flow" of DNA polymerase from cytoplasm to nucleus occurs during active DNA replication is suggested from a consideration of current concepts of DNA structure in chromatin in interphase cells, the propinquity between sites of DNA synthesis and nuclear membranes in mammalian cells (see next section) and the more recent studies of replicative DNA polymerases (17, 19, 83–85). The level of 6–8 S polymerase reflects the state of cell proliferation in various mammalian tissues but the level of 3.39 S enzyme does not (83–85). The activity of smooth membrane-associated polymerase is markedly elevated in proliferating tissues, e.g., hepatomas and fetal and regenerating rat liver (19). The properties of this membrane-associated enzyme are reminiscent of the 6–8 S polymerase. The 6–8 S polymerase—antigenically related to the 3.39 S enzyme—might therefore be membrane-associated. Membrane-associated 6–8 S polymerase may be localized on, or in the vicinity of, the (outer?) nuclear membrane and the nuclear membrane localization of initiation of DNA synthesis (see next section) may reflect the cellular compartmentation of 6–8 S enzyme. Nuclear 3.39 S polymerase which is reasonably tightly bound to DNA (84) may represent a subunit of 6–8 S enzyme involved in DNA repair; 3.39 S enzyme could more or less fortuitously appear in cytoplasm in the course of its synthesis on cytoplasmic polysomes and/or as a result of dissociation or degradation of cytoplasmic (membrane associated?) 6–8 S polymerase.

The possibility of a membrane–DNA–DNA polymerase complex just mentioned may become more interesting since it has been found (20) that the smooth membrane fraction of regenerating rat liver contains (in addition to DNA polymerase that resembles 6–8 S. polymerase) both ribonucleoside diphosphate reductase and thymidine kinase. The presence of deoxythymidylate synthetase in this fraction is also suspected. High salt concentrations do not remove polymerase, reductase, and kinase from the membrane but dissociation can be effected with 2.5% n-butanol:5% Triton X-100 followed by cesium chloride density gradient centrifugation. The material so separated from the membranes is particulate with a diameter of 100–125 Å. Microsomal fraction smooth membranes do not show these enzyme activities. The smooth membrane fraction (from the postmicrosomal supernatant) which does possess polymerase, reductase, and kinase has no detectable mitochondrial enzymes such as monamine oxidase or succinic dehydrogenase. The structural association of these enzymes and increased activities in rapidly dividing cell populations may imply a "concerted action in DNA replication" (20). The evidence available at this time, admittedly scanty and circumstantial, tends to support the existence of a possibly elaborate mammalian DNA replication complex. Definitive characterization of its components, reconstruction, and analysis of its role in DNA replication and/or DNA repair constitutes an important goal (see Section IV,B,4).

IV. DNA Synthesis: Mechanistic Considerations in Higher Organisms

A. Structural Complexities of DNA in Chromatin

The task faced in analyzing the mode of replication of DNA in mammalian cells is formidable. As an illustration, the Novikoff hepatoma cell contains about 10×10^{-12} gm of DNA which represents roughly 200 cm of duplex DNA which is, in turn, packed into a defined nucleus 8–25 μm in diameter (225) or into a volume of about 270–8200 μm^3. Despite the enormous lengths of DNA to be replicated, cells in culture duplicate their genome with precision once every

10–11 hours and distribute exactly the same genetic information to each daughter cell. In this section, a selective review of some aspects of nucleus and chromatin structure will be presented as a prelude to consideration of how DNA in chromatin might be replicated.

1. ASSOCIATION OF DNA WITH THE NUCLEAR ENVELOPE

The logical starting point is to examine the most distinguishing feature of eukaryotes, the nuclear envelope which compartmentalizes the chromatin (Fig. 4.7). The nuclear envelope (Chapter I) consists of outer (interfacing with cytoplasm) and inner (interfacing with nucleoplasm) membranes (each of which appear to be typical unit membranes about 70–80 Å thick) separated by a space 150–300 Å in width (423). The outer nuclear membrane has direct continuity with membranes of the endoplasmic reticulum (475) such that the space between the two membranes of the nuclear envelope is essentially continuous with the space between membranes of the endoplasmic reticulum. With the advent of electron microscopy it became evident that at many points in the nuclear envelope, the inner and outer membranes formed small circular fusions, at the center of which the "pore" was patent (79). The thickened material circumscribing the pore has been termed the annulus (134) and apparently consists of eight structural subunits (146, 155). The diameter of the pore may not be rigidly fixed but can apparently vary from an "open" to a "closed" configuration. Open and closed annuli have been noted in freeze-etched preparations of human liver cells (134) (Fig. 4.8). Fine filaments have been seen (249) to traverse the center of the nuclear envelope pores of Novikoff hepatoma cells. The filaments were easily digestible with pepsin, less so with subtilisin or pronase, and not with RNase or DNase (Fig. 4.9). A "membrane" covering the nuclear envelope pores of honeybee embryonic cells was digested by trypsin solutions (131). A role in control of nuclear–cytoplasmic interchange could be involved in the physical opening and closing of nuclear envelope pores (134, 313) and in the "membranelike" covering of the pores (142, 485).

Another ultrastructural feature of nuclei which has been observed in a Yoshida ascites hepatoma (195, 286), Ehrlich ascites cells (499), Rous sarcoma cells (65), 6C3HED lymphoma cells (276), and Novikoff rat hepatoma cells (225) is the formation, apparently by infolding and invagination of the inner membrane of the nuclear envelope, of an intranuclear canalicular system.

The final aspect of nuclear envelope structure to consider in the replication of DNA is the association of chromatin fibers with the nuclear envelope and, more specifically, with the annuli that circumscribe the nuclear envelope pores. In whole mount preparations of interphase honeybee embryonic cells the chromosome fibers are attached specifically to the edges of the annuli (132). The Chinese hamster interphase nucleus exhibits (Fig. 4.10) dense networks of chromatin fibers which apparently converge at the annuli. A similar phenomenon is exhibited by human testis and Japanese quail testis. The general picture that has developed from studies such as these is schematically illustrated in Fig. 4.11 (107). The specific membrane attachment of chromatin fibers to the

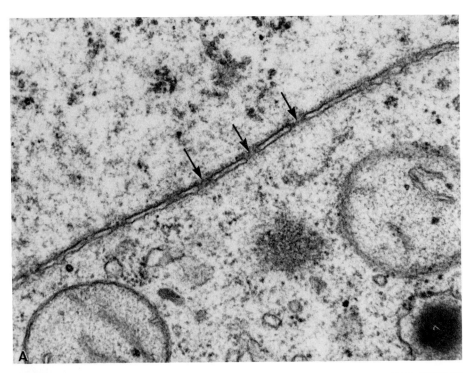

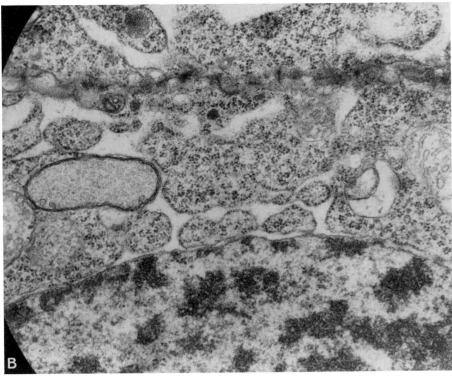

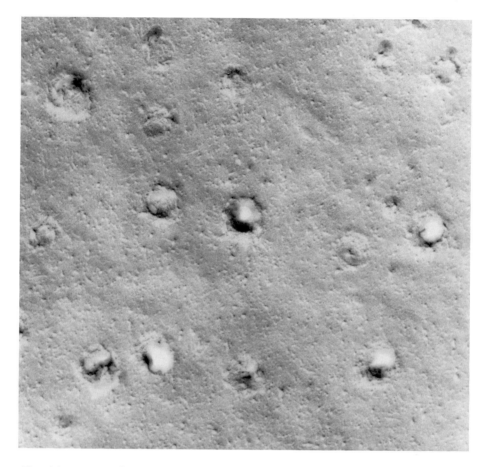

Fig. 4.8. Freeze-etch preparation of a nucleus of a human liver cell showing annuli in the nuclear surface. ×98,200 (from DuPraw, 134).

nuclear envelope will be considered further in Section IV,B with respect to replication of eukaryotic DNA.

2. DNA–Nuclear Protein Interactions

What is the nature of the chromatin fiber attached to the nuclear envelope in the interphase nucleus? The basic component of chromatin from an interphase

Fig. 4.7. Ultrastructural aspects of the nuclear envelope. (A) A thin section passing transversely to the nuclear surface in an oocyte of the spider *Tegenaria* sp. Several nuclear pores (pointers) are sectioned in their median plane. Cytoplasm is at lower portion of the figure and the nucleus at the upper right. Osmium fixed. ×68,800. (B) A thin section normal to the nuclear surface of a tapetal cell from a young anther of *Zea mays*. Extensive communications between the perinuclear space and the endoplasmic reticulum cisternae are observed. Nucleus at lower portion of figure. Gluteraldehyde-osmium. ×43,775 (from Stevens and Andre, 423).

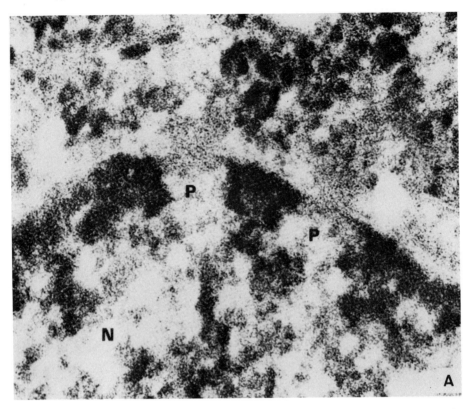

Fig. 4.9. (A) Thin section electron micrograph of a Novikoff hepatoma cell showing nuclear pores (P) the center of which contains fine filaments that are also found within the nucleus (N). ×153,000. (B) Electron micrograph of perpendicular section of nuclear pores in Novikoff hepatoma cell nuclei after treatment with subtilisn for 90 minutes. Most of the fine filaments within the pores have been removed by this treatment. ×30,960 (from Koshiba *et al.*, 249).

nucleus is a 35 Å diameter nucleoprotein fiber composed of a single, long DNA double helix, associated "chromosomal proteins," and presumably nascent messenger RNA's. The chromosomal proteins include "acidic" proteins which possess a ratio of acidic to basic amino acids greater than one and which are soluble in alkali but not solubilized by the acidic conditions used to extract histones, "residual" proteins which are proteins insoluble in alkali after prior acidic extraction of histones, and histones which possess a greater content of basic than acidic amino acids and which are differentially soluble in acidic extraction media (see Chapter VIII). The functional role(s) played by acidic and residual proteins remains largely matters of speculation but a picture has begun to develop concerning the role of the histones (72, 140, 337, 358). Histones can act as repressors of DNA template-directed RNA synthesis (e.g., 41). The small number of chemically different types of histone molecules in given cells as well as controversy over the species and organ specificity of the various histone classes

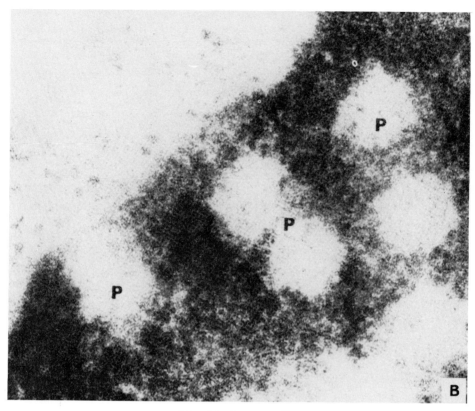

Fig. 4.9. (*Continued*)

(214), the conservation of amino acid sequences in given classes of histones between divergent species (359), and numerous criticisms that can be made concerning experiments on *in vitro* RNA synthesis from eukaryotic DNA or chromatin templates have been taken as evidence that histone repression of transcription does not inherently have the specificity needed for fine control of genomic readout during normal cellular differentiation and/or function.

However, histones do have a distinct role in the structure of chromatin. The fundamental unit of the mammalian chromosome consists of a 100–200 Å diameter fiber (131, 134, 378) which X-ray diffraction studies (353, 354, 376, 488, 505) indicate is in turn composed of a single 35 Å nucleoprotein fiber supercoiled into a fiber of 100 Å diameter and a pitch of 120 Å. Although the exact orientation of DNA in the larger 100–200 Å fibers is still open to interpretation (57, 136, 347), supercoiling of the basic nucleoprotein fiber is decidedly dependent upon the presence or absence of chromosomal proteins. Removal of histones f2a1 and f2a2 (arginine-glycine rich and lysine-arginine rich histones, respectively) results in loss of supercoiling (55). If "naked" DNA is reconstituted with a mixture of histones f2a1, f2a2, f2b (slightly lysine-rich histone), and f3 (arginine-glutamic acid rich histone) or a mixture of histones f2a2 and f3, the resulting nucleohistones again show supercoiling (376). The supercoiling

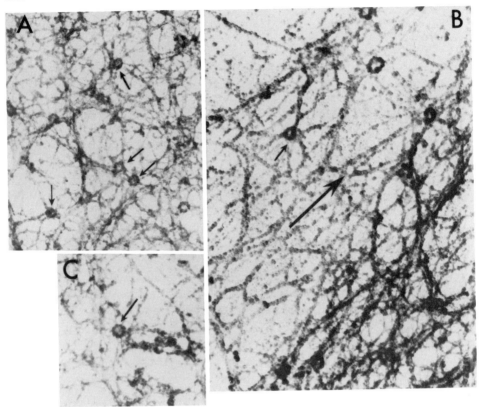

Fig. 4.10. Water-spread preparations of interphase nuclei from Chinese hamster cells. (A) Dense networks of chromatin fibers. Nuclear membrane pulled away but a number of nuclear annuli persist and are seen (arrows) to remain attached to points of convergence of chromatin fibers. ×33,300. (B) The small arrow points to a nuclear annulus attached to convergent chromatin fibers while the large arrow shows a circlelike convergence of chromatin fibers from which nuclear annular material appears to have been removed. ×46,800. (C) A nuclear annulus (arrow) in association with chromatin fibers. Note the eight knoblike protrusions around the periphery of the annulus which might represent the constituent subunits of the annular material. ×61,200 (from Comings and Okada, 107).

effect is not species specific. Identical native nucleohistone X-ray diffraction patterns were obtained when total histones from calf thymus were reconstituted with naked DNA from calf thymus or salmon sperm or T7 phage (159).

The precise means by which certain classes of histones dictate the ultrastructure of the chromatin fiber is not yet clear. The histones as a group seem to occupy the major or deep groove in the 20 Å diameter double helix (346, 406) and the minor groove in DNA is apparently "free" or at least devoid of histones or other proteins that would block interaction of a reporter molecule with DNA-phosphate moieties and/or base intercalation (408). Evidence deduced from melting profiles of free DNA and chromatin (278), from binding studies (91, 207, 208, 236, 346), and from DNase digestion experiments (91, 209) have led to estimates of 1 to 60% of DNA-phosphates being "free" to react in chromo-

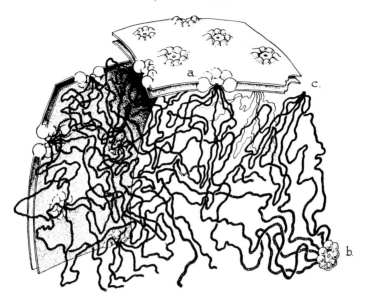

Fig. 4.11. Interpretation of the micrographs in Fig. 4.10. Chromatin fibers in the interphase nucleus converge to attach to the annulus of the nuclear membrane (a). The convergent fibers may attach to the central globule of the annulus and/or the ring portion. With water-spread preparations, the nuclear membrane is disrupted and the annuli may pull away from the membrane yet retain their attachment to the convergent chromatin fibers (b). The annuli might also be pulled away from the chromatin leaving only the convergent fibers (c). Further dispersive forces might disrupt even the convergent chromatin fibers (from Comings and Okada, 107).

somal DNA. Although a large proportion of DNA-phosphates might be accessible for interactions with even large molecular probes, there may be little if any DNA in chromatin present in extensive "free" zones totally devoid of protein (209). It is presently clear (55, 215) that histones are structural proteins only parts of which molecules interact with the DNA, the remainder being available for histone protein interactions, thus controlling the physical state of the chromatin which in turn affects its ability to act as a template for RNA synthesis.

3. CONDENSED AND DIFFUSE CHROMATIN

Since the electron microscopic and X-ray diffraction data all indicate that the physical state of DNA is very markedly altered upon interaction with some classes of histones, it is tempting to speculate that one fundamental difference between euchromatin and heterochromatin resides in DNA–histone interactions. Chromatin can be classified as heterochromatin (chromatin that is condensed and intensely stained in interphase nuclei and which does not unravel from mitotic chromosomes at telophase) and euchromatin (chromatin which is diffuse in interphase and regains this diffuse nature at telophase). Heterochromatin has been further subdivided into constitutive heterochromatin (condensed chromatin presumably always present in homologous chromosomes) and facultative heterochromatin (condensed chromatin resulting from the inactivation of one of the two X chromosomes in females) (503). Heterochromatin—like DNA complexed with certain histones—was believed to be inactive as a template for DNA-directed RNA synthesis (148), although recently euchromatin and heterochromatin from rat liver or Novikoff rat hepatoma were found to support equivalent levels of RNA synthesis using *E. coli* RNA polymerase (120). Does heterochromatin therefore represent DNA maintained in a condensed state because of histone–DNA interactions (211, 284)?

Similar amounts of histones were found in euchromatin and heterochromatin but euchromatin contained more nonhistone proteins and phosphoproteins than heterochromatin (148, 388). Histones present in heterochromatin are apparently also qualitatively similar to the histones in metaphase chromosomes (101) and total interphase chromatin (193). Using synchronized Chinese hamster cell cultures nearly constant proportions of the various histone classes are found (179, 311) throughout the cell cycle which is not consistent with the known propensity of heterochromatin to replicate late in S phase (Section IV,B).

Thus, histones can profoundly affect the ultrastructure of DNA but histone–DNA interactions alone do not seem to account for the observed diffuse versus condensed state of chromatin *in vivo*. The possible role of histone modification (acetylation, methylation, and especially phosphorylation) in determining the active states of chromatin has been the subject of extensive studies but little information exists on the ultrastructural effects of DNA interacted with modified or unmodified histones (4, also see Chapter VIII).

4. SATELLITE AND RAPIDLY REANNEALING DNA's

What factors other than, or perhaps in addition to, DNA–protein interactions might be responsible for the observed tendency of chromatin to exist in both condensed and diffuse states? Recent advances in our knowledge of "satellite DNA's" and repeated sequences in DNA's provide some evidence that the secondary structure of DNA may itself partially account for the varying tertiary structures of DNA in chromatin that underlies the condensed-diffuse states of chromatin.

DNA from mouse cells, when centrifuged to equilibrium in a neutral cesium chloride gradient, exhibits a main peak of DNA of density 1.701 gm/ml but about 10% of the DNA is found in a minor light satellite peak banding at density 1.690 gm/ml (233). Numerous reports of light (AT-rich) or heavy (GC-rich) DNA satellites in bacteria, plants, and animals have subsequently been made in which the observed satellite peaks were said to be "nuclear" in origin, i.e., not merely DNA from mitochondria, chloroplasts, bacterial episomes, or specified or unspecified intracellular parasites (114). A satellite DNA was originally defined as a minor fraction of nuclear DNA molecules separable by neutral CsCl density gradient centrifugation as a result of an overall greater or lesser content of guanine plus cytosine residues. However, DNA fractions of greater, lesser, or even identical GC content can be "rescued" from bulk or main band DNA by several techniques. Thus, heavy metals such as Ag^+ or Hg^{2+} bind differentially to DNA and in so doing alter the buoyant density of DNA (213, 339). This method has been used to reveal the existence of several heavy and light DNA satellite bands in human, guinea pig, and calf thymus DNA's (111–113) and in DNA from African green monkey cell lines (302). It is also possible to "liberate" satellite DNA from main band DNA by decreasing the size of the DNA molecules subjected to isopycnic centrifugation (498).

What properties of satellite DNA's might relate to their function(s), especially insofar as the overall structure of chromatin is concerned? The first property concerns base compositional bias between the two strands of duplex DNA in some satellite DNA. The light satellite of mouse nuclear DNA undergoes strand separation when centrifuged to equilibrium in alkaline gradients of cesium chloride indicating, therefore, a "nonuniform" distribution of all four bases between the two strands. Similar strand separation—and base compositional bias—has been observed in satellite fractions from DNA of guinea pig (113, 143), calf thymus (113), HeLa cells (394), and African green monkey (302). An example of this strand compositional bias is shown in Table 4.5.

The complementary strands of the light satellite from mouse DNA and a heavy satellite from guinea pig DNA were separated and subjected separately to the formic acid-diphenylamine hydrolysis procedure and the resultant pyrimidine clusters were subjected to base sequence analyses (419) using Sanger's (389) techniques. The basic sequence occurring in guinea pig satellite DNA and repeated many times is . . . pCpCpCpTpApA . . . opposed by . . . GpGpGpApTpTp . . . . The heavy strand of light mouse satellite DNA duplex is more complex but the most frequent basic repeating sequences are . . . pTpTpTpTpTpC . . . , . . . pTpTpTpTpCpC . . . , and . . . pTpTpTpCpTpC . . . . The mouse satellite DNA sequences are corroborated by the finding (258) that the light strand of mouse satellite DNA (presumably rich in A-containing sequences) bound large amounts of polyuridylic acid, whereas the separated heavy strand bound none. The same binding technique points to the presence of adenine-cytosine rich clusters in the light strand of a satellite from African green monkey DNA (302).

The possibility that some satellite DNA's consisted of simple repeating sequences had been inferred earlier on the basis of the rates of reassociation of separated strands of satellite DNA duplexes. A large part of mammalian DNA's reanneal as rapidly as simpler bacterial DNA's (310). The concept has developed that within a mammalian genome the fractions of DNA which rapidly

TABLE 4.5

INTERSTRAND BASE COMPOSITIONAL BIAS
IN GUINEA PIG α SATELLITE[a]

	Cytosine	Adenine	Guanine	Thymine
Light α strand	37.8	39.6	4.4	18.3
Heavy α strand	5.2	20.9	30.6	43.3

[a] After Flamm et al. (144); the values are mole %.

reanneal represent families of DNA with repeated, repetitious, or redundant sequences. Thus, in a mammalian genome there are families of highly repetitious DNA containing from 10^3 to 10^6 repeated elements, each element of which is calculated to be around 400 nucleotides in length, which are so similar in base sequence that the separated strands will reanneal with great rapidity. There are also families of DNA sequences with lower degrees of redundancy and even some unique or nonredundant DNA sequences. On the basis of the sequence data mentioned above, the separated strands of light satellite DNA duplex from mouse exhibit an extremely rapid rate of renaturation (463, 469). From a consideration of this rate as well as the length of the DNA fragments analyzed and the amount of DNA per mouse genome, mouse satellite DNA must consist of about a million copies of a repeating nucleotide sequence approximately 300–400 nucleotides in length (469). Since the satellite DNA can be isolated as continuous stretches of DNA 105 base pairs long, several hundred of the basic repeating sequences must be joined in tandem along the polynucleotide strand (462). The base sequence redundancy of mammalian DNA's is not confined to satellite DNA's but the rapid reannealing of separated strands would appear to be a property of many satellite DNA's. The implications of tandemly joined repeating "homopolymerlike" sequences for the ultrastructure of DNA in chromatin will be considered later.

The existence within nuclei from cells of one type of DNA species separable from the bulk of the DNA and possessing unusual properties quite naturally led to the question of whether or not satellite DNA's were distributed uniformly in a cell's genome. Nucleoli from mouse L cells and other cells of mouse origin, which account for no more than 10% of total nuclear DNA in these cells, contain about 30% of total mouse nuclear satellite DNA which suggests that satellite DNA in the mouse might be limited to specific chromosomes, perhaps those involved in the organization and function of the nucleolus. The relative enrichment of nucleolar DNA in satellite DNA has also been noted in mouse liver (106, 309), HeLa cells (303), African green monkey cells (302), and in guinea pig (106, 502).

This association of some DNA satellites with the nucleoli of various cells has been confirmed by in situ autoradiographic hybridization studies which additionally demonstrate an extranucleolar localization of satellite DNA's (216, 355) using interphase mouse cells. Correlation of the time of satellite DNA synthesis in polyoma-infected baby mouse kidney cells with the distribution of autoradiographic grains over the nucleoli in these cells also supports a nucleolar associaton of some satellite DNA's (413). In situ hybridization studies on mouse cells (216, 355), chromosome preparations from Drosophila melanogaster (48, 369), and human lymphocytes (10, 391) also indicate that satellite DNA's and/or highly repetitive DNA's are not restricted solely to the nucleolus.

Some satellite DNA's and/or very rapidly reannealing DNA's hybridize to the heterochromatic centromeric regions of metaphase chromosomes or to condensed blocks of chromatin (nonnucleolar as well as to nucleolar DNA) in interphase nuclei. By use of controlled shearing of DNA followed by differential centrifugation techniques, it has been possible to demonstrate that condensed heterochromatin from nuclei of various murine tissues (129, 309, 495, 496), of guinea pig (502), and of calf thymus (497) is enriched in satellite DNA. The euchromatin fractions are generally very deficient in or devoid of separable satellite DNA's (Fig. 4.12). These studies thus presaged the *in situ* hybridization results since the centromeric localization of heterochromatin had long been noted.

The question of whether or not satellite DNA (other than ribosomal "satellite" DNA's*) codes for RNA remains unclear both for mouse light satellite DNA and many satellites from other species (143, 183). The suggestion has been made by a number of authors (e.g., 462, 464) that satellite DNA's may play a role in chromosome (interphase and mitotic) structure, the establishment and maintenance of which is readily visualized as being of importance in both the transcription and replication of DNA in chromatin. That satellite DNA's per se exhibit unusual configurations can be inferred from several studies. The base composition of many satellite DNA's, when calculated from their buoyant densities in neutral cesium chloride gradients, are significantly in error when chemical base compositions are determined which would indicate that native duplex satellite DNA's have unusual configurations that affect their buoyant densities (258).

* The limitations of space preclude consideration of the significance of satellite DNA's associated with nucleoli and their functions; the interested reader is referred to a monograph on the nucleolus (74).

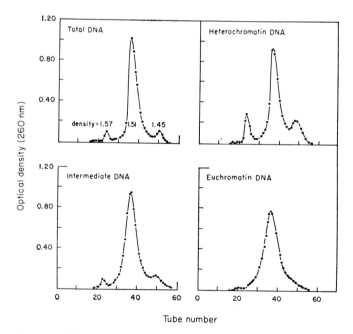

Fig. 4.12. Cesium sulfate-Ag⁺ density gradient sedimentation patterns of total DNA and DNA from the heterochromatin, intermediate, and euchromatin fractions of guinea pig liver. Density increases from right to left. Each gradient loaded with 120 μg of DNA. Note the absence of light or heavy satellite DNA's in the DNA isolated from euchromatin (from Yunis and Yasmineh, 502).

Secondly, each separated strand of the light mouse satellite DNA duplex can, in the known absence of complementary strand, reanneal to itself to the extent of 10–20% hybrid formation (143). The self-annealed single strands, after treatment with single-strand specific nuclease, have an oligonucleotide pattern very similar to the original duplex satellite which may suggest the presence of sequences complementary to other sequences within the same single strand (462). This may relate to the known capability of single strands of AT-rich satellite DNA for looping and self-association (143).

Finally, the secondary structure of DNA depends upon base composition (56). X-Ray scatter patterns show DNA in nucleohistone to be of the "B" type but with a helical pitch of 32 Å per turn compared to 37 Å for fibrous DNA. The X-ray patterns from DNA of low to medium adenine-thymine (AT) content were similar to calf thymus DNA but AT-rich DNA (i.e., AT/GC = 2) had distinctly different scattering patterns which indicated a greater helical pitch (about 42 Å) than DNA of lower AT content. Thus DNA rich in AT could possess a conformation different from low to moderate AT content DNA. X-Ray diffraction studies of synthetic polydeoxynucleotides also support the contention that base sequence can influence the secondary structure of DNA (261).

The structural singularities introduced by AT-rich regions could serve as recognition/control sites for a number of proteins interacting with DNA (56) just as GC-rich regions in DNA in a number of microbial and phage systems might provide the structural basis of promoter-operator regions (437). The influence of large numbers of tandem repeats of "homopolymerlike" regions (i.e., satellite regions) of DNA in mammalian chromatin on the secondary and tertiary structure of that chromatin is not yet known. X-Ray scatter patterns of satellite DNA's or fractions of nonnucleolar heterochromatin will undoubtedly be of interest.

Further information on structural roles for various classes of DNA should also be forthcoming from the recently developed staining techniques for different types of heterochromatin (9, 137). A quinacrine fluorescent staining method shows that late replicating regions of chromosomes (presumably heterochromatic) which stained most intensely also incorporated labeled deoxythymidine but virtually no labeled deoxycytidine (137). Since quinacrine fluorescence is known to be enhanced by AT-rich synthetic polydeoxynucleotides (476), AT-rich heterochromatin might be localized to extracentromeric heterochromatin—a conclusion that hints at some heterogeneity in heterochromatin and satellite DNA's and which was also made on other grounds (106, 391).

The image of DNA in chromatin that is beginning to develop from these diverse studies is that of duplex DNA attached to the annuli of the nuclear membrane pores and extending into the nucleus in the form of supercoils and coiled supercoils folded and held in specific configurations and positions in space by DNA–protein (especially histone) and protein–protein interactions and perhaps by regions of highly repetitious "homopolymerlike" DNA sequences. The influence of structure on function is illustrated by the observation (188) that a euchromatic chromsome segment becomes heterochromatic when translocated to heterochromatic regions of another chromosome.

A number of models of chromosome or chromatin structure have been advanced (e.g., 102, 108, 119, 133, 134, 260, 434) but only three are reproduced here (Figs. 4.13–4.15). The relative featurelessness of the models demonstrates that much remains to be discovered of the ultrastructure or molecular anatomy of DNA in chromatin.

B. The Replication of DNA in Chromatin

The extensive heterogeneity in the molecular anatomy of DNA in chromatin should dispel notions that DNA in the interphase nucleus is a relatively feature-less entity free in solution ready for immediate interaction with and replication by replicative DNA polymerase(s). Replicative heterogeneity also exists for DNA in eukaryotic chromatin.

1. THE CELL CYCLE

Since most nuclei from mitotically active and inactive eukaryotic cells have characteristic and fixed levels of DNA, in these organisms DNA replication

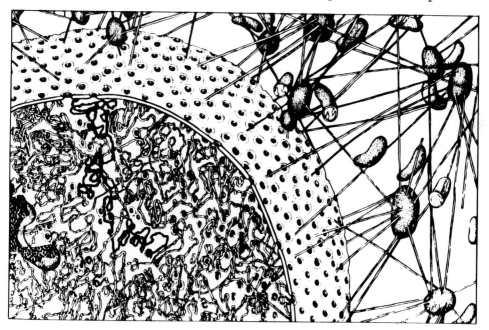

Fig. 4.13. Interpretation of nuclear and chromosome organization in a honeybee embryonic cell. Chromosomal fibers attach to the inside of the nuclear envelope, especially to the edge of the nuclear annuli. The chromosomal fiber shown in black is attached at either end to different annuli. Inside each chromosomal fiber a single DNA double helix is supercoiled into a "type A" fiber about 100 Å in diameter which in turn, is again supercoiled into a "type B" fiber about 230 Å in diameter. The type B fibers predominate in the figure. It is postulated (see text) that histones, and possibly other DNA-associated proteins, help to form and maintain these coiled and coiled-supercoiled configurations (from DuPraw, 134).

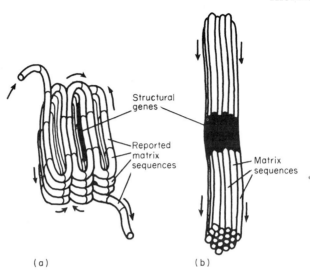

Fig. 4.14. A model for the packing of chromatin strands. Each strand of chromatin is envisaged as a single DNA double helix in association with basic and perhaps other proteins and possibly in coiled or coiled-supercoiled configurations within the one strand. By appropriate folding, the tandemly repeated DNA sequences (see text) might be apposed to yield the "superstructure" shown in (a) for a monotene chromosome. The tandemly repeated segments might be linearly aligned and apposed without folding as shown in (b) for the polytene chromosome (from Sutton, 434).

must be programmed and coordinated with cell division. Microspectrophoto-metric techniques (435, 436) and radioactive labeling of DNA (439) demonstrated duplication of nuclear DNA content during a discrete time period between mitoses in various plant, insect, and mammalian tissues. The eukaryotic cell (life) cycle is divided into four periods (a) M phase or the time during which the chromosomes condense and segregate to opposite poles of the mother cell concluded by reformation of the nuclear envelope, cytokinesis, and redispersion of the chromatin; (b) G_1 phase or the time interval between the end of mitosis and the beginning of DNA replication; (c) S phase or the time during which the nuclear DNA content is replicated; and (d) G_2 phase, the time interval between the end of DNA synthesis and the beginning of mitosis (196). The durations of the phases (determined by following autoradiographically the percent of labeled mitoses at varying times after a pulse label of tritiated thymidine) are both fixed and varied. The S, G_2, and M phases are found to require relatively invariant time intervals for a given cell type whereas the G_1 phase responds to environmental conditions and can be either shorter or longer than usual (328). Generalized estimates of the phases for mammalian cells run 6–10 hours for S phase, 2–5 hours for G_2 phase, and 0.5–1.5 hours for M phase. The G_1 phase can vary from very short times to even days, months, or years. Cells in very prolonged G_1 phase have been referred to as G_0 cells to distinguish them from "true" G_1 cells carrying out preparations for DNA synthesis. Cells in this state can often be recruited back into the cell cycle as witnessed by the proliferation of most hepatocytes in the remaining liver segment 24–36 hours after partial hepatectomy (58, 66). The prereplicative

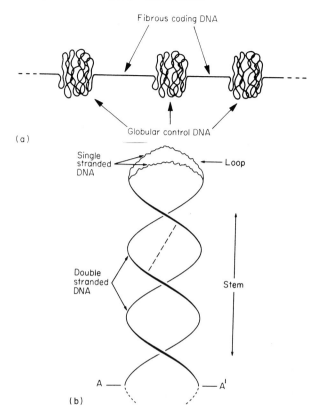

Fig. 4.15. A general model for the chromosomes of higher organisms. (a) A schematic drawing of the postulated general structure of DNA of the chromatid. The line represents part of the continuous DNA in the mononemic chromatid. DNA sequences coding for protein are postulated to be mainly in the extended linear "fibrous" region, whereas the intricately folded "globular" regions are postulated to be sites of control regions. In this model, a genetic complementation group is usually contained in a single fibrous region plus an adjacent globular area or a single fibrous region plus parts of the globular regions at either end of the linear portion. When a gene is active, the globular region is at least partially unfolded. Both the fibrous and globular regions may be complexed with chromosomal proteins. (b) One possible arrangement for DNA folded into globular control regions. A single double helical strand of DNA is pictured as forming a twisted hair pinlike structure which might be formed and/or maintained in that configuration by one or another class of histones bridging the double-helical double helix. The DNA at the turn of the hair pin (the loop) has become unpaired as a result of the untwisting effect produced by the stem. These loops are postulated to be the sites of the actual control elements (sequences) (from Crick, 119).

events that need to occur for subsequent DNA replication are multiple as are the events transpiring within the DNA replicative period itself.

2. THE CHRONOLOGY OF DNA REPLICATION IN S PHASE

After the initial descriptions of a discrete S phase, autoradiography was used (442) to demonstrate the "semiconservative replication" of DNA at the chromatid-chromosomal level and later (396, 440) to show that individual mammalian chromosomes did not replicate randomly in time but followed a distinctly non-random chronological replication pattern. DNA synthesized during a given portion of the S phase is replicated at very close to the same time in the subsequent S phase. Thus, HeLa cells synchronized by amethopterin blockade were allowed to synthesize DNA for a given time in the presence of labeled deoxythymidine (336). After several subsequent generations in unlabeled deoxythymidine, the cells were again synchronized and released in the presence of the density label 5-bromo-2'-deoxyuridine for the same time period as in the labeling period, and subsequent isolation of the DNA was performed. Most of the prelabeled DNA was associated with the density-labeled DNA.

A more detailed analysis of the types of DNA made at varying intervals during S phase was made (45) by pulse labeling synchronized HeLa or mouse L cells with 5-bromodeoxyuridine and [^{14}C]deoxythymidine or ^{32}P$_i$ at various intervals in S phase and subsequently analyzing the DNA by isopycnic centrifugation. By this method, HeLa cells contain GC-rich, early replicating DNA and AT-rich, late replicating DNA. In mouse L cells, the pattern of replication is similar (450, 451). The specific activities of the separable mouse light satellite DNA indicated that about 20% of the satellite DNA replicated in the first two hours of S phase and about 80% after bulk DNA synthesis reached maximum rates and then declined (Fig. 4.16). However, preponderant late replication of mouse satellite DNA has not been universally observed (45, 105, 232, 413). Conversely, in HeLa cells, DNA homologous to 28 S RNA—and thus presumably nucleolar—replicates throughout S phase (130).

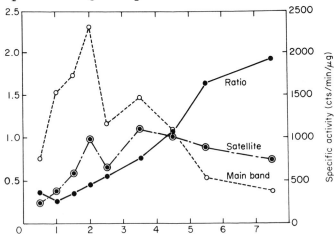

Fig. 4.16. Synthesis of bulk versus satellite DNA in synchronized mouse L cells. Cells were synchronized by a double thymidine blockade of S phase followed by removal of excess TdR. At varying times after removal aliquots of cell suspension were incubated for 30 minutes with ^{32}P$_i$ after which nuclear DNA was extracted and fractionated in preparative cesium chloride density gradients. The specific activities of main band DNA of modal density 1.700 gm/cm^3 and of 85–100% of the satellite DNA for a given time point are illustrated along with the ratios of the specific activities of satellite to main band DNA (from Tobia et al., 450).

In main band DNA, the early replication of GC-rich regions of DNA and the late replication of regions of low GC content has been observed in mouse L cells (45), mouse lymphoma cells (145), and Chinese hamster ovary cells (46). Since heterochromatic regions of eukaryotic chromosomes are more often than not replicated late in S phase (Fig. 4.17) (191, 279, 280, 281), the GC-rich, early replicating regions in main band DNA might represent euchromatin and the relatively AT-rich, late replicating DNA heterochromatin (45). However, purified euchromatin and heterochromatin prepared from nuclei of mouse, Chinese hamster, or rabbit livers have no significant differences in cesium chloride gradient buoyant densities of main peak DNA (47) in contrast to earlier positive findings (105, 309).

Inaccuracies inherent in bulk DNA isolation methods and isopycnic centrifugation techniques may give rise to these conflicting data. Thus, when multiple cesium chloride gradient separations of main band DNA extracted from pulse-labeled synchronized Chinese hamster cell lines harvested at varying times in S phase are performed (103), the early GC-rich/late AT-rich replication pattern still appears (Fig. 4.18). Moreover, very early in S phase, an AT-rich segment of DNA is preferentially synthesized. The observation (218) that 5-bromodeoxy-uridine, a thymidine analogue, greatly decreases the cloning efficiency of HeLa

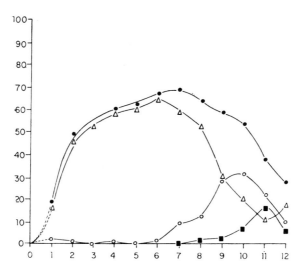

Fig. 4.17. Replication of euchromatin versus heterochromatin in Don-C Chinese hamster cells. Mitotic cells were selected by the monolayer shake technique and resuspended in fresh medium. At hourly intervals individual flasks were labeled with [³H]TdR for 15 minutes then fixed, stained, and subjected to autoradiography. Cells with only diffuse labeling were classed as euchromatin-labeled; cells with discrete heterochromatin labeling were separately scored. Ordinate: percent labeled nuclei *in toto* (●); % of euchromatin-labeled nuclei (△); % of heterochromatin-labeled nuclei (○); % of mitotic nuclei (■). Abcissa: time after removal to fresh medium. Since these curves are based upon percent of cells labeled, the results are qualitative. Analysis of the amount of incorporation of labeled precursor would reveal an S phase having a bimodal incorporation curve the second segment of which would reflect largely heterochromatic DNA synthesis (from Comings, 103).

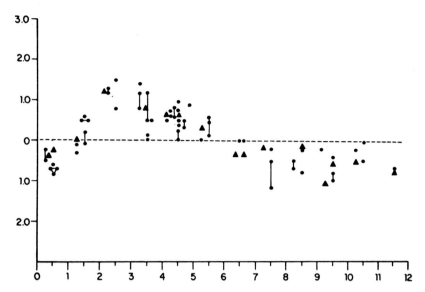

Fig. 4.18. Alterations in the buoyant density of DNA from Don (●) or Don-C (▲) Chinese hamster cells replicated at varying times in the cell cycle. Mitotic cells selected by the shake technique were incubated in fresh media to which, at various times after replating, [³H]TdR was added for 60 minutes. Thus, a data point between 2 and 3 on the abcissa (which is given as hours after replating) means that cells were labeled for one hour between the second and third hour after replating. Cells were harvested and the DNA isolated and subjected to cesium chloride density gradient centrifugation. The ordinate represents the alteration in buoyant density (stated in terms of a tube shift of the peak, one tube shift being the equivalent of a change in density of 0.00164 gm/cm³ or a change in G + C content of 1.77%) of the ³H-pulse-labeled DNA compared to [¹⁴C]TdR-labeled DNA from nonsynchronized cells. Thus, a negative tube shift (values below the dotted line) represents pulse-labeled DNA lighter than control DNA and thus more AT-rich. Values above the line represent DNA richer in GC than control DNA (from Comings, 103).

cells but only if present in the first two hours of S phase may relate to the speculation that the DNA replication initiation regions may be AT rich (103).

Such data point to the replicative heterogeneity of DNA in higher organisms with DNA of varying base compositions and/or varying states of condensation or diffuseness replicating at differing times in the synthetic period of the cell cycle.

3. EUKARYOTIC DNA REPLICONS

A bacterial chromosome under normal growth conditions replicates sequentially at a rate of 20–30 μm/minute through a replication "fork" from an origin to a terminator region (76, 77). This portion of the genome is termed a replicon (12). The average length of double helical DNA per unit chromatid in human cells is 3.8 cm (134). If a single replication origin point for the DNA helix in the chromatid exists, then about 21 hours would be required to replicate the helix at a rate of 30 μm/minute. However, the rate of replication of HeLa cell DNA is not 30 μm/minute but 0.5–1.0 μm/minute (78). Since approximately 6–10 hours suffices for replication of about 200 cm of DNA, there must be multiple replicons in DNA of higher organisms. By analyzing the size of newly synthesized pieces of Chinese hamster cell DNA incorporating [^{3}H-5]bromodeoxyuridine, a rate of chain growth of about 1–2 μm/minute and a length of the replicating unit of 180–360 μm could be calculated (441). Autoradiography of DNA from pulse-labeled Chinese hamster cells showed that long fibers of DNA consist of tandemly joined replication sections (averaging about 300 μm in length) each section of which is replicated by a forklike growing point moving at a rate of about 2.5 μm/min (202) (Fig. 4.19). That DNA is synthesized in opposite directions from adjacent initiation points is inferred from the pattern and density of silver grains following pulse labeling and cold chases with unlabeled deoxythymidine (202) (Fig. 4.20). Neighboring sections can begin replication at different times in S phase such that at any given instant the regions of DNA synthesis may not be distributed equidistantly along the chromosomal DNA fiber. A schematic model for eukaryotic replicon replication is shown in Fig. 4.21.

The process of DNA replication at each fork has been likened to the discontinuous DNA synthesis process postulated to account for synthesis of DNA in bacterial systems using a deoxynucleotidyl transferase having the properties of the E. coli DNA polymerase I (see Section III,A,2). Thus, in a number of mammalian cell types (351, 390, 392, 393, 457) newly synthesized pulse-labeled DNA is present as short segments which "chase" with time into fragments of higher molecular weight.

This simple conception of eukaryotic DNA replication at the level of the DNA double helix raises many questions, e.g., the multiple initiation sites apparently "turn on" at varying times which poses the problem of temporal control mechanisms. The presence of active and inactive "replicons" on a single length of DNA duplex raises anew the need for multiple swivel points upon which the DNA can spin in the process of unwinding and rewinding. Added to these questions are recent findings indicating that experimental protocols used in earlier studies might have generated serious artifacts. The rate of DNA chain growth in HeLa cells synchronized by either the mitotic cell selection method (449) or by double S-phase blockade was five times greater 5 to 6 hours after the onset of S phase than the rate at the beginning of S phase (352). The specific activity of DNA made in "early" S phase was one-fifth that found in "middle" S-phase DNA in cells synchronized by mitotic selection. No difference in specific activities of "early" and "middle" S-phase DNA was observed in cells synchronized by S-phase blockade. It is possible that many "replicons" not usually initiated at the onset of S phase were "aligned" by the double block such that they were able, upon reversal of blocking conditions, to begin replication out of their "normal sequence." Thus, use of S-phase blockade synchronized cells (202) might induce artifacts concerning the number and perhaps localization of mammalian DNA replication regions.

The number of replication forks per replicon may also be considered an open question. Recently (266), Chinese hamster cells synchronized with 5-fluorode-

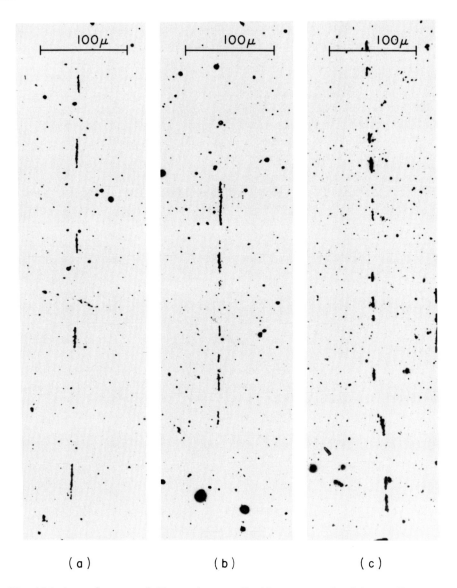

(a)   (b)   (c)

Fig. 4.19. Autoradiograms of Chinese hamster fibroblast DNA isolated from cells pretreated with 5-fluorodeoxyuridine for 12 hours followed by a 30-minute labeling period with [³H]TdR and ending with a cold chase with unlabeled TdR for 45 minutes. Cells were lysed by dialysis against SDS and the lysate further dialyzed against saline-EDTA. Released DNA was trapped on Millipore VM filters then subjected to autoradiography using stripping film (from Huberman and Riggs, 202).

oxyuridine were initially labeled with low specific [³H]TdR (more or less the inverse of an experiment discussed earlier). According to the bidirectional model, a lightly labeled segment of DNA should be bordered at each end by a heavily labeled segment. The results, however, were the observation of a region of

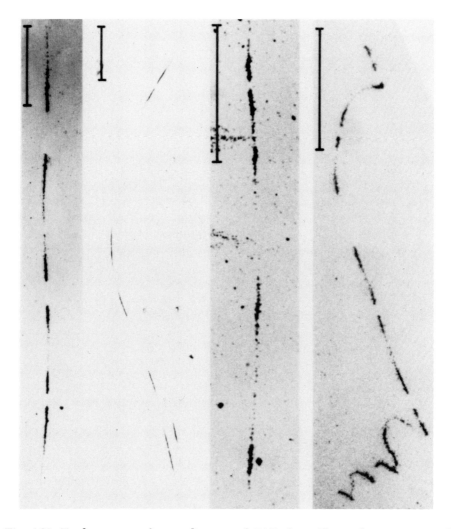

Fig. 4.20. Tandem arrays of autoradiograms of DNA from Chinese hamster ovary cells pretreated with 5-fluorodeoxyuridine for 12 hours then labeled for 30 minutes either with [³H]TdR (51 Ci/mmole) followed by a 45-minute "chase" in unlabeled TdR or with [³H]TdR (20 Ci/mmole) followed by a 45-minute "chase" with [³H]TdR at 51 Ci/mmole (the two left-hand panels). The two right-hand panels represent similar studies except that the low specific activity to high specific activity "chase" study utilized [³H]TdR at 8 Ci/mmole and 51 Ci/mmole. The density gradients of silver grains in all cases unambiguously suggest bidirectional replication in each replicon. These results also suggest that a recent inability to detect bidirectional replication (266) might have been due to the low difference in specific activities of [³H]TdR used earlier in the low labeling-high specific activity "chase" study (from Huberman and Tsai, 202a). Scale represents 50 μm.

light labeling bordered on only one end by a heavily labeled segment, which suggests a single replication fork per replicon (see legend of Fig. 4.20 for a recent criticism of this experiment).

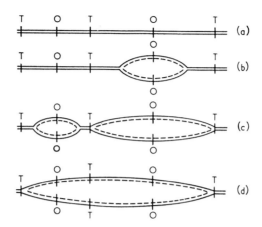

Fig. 4.21. Bidirectional model for DNA replication. Diagrams (a) through (d) represent different steps in the replication of two different adjacent replication units (replicons): (a) prior to replication; (b) replication has begun in right-hand unit; (c) replication has begun in left-hand unit and is completed at the terminus of the right-hand unit; (d) replication is completed in both units with sister helices separated at the shared terminus. The solid line represents parental DNA chains and the dotted line, newly synthesized DNA chains. O and T represent origin and termination sites (from Huberman and Riggs, 202).

4. *In Vivo* DNA Replication and the Nuclear Envelope

One of the earliest reports linking DNA replication with nuclear membrane in mammalian systems was that newly synthesized DNA from rabbit kidney cells was refractory to chloroform-isoamyl alcohol deproteinization and could be found at the interphase after phase separation (25; see also 151, 277). Pulse-labeled HeLa DNA is associated with nuclear membrane(s) separated by zonal sedimentation in sucrose density gradients containing sodium lauryl sarcosinate and can be "chased" into bulk DNA which is easily sheared away from the "membrane" band (182). The results point to membrane localization of replicator sites. In regenerating rat liver both initiation and replication of DNA is intimately associated with the nuclear envelope, more specifically, with the inner membrane of the nuclear envelope (326, 327).

Autoradiogaphic evidence that initiation of DNA replication in mammalian cells might occur on or at the nuclear envelope derives from studies on human amnion cells synchronized with excess thymidine and amethopterin and, following release from the S-phase blockade, exposed to [³H]TdR for 5, 10, or 20 minutes (104). Label in the short-term exposure synchronized cells was confined to the periphery of the nuclear membrane and to the nucleolus (Fig. 4.22). After a 20-minute labeling period, the distribution of label becomes less localized and occurs more interiorly in the nucleus (Fig. 4.23).

The nuclear envelope localization of DNA replication sites may also be subject to experimentally introduced artifacts. The nuclear peripheral localization of silver grains after pulse labeling synchronized cells with [³H]TdR may not represent normal replication but rather the accumulation of small replicating frag-

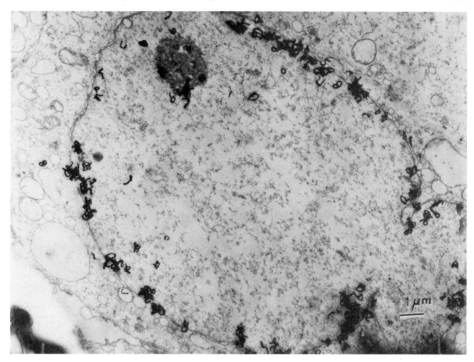

Fig. 4.22. Electron microscopic autoradiograph of a human amnion cell labeled with [³H]TdR for 10 minutes at the beginning of the S phase. Cells were synchronized by excess thymidine and amethopterin S-phase blockade. Autoradiographic silver grains are generally restricted to the nuclear membrane region and the periphery of the nucleus. ×7600 (from Comings and Kakefuda, 104).

ments of DNA as an artifactual response to being held in the "thymineless state" by S-phase blocking agents (342, 489). Chinese hamster cells, synchronized by mitotic selection and hydroxyurea treatment, show a very low percentage of silver grains at the nuclear periphery when pulse-labeled at early times after the onset of S phase.° Similar findings have very recently been published (202b, 492a). Thus, the earlier contention (104) that DNA replication is initiated at the nuclear membrane may not be correct.

Whether the replication forks move from the membrane initiation site along the unreplicated DNA into the interior of the nucleus or whether the yet to be replicated DNA moves through a membrane bound replication site seems not to be settled since it is possible to autoradiographically demonstrate "cold chasing" of silver grains from the nuclear membrane to the interior of the nucleus (341). High isotope contents of DNA (pulse-labeled at varying times into S phase) with the inner nuclear envelope tend to support the second alternative (326), but the suggestion has been made (139a) that the association of newly synthesized DNA with membrane(s) may be artifactual.

The cytoplasmic localization of a mammalian DNA polymerase, the activity

° Personal communication from D. E. Comings.

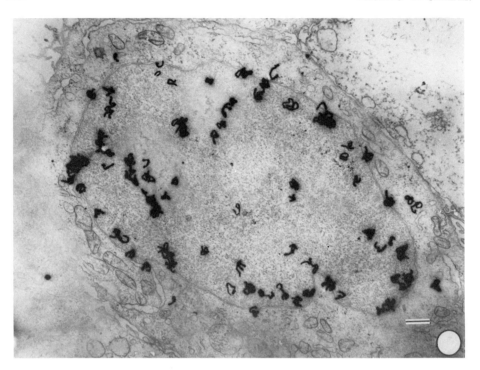

Fig. 4.23. Electron microscope autoradiograph of a synchronized human amnion cell labeled with [³H]TdR for 20 minutes after the beginning of the S phase. ×7700 (from Comings and Kakefuda, 104).

of which varies with the proliferative status of the tissue, and the association of deoxynucleotidyl transferases with cytoplasmic (Section III,B,2) and nuclear (501) membrane fractions has already been noted. What has not yet been remarked on is the association of DNA in higher organisms with cytoplasmic membranes. Cytoplasmic and/or cytoplasmic membrane-associated DNA has been described in adult rat liver (40, 397), embryonic muscle cells (23), embryonic mouse liver cells (490), and cultured diploid human lymphocytes (181, 275). The membrane-associated cytoplasmic DNA resembles nuclear DNA in many respects but has different labeling characteristics (181, 275, 490). Although degradation of nuclear DNA has been proposed to account for some cytoplasmic membrane-associated DNA (490), precise interrelationships between nuclear and cytoplasmic membrane DNA remain to be established.

V. Modification of DNA

A. Normal DNA Modification

One of the earlier problems in elucidating the structure of DNA lay in accounting for the presence of minor bases in DNA. Although the DNA polymerase

I of *E. coli* can polymerize 5-methyl-deoxycytidine triphosphate into DNA, no mechanism could explain the specific nonrandom localization of 5-methylcytosine in a variety of DNA's (70, 71, 404, 420) until it was discovered that in *E. coli* an enzyme utilizing S-adenosylmethionine as the methyl donor methylated specific DNA bases after synthesis of the polymer. Such bacterial DNA methylases catalyzing the formation of N^6-methyladenine and 5-methylcytosine have been purified (44, 422). An enzyme from rat liver catalyzing the methylation of DNA-cytosine residues (the only modified base in mammalian DNA's) has been purified to some extent (127, 128, 331).

The biological function(s) of DNA methylation remains unclear. A multiauxotroph of *E. coli*, when deprived of methionine, can complete DNA synthesis in progress but cannot initiate new rounds of DNA synthesis until the unmethylated DNA is properly methylated (28, 262, 263). It has been suggested (264) that methylated bases serve as "flags" for enzymic recognition of replication initiation sites and this concept has also been included in the "prefork" model for DNA synthesis (186). *In vivo* studies on DNA methylation in mammalian cells (2, 67, 223, 407, 415–417, 458) have pointed to a temporal association of DNA methylation and DNA synthesis but the function of mammalian DNA methylation remains unknown.

The only known functional role for DNA methylation is the modification-restriction process in which certain bacterial strains detect the entry of "foreign" DNA into the cell and subsequently degrade it. Host-directed enzymes methylate specific residues in host and nonrestricted foreign DNA's such that the specifically methylated DNA's are protected against host-produced endonucleases (8).

The consistent correlation of DNA methylation and DNA synthesis in many mammalian systems suggests an important role for the process in normal DNA "metabolism." Proposals have been made that altered methylation of nucleic acids generally—but especially of tRNA's (43)—may be involved in the etiology of neoplasia (119a) but these suggestions remain without definitive experimental support (Chapter VI).

B. Modification of DNA by Chemical Carcinogens

Studies on the molecular mechanism(s) of chemical carcinogenesis stem from experiments demonstrating the covalent interaction of aminoazo dyes with cellular proteins (318, 319) and the covalent interaction of nitrogen mustard with nucleic acids (481) of various animal tissues. Because of the heritable nature of neoplastic transformation, much effort has subsequently been expended in attempts to correlate covalent interaction of various chemical carcinogens with DNA of target tissues. Thus, in a series of polycyclic hydrocarbons of increasing carcinogenicity, there was no correlation of carcinogenic potency with binding to proteins or RNA but a good positive correlation with DNA binding was found (60). Only DNA-bound carcinogen persisted over 48 hours after injection of the hydrocarbons. Radioactive ^{14}C-labeled 2-acetamidofluorene covalently bound to rat liver DNA, whereas 3-methylcholanthrene which does not induce hepatic tumors did not bind to rat liver DNA (44). Persistent (>3 months) covalent binding of ^{3}H-labeled 4-dimethylaminoazobenzene or its metabolites to rat liver DNA was noted, whereas label associated with RNA or protein fractions fell to undetectable levels in 4 weeks (470). A positive correlation also exists between carcinogenic potency of a series of azo dyes and rat liver DNA-binding (123). The ability of certain alkylating agents (including β-propriolactone) to initiate skin tumorigenesis correlates with their ability to covalently interact with mouse skin DNA (100).

The general inference from studies of this type is that interaction of chemical carcinogens with cellular DNA constitutes a primary reaction from whence all subsequent manifestations of neoplastic transformation directly or indirectly flow. This statement is not meant to rule out the possibility of etiologically important interactions with RNA's, proteins, or other cellular components. For example, there is a profound *in vitro* inhibition of hamster fibroblast "DNA polymerase" by the agent N-methyl-N'-nitro-N-nitrosoguanidine (7). Modification of the structure and function of other important cellular proteins by reactive carcinogens undoubtedly occurs *in vivo*. Additionally, interaction of 2-acetylaminofluorene and β-propriolactone with cellular membranes alters the ability of DNA or synthetic polynucleotides to bind to membrane (257). In view of the intimate association of mammalian DNA with nuclear envelope membranes (Sections IV,A,1 and IV,B,4) such membrane–carcinogen interactions may be quite significant.

1. THE NATURE OF CARCINOGEN–DNA INTERACTIONS

a. "ALKYLATING" AGENTS. It was clear for many years that certain highly reactive chemical carcinogens (e.g., classic alkylating agents such as sulfur or nitrogen mustards) could form covalent chemical bonds with a variety of biological macromolecules or their reactive moieties (Chapter IX). The products of alkylation of DNA were shown to be primarily guanine residues possessing an alkyl substitution on the N-7 of the purine nucleus; adenine bases in DNA were alkylated at the N-3 position of the purine nucleus but not at N-1 which presumably reflects the unavailability of that ring nitrogen due to its participation in hydrogen-bonding in duplex DNA. Sulfur and nitrogen mustards having two functional or reactive groups can cross-link DNA by reacting with target bases on each strand of a duplex. Alkane sulfonates (such as methylmethanesulfonate, ethylmethanesulfonate), and, after appropriate metabolic "activation," a wide variety of alkylnitroso compounds such as dimethylnitrosamine, diethylnitrosamine, N-methyl-N'-nitro-N-nitrosoguanidine, N-methyl-N-nitrosourea, N-ethyl-N-nitrosourea, and N-nitrosomethylurethane also form adducts with purine bases in DNA (267, 298, 405).

The identity of the alkyl substituent covalently linked to the DNA base depends on the alkylating agent used. β-Propriolactone reacts with free guanosine or guanine in RNA and DNA to form a 2-carboxyethyl substituent on the N-7 of the purine (380). Methylation or ethylation of reactive sites in DNA-guanine

(N-7) and DNA-adenine (N-3) by alkylating agents or potential alkylating agents possessing, respectively, methyl or ethyl groups (e.g., dimethylnitrosamine and diethylnitrosamine) has been well demonstrated (59, 267, 298). The production of O^6-alkylguanine was shown by reacting deoxyguanosine with N-methyl- or N-ethyl-N-nitrosourea or ethylmethanesulfonate (291) but not methyl-methanesulfonate—an alkyl sulfonate that does not mutagenize T-even phage (292). DNA treated *in vitro* with N-methyl-N'-nitro-N-nitrosoguanidine or methylmethanesulfonate yields the usual distribution of methylated purines (N^7-methylguanine, N^3-methyladenine), but only the N-methyl-N'-nitro-N-nitro-soguanidine-treated DNA yielded O^6-methylguanine (271).

The pyrimidine bases in duplex DNA are not believed to react at neutral pH with alkylating agents or potential alkylating agents (267, 268, 270, 272), whereas the N-3 position of the pyrimidine ring in RNA's or free bases, nucleosides, or nucleotides is free to react (267, 272). However, if rats are treated with [^{14}C]dimethylnitrosamine and DNA extracted from the livers of the animals is subsequently hydrolyzed and analyzed, label is found in the pyrimidine breakthrough peak from a Dowex-50 column. The identity of the compound remains to be established (117).

Alkylating agents may also react with the diesterified phosphate residues in nucleic acids yielding a phosphotriester linkage. Radioisotopically labeled methylmethanesulfonate or ethylmethanesulfonate incubated at pH 7.4 with thymine or deoxythymidine yields no reaction of this pyrimidine with the reagent. When deoxythymidylyl ($3' \rightarrow 5'$) deoxythymidine is treated, a phosphotriester formation of 10% of available phosphodiesters is observed (375). It is not known if phosphotriester formation occurs to a significant extent during *in vivo* DNA alkylation (267).

b. AROMATIC AMINES, AMIDES, AND AZO DYES. The covalent interactions of aromatic amines and amides, azo dyes, and polycyclic hydrocarbons as well as the nature of the products formed with DNA constituents have been less easy to visualize due to the complexity of the carcinogen molecules and, in the case of the polycyclic hydrocarbons, a relative lack of chemical reactivity. Much light has been shed on this, however, by a theory advanced by the Millers (321–323, Chapter IX).

The "electrophilic reactant theory" presumes that most chemical carcinogens are either enzymatically or nonenzymatically converted *in vivo* to electrophilic forms which are the ultimate reactive forms of the carcinogen. As electrophilic reactants, the compounds can attack important intracellular nucleophilic sites including several amino acid residues (e.g., methionine, cystine, tyrosine, histidine) or nucleic acid bases (e.g., N-7, C-8, and O-6 of guanine, N-3 and N-1 of adenine, N-3 of cytosine). When N-acetoxy-2-acetylaminofluorene is reacted with guanosine *in vitro,* N-(guanosin-8-yl)-acetylaminofluorene is formed (256, 320). The corresponding deoxyguanosine adduct is also formed when deoxyguanosine is used. Radioisotopically labeled N-hydroxy-2-acetylaminofluorene formed N-(deoxyguanosin-8-yl)-acetylaminofluorene and N-(deoxyguanosin-8-yl)-aminofluorene adducts *in vivo* with rat liver DNA (206, 253). Metabolism of 2-acetylaminofluorene generates an esterified or glucuronidated *N*-hydroxy-2-acetylaminofluorene which can attack the C-8 of guanine residues. An azo dye, *N*-methyl-4-aminoazobenzene, has also been reported to yield an adduct at the C-8 position of the guanine residues in rat liver DNA (320). Whether *N*-hydroxylation and esterification of azo dyes (365) or metabolism of *N*-methyl groups on azo dyes (124) generates the "ultimate" carcinogenic reactant in this series of carcinogens is still not clear.

Less well defined is the nature of the adduct formed between the carcinogen 4-nitroquinoline-1-oxide and DNA. One molecule of 4-nitroquinoline-1-oxide (or a metabolite thereof) is found per 104 DNA base pairs in treated Ehrlich ascites cells. Depurination of the DNA releases almost all labeled carcinogen suggesting association with purine bases (204, 438).

c. POLYCYCLIC HYDROCARBONS. Many of the earlier isolates of carcinogenic substances were polycyclic hydrocarbons, e.g., 3,4-benzo(*a*)pyrene, 3-methyl-cholanthrene, dibenz(*a,h*)anthracene, and 7,12-dimethylbenzanthracene. Most polycyclic hydrocarbons are relatively nonreactive chemically, yet polar metabolites of these compounds are found *in vivo* as well as covalently linked adducts to DNA. *In vivo* observations on metabolism of polycyclic hydrocarbons were followed by demonstrations *in vitro* of microsomal enzyme systems catalyzing the oxidation of these compounds (109). Before this time, however, the nature of the dihydrodihydroxy metabolites of a number of polycyclic hydrocarbons led to the proposal that epoxides

of polycyclic hydrocarbons were intermediates in their metabolism and as such might interact with cellular molecules in the manner of alkylating agents (51, 52). The regions on the polycyclic hydrocarbons most likely to react were deduced from quantum chemical calculations and called the "K regions" (366). The reactive nature of the K-region epoxides has prevented their actual demonstration *in vivo* in addition to which it must be noted that artifically synthesized epoxides of polycyclic hydrocarbons always had lesser carcinogenic activity than their parent compound (52).

Radicals or ions of hydrocarbons formed prior to the actual epoxides might thus represent the reactive species (52, 124). It has been proposed that polycyclic hydrocarbons are metabolized *in vivo* ultimately to reactive aralkyl carbonium ions which could be located in the K region of the rings for unsubstituted hydrocarbons or which could be extranuclear methyl group carbons (as in 7,12-dimethylbenzenthracene) (124). Thus, 7-bromomethylbenzanthracene, an "artificial" reactive species, was used for *in vitro* study of covalent binding to nucleic acids (61).° *In vitro*, the 7-bromomethylbenzanthracene reacts with the C-8 of guanine residues through the methyl group at the 7-position of the hydrocar-

° The 7-bromomethylbenzanthracene, at appropriate dose levels, has been reported to induce tumors in rat and mouse (125).

bon (363). A model with the covalently linked hydrocarbon lying in the major groove of DNA parallel to the DNA-helix axis and perpendicular to the base pairs best fits the physicochemical data from natural DNA's reacted with the 7-bromomethylbenzanthracene (364).

7-Bromomethylbenzanthracene reacted *in vitro* with DNA in aqueous solution at pH 5.5 yields substantial levels of substitution of extranuclear amino groups in DNA-guanine (N-2 amino), DNA-adenine (N-6 amino), and possibly in DNA-cytosine (*N*-4 amino) (125). The involvement of these amino groups in base-pairing dictates that their substitution may have profound functional implications. Additionally, 85% of the DNA reacted with 7-bromomethylbenzanthracene reversibly denatures (316). A cross-linked dimer was isolated in which the methyl group of the 7-bromomethylbenzanthracene was probably linked to the C-8 of guanine or adenine and some other portion of the hydrocarbon was linked to the DNA-pyrimidine residue on the opposite strand of the double helix. The N-4 amino of DNA-cytosine might be involved in the cross-linking (316). The formation of cross-linked DNA has also been noted after treatment with *N*-acetoxy-2-acetylaminofluorene followed by irradiation of the adducted DNA with light of wavelength 310 nm (317).

2. INFLUENCE OF DNA STRUCTURE AND COMPOSITION ON MODIFICATION BY CARCINOGENS

Although a number of carcinogens interact with most possible sites on monomeric nucleic acid bases, a number of reactive sites are not accessible in duplex DNA by virtue of base-pair formation. In addition, the C-8 position of purines is subject to stereochemical blocking by the 2'-carbon of deoxyribose in duplex DNA (224, 363). Since both 2-acetylaminofluorene and 7-bromomethylbenzanthracene react at the C-8 of guanine, dynamic "breathing" of duplex DNA (312) may permit sufficient deformation of the structure of duplex DNA to allow reaction at stereochemically restricted loci. Conformational dependence of the reaction of 2-acetylaminofluorene with polynucleotides has been described (255). As another example, polydeoxyribocytidylic acid, which has a high degree of secondary structure, is alkylated to a much lesser extent (1.3% of residues alkylated) by dimethylsulfate at 25°C and pH 7 than polyribocytidylic acid (18.6% of residues methylated) (296). The influence of tertiary structure upon carcinogen modifications is not clear but it may be that supercoiling of the DNA helix enhances the ability of at least some chemicals to physically bind to DNA, which presumably might increase the probability of covalent interactions. Planar polycyclic hydrocarbons might well preferentially interact with supercoiled mitochondrial DNA in a manner similar to ethidium bromide and acridine dyes (493, 494). The intracellular localization of tritiated dimethylbenzanthracene by electron microscopic autoradiography of mouse prostate cells shows no unusual nuclear localization of autoradiographic grains but significant numbers of cytoplasmic grains (210), perhaps reflecting preferential binding of the hydrocarbon to mitochondrial DNA.

The influence of nucleoproteins on DNA–carcinogen interactions has not received detailed attention. The presence *in vitro* of nuclear proteins or the addition of nuclear histones to DNA reduces the interactions of carcinogens with DNA (386, 456), perhaps by direct steric blocking of reactive sites or by inducing higher orders of folding and structuring of the DNA molecule. However, there are no demonstrated differences in template activity of Ehrlich ascites cells chromatin versus deproteinized DNA when both are alkylated *in vitro* with an ethyleneimino compound (367).

Related to this aspect of chromatin structure is the interaction of carcinogens with one or another of the structural or functional classes of DNA discussed in Section IV. As studied by electron microscopic autoradiography, there is no preferential localization of tritiated dimethylbenzanthracene on any chromosomes in cultured mouse prostate cells (210). After application of tritiated dimethylbenzanthracene to mouse skin, labeled carcinogen was bound to main band and satellite DNA to the same extent per unit weight of DNA (504). The functional significance of condensed and diffuse chromatin, the possible importance of GC- or AT-rich regions in DNA as recognition sites for replication or transcriptional controls, and the possible suprastructural role played by highly repetitive DNA sequences, must all be examined from the standpoint of how such structural chracteristics of DNA influence the modification of DNA by carcinogens.

3. EFFECTS OF CARCINOGEN MODIFICATION OF DNA

a. STRUCTURAL EFFECTS. The structural defects introduced into DNA by modification with carcinogens can generally be classed into five categories: (a) cross-linking of the two strands of duplex DNA, (b) "spontaneous" removal of adducted bases from the deoxyribose phosphate "backbone" of the polynucleotide strand, (c) scissions of phosphodiester linkages in the "backbone", (d) deformation of the three-dimensional structure of the DNA double helix, and (e) alteration of the chemical characteristics of the modified bases.

Interstrand cross-links can be formed between guanine residues substituted at the C-8 position with 7-bromomethylbenzanthracene and a pyrimidine base (presumably the N-4 amino group of cytosine) on the opposite strand. N-Acetoxy-2-acetylaminofluorene can also form interstrand cross links under appropriate conditions. Difunctional alkylating agents can form diguanyl derivatives linked via substitution at the N-7 position of the purine bases (267) and methylmethanesulfonate, a monofunctional alkylating agent, can induce interstrand cross-links in DNA after moderate (50°C) heating at pH 7 (69). Cross-linked DNA is reversibly denaturable; inability to separate the two strands of the double helix can be expected to seriously impair the ability of DNA to replicate.

The substitution of an alkyl group at the N-7 of guanine or the N-3 of adenine labilizes the glycosidic linkage between the N-9 of the purines and the C-1 of the deoxyribose making it more susceptible to hydrolysis at neutral pH than unsubstituted purines. The rate of depurination of methylated adenine residues is approximately five times the rate for methylated guanine residues (254, 270), but the major depurination reaction observed in alkylated DNA involves substituted guanines since these account for the greatest percentage of alkylated bases. The net result of purine alkylation is the formation of apurinic sites in DNA followed by the formation of single strand scissions in the polynucleotide strands. Single strand scissions might also be introduced into polynucleotide strands as a result of alkylation of the internucleotide phosphodiester (375).

The ability of carcinogen modification to induce conformational alterations in DNA structure depends on the type of carcinogen used. DNA's from various bacterial and mammalian sources treated with dimethylsulfate give products in which up to 40% of the guanine residues are methylated (274). No loss of secondary structure of the DNA's could be detected by light scattering, intrinsic viscosity, sedimentation, or melting characteristics. Profound changes in structure of alkylated DNA do occur upon extended incubation perhaps due to depurination of alkylated bases and subsequent single strand scissions (459). Dimethysulfate alkylation of DNA's of varying GC content demonstrates a reduction in the ability of poly-L-lysine to bind to AT-rich regions of DNA, but since the N-7 of guanine when methylated possesses a positive charge, the reduced poly-L-lysine interaction might reflect electrostatic effects (370). Fluorescence spectra of DNA methylated at the N-7 of guanine reflected strong interactions between the modified base residues and their neighboring stacked bases which can be taken as evidence of little or no local denaturation of alkylated regions in DNA (370).

That some structural effect of alkylation might occur is suggested by the observation that 7-bromomethylbenzanthracene-induced cross-linking of DNA (involving the C-8 of guanine residues and possibly the N-4 amino of cytosine) was completely inhibited by prior methylation at N-7 of 10% of the guanines in *Micrococcus lysodeikticus* DNA (316). Covalent modification of DNA-guanine residues by 7-bromomethylbenzanthracene does not apparently cause distortion or denaturation of the secondary structure of the DNA helix (364), whereas adduction of N-acetoxy-2-acetylaminofluorene to the C-8 of guanine residues yields local regions of denaturation in duplex DNA (152, 224).

b. EFFECTS ON TEMPLATE FUNCTIONS. One of the more profound effects of carcinogen modification—at least from the standpoint of the template functions of DNA—is the alteration of the chemical characteristics of modified bases especially as related to their base-pairing properties. The introduction of alkyl groups on the N-7 of guanine lowers the pK_a of the N-1 hydrogen from 9.2 to 7.0 (269) as well as imparting an acidic function to the C-8 position (452).* The former effect may properly tend to make the N-7 substituted guanine mispair as though it were adenine (269), but the alkylation of adenine at N-3 does not appear to induce protonation at N-1 with an imino function at N-6 (267). Although the N-3 position of cytosine in DNA is "protected" by its participation in base-pairing, local regions of DNA helix "breathing" or denaturation might permit some cytosine residues to be alkylated which might then affect subsequent base-pairing. The O-6-alkylation of guanine as well as the adduction of free

---

* Although it has been considered that the primary alkylation of deoxyguanylic acid could be at the N-7 position, recent reports have indicated that the primary site of alkylation may be at the C-8 position. It is uncertain whether these major points of alkylation are the most critical ones in carcinogenesis. It is possible that some other point of alkylation may be even more significant for carcinogenesis.

amino groups of adenine, guanine, and cytosine residues in DNA by 7-bromo-methylbenzanthracene (described in Section V,B) may also influence accurate formation of complementary base pairs.

The effects of certain alterations on base-pairing in RNA and DNA synthesizing systems have been studied. The alternating copolymer ribouridylic-riboguanylic acid (in which the guanine residues were methylated at the N-7 position) in a cell-free protein-synthesizing system caused no misincorporation of amino acids into newly synthesized polypeptides (486). The products formed from incubations of either riboguanylic-ribouridylic copolymers or ribo-7-methyl-guanylic-ribouridylic copolymers with *Micrococcus lysodeikticus* RNA polymerase and ATP and CTP were compared (294). The alkylated template base-paired normally to produce adenylic-cytidylic copolymer. Mispairing of alkylated guanine with uracil was also not detected using a polymer of ribo-7-methyl-guanylic-ribocytidylic acid and GTP plus UTP in the reaction mixture. Moreover, 7-methyldeoxyguanosine triphosphate substitutes for deoxyguanosine triphosphate in an *in vitro* DNA-synthesizing system—albeit at lower efficiency than the nonalkylated monomer—but does not substitute for any other deoxynucleoside triphosphate including deoxyadenosine triphosphate (189). N-7 Alkylation (methylation) of guanine therefore seems to have little influence on the *in vitro* base-pairing characteristics of the modified guanine residues. The known mutagenicity of methylating and ethylating agents (see 267, 409) yielding apparent G:C to A:T transitions is difficult to reconcile with this suggestion. Ethylated guanine residues are much more stable than methylated guanines in DNA (267); their longer survival in DNA, assuming the lesions are not repaired, may permit the expression of aberrant base-pairing *in vivo* which is not detectable *in vitro* for reasons that might include pH at site of reaction and specificity of the enzyme systems used to test for mispairing.

Distinct alterations in the properties of alkylated cytosine residues in ribo- and deoxyribonucleotide polymers have been noted. Ribopolymer templates containing randomly or regularly spaced 3-methylcytosine residues directed the misincorporation of UTP into polymer product (295, 297, 410). Misincorporation of UTP also occurs with ethylated templates (410). Dimethyl sulfate-modified polydeoxycytidylic acid also directed misincorporation of UTP and ATP when used as "DNA" template for *in vitro* RNA synthesis (296). Cytosine residues methylated at the N-3 position may not in reality direct the misincorporation of bases but perhaps any base can fill the gap opposite this modified base. This is in contrast to cytosine residues modified at the N-4 position with hydroxylamine or methoxyamine which behave like uracil and misincorporate only ATP in *in vitro* RNA synthesis (410).

Escherichia coli or *Micrococcus lysodeiktius* DNA methylated *in vitro* with dimethyl sulfate is only 10% as effective a template for *in vitro* RNA synthesis using either labeled cytidylic or guanylic acids as precursors (248, 274). Such decreases could result from depurination or strand scission reactions that accompany alkylation of DNA. However, when coliphage T7 DNA was treated with either methylmethanesulfonate or ethylmethanesulfonate under conditions in which depurination and chain breakage were minimized (a fact which was experimentally verified), the alkylated DNA was 30 (methylated) to 50% (ethylated) less effective a template with *E. coli* RNA polymerase than untreated T7 DNA (304).

The effects of modification of DNA's by carcinogens other than "classic" alkylating agents on template characteristics of the DNA's have not been extensively analyzed. The ability of calf thymus DNA to serve as a template for *in vitro* RNA synthesis using *Micrococcus lysodeikticus* RNA polymerase after reacting the DNA with N-acetoxy-2-acetylaminofluorene was reduced to 40% of control after one minute of reaction with the carcinogen and completely abolished after one hour (453). Since arylamidation of guanine residues at the C-8 position does not labilize the purine–deoxyribose linkage (thus does not yield depurination strand scission) and does not influence appreciably the pK_a of the N-1 hydrogen (256), the decreased template ability might be ascribed to projection of the bulky fluorene molecule in the major groove of the DNA (Section V,B,1). The importance of the major groove of DNA in RNA transcription has been stressed (293) and bulky substituents in this groove may well adversely influence transcription.

c. MUTAGENESIS. A crucial question, not yet unequivocally answered, is whether or not carcinogen-induced modifications of DNA do in fact constitute mutational events in regions of the genome critical for control of cell proliferation. Identity and localization of such regions are not known but it has been possible to test to some extent whether or not carcinogens can be mutagenic agents.

Bacillus subtilis transforming DNA was reacted *in vitro* with reactive forms of 2-acetylaminofluorene and N-methyl-4-aminoazobenzene and its ability to transform a *B. subtilis* strain blocked for tryptophan synthesis was measured (300). The results suggest the production of point mutations by the interaction of both types of carcinogen with transforming DNA. The mutagenicity of a number of chemical carcinogens of different classes was examined by treatment of T4 coliphage and subsequent analysis of the growth of phage on certain bacterial strains (110). Some chemically reactive species yielded mutations of varying types. Two alkylating agents, nitrogen mustard and β-propriolactone, induced apparent base pair transitions of the G:C to A:T type, whereas N-acetoxy-2-acetylaminofluorene induced A:T to G:C base pair transitions. *Bacillus subtilis* transforming DNA modified by the covalent linkage of either 3,4-benzo(*a*) pyrene or dimethylbenzanthracene, exhibited an increased number of mutations compared to control DNA (301). The mutations did not readily revert suggesting that the modification resulted in deletion-type mutants. By measuring the effect of various carcinogens on the frequency of reversion of histidine-requiring strains of *Salmonella typhimurium*, epoxides of polycyclic hydrocarbons (5) as well as several nitroso derivatives of carcinogenic aromatic amines (6) were found to be potent frameshift mutagens.

The ability of a series of alkylating and nitroso compounds and a series of compounds of lesser reactivity (such as the polycyclic hydrocarbons, the aromatic amines, and azo dyes) to interact with and mutate specific genome regions associated with ribosomal RNA formation as compared to "nonspecific" genetic damage to X-linked genes was analyzed in *Drosophila* (138, 139). Carcinogens in both series of compounds proved particularly active for ribosomal RNA-forming loci. "Generalized" mutagenic activity was high for the alkylating and nitroso series but low with the compounds of low reactivity. Beyond demonstrating carcinogen-induced mutagenesis in an *in vivo* eukaryotic system, the significance of the seemingly preferential mutation of ribosomal RNA genetic loci with respect to carcinogenesis is not known.

In summary, many, if not all, carcinogens covalently interact with DNA. DNA thus modified with carcinogens can exhibit alterations in the basic content and expression of the encoded genetic information. Possible steps from a carcinogen-modified DNA to a neoplastic cell will be considered in Section VII.

VI. The Repair of DNA

A. Mechanisms of DNA Repair

The elucidation of DNA repair processes was a natural outgrowth of earlier studies on the genetic effects of various chemical and physical agents on living organisms, one of the more intensively studied agents being short-wave ultraviolet radiation known to be mutagenic for many prokaryotes. The principal effect of UV light on DNA is the dimerization of adjacent pyrimidine bases in DNA formed via the covalent linkage of the 5 and 6 pyrimidine ring carbons on one pyrimidine to the 5 and 6 carbons on the adjacent pyrimidine yielding a cyclobutane configuration (27, 402, 461). A dose of 254 nm radiation of 1 erg/mm^2 will produce about six pyrimidine dimers in a DNA molecule of 10^7 nucleotide residues using *E. coli* DNA (197). The removal of ultraviolet radiation-induced pyrimidine dimers from DNA forms the basis of most studies on DNA repair (see reviews in 21, 197, 400, 427).

Ultraviolet radiation damage to DNA is repaired by at least three processes: photoreactivation, excision repair, and postreplication or recombinational repair. Photoreactivation repair involves the reversal of pyrimidine dimer formation rather than the replacement of "damaged" or altered DNA bases (109a, 185, 387). Since repair of chemically modified DNA apparently involves replacement mechanisms, no further treatment of photoreactivation will be given here.

1. EXCISION REPAIR

Excision repair of UV-damaged DNA was first noted during an investigation of the nature of the biochemical difference between a mutant strain of *E. coli* that was extremely sensitive to UV irradiation and the more resistant wild-type *E. coli* (50, 401). With time pyrimidine dimers were lost from DNA of the wild-type *E. coli* but pyrimidine dimers in the radiation-sensitive mutant strain always remained in the acid-precipitable fraction, presumably unexcised from DNA. Further *in vivo* studies demonstrated that a nonsemiconservative synthesis of DNA follows UV irradiation suggesting that, following excision of pyrimidine dimers, the resultant gaps in both DNA strands were filled (357).

The more detailed picture of excision repair developed since these germinal observations is depicted in Fig. 4.24. The pyrimidine dimer-containing region of the DNA (or DNA containing alkylated bases) is recognized by an endonuclease (by an as yet little understood mechanism) which then specifically hydrolyzes single phosphodiester links 5' to the pyrimidine dimer region yielding a 3'-phosphoryl terminus and a 5'-hydroxyl terminus which is at, or one nucleotide 5' to, the photoproduct. The number of single strand incisions made by the enzyme is directly correlated with the number of pyrimidine dimers in the substrate DNA. Endonucleases specific for UV-damaged DNA (221, 259) or for DNA containing covalently bound alkyl group "lesions" (149) have been described suggesting that different enzymes may be required to recognize and incise DNA regions with structurally quite different lesions (221). Following

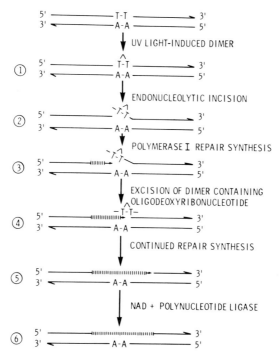

Fig. 4.24. A model for excision repair of DNA. Step 1: A UV-irradiated double helix of DNA is shown as containing one pyrimidine dimer. Step 2: A specific endonuclease recognizes the dimer-containing region and incises the polynucleotde strand on the 5' side of the photoproduct. Step 3: DNA polymerase I binds to the nicked DNA and, using the opposing strand as template, starts repair polymerization of the damaged strand displacing the dimer-containing region in the process. Step 4: When the 5' to 3' exonuclease site of the polymerase reaches the next hydrogen-bonded base pair, the phosphodiester linkage is hydrolyzed releasing the dimer within a short oligodeoxyribonucleotide. Steps 5 and 6: Polymerization and hydrolytic activities may continue in the 5' to 3' direction until step 6 when the polymerase is displaced by polynucleotide ligase which together with NAD restores the integrity of the phosphodiester backbone of DNA. Model drawn on the basis of concepts presented by Boyle (53).

incision an exonucleolytic activity (259) removes the photoproduct-containing region leaving a 5′-phosphoryl group on the DNA and a 3′-hydroxyl on the excised fragment and then exonucleolytically degrades the excised fragment. The newly liberated 3′-hydroxyl DNA terminus at the gap can serve as a primer site for repair replication by DNA polymerase I. The process is completed by the action of polynucleotide ligase. Thus, the mechanism conforms to the "cut and patch" model of repair (198).

However, studies on the *polA1* mutants (see Section III,A,4) indicate that the "patch then cut" model (187) may more closely approximate the mechanism of excision repair (at least in *E. coli*). This model also invokes initial recognition and endonuclease action. DNA polymerase I covalently adds nucleotides to the 3′-hydroxyl group, using the opposing undamaged strand as a template and displacing the 5′-terminus photoproduct-containing strand until the dimer is reached. The dimer itself is not hydrogen-bonded to the opposite strand so that the damaged strand peels away as far as the next hydrogen-bonded base pair. The polymerase continues filling in the resultant gap up to the next hydrogen-bonded base pair and then the 5′ to 3′ exonuclease activity of the polymerase excises the damaged section of DNA as an oligonucleotide which will either be recovered as such or be subject to more complete nucleolytic cleavages. The DNA polymerase I continues its translation in a 5′ → 3′ direction (thus accounting for the incorporation of 50 or more nucleotides per dimer, see ref. 29) until displaced by polynucleotide ligase which catalyzes formation of the final phosphodiester linkage (231). Consistent with this role for DNA polymerase I in DNA repair is the observation that the *polA1* mutant could excise UV-induced pyrimidine dimers from their DNA but could apparently not fill the resultant gaps (54, 220).

3. RECOMBINATIONAL REPAIR

The existence of recombinational or postreplication repair was inferred from the observation that *E. coli* mutants unable to excise dimers survive and form colonies after UV doses that produce 50 pyrimidine dimers per bacterial chromosome (197). They must, therefore, replicate their DNA in spite of these defects. Mechanisms of recombinational repair have been postulated (see 197, 199) and one such model is depicted in Fig. 4.25; template containing the unexcised lesion (pyrimidine dimer, apurinic or apyrimidinic site, alkylated bases, "mutagenized" bases) is replicated semiconservatively yielding one undamaged daughter double helix and a second daughter double helix with a gap in the newly synthesized strand opposite the unexcised lesion (in "wild-type" cells with intact excision-repair processes the lesion could escape excision if normal semiconservative DNA replication occurred before the excision repair process "discovered" and repaired the lesion). Since the lesion, after normal replication, is opposite a gap, the excision-repair process cannot then function inasmuch as the required template is lacking. Thus, it is postulated that recombinational type of genetic exchanges occur between daughter duplexes such that both the lesion and the gap are opposite their appropriate templates. The gap can

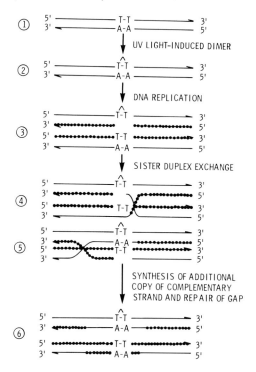

Fig. 4.25. A model for recombinational repair by sister duplex exchanges following DNA replication. Steps 1 and 2: Duplex DNA is exposed to UV light inducing the formation of a pyrimidine dimer. Step 3: The unexcised dimer-containing DNA is replicated resulting in production of one normal DNA duplex and a second duplex that contains a gap in the daughter strand opposite the dimer. Steps 4 and 5: Recombinational genetic exchanges occur between sister duplexes. Step 6: Damaged parental strand is now opposite a daughter strand that contains no gap (filled by recombinational events) and can thus be repaired by the excision repair process (modified from a figure by Howard-Flanders and Rupp, 199).

then be accurately filled (by polymerase I) and the lesion can be repaired by the template requiring excision-repair process.

B. The Repair of Mammalian DNA

In contrast to detailed studies of microbial DNA repair, the depth of knowledge of mammalian DNA repair is not great. The nature of the lesions introduced into mammalian DNA are incompletely elucidated. Additionally, the damage and repair of free, apparently noncompartmentalized bacterial DNA is relatively easy to visualize compared to the very complex picture presented by damage and repair of mammalian DNA's packaged in chromatin fibers of differing states of condensation which interact with the nuclear membrane in some organized but as yet unknown manner (see Section IV). The available methods for analysis of high molecular weight mammalian DNA's with attendant shear and nucleolytic degradation of DNA and formidable problems of interpretation of "pulse labeling" studies with mammalian cells introduce multiple uncertainties into studies of mammalian DNA repair.

1. EXCISION REPAIR OF UV LIGHT-INDUCED DNA LESIONS

Although UV irradiation can effect multiple changes in DNA (e.g., photohydration, DNA-protein cross-links), pyrimidine dimer formation is the most important molecular lesion. In mammalian cells (Chinese hamster cell line) about 150,000 pyrimidine dimers per nucleus are formed upon exposure to 265 nm radiation at 100 ergs/mm² (455). No excision of UV-induced pyrimidine dimers into trichloracetic acid soluble fragments was detected in irradiated Chinese hamster cells (424, 454, 455), mouse L cells (194, 239), or porcine kidney cells (194). On the other hand, 50% of the pyrimidine dimers were excised from DNA 12–24 hours after UV irradiation of human amnion cells (372). With the exception of bovine fibroblasts (98) most nonprimate mammalian cells do not excise pyrimidine dimers at least as determined by the usual criterion of acid solubilization of such dimers from DNA. Since the nonprimate cell lines can carry out excision repair (see below), the inability to detect dimer excision by the usual methodology is regarded as artifactual.

UV-induced "unscheduled DNA synthesis" (defined as autoradiographically detected incorporation of [³H]TdR into DNA of cells not in S phase) correlates with "repair replication" of DNA (studied by density labeling techniques, 357) and both are probably manifestations of the same repair process. More rigorous techniques (rebanding of nonsemiconservatively replicated DNA regions of density gradients as well as long exposure times for autoradiographs) reveal a low level of repair replication in Chinese hamster cells and mouse L cells (350).

Greater insight into the process of repair replication in mammalian cells has come from studies of DNA repair in cells cultured from patients with xerodema pigmentosum. Such patients exhibit a recessive hereditary tendency to develop various types of skin cancers on exposure to sunlight. One form of the syndrome is restricted to skin symptoms while a second form, the de Sanctis-Cacchione syndrome, additionally involves mental retardation. Fibroblasts cultured from skin biopsies demonstrate enhanced sensitivity to UV irradiation as measured by colony formation compared to control cells (96) and are much less able to support multiplication of UV-damaged herpes simplex or SV40 virus (1, 368).*

Xerodema cells apparently have a low or negligible ability to excise pyrimidine dimers (96, 98) and are deficient in autoradiographic "unscheduled DNA synthesis" and density labeling-determined "repair replication" (92, 93, 96, 98) (Table 4.6). However, xeroderma cells subjected to X-irradiation, which produces polynucleotide chain scissions, perform normal levels of repair (93). Since strand breaks induced by X-irradiation are not repairable by simple reformation of a phosphodiester link between apposed termini implying loss of DNA bases as well as simple phosphodiester bond scission (222), and since X irradiation damage

---

* Recent studies (378a) have shown that at least in some patients with xeroderma pigmentosum there was no detectable abnormality in UV-induced [³H]thymidine incorporation into DNA.

TABLE 4.6
RELATIVE LEVELS OF EXCISION REPAIR
FOUR HOURS AFTER UV IRRADIATION

Cell type	Percent of normal
Normal skin fibroblasts	100
Fibroblasts from 3 amniocenteses	103
HeLa cells (cervical carcinoma)	94
Xeroderma pigmentosum fibroblasts	
Heterozygotes	
XPHK[b]	100
XPH11 male	44,48
XPH11 female	47,42
XPH1	67,84,87
Homozygotes	
XPK male[b] } siblings	0
XPK female[b] } siblings	0
XP11	<4
XP1A[b] } siblings	9
XP1B } siblings	25
XP1W	0
XP7	5
XPJ	6
XP6	5

[a] Modified from Cleaver (95).
[b] deSanctis-Cacchione syndrome.

of DNA is also accompanied by repair replication, the inference made is that xeroderma cells possess the enzymes necessary for repair polymerization and joining of repaired stretches of DNA but lack the enzyme(s) needed to incise UV-damaged DNA near the photoproducts. Xerodema cells can repair X-irradiation damage since the DNA chains are already "open" at the point of damage but, lacking appropriate recognition-incision enzymes, are unable to perform UV-induced excision repair on DNA containing pyrimidine dimers (42, 93, 98, 235).

That the defect may be slightly more complicated than the above model is perhaps indicated by the fact that somatic cell hybrids between xeroderma and deSanctis-Cacchione syndrome fibroblasts can carry out repair synthesis (122) (Table 4.7). Since the data are based on labeled binucleated cells, and since there could be three classes of binucleated cells in a given fusion experiment, xeroderma cells from a female patient were fused with cells from a male deSanctis-Cacchione patient and subsequently binucleated cells in the hybrids were scored after atebrin staining to identify the truly hybrid binucleated cell. These data (last three lines in Table 4.7) demonstrate that most truly heterologous hybrid cells carry out repair synthesis; grain counts in the heterologous hybrids were similar to those in control irradiated cells. The data are reminiscent of intergenic complementation and suggest that two different genes might be involved in the basic defect in xeroderma pigmentosum and the deSanctis-Cacchione syndrome (122).

TABLE 4.7

DNA Repair in Repair Defective Somatic Human Cell Hybrids[a]

Strain	Origin	Labeled nuclei[b] post-UV-irradiation (%)
C2	Normal male	96
C3	Normal female	94
XP4	Xeroderma pigmentosum female	3
XP9	Xeroderma pigmentosum male	15
XP12	deSanctis-Cacchione syndrome male	3
XP16	Xeroderma pigmentosum male	4

Fusion	Labeled[b] binuclear cells (%)	
	Unirradiated	UV-irradiated
XP4 cells with XP4 cells	0	5
XP12 cells with XP12 cells	<2	0
XP4 cells with XP9 cells	<1	8
XP4 cells with XP16 cells	<1	2
XP9 cells with XP16 cells	<1	4
XP4 cells with XP12 cells	1	36[c]
XP9 cells with XP12 cells	<1	30[c]
XP16 cells with XP12 cells	<1	36[c]
XP4 cells with XP12 cells	—	8[d]
XP4 cells with XP12 cells	—	2[e]
XP4 cells with XP12 cells	—	87[f]

[a] From DeWeerd-Kastelein *et al.* (122).
[b] Grain counts exclude nuclei labeled by normal semiconservative synthesis.
[c] Based on percent of *all* labeled binucleated cells.
[d] Based on binucleated cells with both nuclei XX.
[e] Based on binucleated cells with both nuclei XY.
[f] Based on binucleated cells with one XX and one XY nucleus.

2. Postreplication Repair of UV-Damaged DNA

The evidence for postreplication repair of UV-lesions in mammalian DNA is not voluminous. Acriflavine inhibits repair replication in a number of systems (94) but has no specific effect on survival of UV-irradiated mouse L cells (371) which do not excise pyrimidine dimers (239). Caffeine, which has no effect on repair replication in HeLa cells, decreases the survival of UV-treated L cells only if present during the first S phase after irradiation despite the fact that repair replication can occur throughout the cell cycle. In Chinese hamster cells, which have only a very low level of dimer excision, the size of the single strands of DNA synthesized after irradiation decreases as a function of UV dose (99). In both control and irradiated cells, the pulse-labeled DNA is increasingly found in longer and longer lengths of DNA but the mechanisms for this probably differ since caffeine inhibits the "chase" into higher molecular weight DNA only in irradiated cells.

DNA synthesized after UV irradiation in mouse L5178 strain lymphoma cells, which cannot excise pyrimidine dimers, is smaller than "pulse DNA" made in unirradiated control cells (273). At a UV dose of 110 ergs/mm^2 randomly introduced pyrimidine dimers would be spaced apart about 9.5×10^6 daltons of DNA. The average molecular weight of the low molecular weight newly synthessized DNA fragments from the irradiated cells is about 12×10^6 daltons suggesting that the observed gaps in newly synthesized DNA might indeed be opposite pyrimidine dimers. If the irradiated cells are incubated for longer times after irradiation, the labeled DNA is "chased" into higher molecular weight DNA which indicates that the gaps resulting from replication of a dimer-containing template were somehow filled. The gaps could be closed by either a recombinational repair mechanism or by *de novo* synthesis utilizing the damaged template strand.

To determine which mechanism operates, irradiated cells were pulse labeled with TdR then incubated in 5-bromodeoxyuridine followed by exposure to light of wavelength 313 nm (273). DNA is selectively disrupted at bromouracil loci by exposure to 313 nm radiation. If recombination is responsible for the observed repair, the gap will be closed with parental thymidine-containing DNA and the molecular weight distribution after 313 nm irradiation will be the same in control and irradiated cultures. If gap closure proceeds by *de novo* synthesis, then the labeled gapped DNA will be closed with newly synthesized bromouracil-containing DNA. After 313 nm radiation, the UV-irradiated DNA will again be disrupted into low molecular weight segments as if no gap closure had occurred. The results indicate that gap closure occurs via *de novo* synthesis utilizing the damaged strand of DNA as template, that recombination with sister duplex parental strand DNA does not occur, and that gaps of about 800 nucleotides in length are formed opposite pyrimidine dimers (273).

This study raises several questions, e.g., how does the *de novo* gap closure mechanism replicate the dimer? If gap closure occurs via *de novo* synthesis utilizing the damaged template, why is a gap produced at all during the initial semiconservative replication, e.g., is gap closure, therefore, accomplished by an enzyme system different from the enzyme system responsible for normal semiconservative replication?

3. Repair of Carcinogen-Modified DNA's

The relationship of DNA repair processes to carcinogenesis is most clearcut and direct in the case of xeroderma pigmentosum. The role of DNA repair in protection against or causation of cancer by chemical agents is, at this time, largely conjectural since the mechanism(s) of chemical carcinogenesis has not yet been delineated. However, a substantial body of evidence implicates the covalent interaction of chemical carcinogens with DNA as a necessary prerequisite for induction of neoplasia by these agents (Section V). Therefore, the ability of mammalian cells to detect and repair DNA covalently modified by chemical carcinogens may be of importance in the etiology and, conceivably, the prevention of neoplasia. Additionally, a large number of "classic" alkylating agents used in cancer chemotherapy are thought to be effective by virtue of their ability to form covalent cross-links between DNA bases and thus inhibit DNA synthesis in the dividing neoplastic cells. The ability of the neoplastic mammalian cell to repair alkylated DNA may, in these instances, influence the efficacy of chemotherapy. Most studies on repair of chemically modified mammalian DNA have been carried out using "direct" alkylating agents but a study of the repair of DNA modified with simple alkylating agents may be directly applicable to DNA covalently modified with more complex carcinogens such as 2-acetylaminofluorene and 4-nitroquinoline-1-oxide.

a. Evidence for Excision Repair and Recombinational Repair. The excision of alkylation products from DNA has been demonstrated in HeLa cells (118) and in a resistant line of mouse L cells (373) after treatment with sulfur mustard. Nonsemiconservative repair replication was noted following alkylation of DNA of HeLa cells (381) or mouse leukemic P388 cells (12) by methylmethanesulfonate. The autoradiographic equivalent of repair replication, i.e., "unscheduled DNA synthesis," has also been noted (180) following treatment of Chinese hamster cells with methylmethanesulfonate. A Chinese hamster cell line treated with either N-methyl-N'-nitro-N-nitrosoguanidine, N-methyl-N-nitrosourea, or methylmethanesulfonate (all of which give equal levels of reaction with DNA for equal levels of cell survival) exhibits the same degree of repair replication for all three agents (382). The loss of labeled methyl groups from the DNA of hamster cells treated with tritiated N-methyl-N'-nitro-N-nitrosoguanidine parallels the time course of repair replication and for each alkyl group excised, approximately 100 nucleotides were incorporated into DNA (382).

The exact mode of excision of alkyl lesions is not known with certainty. The great lability of the N-9 to C'-1 glycosidic linkage in N-7-substituted DNA-guanine and N-3-substituted DNA-adenine implies the "spontaneous" production of apurinic sites in alkylated DNA which can then undergo chain scission. Chains so broken might then be subject to the concerted action of exonucleases and gap-filling polymerase or the multiple actions of type I DNA polymerase. Endo-nucleases that specifically recognize alkylated sites in DNA and incise the DNA at or near these sites have been described in microbial systems (149, 428, 429). These observations in conjunction with studies of xeroderma cells cited below lead to the conclusion that alkylation lesions in DNA are repaired by an excision repair process like that demonstrable for UV lesions in mammalian DNA.

That yet another repair process is operative has been inferred from the observation that Yoshida sarcoma cells treated with difunctional alkylating agents had identical levels of excision of alkyl groups and identical levels of semiconservative repair synthesis even though one strain of cells was 20 times more sensitive to the alkylating agent (15). Furthermore, although HeLa cells and hamster cells have equivalent responses to sulfur mustard, they differ markedly in their biological response to N-methyl-N'-nitro-N-nitrosoguanidine and N-methyl-nitrosourea (383). The greater sensitivity of HeLa cells to these agents, however, does not reside in a lesser capacity for excision repair in HeLa cells since both the HeLa cells and hamster cells have equal levels of alkyl excision and nonsemiconservative repair synthesis for DNA containing equal levels of alkylation (382). The normal semiconservative replication of unrepaired or incompletely repaired alkylated DNA may be involved in the different sensitivities observed, and, in addition to excision repair, postreplication repair may be operative (361, 362, 379). A similar conclusion has been drawn on the basis of studies of HEp-2 cells treated with methylmethanesulfonate or various S-phase inhibitors of DNA synthesis (115, 430). Interestingly, caffeine increases the sensitivity of hamster cells to the effects of N-methylnitrosourea but has no detectable effect on nonsemiconservative repair replication (379). These results are reminiscent of the findings (see previous section) which pointed to postreplication repair mechanisms for UV-damaged mammalian DNA.

b. STUDIES IN XERODERMA PIGMENTOSUM CELLS. Additional insight into the repair of DNA modified with carcinogenic chemicals has recently come from *in vitro* studies with cells from xeroderma pigmentosum patients. Using autoradiographic (unscheduled DNA synthesis) and density labeling (repair replication) techniques, the response of normal human skin fibroblasts and xeroderma fibroblasts to methylmethanesulfonate and N-methyl-N'-nitro-N-nitrosoguanidine was studied (97). Xeroderma cells performed normal levels of repair replication after DNA alkylation. Since both alkylating agents induce nonenzymic breakage of DNA, it was concluded that the initial step in excision repair (recognition and endonucleolytic incision of DNA strands in the vicinity of damaged regions) was bypassed and the xeroderma cells were fully capable of carrying out subsequent steps in excision repair. However, other types of chemical modification are not repairable in xeroderma cells.

When normal human skin fibroblasts or cells from xeroderma patients were treated with N-acetoxy-2-acetylaminofluorene and then incubated with 5-bromodeoxyuridine, exposure of DNA from normal cells to 313 nm radiation resulted in extensive photolytic fragmentation of the DNA indicating the incorporation of 5-bromodeoxyuridine via repair synthesis. DNA from xeroderma cells exhibited no photolysis-induced DNA fragments suggesting that little or no repair replication occurred (403). "Unscheduled DNA synthesis" in skin fibroblasts from normal and xeroderma patients was studied after exposure to UV irradiation, 4-nitroquinoline-1-oxide, 2-acetylaminofluorene, N-hydroxy-2-acetylaminofluorene, N-acetoxy-2-acetylaminofluorene, and N-methyl-N'-nitro-N-nitrosoguanidine (426). Xeroderma cells, unlike normal control fibroblasts, were defective in "unscheduled DNA synthesis" elicited by UV irradiation, 4-nitroquinoline-1-oxide, or N-acetoxy-2-acetyl-aminofluorene. All xeroderma cell lines were able to respond to exposure to N-methyl-N'-nitro-N-nitrosoguanidine. The results confirm earlier work (97, 425) and again indicate that repair of some types of modification of DNA by carcinogens requires a recognition and polynucleotide strand incision step prior to repair synthesis.

4. RELEVANCE TO CARCINOGENESIS

Mammalian cells possess at least two mechanisms for repair of damage to their DNA induced by agents that cause strand breaks, abnormal photoproducts in DNA, or chemically modified bases in DNA. In the case of xeroderma pig-

mentosum, defective DNA repair is associated with heightened susceptibility
to UV-induced skin carcinogensis. Whether or not defective DNA repair mechanisms are the *sine qua non* for neoplastic transformation by a variety of oncogenic agents is uncertain. Established lines of neoplastic cells have apparently
normal DNA repair processes, but it is not difficult to imagine that in a population of cells exposed to carcinogenic chemicals or ionizing radiation, a lesion
in a crucial DNA site might escape repair and permit the establishment of
a stable alteration in DNA that in some unknown manner leads to transformation.
That defective DNA repair could also be involved in oncogenesis in the absence
of exogenous agents is suggested by the calculation that in the normal course
of existence at pH 7.4 and 37°C, as many as 100,000 purine bases might be
spontaneously "lost" from a mammalian cell's genome per cell generation (282).
The unscheduled repair seen in "normal" untreated HeLa cells (126) could
reflect the repair necessitated by "spontaneous" purine losses in normal cells.
It has also been suggested that DNA repair could conceivably enhance neoplastic
transformation by integration of oncogenic viral DNA into the host cell genome
(96).

VII. Reprise: DNA and Carcinogenesis

A. A Heuristic Model

This review of DNA "metabolism" clearly illustrates the still primitive state
of knowledge of the molecular biology of DNA synthesis, structure, and repair
even in "simpler" viral, bacteriophage, and microbial systems. Sections III,B
and IV reveal the very substantial gaps in our knowledge and the formidable
task of grappling with molecular aspects of "metabolism" in normal cells from
higher organisms.

It is, nevertheless, possible to address the issue of whether or not there
is a "cancer DNA" (73) as long as the reader is aware of the complexities
which such a simplifying concept inherently ignores. In fact, recent advances
in viral oncology (see below) tend to support the existence of DNA in the
genome of the neoplastic cell, the expression of which is the *sine qua non*
of the transformed state in those systems. One can speak of a "cancer DNA"
in the general sense of a heritable alteration induced in a cell genome by oncogenic agents resulting in the loss of control of those portions of the cell's genome
that specify and control the multiple processes that operate in cell division.
The "simple" act of one cell dividing into two genetically identical cells requires
the temporally coordinated interactions of hundreds of distinctly different metabolic pathways during the course of the cell cycle. How these coordinated
processes are controlled at the genomic level is not known. In a continuously
dividing cell population, one could construct a theoretical model in which, by a
kind of cyclical cascade effect, all the required processes are turned on and

off by positive and negative feedback networks at the appropriate times yielding two daughter cells in condition to begin another "cascade" through the cell cycle. Such a "semiautomatic" cascading system could be controlled at one or two crucial steps.

Chemical carcinogens might induce heritable neoplastic alterations by direct (protein modification) or indirect (modification of the cistron) production of "faulty" replicative DNA polymerase which in turn might produce DNA with heritable defects in the appropriate controlling segments. Direct chemical carcinogen modification of those control segments could establish a cell clone unresponsive to normal regulation and which would constantly generate new cells.

The probability of introducing chemical lesions into only a few critical base pairs in control regions out of perhaps 10^{10} base pairs in total human DNA may be vanishingly small at low doses of carcinogens, if (a) very few portions of the genome are involved at the control steps, (b) these portions do not show preferential interaction with chemical carcinogens, and (c) there are structural restraints that would preclude the random interaction of carcinogens with all target bases in DNA. One must add into this equation the knowledge that carcinogen-modified DNA may well be "detected" and repaired thus obviating the lesion. It is also possible that an innocuous base modification in or near critical control segments of the genome might be "detected" and repaired in an inaccurate manner in which case the repair processes might be termed the "ultimate carcinogen."

If very high doses are employed, the probability of hitting the critical targets is increased, but at the same time the incidence of additional lesions inimical to continued existence of the cell is also greatly increased. High doses of chemical carcinogens can elicit cellular proliferaton (see, e.g., 418) which could heritably "fix" base modifications into altered base sequences, as well as massive DNA repair (165) which could introduce heritable alterations by inaccurate repair. If there are no lethal ontogenetic alterations induced by the agent, and if repair processes have not detected and accurately repaired the critical adducted base(s) prior to their "transformation" into usual DNA bases, the quiescent cell can "cascade" with impunity.

The model predicts that neoplastic transformation may or may not be accompanied by alterations in cell karyotypes, depending on the extent of genomic alterations and subsequent repair, which thus accommodate those situations in which karyotypic changes occur and those in which neoplastic cells have normal karyotypes (e.g., 340).

B. Oncogenic Viruses and Host Cell DNA

A number of DNA-containing viruses—polyoma virus, simian virus 40 (SV40), and certain human adenoviruses—can nonlytically infect suitable host cells and, in so doing, alter the growth properties of the cells, changing their morphology, and, if the transformed cells are inoculated into a suitable host, result in tumor formation. The nonlytically infected cells do not produce virus yet the progeny of the infected cells maintain the transformed state, i.e., the oncogenic change wrought by the virus becomes heritable. Several lines of evidence have indicated that the viral genome or portions thereof persist in the nonlytically infected cell and its progeny in a manner akin to that observed in the lysogenic state of temperate bacteriophages. This evidence (492) includes: the detection of viral specific antigens in the nuclei of all transformed cells; the ability to recover infectious SV40 or polyoma virus (but not adenoviruses) from some transformed cells; and the identification by molecular hybridization techniques of the number of viral genome equivalents integrated into host cell DNA as well as the extent to which the integrated viral genetic material is transcribed. Although the mechanisms of integration of viral genetic material into host DNA and of the precise manner in which viral genetic expression transforms host cells such that control of cell replication is lost are not known, the oncogenicity of viral DNA integrated into host DNA could be accommodated by the model discussed above (see also Chapter XI).

Until quite recently the oncogenic transformation wrought by RNA tumor virions (oncornaviruses) was much more difficult to analyze. Viruses in this class include Rous sarcoma virus, murine leukemia virus, mouse mammary tumor virus, feline leukemia virus, and hamster leukemia virus among others. These viruses too can nonlytically infect cells, effect their transformation, and produce infectious virus. The infected cells appear capable of passing on to their progeny the information required for virus production and cell transformation. The "transferral" of viral RNA information into a DNA template was inferred from experiments demonstrating a requirement for DNA synthesis shortly after infection of the cells with Rous sarcoma virus (443, 444) and from nucleic acid hybridization studies which suggested homology between viral RNA and the DNA made soon after infection (444). Definitive proof of "transferral" was obtained by treating cells with 5-bromodeoxyuridine shortly after infection with the oncogenic RNA virus and subsequently exposing the cells to 313 nm radiation which destroys DNA containing the 5-bromodeoxyuridine. The "provirus" DNA was inactivated but not cellular DNA (14, 30).

RNA to DNA information transfer is catalyzed by an enzyme which catalyzes the polymerization of deoxyribonucleoside triphosphate precursors using RNA as a template (16, 447). Such RNA-dependent (or directed) DNA polymerase activity—also termed reverse transcriptase—has been detected in leukemia and sarcoma virions from various animals, from mammary tumor virions from mice, rats, and monkeys, as well as in cells from patients with acute lymphocytic leukemia (156, 157). The occurrence of RNA-directed DNA polymerase has been noted in a number of normal nonneoplastic human cell lines (e.g., 398) and it has been proposed that RNA-directed DNA synthesis in uninfected cells might represent a normal cellular mechanism for amplification of DNA and could play a role in cell differentiation (446, 448).

With respect to viral oncogenesis, however, the virion-associated reverse transcriptase catalyzes the synthesis of a DNA complementary to the single-stranded RNA forming a RNA-DNA hybrid which in turn is used as template for synthesis of a duplex DNA. The duplex DNA is then presumably integrated into the host genome where it is inherited, can direct synthesis of new viral RNA, and can somehow alter the normal controls on cell replication. As was the case with oncogenic DNA viruses, little is known of the exact mechanisms of integration and of the cell-transforming functions (see Chapter XI).

Recent studies with temperature-sensitive mutants of oncogenic viruses tend to support a specific mechanism of transformation (130, 307). Suitable host cells when infected by the temperature-sensitive mutant exhibit all the manifestations of transformation at the permissive temperature of growth, but when shifted to the restrictive temperature, revert to the nontransformed state. The mutant virus apparently codes for a temperature-sensitive factor which at the permissive temperature, somehow interacts with the normal regulatory mechanisms to elicit the transformed state. At the restrictive temperature, viral gene product is defective and unable to effect this alteration of control mechanisms.

Whether or not there is a direct relationship between chemical and viral carcinogenesis is still open to question. DNA repair processes, perhaps stimulated by carcinogen-induced lesions, might accidentally result in integration of the available oncogenic DNA (from DNA or RNA viruses) (96). Others (203) have postulated the existence of a vertically transmitted "oncogene" in every cell which, when derepressed in some unknown manner by a virus, carcinogen, or radiation, produces gene products that elicit transformation. Infectious viruses

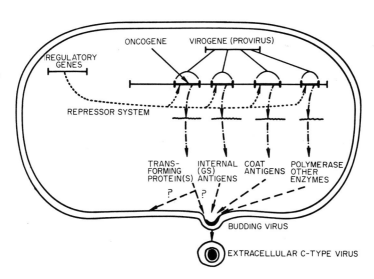

Fig. 4.26. A model illustrating the oncogene hypothesis which proposes that tumors are produced by transforming proteins which are coded for by an oncogene which in turn is part of a larger structure termed the virogene. The entire unit is postulated to be integrated in the DNA of most, if not all, cells and vertically passed from generation to generation. Derepression of the virogene yields a cell that produces a complete tumor virus; derepression of the oncogene portion of the virogene yields protein(s) that transform the cell into a neoplastic state. Normal cells produce repressor(s) that maintain the integrated onco/virogene in a repressed state. Presumably, induced or spontaneous neoplasia results from disruption of this repressor system. From Science **177,** 45 (1972) and reproduced with permission.

need not necessarily be produced (Fig. 4.26). Further studies on possible relationships between viral and chemical carcinogenesis will be highly interesting from the standpoint of mechanisms of carcinogenesis (Chapters X and XI).

References

1. Aaronson, S. A., and Lytle, C. D. (1970). *Nature. (London)* **228**, 359–361.
2. Adams, R. L. P. (1971). *Biochim. Biophys. Acta* **254**, 205–212.
3. Alberts, B. M. (1971). *In* "Nucleic Acid-Protein Interactions. Nucleic Acid Synthesis in Viral Infection" (D. W. Ribbons, J. F. Woessner, and J. Schultz, eds.), pp. 128–143. North Holland Publ., Amsterdam.
4. Allfrey, V. G. (1971). *In* "Histones and Nucleohistones" (D. M. P. Phillips, ed.), pp. 241–294. Plenum Press, London.
5. Ames, B. N., Sims, P., and Grover, P. L. (1972). *Science* **176**, 47–48.
6. Ames, B. N., Gurney, E. G., Miller, J. A., and Bartsch, H. (1972). *Proc. Nat. Acad. Sci. U.S.* **69**, 3128–3133.
7. Anderson, T. J., and Burdon, R. H. (1970). *Cancer Res.* **30**, 1773–1781.
8. Arber, W., and Linn, S. (1969). *Annu. Rev. Biochem.* **38**, 467–500.
9. Arrighi, F. E., and Hsu, T. C. (1971). *Cytogenetics* **10**, 81–86.
10. Arrighi, F. E., Saunders, P. P., Saunders, G. F., and Hsu, T. C. (1971). *Experientia* **27**, 964–966.
11. Avery, O. T., MacLeod, C. M., and McCarty, M. (1944). *J. Exp. Med.* **79**, 137–158.
12. Ayad, S. R., Fox, M., and Fox, B. W. (1969). *Mutat. Res.* **8**, 639–645.
13. Bach, M. K. (1962). *Proc. Nat. Acad. Sci. U.S.* **48**, 1031–1035.
13a. Balazs, I., and Schildkraut, C. L. (1971). *J. Mol. Biol.* **57**, 153–158.
14. Balduzzi, P., and Morgan, H. R. (1970). *J. Virol.* **5**, 470–477.
15. Ball, C. R., and Roberts, J. J. (1970). *Chem. Biol. Interact.* **2**, 321–329.
16. Baltimore, D. (1970). *Nature (London)* **226**, 1209–1211.
17. Baril, E. F., Jenkins, M. D., Brown, O. E., and Laszlo, J. (1970). *Science* **169**, 87–89.
18. Baril, E. F., Brown, O. E., and Laszlo, J. (1971). *Biochem. Biophys. Res. Commun.* **43**, 754–759.
19. Baril, E. F., Brown, O. E., Jenkins, M. D., and Laszlo, J. (1971). *Biochemistry* **10**, 1981–1992.
20. Baril, E. F., Baril, B., and Elford, H. (1972). *Proc. Amer. Ass. Cancer Res.* **13**, 84.
21. Beers, R. F., Herriott, R. M., and Tilgham, R. C. (eds.) (1972). "Molecular and Cellular Repair Processes." Johns Hopkins Univ. Press, Baltimore, Maryland.
22. Behki, R. M., and Schneider, W. C. (1963). *Biochim. Biophys. Acta* **68**, 34–44.
23. Bell, E. (1969). *Nature (London)* **224**, 326–328.
24. Bellair, J. T. (1968). *Biochim. Biophys. Acta* **161**, 119–124.
25. Ben-Porat, T., Stere, A., and Kaplan, A. S. (1962). *Biochim. Biophys. Acta* **61**, 150–152.
26. Berger, H., Huang, R. C. C., and Irvine, J. L. (1971). *J. Biol. Chem.* **246**, 7275–7283.
27. Beukers, R., Ijlstra, J., and Berends, W. (1960). *Rec. Trav. Chim.* **79**, 101–104.
28. Billen, D. (1968). *J. Mol. Biol.* **31**, 477–486.
29. Billen, D., Hewitt, R. R., Lapthisophon, T., and Achey, P. M. (1967). *J. Bacteriol.* **94**, 1538–1545.
30. Boettiger, D., and Temin, H. M. (1970). *Nature (London)* **228**, 622–624.
31. Boivin, A., Vendrely, R., and Vendrely, C. (1948). *C. R. Sci. Acad. Sci.* **226**, 1061–1063.
32. Bollum, F. J. (1960). *J. Biol. Chem.* **235**, 2399–2403.
33. Bollum, F. J. (1962). *J. Biol. Chem.* **237**, 1945–1949.
34. Bollum, F. J. (1963). *Cold Spring Harbor Symp. Quant. Biol.* **28**, 21–26.
35. Bollum, F. J. (1963). *J. Cell. Comp. Physiol. Suppl.* 1 **62**, 61–71.

36. Bollum, F. J., and Potter, V. R. (1957). *J. Amer. Chem. Soc.* **79**, 3603–3604.
37. Bollum, F. J., and Potter, V. R. (1958). *J. Biol. Chem.* **233**, 478–482.
38. Bollum, F. J., and Potter, V. R. (1959). *Cancer Res.* **19**, 561–565.
39. Bollum, F. J., Groeniger, E., and Yoneda, M. (1964). *Proc. Nat. Acad. Sci. U.S.* **51**, 853–859.
40. Bond, H. E., Cooper, J. A., Courington, D. P., and Wood, J. S. (1969). *Science* **165**, 705–706.
41. Bonner, J., Dahmus, M. E., Fambrough, D., Huang, R. C., Marushige, K., and Tuan, D. Y. H. (1968). *Science* **159**, 47–56.
42. Bootsma, D., Mulder, M. P., Pot, F., and Cohen, J. A. (1970). *Mutat. Res.* **9**, 507–516.
43. Borek, E. (Ed.) (1971). *Cancer Res.* **31**, 591–721.
44. Borek, E., and Srinivasan, P. R. (1966). *Ann. Rev. Biochem.* **35**, 275–298.
45. Bostock, C. J., and Prescott, D. M. (1971). *Exp. Cell Res.* **64**, 267–274.
46. Bostock, C. J., and Prescott, D. M. (1971). *Exp. Cell Res.* **64**, 481–484.
47. Bostock, C. J., and Prescott, D. M. (1971). *J. Mol. Biol.* **60**, 151–162.
48. Botchan, M., Kram, R., Schmid, C. W., and Hearst, J. E. (1971). *Proc. Nat. Acad. Sci. U.S.* **68**, 1125–1129.
49. Boveri, T. (1929). "The Origin of Malignant Tumors." Williams and Wilkins, Baltimore, Maryland.
50. Boyce, R. P., and Howard-Flanders, P. (1964). *Proc. Nat. Acad. Sci. U.S.* **51**, 293–300.
51. Boyland, E. (1950). *Symp. Biochem. Soc.* **5**, 40–54.
52. Boyland, E. (1969). *In* "Physico-Chemical Mechanisms in Carcinogenesis" (E. D. Bergmann and B. Pullman, eds.), pp. 25–44. Israeli Acad. of Sci. and Humanities, Jerusalem.
53. Boyle, J. M. (1972). *In* "Molecular and Cellular Repair Processes" (R. F. Beers, R. M. Herriott, and R. C. Tilgham, Eds.), pp. 14–33. Johns Hopkins Univ. Press, Baltimore, Maryland.
54. Boyle, J. M., Patterson, M. C., and Setlow, R. B. (1970). *Nature (London)* **226**, 708–710.
55. Bradbury, E. M., and Crane-Robinson, C. (1971). *In* "Histones and Nucleohistones" (D. M. Phillips, ed.), pp. 85–134. Plenum Press, New York.
56. Bram, S. (1971). *Nature New Biol.* **232**, 174–176.
57. Bram, S., and Ris, H. (1971). *J. Mol. Biol.* **55**, 325–336.
58. Bresnick, E. (1971). *In* "Methods in Cancer Research" (H. Busch, ed.), Vol. VI, pp. 347–397. Academic Press, New York.
59. Brookes, P. (1971). *Biochem. Pharm.* **20**, 999–1003.
60. Brookes, P., and Lawley, P. D. (1964). *Nature (London)* **202**, 781–784.
61. Brookes, P., and Dipple, A. (1969). *In* "Physicochemical Mechanisms in Carcinogenesis" (E. D. Bergmann and B. Pullman, eds.), pp. 139–148. Israeli Acad. of Sci. and Humanities, Jerusalem.
62. Brutlag, D., and Kornberg, A. (1972). *J. Biol. Chem.* **247**, 241–248.
63. Brutlag, D., Atkinson, M. R., Setlow, P., and Kornberg, A. (1969). *Biochem. Biophys. Res. Commun.* **37**, 982–989.
64. Brutlag, D., Schekman, R., and Kornberg, A. (1971). *Proc. Nat. Acad. Sci. U.S.* **68**, 2826–2829.
65. Bucciarelli, E. (1966). *J. Cell. Biol.* **30**, 664–665.
66. Bucher, N. L. R. (1963). *Int. Rev. Cytol.* **15**, 245–300.
67. Burdon, R. H., and Adams, R. L. P. (1969). *Biochim. Biophys. Acta* **174**, 322–329.
68. Burgoyne, L. A., Waquar, M. A., and Atkinson, M. R. (1970). *Biochem. Biophys. Res. Commun.* **39**, 254–259.
69. Burnotte, J., and Verly, W. E. (1972). *Biochim. Biophys. Acta* **262**, 449–452.
70. Burton, K. (1960). *Biochem. J.* **77**, 547–552.
71. Burton, K., and Peterson, G. B. (1960). *Biochem. J.* **75**, 17–27.
72. Busch, H. (1965). "The Histones and Other Nuclear Proteins." Academic Press, New York.
73. Busch, H. (1965). "Biochemistry of the Cancer Cell." Academic Press, New York.

74. Busch, H., and Smetana, K. (1970). "The Nucleolus." Academic Press, New York.
75. Buttin, G., and Wright, M. (1968). *Cold Spring Harbor Symp. Quant. Biol.* **33**, 259–268.
76. Cairns, J. (1963). *J. Mol. Biol.* **6**, 208–213.
77. Cairns, J. (1963). *Cold Spring Harbor Symp. Quant. Biol.* **28**, 43–46.
78. Cairns, J. (1966). *J. Mol. Biol.* **15**, 372–373.
79. Callan, H. G., and Tomlin, S. G. (1950). *Proc. Roy. Soc. London B* **137**, 367–378.
80. Chang, L. M. S. (1971). *Biochem. Biophys. Res. Commun.* **44**, 124–131.
81. Chang, L. M. S., and Bollum, F. J. (1970). *Proc. Nat. Acad. Sci. U.S.* **65**, 1041–1048.
82. Chang, L. M. S., and Bollum, F. J. (1971). *J. Biol. Chem.* **246**, 909–916.
83. Chang, L. M. S., and Bollum, F. J. (1971). *J. Biol. Chem.* **246**, 5835–5837.
84. Chang, L. M. S., and Bollum, F. J. (1972). *Biochemistry* **11**, 1264–1272.
85. Chang, L. M. S., and Bollum, F. J. (1972). *Science* **175**, 1116–1117.
86. Chargaff, E. (1950). *Experientia* **6**, 201–209.
87. Chargaff, E. (1955). *In* "The Nucleic Acids" (E. Chargaff and J. N. Davidson, eds.), Vol. 1, pp. 307–371. Academic Press, New York.
88. Chargaff, E. (1971). *Science* **172**, 637–642.
89. Chiu, J.-F., and Sung, S. C. (1970). *Biochim. Biophys. Acta* **209**, 34–42.
90. Chiu, J.-F., and Sung, S. C. (1972). *Biochem. Biophys. Res. Commun.* **46**, 1830–1836.
91. Clark, R. J., and Felsenfeld, G. (1971). *Nature New Biol.* **229**, 101–106.
92. Cleaver, J. E. (1968). *Nature (London)* **218**, 652–656.
93. Cleaver, J. E. (1969). *Proc. Nat. Acad. Sci. U.S.* **63**, 428–435.
94. Cleaver, J. E. (1969). *Radiat. Res.* **37**, 334–348.
95. Cleaver, J. E. (1970). *Int. J. Radiat. Biol.* **18**, 557–565.
96. Cleaver, J. E. (1971). *In* "Nucleic Acid Protein Interactions—Nucleic Acid Synthesis in Viral Infections" (D. W. Ribbons, J. F. Woessner and J. Schultz, eds.), pp. 87–111. North Holland Publ., Amsterdam.
97. Cleaver, J. E. (1971). *Mutat. Res.* **12**, 453–462.
98. Cleaver, J. E. (1972). *In* "Molecular and Cellular Repair Processes" (R. F. Beers, R. M. Herriott, and R. C. Tilgham, eds.), pp. 195–211. Johns Hopkins University Press, Baltimore, Maryland.
99. Cleaver, J. E., and Thomas, G. H. (1969). *Biochem. Biophys. Res. Commun.* **36**, 203–208.
100. Colburn, N. H., and Boutwell, R. K. (1968). *Cancer Res.* **28**, 653–660.
101. Comings, D. E. (1967). *J. Cell. Biol.* **35**, 699–708.
102. Comings, D. E. (1968). *Amer. J. Human Genet.* **20**, 440–460.
103. Comings, D. E. (1972). *Exp. Cell Res.* **71**, 106–112.
104. Comings, D. E., and Kakefuda, T. (1968). *J. Mol. Biol.* **33**, 225–229.
105. Comings, D. E., and Mattoccia, E. (1970). *Proc. Nat. Acad. Sci. U.S.* **67**, 448–455.
106. Comings, D. E., and Mattoccia, E. (1972). *Exp. Cell Res.* **71**, 113–131.
107. Comings, D. E., and Okada, T. A. (1970). *Exp. Cell Res.* **62**, 293–302.
108. Comings, D. E., and Riggs, A. D. (1971). *Nature (London)* **223**, 48–50.
109. Conney, A. H., Miller, E. C., and Miller, J. A. (1957). *J. Biol. Chem.* **228**, 753–766.
109a. Cook, J. S. (1972). *In* "Molecular and Cellular Repair Processes" (R. F. Beers, R. M. Herriott, and R. C. Tilgham, eds.), pp. 79–94. Johns Hopkins Univ. Press, Baltimore, Maryland.
110. Corbett, T. H., Heidelberger, C., and Dove, W. F. (1970). *Mol. Pharmacol.* **6**, 667–679.
111. Corneo, G., Ginelli, E., and Polli, E. (1968). *J. Mol. Biol.* **33**, 331–335.
112. Corneo, G., Ginelli, E., Soave, C., and Bernardi, G. (1968). *Biochemistry* **7**, 4373–4379.
113. Corneo, G., Ginelli, E., and Polli, E. (1970). *Biochemistry* **9**, 1565–1571.
114. Coudray, Y., Quetier, F., and Guille, E. (1970). *Biochim. Biophys. Acta* **217**, 259–267.
115. Coyle, M. B., and Strauss, B. S. (1969/1970). *Chem.-Biol. Interactions* **1**, 89–98.
116. Cozarelli, N. R., Kelly, R. B., and Kornberg, A. (1969). *J. Mol. Biol.* **45**, 513–531.
117. Craddock, V. M. (1971/1972). *Chem.-Biol. Interactions* **4**, 149–154.
118. Crathorn, A. R., and Roberts, J. J. (1969). *Nature (London)* **211**, 150–153.
119. Crick, F. H. C. (1971). *Nature (London)* **234**, 25–27.

119a. Datta, R. K., and Datta, B. (1969). *Exp. Mol. Pathol.* **10**, 129–140.
120. DeBellis, R. H., Benjamin, W., and Gellhorn, A. (1969). *Biochem. Biophys. Res. Commun.* **36**, 166–173.
121. DeLucia, P., and Cairns, J. (1969). *Nature (London)* **224**, 1164–1166.
122. De-Weerd-Kastelein, E. A., Keijzer, W., and Bootsma, D. (1972). *Nature New Biol.* **238**, 80–83.
123. Dingman, C. W., and Sporn, M. B. (1967). *Cancer Res.* **27**, 938–944.
124. Dipple, A., Lawley, P. D., and Brookes, P. (1968). *Eur. J. Cancer* **4**, 493–506.
125. Dipple, A., Brookes, P., Mackintosh, D. S., and Rayman, M. P. (1971). *Biochemistry* **10**, 4323–4330.
126. Djordevic, B., Evans, R. G., Perez, A. G., and Weill, M. K. (1969). *Nature (London)* **224**, 803–804.
127. Drahovsky, D., and Morris, N. R. (1971). *J. Mol. Biol.* **57**, 475–489.
128. Drahovsky, D., and Morris, N. R. (1971). *J. Mol. Biol.* **61**, 343–356.
129. Duerksen, J. D., and McCarthy, B. J. (1971). *Biochemistry* **10**, 1471–1478.
130. Dulbecco, R., and Eckhart, W. (1970). *Proc. Nat. Acad. Sci. U.S.* **67**, 1775–1781.
131. DuPraw, E. J. (1965). *Nature (London)* **206**, 338–343.
132. DuPraw, E. J. (1965). *Proc. Nat. Acad. Sci. U.S.* **53**, 161–168.
133. DuPraw, E. J. (1968). "Cell and Molecular Biology." Academic Press, New York.
134. DuPraw, E. J. (1970). "DNA and Chromosomes." Holt, New York.
135. Dürwald, H., and Hoffman-Berling, H. (1971). *J. Mol. Biol.* **58**, 755–773.
136. Dusenberg, D. B., and Uretz, R. B. (1972). *J. Cell. Biol.* **52**, 639–642.
137. Ellison, J. R., and Barr, H. V. (1972). *Chromosoma* **36**, 375–390.
138. Fahmy, O. G., and Fahmy, M. J. (1972). *Int. J. Cancer* **9**, 284–298.
139. Fahmy, O. G., and Fahmy, M. J. (1972). *Cancer Res.* **32**, 550–557.
139a. Fakan, S., Turner, G. N., Pagano, J. S., and Hancock, R. (1972). *Proc. Nat. Acad. Sci. U.S.* **69**, 2300–2305.
140. Fambrough, D. M. (1969). *In* "Handbook of Molecular Cytology" (A. Lima-de-Faria, ed.), pp. 437–471. North Holland Publ., Amsterdam.
141. Fansler, B., and Loeb, L. A. (1969). *Exp. Cell Res.* **57**, 305–310.
142. Feldherr, C. M. (1965). *J. Cell. Biol.* **25**, 43–53.
143. Flamm, W. G., Walker, P. M. B., and McCallum, M. (1969). *J. Mol. Biol.* **40**, 423–443.
144. Flamm, W. G., Walker, P. M. B., and McCallum, M. (1969). *J. Mol. Biol.* **42**, 441–455.
145. Flamm, W. G., Bernheim, J. M., and Brubaker, P. E. (1971). *Exp. Cell Res.* **64**, 97–104.
146. Franke, W. W. (1966). *J. Cell. Biol.* **31**, 619–623.
147. Franklin, R. E., and Gosling, R. G. (1953). *Nature (London)* **171**, 740–741.
148. Frenster, J. H. (1965). *Nature (London)* **206**, 680–683.
149. Friedberg, E. C., Hadi, S.-M., and Goldthwait, D. A. (1969). *J. Biol. Chem.* **244**, 5879–5889.
150. Freidman, D. L. (1970). *Biochem. Biophys. Res. Commun.* **39**, 100–109.
151. Friedman, D. L., and Mueller, G. C. (1969). *Biochim. Biophys. Acta* **174**, 253–263.
152. Fuchs, R., and Daune, M. (1971). *FEBS Lett.* **14**, 206–208.
153. Furlong, N. B. (1960). *Arch. Biochem. Biophys.* **87**, 154–155.
154. Furlong, N. B., and Gresham, C. (1971). *Tex. Rep. Biol. Med.* **29**, 75–82.
155. Gall, J. G. (1967). *J. Cell. Biol.* **32**, 391–399.
156. Gallo, R. C., Yang, S. S., and Ting, R. C. (1970). *Nature (London)* **228**, 927–929.
157. Gallo, R. C., Yang, S. S., Smith, R. G., Herrera, F., Ting, R. C., and Fujioka, S. (1971). *In* "Nucleic Acid Protein Interactions—Nucleic Acid Synthesis in Viral Infections" (D. W. Ribbons, J. F. Woessner, and J. Schultz, eds.), pp. 353–376. North Holland Publ., Amsterdam.
158. Ganesan, A. T. (1968). *Cold Spring Harbor Symp. Quant. Biol.* **33**, 45–57.
159. Garret, R. A. (1968). *J. Mol. Biol.* **38**, 249–250.
160. Gefter, M. L., Hirota, Y., Kornberg, T., Weschsler, J. A., and Barnoux, C. (1971). *Proc. Nat. Acad. Sci. U.S.* **68**, 3150–3153.

161. Gefter, M. L., Molineux, I. J., Kornberg, T., and Khorana, H. G. (1972). *J. Biol. Chem.* **247**, 3321–3326.
162. Gellert, M., Little, J. W., Oshinski, C. K., and Zimmerman, S. B. (1968). *Cold Spring Harbor Symp. Quant. Biol.* **33**, 21–26.
163. Gilbert, W. G., and Dressler, D. (1968). *Cold Spring Harbor Symp. Quant. Biol.* **33**, 473–484.
164. Gold, M., and Helleiner, C. W. (1964). *Biochim. Biophys. Acta* **80**, 193–203.
165. Goodman, J. I., and Potter, V. R. (1972). *Cancer Res.* **32**, 766–775.
166. Gottesman, M. E., and Canellakis, E. S. (1966). *J. Biol. Chem.* **241**, 4339–4352.
167. Goulian, M. (1968). *Cold Spring Harbor Symp. Quant. Biol.* **33**, 11–20.
168. Goulian, M. (1971). *Ann. Rev. Biochem.* **40**, 855–898.
169. Goulian, M. (1972). *In* "Progress in Nucleic Acid Research and Molecular Biology" (J. N. Davidson and W. E. Cohn, eds.), Vol. 12, pp. 29–48. Academic Press, New York.
170. Goulian, M., and Kornberg, A. (1967). *Proc. Nat. Acad. Sci. U.S.* **58**, 1723–1730.
171. Goulian, M., Kornberg, A., and Sinsheimer, R. L. (1967). *Proc. Nat. Acad. Sci. U.S.* **58**, 2321–2328.
172. Green, M., and Piña, M. (1962). *Virology* **17**, 603–604.
173. Green, M., Piña, M., and Chagoya, V. (1964). *J. Biol. Chem.* **239**, 1188–1197.
174. Greene, R., and Korn, D. (1970). *J. Biol. Chem.* **245**, 254–261.
175. Griffith, F. (1928). *J. Hyg.* **27**, 113–139.
176. Gross, J., and Gross, M. (1969). *Nature (London)* **224**, 1166–1168.
177. Gross, J. D., Karamata, P., and Hempstead, P. G. (1968). *Cold Spring Harbor Symp. Quant. Biol.* **33**, 307–312.
178. Guild, W. R. (1968). *Cold Spring Harbor Symp. Quant. Biol.* **33**, 142–143.
179. Gurley, L. R., and Hardin, J. M. (1968). *Arch. Biophys. Biochem.* **128**, 285–292.
180. Hahn, G. M., Yang, S.-J., and Parker, V. (1968). *Nature (London)* **220**, 1142–1144.
181. Hall, M. R., Meinke, W., Goldstein, D. A., and Lerner, R. A. (1971). *Nature New Biol.* **234**, 227–229.
182. Hanaoka, F., and Yamada, M. (1971). *Biochem. Biophys. Res. Commun.* **42**, 647–653.
183. Harel, J., Hanania, N., Tapiero, H., and Harel, L. (1968). *Biochem. Biophys. Res. Commun.* **33**, 696–701.
184. Harford, C. G., and Kornberg, A. (1958). *Fed. Proc.* **17**, 515.
185. Harm, W., Rupert, C. S., and Harm, H. (1972). *In* "Molecular and Cellular Repair Processes" (R. F. Beers, R. M. Herriott, and R. C. Telgham, eds.), pp. 53–63. Johns Hopkins Univ. Press, Baltimore, Maryland.
186. Haskell, E. H., and Davern, C. I. (1969). *Proc. Nat. Acad. Sci. U.S.* **64**, 1065–1071.
187. Haynes, R. H. (1966). *Radiat. Res. Suppl.* **6**, 1–24.
188. Hearst, J. E., and Botchan, M. (1970). *Ann. Rev. Biochem.* **39**, 151–182.
189. Hendler, S., Fürer, E., and Srinivasan, P. R. (1970). *Biochemistry* **9**, 4141–4153.
190. Hershey, A. D., and Chase, M. (1952). *J. Gen. Physiol.* **36**, 39–56.
191. Hill, R. N., and Yunis, J. J. (1967). *Science* **155**, 1120–1121.
192. Hirota, Y., Ryter, A., and Jacob, F. (1968). *Cold Spring Harbor Symp. Quant. Biol.* **33**, 677–693.
193. Hnilica, L. S., McClure, M. E., and Spelsberg, T. C. (1971). *In* "Histones and Nucleohistones" (D. M. Phillips, ed.), pp. 187–240. Plenum Press, New York.
194. Horikawa, M., Nikaido, O., and Sugahara, T. (1968). *Nature (London)* **218**, 489–491.
195. Hoshino, M. (1961). *Exp. Cell. Res.* **24**, 606–609.
196. Howard, A., and Pelc, S. R. (1953). *Heredity Suppl.* **6**, 261–273.
197. Howard-Flanders, P. (1968). *Ann. Rev. Biochem.* **37**, 175–200.
198. Howard-Flanders, P., and Boyce, R. P. (1966). *Radiat. Res. Suppl.* **6**, 156–184.
199. Howard-Flanders, P., and Rupp, W. P. (1972). *In* "Molecular and Cellular Repair Processes" (R. F. Beers, R. M. Herriott, and R. C. Tilgham, eds.), pp. 212–225. Johns Hopkins Univ. Press, Baltimore, Maryland.

200. Howk, R., and Wang, T. Y. (1969). *Arch. Biochem. Biophys.* **133**, 238–246.
201. Howk, R., and Wang, T. Y. (1970). *Arch. Biochem. Biophys.* **136**, 422–429.
202. Huberman, J. A., and Riggs, A. D. (1968). *J. Mol. Biol.* **32**, 327–341.
202a. Huberman, J. A., and Tsai, A. (1973). *J. Mol. Biol.* **75**, 5–12.
202b. Huberman, J. A., Tsai, A., and Deich, R. A. (1973). *Nature (London)* **241**, 32–36.
203. Huebner, R. J., and Todaro, G. J. (1969). *Proc. Nat. Acad. Sci. U.S.* **64**, 1087–1094.
204. Ikegami, S., Nemoto, N., Sato, S., and Sugimura, T. (1969/1970). *Chem.-Biol. Int.* **1**, 321–330.
205. Inman, R., Schildkraut, C. L., and Kornberg, A. (1965). *J. Mol. Biol.* **11**, 285–292.
206. Irving, C. C., Veazey, R. A., and Russell, L. T. (1969/1970). *Chem.-Biol. Int.* **1**, 19–26.
207. Itzhaki, R. (1971). *Biochem. Biophys. Res. Commun.* **41**, 25–32.
208. Itzhaki, R. (1971). *Biochem. J.* **122**, 583–592.
209. Itzhaki, R. (1971). *Biochem. J.* **125**, 221–224.
210. Iype, P. T., and Ockey, C. H. (1971/1972). *Chem.-Biol. Int.* **4**, 71–74.
211. Izawa, M., Allfrey, V. G., and Mirsky, A. E. (1963). *Proc. Nat. Acad. Sci. U.S.* **49**, 544–551.
212. Jacob, F., Brenner, S., and Cuzin, F. (1963). *Cold Spring Harbor Symp. Quant. Biol.* **28**, 329–348.
213. Jensen, R. H., and Davidson, N. (1966). *Biopolymers* **4**, 17–32.
214. Johns, E. W. (1971). *In* "Histones and Nucleohistones" (D. M. Phillips, ed.), pp. 1–45. Plenum Press, New York.
215. Johns, E. W. (1972). *Nature New Biol.* **237**, 87–88.
216. Jones, K. W. (1970). *Nature (London)* **225**, 912–915.
217. Josse, J., Kaiser, A. D., and Kornberg, A. (1961). *J. Biol. Chem.* **236**, 864–875.
218. Kajiwara, K., and Mueller, G. C. (1964). *Biochim. Biophys. Acta* **91**, 486–493.
219. Kalf, G. F., and Chih, J. J. (1968). *J. Biol. Chem.* **243**, 4904–4916.
220. Kanner, L., and Hanawalt, P. (1970). *Biochem. Biophys. Res. Commun.* **39**, 149–155.
221. Kaplan, J. C., Kushner, S. R., and Grossman, L. (1971). *Biochemistry* **10**, 3315–3324.
222. Kapp, D. S., and Smith, K. C. (1968). *Radiat. Res.* **35**, 515–516.
223. Kappler, J. W. (1969). *J. Cell. Physiol.* **75**, 21–32.
224. Kapuler, A. M., and Michelson, A. M. (1971). *Biochim. Biphys. Acta* **232**, 436–450.
225. Karasaki, S. (1970). *Cancer Res.* **30**, 1736–1742.
226. Kato, K.-I., Goncalves, J. M., Houts, G. F., and Bollum, F. J. (1967). *J. Biol. Chem.* **242**, 2780–2789.
227. Keir, H. M. (1965). *In* "Progress in Nucleic Acid Research and Molecular Biology" (J. N. Davidson and W. E. Cohn, eds.), Vol. 4, p. 81–128. Academic Press, New York.
228. Keir, H. M., and Gold, E. (1963). *Biochim. Biophys. Acta* **72**, 263–276.
229. Keir, H. M., and Smith, Sr. M. J. (1963). *Biochim. Biophys. Acta* **68**, 589–598.
230. Keir, H. M., Smellie, R. M. S., and Siebert, G. (1962). *Nature (London)* **196**, 752–754.
231. Kelly, R. B., Atkinson, M. R., Huberman, J. A., and Kornberg, A. (1969). *Nature (London)* **224**, 495–501.
232. Kidwell, W. R. (1972). *Biochim. Biophys. Acta* **269**, 51–61.
233. Kit, S. (1961). *J. Mol. Biol.* **3**, 711–716.
234. Kit, S. (1970). *In* "Metabolic Pathways" (D. M. Greenberg, ed.), 3rd ed., Vol. IV, pp. 69–275. Academic Press, New York.
235. Kleijer, W. J., Lohman, P. H. M., Mulder, M. P., and Bootsma, D. (1970). *Mutat. Res.* **9**, 517–523.
236. Kleinman, L., and Huang, R. C. C. (1971). *J. Mol. Biol.* **55**, 503–521.
237. Klenow, H., and Henningsen, I. (1970). *Proc. Nat. Acad. Sci. U.S.* **65**, 168–175.
238. Klenow, H., and Overgaard-Hansen, K. (1970). *FEBS Lett.* **6**, 25–27.
239. Klimek, M. (1966). *Photochem. Photobiol.* **5**, 603–607.
240. Knippers, R., and Strätling, W. (1970). *Nature (London)* **226**, 713–717.
241. Knippers, R., Ferdinand, F. J., and Strätling, W. (1972). *In* "Molecular and Cellular

Repair Processes" (R. F. Beers, R. M. Herriott, and R. C. Tilgham, eds.), pp. 34–44. Johns Hopkins Univ. Press, Baltimore, Maryland.

242. Kornberg, A. (1969). *Science* **163**, 1410–1418.
243. Kornberg, A. (1971). *In* "Nucleic Acid Protein Interactions. Nucleic Acid Synthesis in Viral Infection" (D. W. Ribbons, J. F. Woessner, and J. Schultz, eds.), pp. 3–24. North Holland Publ., Amsterdam.
244. Kornberg, A., Lehman, I. R., and Simms, E. S. (1956). *Fed. Proc.* **15**, 291–292.
245. Kornberg, A., Lehman, I. R., Bessman, M. J., and Simms, E. S. (1956). *Biochim. Biophys. Acta* **21**, 197–198.
246. Kornberg, T., and Gefter, M. L. (1970). *Biochem. Biophys. Res. Commun.* **40**, 1348–1355.
247. Kornberg, T., and Gefter, M. L. (1971). *Proc. Nat. Acad. Sci. U.S.* **68**, 761–764.
248. Kornprobst, M., Ramstein, J., and Leng, M. (1971). *Eur. J. Biochem.* **21**, 134–136.
249. Koshiba, K., Smetana, K., and Busch, H. (1970). *Exp. Cell Res.* **60**, 199–209.
250. Krakow, J. S., and Kammen, H. O. (1960). *Fed. Proc.* **19**, 307.
251. Krakow, J. S., Kammen, H. O., and Canellakis, E. S. (1961). *Biochim. Biophys. Acta* **53**, 52–64.
252. Krakow, J. S., Coutsogeorgopoulos, C., and Canellakis, E. S. (1962). Biochim. Biophys. Acta **55**, 639–650.
253. Kriek, E. (1969–1970). *Chem.-Biol. Int.* **1**, 3–17.
254. Kreik, E., and Emmelot, P. (1964). *Biochim. Biophys. Acta* **91**, 59–66.
255. Kriek, E., and Reitsma, J. (1971). *Chem.-Biol. Int.* **3**, 397–400.
256. Kriek, E., Miller, J. A., Juhl, U., and Miller, E. C. (1967). *Biochemistry* **6**, 177–182.
257. Kubinski, H., and Kasper, C. B. (1971). *Science* **171**, 201–203.
258. Kurnit, D. M., Schildkraut, C. L., and Maio, J. (1972). *Biochim. Biophys. Acta* **259**, 297–312.
259. Kushner, S. R., Kaplan, J. C., Ono, H., and Grossman, L. (1971). *Biochemistry* **10**, 3325–3334.
260. Lampert, F. (1971). *Nature New Biol.* **234**, 187–188.
261. Langridge, R. (1969). *J. Cell. Physiol.* **74**, Suppl. 1, 1–20.
262. Lark, C. (1968). *J. Mol. Biol.* **31**, 389–399.
263. Lark, C. (1968). *J. Mol. Biol.* **31**, 401–414.
264. Lark, K. G. (1969). *Ann. Rev. Biochem.* **38**, 569–604.
265. Lark, K. G. (1972). *J. Mol. Biol.* **64**, 47–60.
266. Lark, K., Consigli, R., and Toliver, A. (1971). *J. Mol. Biol.* **58**, 873–875.
267. Lawley, P. D. (1966). *In* "Progress in Nucleic Acid Research and Molecular Biology" (J. N. Davidson and W. E. Cohn, eds.), Vol. 5, pp. 89–131. Academic Press, New York.
268. Lawley, P. D. (1968). *Nature (London)* **218**, 580–581.
269. Lawley, P. D., and Brookes, P. (1961). *Nature (London)* **192**, 1081–1082.
270. Lawley, P. D., and Brookes, P. (1963). *Biochem. J.* **89**, 127–138.
271. Lawley, P. D., and Thatcher, C. J. (1970). *Biochem. J.* **116**, 693–707.
272. Lawley, P. D., Brookes, P., Magee, P. N., Craddock, V. M., and Swann, P. P. (1968). *Biochim. Biophys. Acta* **157**, 646–648.
273. Lehmann, A. R. (1972). *J. Mol. Biol.* **66**, 319–337.
274. Leng, M., Rosilio, C., and Boudet, J. (1969). *Biochim. Biophys. Acta* **174**, 574–584.
275. Lerner, R. A., Meinke, W., and Goldstein, D. A. (1971). *Proc. Nat. Acad. Sci. U.S.* **68**, 1212–1216.
276. Levine, A. S., Nesbit, N. E., White, J. G., and Yarbro, J. W. (1968). *Cancer Res.* **28**, 831–844.
277. Levis, A. G., Krsmanovic, V., Miller-Faures, A., and Errera, M. (1967). *Eur. J. Biochem.* **3**, 57–69.
278. Li, H. J., and Bonner, J. (1971). *Biochemistry* **10**, 1461–1470.
279. Lima-de-Faria, A. (1969). *In* "Handbook of Molecular Cytology" (A. Lima-de-Faria, ed.), pp. 277–325. North Holland Publ., Amsterdam.
280. Lima-de-Faria, A., and Jaworska, H. (1968). *Nature (London)* **217**, 138–142.

281. Lima-de-Faria, A., and Reitalu, J. (1963). *J. Cell Biol.* **16**, 315–322.
282. Lindahl, T. (1972). *In* "Molecular and Cellular Repair Processes" (R. F. Beers, R. M. Herriott, and R. C. Tilgham, eds.), pp. 3–13. Johns Hopkins Univ. Press, Baltimore, Maryland.
283. Lindahl, T., and Edelman, G. M. (1968). *Proc. Nat. Acad. Sci. U.S.* **61**, 680–687.
284. Littau, V. C., Burdick, C. J., Allfrey, V. G., and Mirsky, A. E. (1965). *Proc. Nat. Acad. Sci. U.S.* **54**, 1204–1212.
285. Littlefield, J. W., McGovern, A. P., and Margerson, K. B. (1963). *Proc. Nat. Acad. Sci. U.S.* **49**, 102–107.
286. Locher, J., Goldblatt, P. J., and Leighton, J. (1968). *Cancer Res.* **28**, 2039–2050.
287. Loeb, L. A. (1969). *J. Biol. Chem.* **244**, 1672–1681.
288. Loeb, L. A., and Fansler, B. (1970). *Biochim. Biophys. Acta* **217**, 50–55.
289. Loeb, L. A., Fansler, B., Williams, R., and Mazia, D. (1969). *Exp. Cell Res.* **57**, 298–304.
290. Long, G. L., and Garren, L. D. (1972). *Biochem. Biophys. Res. Commun.* **46**, 1228–1235.
291. Loveless, A. (1959). *Proc. Roy. Soc. London B.* **150**, 497–508.
292. Loveless, A. (1969). *Nature (London)* **223**, 206–207.
293. Löwdin, P. O. (1969). *In* "Physico-Chemical Mechanisms of Carcinogenesis" (E. D. Bergman and B. Pullman, eds.), pp. 203–207. Israeli Acad. of Sci. and Humanities, Jerusalem.
294. Ludlum, D. B. (1970). *J. Biol. Chem.* **245**, 477–482.
295. Ludlum, D. B. (1970). *Biochim. Biophys. Acta* **213**, 142–148.
296. Ludlum, D. B. (1971). *Biochim. Biophys. Acta* **247**, 412–418.
297. Ludlum, D. B., and Wilhelm, R. C. (1968). *J. Biol. Chem.* **243**, 2750–2753.
298. Magee, P. N., and Barnes, J. M. (1967). *Advan. Cancer Res.* **10**, 163–246.
299. Magee, W. E. (1962). *Virology* **17**, 604–607.
300. Maher, V. M., Miller, E. C., Miller, J. A., and Szybalski, W. (1968). *Mol. Pharm.* **4**, 411–426.
301. Maher, V. M., Lesko, S. A., Straat, O. A., and Tso, P. O. P. (1971). *J. Bact.* **108**, 202–212.
302. Maio, J. (1971). *J. Mol. Biol.* **56**, 579–595.
303. Maio, J., and Schildkraut, C. L. (1969). *J. Mol. Biol.* **40**, 203–216.
304. Mamet-Bratley, M. P. (1971). *Biochim. Biophys. Acta* **247**, 233–242.
305. Mantsavinos, R. (1964). *J. Biol. Chem.* **239**, 3431–3435.
306. Mantsavinos, R., and Canellakis, E. S. (1959). *J. Biol. Chem.* **234**, 628–635.
307. Martin, G. S. (1970). *Nature (London)* **227**, 1021–1023.
308. Masui, H. and Garren, L. D. (1970). *J. Biol. Chem.* **245**, 2627–2632.
309. Mattoccia, E., and Comings, D. E. (1971). *Nature New Biol.* **229**, 175–176.
310. McCarthy, B. J. (1967). *Bact. Rev.* **31**, 215–229.
311. McClure, M. E., and Hnilica, L. S. (1970). *Abstract, Int. Cancer Congr. 10th Houston* #441.
312. McConnell, B., and von Hippel, P. H. (1970). *J. Mol. Biol.* **50**, 317–332.
313. Merriam, R. W. (1962). *J. Cell. Physiol.* **12**, 79–90.
314. Meselson, M. S., and Stahl, F. W. (1958). *Proc. Nat. Acad. Sci. U.S.* **44**, 671–682.
315. Meyer, R. R., and Simpson, M. V. (1968). *Proc. Nat. Acad. Sci. U.S.* **61**, 130–137.
316. Michelson, A. M., and Pochon, F. (1972). *Biochimie* **51**, 17–24.
317. Michelson, A. M., Kapuler, A. M., and Pochon, F. (1972). *Biochim. Biophys. Acta* **262**, 441–448.
318. Miller, E. C., and Miller, J. A. (1947). *Cancer Res.* **7**, 468–480.
319. Miller, E. C., and Miller, J. A. (1952). *Cancer Res.* **12**, 547–556.
320. Miller, E. C., Juhl, U., and Miller, J. A. (1966). *Science* **153**, 1125–1127.
321. Miller, J. A. (1970). *Cancer Res.* **30**, 559–576.
322. Miller, J. A., and Miller, E. C. (1969). *In* "Physico-Chemical Mechanisms of Carcinogenesis" (E. D. Bergmann and B. Pullman, eds.), pp. 237–261. Israeli Acad. of Sci. and Humanities, Jerusalem.

323. Miller, J. A., and Miller, E. C. (1971). *J. Nat. Cancer Inst.* **47**, v–xiv.
324. Mirsky, H. E., and Ris, H. (1949). *Nature (London)* **163**, 666–667.
325. Mitra, S., and Kornberg, A. (1966). *J. Gen. Physiol.* **49**, 59–78.
326. Mizuno, N. S., Stoops, C. E., and Pfeiffer, R. L. (1971). *J. Mol. Biol.* **59**, 517–525.
327. Mizuno, N. S., Stoops, C. E., and Sinha, A. A. (1971). *Nature New Biol.* **229**, 22–24.
328. Monesi, V. (1969). *In* "Handbook of Molecular Cytology" (A. Lima-de-Faria, ed.), pp. 472–499. North-Holland Publ., Amsterdam.
329. Mordoh, J., Hirota, Y., and Jacob, F. (1970). *Proc. Nat. Acad. Sci. U.S.* **67**, 773–778.
330. Morgan, A. R. (1970). *Nature* **227**, 1310–1313.
331. Morris, N. R., and Pih, K. D. (1971). *Cancer Res.* **31**, 433–440.
332. Moses, R. E., and Richardson, C. C. (1970). *Proc. Nat. Acad. Sci. U.S.* **67**, 674–681.
333. Moses, R. E., and Richardson, C. C. (1970). *Biochem. Biophys. Res. Commun.* **41**, 1557–1564.
334. Moses, R. E., and Richardson, C. C. (1970). *Biochem. Biophys. Res. Commun.* **41**, 1565–1571.
335. Moses, R. E., Campbell, J. L., Fleischman, R. A., and Richardson, C. C. (1971). *In* "Nucleic Acid-Protein Interaction. Nucleic Acid Synthesis in Viral Infection" (D. W. Ribbons, J. F. Woessner and J. Schultz, eds.), pp. 48–66. North Holland Publ., Amsterdam.
336. Mueller, G. C., and Kajiwara, K. (1966). *Biochem. Biophys. Acta* **114**, 108–115.
337. Murray, K. (1965). *Ann. Rev. Biochem.* **34**, 209–246.
338. Nagata, T. (1963). *Cold Spring Harbor Symp. Quant. Biol.* **28**, 55–57.
339. Nandi, U. S., Wang, J. C., and Davidson, N. (1965). *Biochemistry* **4**, 1687–1696.
340. Nowell, P. C., Potter, V. R., and Morris, H. P. (1967). *Cancer Res.* **27**, 1565–1579.
341. O'Brien, R. L., Sanyal, A. B., and Stanton, R. H. (1972). *Exp. Cell Res.* **70**, 106–112.
342. Ockey, C. H. (1972). *Exp. Cell Res.* **70**, 203–213.
343. Okazaki, R., Okazaki, T., Sakabe, K., Sugimoto, K., and Sugino, A. (1968). *Proc. Nat. Acad. Sci. U.S.* **59**, 598–605.
344. Okazaki, R., Okazaki, T., Sukabe, K., Sugimoto, K., Kainuma, R., Sugino, A., and Iwatsuki, N. (1968). *Cold Spring Harbor Symp. Quant. Biol.* **33**, 129–142.
345. Okazaki, R., Sugimoto, K., Okazaki, T., Imae, Y., and Sugino, A. (1970). *Nature (London)* **228**, 223–226.
346. Olins, D. E. (1969). *J. Mol. Biol.* **43**, 439–460.
347. Olins, D. E., and Olins, A. L. (1972). *J. Cell Biol.* **53**, 715–736.
348. Ove, P., Jenkins, M. D., and Laszlo, J. (1969). *Biochem. Biophys. Acta* **174**, 629–635.
349. Ove, P., Jenkins, M. D., and Laszlo, J. (1970). *Cancer Res.* **30**, 535–539.
350. Painter, R. B., and Cleaver, J. E. (1969). *Radiat. Res.* **37**, 451–466.
351. Painter, R. B., and Schaeffer, A. W. (1969). *Nature (London)* **221**, 1215–1217.
352. Painter, R. B., and Schaeffer, A. W. (1971). *J. Mol. Biol.* **58**, 289–295.
353. Palau, J., Pardon, J. F., and Richards, B. M. (1967). *Biochim. Biophys. Acta* **138**, 633–636.
354. Pardon, J. F., Wilkins, M. H. F., and Richards, B. M. (1967). *Nature (London)* **215**, 508–509.
355. Pardue, M. L., and Gall, J. G. (1970). *Science* **168**, 1356–1358.
356. Patel, G., Howk, R., and Wang, T. Y. (1967). *Nature (London)* **215**, 1488–1489.
357. Pettijohn, D., and Hanawalt, P. (1964). *J. Mol. Biol.* **9**, 395–410.
358. Phillips, D. M. (ed.) (1971). "Histones and Nucleohistones." Plenum Press, New York.
359. Phillips, D. M. (1971). *In* "Histones and Nucleohistones" (D. M. Phillips, ed.), pp. 47–83. Plenum Press, New York.
360. Pitot, H., and Heidelberger, C. (1963). *Cancer Res.* **23**, 1694–1700.
361. Plant, J. E., and Roberts, J. J. (1971). *Chem.-Biol. Int.* **3**, 337–342.
362. Plant, J. E., and Roberts, J. J. (1971). *Chem.-Biol. Int.* **3**, 343–351.
363. Pochon, F., and Michelson, A. M. (1971). *Eur. J. Biochem.* **21**, 144–153.
364. Pochon, F., Brookes, P., and Michelson, A. M. (1971). *Eur. J. Biochem.* **21**, 154–160.
365. Poirer, L. A., Miller, J. A., Miller, E. C., and Sato, K. (1967). *Cancer Res.* **27**, 1600–1613.
366. Pullman, A., and Pullman, B. (1969). *In* "Physicochemical Mechanisms of Carcinogene-

sis" (E. D. Bergmann and B. Pullman, eds.), pp. 9–24. Israeli Acad. Sci. and Humanities, Jerusalem.

367. Puschendorf, B., Wolf, H., and Grünicke, H. (1971). *Biochem. Pharm.* **20**, 3039–3050.
368. Rabson, A. S., Tyrell, S. A., and Legallais, F. Y. (1969). *Proc. Soc. Exp. Biol. Med.* **132**, 802–806.
369. Rae, P. M. M. (1970). *Proc. Nat. Acad. Sci. U.S.* **67**, 1018–1025.
370. Ramstein, J., Helene, C., and Leng, M. (1971). *Eur. J. Biochem.* **21**, 125–136.
371. Rauth, A. M. (1967). *Radiat. Res.* **31**, 121–138.
372. Regan, J. D., Trosko, J. E., and Carrier, W. L. (1968). *Biophys. J.* **8**, 319–325.
373. Reid, B. D., and Walker, I. G. (1969). *Biochim. Biophys. Acta* **179**, 179–188.
374. Research News (1972). *Science* **177**, 44–47.
375. Rhaese, H. J., and Freese, E. (1969). *Biochim. Biophys. Acta* **190**, 418–433.
376. Richards, B. M., and Pardon, J. F. (1970). *Exp. Cell Res.* **62**, 184–196.
377. Richardson, C. C. (1969). *Ann. Rev. Biochem.* **38**, 795–840.
378. Ris, H. (1961). *Can. J. Genet. Cytol.* **3**, 95–120.
378a. Robbins, J. H., and Burk, P. G. (1973). *Cancer Res.* **33**, 929–935.
379. Roberts, J. J. (1972). In "Molecular and Cellular Repair Processes" (R. F. Beers, R. M. Herriott, and R. C. Tilgham, eds.), pp. 226–238. Johns Hopkins Univ. Press, Baltimore, Maryland.
380. Roberts, J. J., and Warwick, G. P. (1963). *Biochem. Pharm.* **12**, 1441–1442.
381. Roberts, J. J., Crathorn, A. R., and Brent, J. P. (1968). *Nature (London)* **218**, 970–972.
382. Roberts, J. J., Pascoe, J. M., Smith, B. A., and Crathorn, A. R. (1971). *Chem.-Biol. Int.* **3**, 49–68.
383. Roberts, J. J., Pascoe, J. M., Plant, J. E., Sturrock, J. E., and Crathorn, A. R. (1971). *Chem.-Biol. Int.* **3**, 29–47.
384. Roychoudhury, R., and Bloch, D. P. (1969). *J. Biol. Chem.* **244**, 3359–3368.
385. Roychoudhury, R., and Bloch, D. P. (1969). *J. Biol. Chem.* **244**, 3369–3374.
386. Ruddon, R. W., and Johnson, J. M. (1968). *Mol. Pharm.* **4**, 258–273.
387. Rupert, C. S., Harm, W., and Harm, W. (1972). In "Molecular and Cellular Repair Processes" (R. F. Beers, R. M. Herriott and R. C. Tilgham, eds.), pp. 64–78. Johns Hopkins Univ. Press, Baltimore, Maryland.
388. Salganik, R. I., Morozora, T. M., and Zakharov, M. A. (1969). *Biochim. Biophys. Acta* **174**, 755–757.
389. Sanger, F., Brownlee, G. G., and Barrell, B. G. (1965). *J. Mol. Biol.* **13**, 373–398.
390. Sato, S., Tanaka, M., and Sugimura, T. (1970). *Biochim. Biophys. Acta* **209**, 43–48.
391. Saunders, G. F., Shirakawa, S., Saunders, P. P., Arrighi, F. E., and Hsu, T. C. (1972). *J. Mol. Biol.* **63**, 323–334.
392. Schandl, E. K., and Taylor, J. H. (1969). *Biochem. Biophys. Res. Commun.* **34**, 291–300.
393. Schandl, E. K., and Taylor, J. H. (1971). *Biochim. Biophys. Acta* **228**, 595–609.
394. Schildkraut, C. L., and Maio, J. J. (1969). *J. Mol. Biol.* **46**, 305–312.
395. Schlabach, A., Fridlender, B., Bolden, A., and Weissbach, A. (1971). *Biochem. Biophys. Res. Commun.* **44**, 879–885.
396. Schmid, W. (1963). *Cytogenetics* **2**, 175–193.
397. Schneider, W. C., and Kuff, E. L. (1969). *J. Biol. Chem.* **244**, 4843–4851.
398. Scolnick, E. M., Aaronson, S. A., Todaro, G. J., and Parks, W. P. (1971). *Nature (London)* **229**, 318–321.
399. Setlow, P., Brutlag, D., and Kornberg, A. (1972). *J. Biol. Chem.* **247**, 224–231.
400. Setlow, R. B. (1968). In "Progress in Nucleic Acid Research and Molecular Biology" (J. N. Davidson and W. E. Cohn, eds.), Vol. 8, pp. 257–295. Academic Press, New York.
401. Setlow, R. B., and Carrier, W. L. (1964). *Proc. Nat. Acad. Sci. U.S.* **51**, 226–231.
402. Setlow, R. B., and Carrier, W. L. (1966). *J. Mol. Biol.* **17**, 237–254.
403. Setlow, R. B., and Regan, J. D. (1972). *Biochem. Biophys. Res. Commun.* **46**, 1019–1024.
404. Shapiro, H. S., and Chargaff, E. (1960). *Biochim. Biophys. Acta* **39**, 68–82.
405. Shapiro, R. (1968). In "Progress in Nucleic Acid Research and Molecular Biology" (J. N. Davidson and W. E. Cohn, eds.), Vol. 8, pp. 73–112. Academic Press, New York.

406. Shih, T. Y., and Bonner, J. (1970). *J. Mol. Biol.* **48**, 469–487.
407. Shirakawa, S., and Saunders, G. F. (1971). *Proc. Soc. Exp. Biol. Med.* **138**, 364–372.
408. Simpson, R. T. (1970). *Biochemistry* **9**, 4814–4818.
409. Singer, B., and Fraenkel-Conrat, H. (1969). In "Progress in Nucleic Acid Research and Molecular Biology" (J. N. Davidson and W. E. Cohn, eds.), Vol. 9, pp. 1–29. Academic Press, New York.
410. Singer, B., and Fraenkel-Conrat, H. (1970). *Biochemistry* **9**, 3694–3701.
411. Smellie, R. M. S., Keir, H. M., and Davidson, J. N. (1959). *Biochim. Biophys. Acta* **35**, 389–404.
412. Smellie, R. M. S., Grey, E. D., Keir, H. M., Richards, J., Bell, D., and Davidson, J. N. (1960). *Biochim. Biophys. Acta* **37**, 243–250.
413. Smith, B. J. (1970). *J. Mol. Biol.* **47**, 101–106.
414. Smith, D. W., Schaller, H. E., and Bonhoefer, F. J. (1970). *Nature (London)* **226**, 711–713.
415. Sneider, T. W. (1971). *J. Biol. Chem.* **246**, 4774–4783.
416. Sneider, T. W. (1972). *J. Biol. Chem.* **247**, 2872–2875.
417. Sneider, T. W., and Potter, V. R. (1969). *J. Mol. Biol.* **42**, 271–284.
418. Sneider, T. W., Bushnell, D. E., and Potter, V. R. (1970). *Cancer Res.* **30**, 1867–1873.
419. Southern, E. M. (1970). *Nature (London)* **227**, 794–798.
420. Spencer, J. H., and Chargaff, E. (1963). *Biochim. Biophys. Acta* **68**, 9–17.
421. Sporn, M. B., and Dingman, C. W. (1966). *Nature (London)* **210**, 531–532.
422. Srinivasan, P. R., and Borek, E. (1966). In "Progress in Nucleic Acid Research and Molecular Biology" (J. N. Davidson and W. E. Cohn, eds.), Vol. 5, pp. 159–189. Academic Press, New York.
423. Stevens, B. J., and Andre, J. (1969). In "Handbook of Molecular Cytology" (A. Lima-de-Faria, ed.), pp. 837–871. North-Holland Publ., Amsterdam.
424. Steward, D. L., and Humphrey, R. M. (1966). *Nature (London)* **212**, 298–300.
425. Stich, H. F., and San, R. H. C. (1970). *Mutat. Res.* **10**, 389–404.
426. Stich, H. F., San, R. H. C., Miller, J. A., and Miller, E. C. (1972). *Nature New Biol.* **238**, 9–10.
427. Strauss, B. S. (1968). *Current Topics Microbiol Immunol.* **44**, 1–85.
428. Strauss, B. S., and Robbins, M. (1968). *Biochim. Biophys. Acta* **161**, 68–75.
429. Strauss, B., Coyle, M., and Robbins, M. (1968). *Cold Spring Harbor Symp. Quant. Biol.* **33**, 227–287.
430. Strauss, B., Coyle, M., McMahon, M., Kato, K., and Dolyniuk, M. (1972). In "Molecular and Cellular Repair Processes" (R. F. Beers, R. M. Herriott, and R. C. Tilgham, eds.), pp. 111–124. Johns Hopkins Univ. Press, Baltimore, Maryland.
431. Sueoka, N., and Quinn, W. G. (1968). *Cold Spring Harbor Symp. Quant. Biol.* **33**, 695–705.
432. Sueoka, N., and Yoshikawa, H. (1963). *Cold Spring Harbor Symp. Quant. Biol.* **28**, 47–54.
433. Sugino, A., Hirose, S., and Okazaki, R. (1971). *Proc. Nat. Acad. Sci. U.S.* **69**, 1863–1867.
434. Sutton, W. D. (1972). *Nature New Biol.* **237**, 70–71.
435. Swift, H. (1950). *Physiol. Zool.* **26**, 169–198.
436. Swift, H. (1950). *Proc. Nat. Acad. Sci. U.S.* **36**, 643–654.
437. Szybalski, W., Bovre, K., Fiandt, M., Guha, A., Hradecna, Z., Kumar, S., Lozeron, H. A., Maher, V. M., Nijkamp, H. J. J., Summers, W. C., and Taylor, K. (1969). *J. Cell. Physiol. Suppl. 1* **74**, 33–70.
438. Tada, M., and Tada, M. (1971). *Chem.-Biol. Int.* **3**, 225–229.
439. Taylor, J. H. (1953). *Exp. Cell Res.* **4**, 164–173.
440. Taylor, J. H. (1960). *J. Biophys. Biochem. Cytol.* **7**, 455–463.
441. Taylor, J. H. (1968). *J. Mol. Biol.* **31**, 579–594.
442. Taylor, J. H., Woods, P. S., and Hughes, W. L. (1957). *Proc. Nat. Acad. Sci. U.S.* **43**, 122–128.
443. Temin, H. M. (1963). *Virology* **20**, 577–582.

444. Temin, H. M. (1964). *Virology* **23**, 486–494.
445. Temin, H. M. (1964). *Proc. Nat. Acad. Sci. U.S.* **52**, 323–329.
446. Temin, H. M. (1970). *Perspect. Biol. Med.* **14**, 11–26.
447. Temin, H. M., and Mizutani, S. (1970). *Nature* (*London*) **226**, 1211–1213.
448. Temin, H. M., Mizutani, S., and Coffin, J. (1971). *In* "Nucleic Acid Protein·Interactions. Nuclei Acid Synthesis in Viral Infections" (D. W. Ribbons, J. F. Woessner, and J. Schultz, eds.), pp. 291–308. North-Holland Publ., Amsterdam.
449. Terasima, T., and Tolmach, L. J. (1963). *Exp. Cell Res.* **30**, 344–362.
450. Tobia, A. M., Schildkraut, C. L., and Maio, J. (1970). *J. Mol. Biol.* **54**, 499–515.
451. Tobia, A. M., Schildkraut, C. L., and Maio, J. (1971). *Biochim. Biophys. Acta* **246**, 258–262.
452. Tomasz, M. (1970). *Biochim. Biophys. Acta* **19**, 18–28.
453. Troll, W., Rinde, E., and Day, P. (1969). *Biochim. Biophys. Acta* **174**, 211–219.
454. Trosko, J. E., and Kasschan, M. R. (1967). *Photochem. Photobiol.* **6**, 215–219.
455. Trosko, J. E., Chu, E. H. Y., and Carrier, W. L. (1965). *Radiat. Res.* **24**, 667–672.
456. Tso, P. O. P., Lesko, S. A., and Umans, R. S. (1969). *In* "Physico-Chemical Mechanism of Carcinogenesis" (E. D. Bergmann and B. Pullman, eds.), pp. 106–135. Israeli Acad. of Sci. and Humanities, Jerusalem.
457. Tsukada, K., Moriyama, T., Lynch, W. E., and Lieberman, I. (1968). *Nature* (*London*) **220**, 162–164.
458. Turkington, R. W., and Spielvogel, R. L. (1971). *J. Biol. Chem.* **246**, 3835–3840.
459. Uhlenhopp, E. L., and Krasna, A. I. (1971). *Biochemistry* **10**, 3290–3295.
460. Vosberg, H. P., and Hoffman-Berling, H. (1971). *J. Mol. Biol.* **58**, 739–753.
461. Wacker, A., Dellweg, H., and Weinblum, D. (1961). *J. Mol. Biol.* **3**, 787–789.
462. Walker, P. M. B. (1971). *Progr. Biophys. Mol. Biol.* **23**, 147–190.
463. Walker, P. M. B., and McLaren, A. (1965). *Nature* (*London*) **208**, 1175–1179.
464. Walker, P. M. B., Flamm, W. G., and McLaren, A. (1969). *In* "Handbook of Molecular Cytology" (A. Lima-de-Faria, ed.), pp. 52–66. North-Holland Publ., Amsterdam.
465. Wallace, P. F., Hewish, D. R., Venning, M. M., and Burgoyne, L. A. (1971). *Biochem. J.* **125**, 47–54.
466. Walwick, E. R., and Main, R. K. (1962). *Biochim. Biophys. Acta* **61**, 876–884.
467. Wang, T. Y. (1968). *Proc. Soc. Exp. Biol. Med.* **129**, 469–472.
468. Waquar, M. A., Burgoyne, L. A., and Atkinson, M. R. (1971). *Biochem. J.* **121**, 803–809.
469. Waring, M., and Britten, R. J. (1966). *Science* **154**, 791–794.
470. Warwick, G. P., and Roberts, J. J. (1967). *Nature* (*London*) **213**, 1206–1207.
471. Watson, J. D. (1968). "The Double-Helix." Atheneum Press, New York.
472. Watson, J. D., and Crick, F. H. C. (1953). *Nature* (*London*) **171**, 737–738.
473. Watson, J. D., and Crick, F. H. C. (1953). *Nature* (*London*) **171**, 964–967.
474. Watson, J. D., and Crick, F. H. C. (1953). *Cold Spring Harbor Symp. Quant. Biol.* **18**, 123–131.
475. Watson, M. L. (1955). *J. Biophys. Biochem. Cytol.* **1**, 257–270.
476. Weisblum, B., and de Haseth, P. L. (1972). *Proc. Nat. Acad. Sci. U.S.* **69**, 629–632.
477. Weiss, B., and Richardson, C. C. (1967). *Proc. Nat. Acad. Sci. U.S.* **57**, 1021–1028.
478. Weissbach, A., Schlabach, A., Fridlender, B., and Bolden, A. (1971). *Nature New Biol.* **231**, 167–170.
479. Werner, R. (1971). *Nature New Biol.* **233**, 99–103.
480. Werner, R. (1971). *In* "Nucleic Acid-Protein Interactions. Nucleic Acid Synthesis in Viral Infections" (D. W. Ribbons, J. F. Woessner, and J. Schultz, eds.), pp. 25–45. North-Holland Publ., Amsterdam.
481. Wheeler, G. R., and Skipper, H. E. (1957). *Arch. Biochem. Biophys.* **72**, 465–475.
482. Wickner, R. B., Ginsberg, B., and Hurwitz, J. (1972). *J. Biol. Chem.* **247**, 498–504.
483. Wickner, R. B., Ginsberg, B., Berkower, I., and Hurwitz, J. (1972). *J. Biol. Chem.* **247**, 489–492.
484. Wickner, W., Brutlag, D., Schekman, R., and Kornberg, A. (1972). *Proc. Nat. Acad. Sci. U.S.* **69**, 965–969.

485. Wiener, J., Spiro, D., and Loewenstein, W. J. (1965). *J. Cell. Biol.* **27**, 107–117.
486. Wilhelm, R. C., and Ludlum, D. B. (1966). *Science* **153**, 1403–1405.
487. Wilkins, M. H. F., Stokes, A. R., and Wilkins, H. R. (1953). *Nature (London)* **171**, 738–740.
488. Wilkins, M. H. F., Zubay, G., and Wilson, H. R. (1959). *J. Mol. Biol.* **1**, 179–185.
489. Williams, C. H., and Ockey, C. H. (1970). *Exp. Cell Res.* **63**, 365–372.
490. Williamson, R. (1970). *J. Mol. Biol.* **51**, 157–168.
491. Wilson, E. B. (1900). "The Cell in Development and Inheritance." Macmillian, New York.
492. Winocour, E. (1971). *Advan. Cancer Res.* **14**, 37–70.
492a. Wise, G. E., and Prescott, D. M. (1973). *Proc. Nat. Acad. Sci. U.S.* **70**, 714–717.
493. Wunderlich, V., Schütt, M., Böttger, M., and Graffi, A. (1970). *Biochem. J.* **118**, 99–109.
494. Wunderlich, V., Tetzlaff, I., and Graffi, A. (1971/1972). *Chem.-Biol. Int.* **4**, 81–89.
495. Yasmineh, W. G., and Yunis, J. J. (1969). *Biochem. Biophys. Res. Commun.* **35**, 779–782.
496. Yasmineh, W. G., and Yunis, J. J. (1970). *Exp. Cell Res.* **59**, 69–75.
497. Yasmineh, W. G., and Yunis, J. J. (1971). *Exp. Cell Res.* **64**, 41–48.
498. Yasmineh, W. G., and Yunis, J. J. (1971). *Biochem. Biophys. Res. Commun.* **43**, 580–587.
499. Yasuzumi, G., and Sugihara, R. (1965). *Exp. Cell Res.* **37**, 207–229.
500. Yoneda, M., and Bollum, F. J. (1965). *J. Biol. Chem.* **240**, 3385–3391.
501. Yoshikawa-Fukada, M., and Ebert, J. D. (1971). *Biochem. Biophys. Res. Commun.* **43**, 133–141.
502. Yunis, J. J., and Yasmineh, W. G. (1970). *Science* **168**, 263–265.
503. Yunis, J. J., and Yasmineh, W. G. (1971). *Science* **174**, 1200–1209.
504. Zeiger, R. S., Salomon, R., Kinoshita, N., and Peacock, A. C. (1972). *Cancer Res.* **32**, 643–647.
505. Zubay, G., and Wilkins, M. H. F. (1964). *J. Mol. Biol.* **9**, 246–249.

CHAPTER V

Messenger RNA and Other High Molecular Weight RNA

HARRIS BUSCH

I. Introduction*

The evolution of the concept of messenger RNA of viruses and bacterial and mammalian cells has been one of the most remarkable developments of the last decade (107, 303, 350). Beginning with the suggestion (155) that such RNA species were important in the transmission of genetic information from the genome to the protein synthesizing machinery of cells (Fig. 5.1a, b) and the discovery of the genetic code, many studies have been made on the origin and fate of mRNA's and their functional roles. Several types of mRNA molecules have been intensively studied, and at present most is known about those of viral or phage origin. Although some mRNA molecules are monocistronic, i.e., they code for only one protein, most viral and some mammalian mRNA's are polycistronic messengers (2, 3, 165, 203, 280, 343, 368); all function as components of polysomes or polyribosomes (Fig. 5.1).

Recently, highly purified mRNA molecules for synthesis of hemoglobin (182), silk fibroin (324), myoglobin (141), ovalbumin (236–239), and other proteins have been isolated (Table 5.1). Accordingly, much more definitive experiments on their actual template function have been possible. Demonstration of *in vitro* synthesis of specific protein species has been achieved by immunological studies, chromatographic behavior of the products, and peptide analysis. In addition, it has been possible to demonstrate specific effects of hormones on biosynthetic systems both *in vivo* and *in vitro* (344).

Synthesis of messenger RNA has been attempted *in vitro* using RNA polymerases. Recently, synthesis of specific hemoglobin mDNA has been reported in systems using reverse transcriptases (21, 348). After transcription of the mRNA on DNA templates *in vivo*, polyadenylic acid sequences are added to the 3' terminus before transport of the mRNA to the cytoplasm (see Section III,D). Moreover, specific proteins or ribonucleoprotein (RNP) particles are essential for this transport and it now seems that even in the polysomes of the cytoplasm, where mRNA functions, it is specifically bound to proteins (32–34, 235).

mRNA of Cancer Cells

A key problem of the molecular biology of cancer is to define differences in the mRNA's of tumors and other cells (52, 68, 69, 195, 369). The positive

---

* Abbreviations: A + U/G + C = the ratio of either total isotope or total amounts of nucleotide in adenylic acid (A), uridylic acid (U), guanylic acid (G) and cytidylic acid (C); AU-rich RNA = RNA rich in adenylic and uridylic acids; GC-rich RNA = RNA rich in guanylic and cytidylic acids. D-RNA = RNA presumably more closely related to DNA because of its higher AU content and lower GC content; like DNA, it is extracted at higher temperatures or pH than rRNA; mRNA = messenger RNA; mDNA = DNA which codes for a specific mRNA; ^{32}P-nucleotide composition = nucleotide composition based upon post-labeling isotope content of each of the four nucleotides in RNA; UV nucleotide composition = nucleotide composition based upon analysis of content of nucleotides in RNA by ultraviolet absorption of the bases, HnRNA = rapidly labeled high molecular weight nuclear RNA.

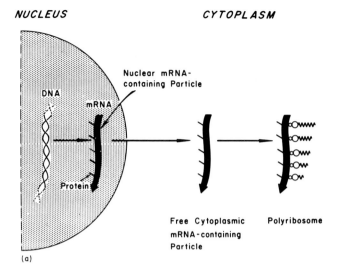

Fig. 5.1a. Scheme of synthesis and transport of mRNA from the nucleus to the cytoplasm where it functions as part of the polyribosome complex. (Courtesy of Dr. Edgar C. Henshaw, Harvard University Medical School.)

MODEL OF RIBOSOME – SUBUNIT CYCLE

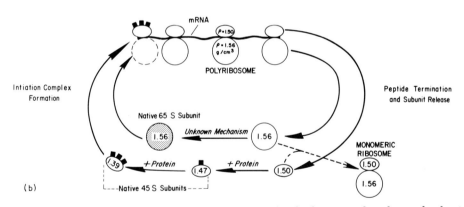

Fig. 5.1b. Scheme of dissociation and reformation of polyribosomes, the ribosomal subunit cycle. (Courtesy of Dr. Edgar C. Henshaw, Harvard University Medical School.)

hypothesis of the biochemistry of cancer is that there are new "cancer-specific" gene readouts in cancer cells. Although high hopes were held that appropriate technology might quickly be developed to test this hypothesis, many problems have become apparent that have not been resolved. In some respects, the difficulties in these problems resemble those of DNA chemistry of cancer cells that have not been amenable to solution. For example, it has not been possible to separate cancer- or growth-specific messenger RNA from other mRNA species although products of oncogenic viruses have been suggested to be quite specific readouts of genome-integrated viral DNA. Some of the requirements that are very important in this field include the need to work with intact, undegraded molecular species (59, 316, Fig. 5.2) and the need for development of methods

TABLE 5.1 Some Messenger RNA Species Studied

Protein products	Tissue or origin	Characteristics	Ref.
I. Eukaryotic mRNA			
A. Known products of mammalian cells			
Albumin	Liver		191
Antibodies (immunoglobulins)	Mouse spleen, rabbit lymph nodes, rat spleen, liver		25, 70, 84, 173, 184, 260, 270
Catalase	Liver		345
Hemoglobin	See Table 5.5		
Histones	HeLa cells	7–9 S	38, 156, 161
Lens protein (α-crystallin)	Lens		191a, 321, 322
Myeloma proteins	Plasmacytomas		116, 325
Myosin	Muscle		141
Tdr kinase	Novikoff hepatoma	Half-life of 3.5 hours	41
B. Unknown products of mammalian cells			
	Cerebral tissue		372
	Kidney, thymus	High molecular weight RNA: A 28, U 28, G 21, C 21; much higher hybridization than with ribosomal RNA	361
	Liver nuclei	High stimulation of amino acid incorporation into proteins; liver: A 30, U 25, G 25, C 23	87, 361
	Liver	10 S RNA; high AU; A 23, U 20, G 28, C 28; A 29, U 22, G 24, C 25.	124
	Liver-extranucleolar Nuclear RNA	Nucleolar RNA: A 20, U 16, G 38, C 25; extranucleolar nuclear RNA: A 30, U 21, G 24, C 23.	212
	Liver polysomal mRNA	A 32, U 20, G 22, C 25	138
	Liver mRNA, total	A 32, U 29, G 22, C 17	287, 320, 345
	Pancreas and liver	A 29, U 33, G 26, C 13; 8–18 S; used polyacrylamide gels for 1st time	74
	Thyroid	A 29, U 33, G 26, C 13; 8–18 S	61–64
C. mRNA of other species			
Avidin	Chick oviduct		236–239
Chromosomal mRNA	Chromosomes, salivary cells		78

TABLE 5.1 (*Continued*)

Protein products	Tissue or origin	Characteristics	Ref.
Embryogenesis	*Xenopus laevis*		46
	Wheat polysomes		286
"Informational RNA"	Sea urchin		151, 223
Microtubule protein	Oocyte		82, 259
Ovalbumin	Chick oviduct mRNA	A 26, U 20, G 27, C 26	72, 201, 236– 239, 244, 269, 310
Salivary gland proteins	*Chironomus* sp.	70 S mRNA	77a, 78, 93a
Silk fibroin	*Bombyx mori*		324
II. Prokaryotic mRNA			
β-Galactosidase synthesis	β-Galactosidase of *E. coli*	Stimulated by IPTG	24, 165
	Bacteria	Long-lived mRNA	371
	R17 virus	Untranslated 74	2, 3
	Qβ	Nucleotides on 5′ terminal	
	MS2 RNA	Untranslated: 129 residues; A protein begins at 130	86, 102, 125, 203

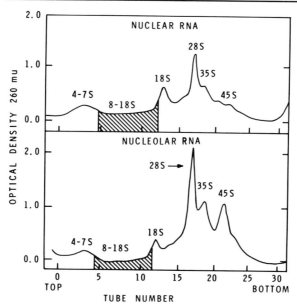

Fig. 5.2. Sucrose density gradient (5–47%) of nuclear and nucleolar RNA of Novikoff hepatoma ascites cells. The low molecular weight RNA is generally considered to be 4–7 S RNA. These gradients were centrifuged in an SW-27 rotor at 25,000 rpm for 16 hours. The nucleolar 28 S, 35 S, and 45 S RNA contained largely precursors of ribosomal RNA. The 8–18 S RNA of these gradients (shaded) was collected and subjected to gel electrophoresis shown in Figs. 5.3a and 5.3b. This RNA has been found to contain "messenger" activity.

that adequately separate individual messenger species from what must be a large group of molecules, i.e., perhaps 10–50 thousand molecular species (52, 303) (Fig. 5.3). Within the limits of the methods for studies on such molecules, few meaningful differences have been found in a variety of characteristics of the high, intermediate, and low molecular weight types of HnRNA's of tumors and other tissues (296).

The problem of isolation and demonstration of differences of "cancer-specific" mRNA has proven to be exceedingly difficult. The situation now for such RNA of cancer cells is similar to that several years ago when Singer and Leder (303) commented that mRNA was as elusive as the Scarlet Pimpernel:

> We seek him here, we seek him there,
> Those Frenchies seek him everywhere.
> Is he in heaven?—Is he in hell?
> That demmed elusive Pimpernel.

NOVIKOFF HEPATOMA NUCLEAR 8-18 S RNA

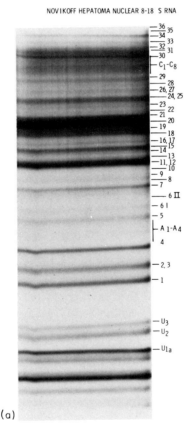

(a)

Fig. 5.3a. Separation of many bands of nuclear and nucleolar intermediate molecular weight RNA (8–18 S RNA) on 4.6% polyacrylamide gels. This figure provides an indication of the complexity of nucleolar and nuclear RNA species. Some of these bands may contain mRNA and others degradation products of higher molecular weight RNA species. (Courtesy of Dr. H. Savage, Baylor College of Medicine.)

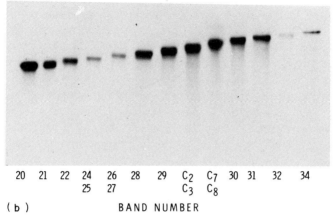

(b) BAND NUMBER

Fig. 5.3b. Purification of some of the RNA bands shown in Fig. 5.3a. (Courtesy of Dr. H. Savage, Baylor College of Medicine.)

II. The Complexity of the Problem

Among the important questions about mRNA that are unanswered are

1. What is the actual number of genes read in a given cell?
2. What are the numbers of RNA species that are transcribed into proteins or used in other ways?
3. Are the RNA readouts from chromatin in various types of cells the same or different ?
4. If they are the same, what types of systems determine which gene readouts are transmitted to the cytoplasm or are translated in the cytoplasm?
5. If they are different, what are the control mechanisms that define their similarities and differences?
6. What types of techniques are required to demonstrate the similarities and differences of the types of RNA in various tissues?

A. Numbers of Messenger RNA Molecules Produced per Cell

In theory, the amount of gene information in nuclear DNA is tremendously excessive for any given cell (44, 45, 52). Despite their origin from a single germ cell, only some cells produce hair, have visual pigment, exhibit contractility, are affected by hormones, produce albumin, stimulate motor function, etc. There is such an immense specialization of mammalian cells that the order of magnitude of differences for special characteristics in cells must approach thousands. Although such numbers are probably only valid as estimates, it seems likely that approximately 95–98% of the genes are "phenotypically silent" in any given cell type (52). Most genes are permanently silent as reflected by the fact that regenerating liver produces only liver tissue and no errors are made such as the production of kidney, intestine, lung, or other specialized cells in the regenerating liver. Such results indicate that the gene control mechanisms, at least with respect to phenotypic aspects of gene expression, are permanently fixed in some cell types.

Theoretically, several million proteins could be coded for by the genome (Chapter I), and if 5% of these genes are read or expressed (47), approximately 10^5 messages or "mRNA's" may be produced in any given cell (44, 45, 52). Such a calculation is very approximate because of the possibility that many genes are expressed in smaller or larger protein entities than the mean molecular weight of 50,000 and there are intergene interactions involving control mechanisms that are not defined at present.

It is still not clear how much of the genome is available for transcription in any given cell, but it seems unlikely that there is total readout and subsequent translational selection. Early work (36) showed that only about 20% of DNA can be transcribed when freed of histones and other nuclear proteins. Of course, in cells there are both restriction and/or derepression of genes by DNA-associated proteins. Many recent studies have provided evidence that nonhistone nuclear proteins (6, 21a, 23, 36, 37, 59, 247, 310) play a key role in defining gene readouts (see Chapter VII).

B. Satellite DNA

Recent reports have indicated that huge amounts, i.e., up to 50%, of DNA may be composed of noninformative sequences, much of which may be in "spacer" regions. Although "satellite DNA," which sediments differently from the main DNA mass, has been found, it contains little "messenger" information (44, 45, 159). Some satellite DNA is uniquely localized in the centromeric region of the chromosome where it apparently serves as the attachment site for the mitotic spindle rather than as a specific gene functional region of the chromosome (44, 159). Other types of "satellites" have been found such as the rDNA satellite of the toad nucleus that serves for synthesis of rRNA (44, 45). Satellites for other purposes are becoming specified in other species (59).

C. Is the Whole mRNA Read for Protein Synthesis?

Just as the whole DNA does not serve specifically for synthesis of mRNA, there is conclusive evidence that the whole mRNA is not read for protein synthesis. In R17, MS2, f2, and Qβ phage, there are regions that are not translated, at least on the 5'-terminal segment of the molecules (2, 3, 26, 27, 85, 102, 115, 157, 224, 278, 318). In the R17 phage, 74 nucleotides are not translated and there are nucleotides that are not translated in the Qβ RNA. A "leader sequence" of 129 nucleotides was found (86) in the MS2 virus preceding the AUG initiator codon at nucleotide 130. Thus far, no definitive function has been established for these portions of these RNA molecules.

D. Messenger Test-Systems

In determination of the genetic code (192, 227, 303), an *in vitro* system was used that employed a series of soluble factors and ribosomes of *E. coli* (227, 228, 303, 332); this test was initially limited to an analysis of uptake of labeled amino acid into protein. Synthetic oligonucleotides and polynucleotides, e.g., poly U (polyuridylic acid), that produce increases of uptake of labeled amino acids into proteins aided in definition of the "genetic code."

The recent isolation of a host of proteins involved in the intermediary reactions of protein synthesis has permitted a greater understanding of the operation of this system (see Chapter IX). However, demonstration of messenger activity has required techniques such as isolation of the newly synthesized protein either by chromatography or other methods, demonstration of its structural identity with the intended product by analysis of its constituent peptides, and immuno-assays to demonstrate its interaction with specific antibodies such as hemoglobin mRNA. More recently, injection of mRNA into oocytes has been shown to result in formation of specific protein products (121, 205). Such methods are markedly advanced over the initial efforts that employed systems that enhanced incorporation of labeled amino acids or aminoacyl-tRNA into protein residues.

Enhancement of uptake of amino acids reflects the presence of specific information in various RNA molecules. However, nonmessenger RNA may produce a similar effect when it is single-stranded (134, 135, 146, 160). For precise demonstration of messenger activity, only the synthesis of hemoglobin and a few other proteins has provided adequate evidence for protein synthesis.

E. Other Characteristics of mRNA

Early descriptions of messenger RNA (120) suggested that it (a) turned over rapidly, (b) banded in specific intermediate molecular weight positions on sucrose density gradients, and (c) contained a number of species rich in AMP and UMP, i.e., its nucleotide composition was "DNA-like." These suggestions were oversimplified but provocative. With regard to metabolic turnover, the best known mRNA species, the reticulocyte hemoglobin mRNA, a 9 S species, has a slow turnover rate (288). Although some controversy has existed, it is now clear that many species of mRNA in mammalian cells turn over very slowly if at all (118a, 303a).

With regard to sedimentation characteristics, it now appears that mRNA has a range of sizes that reflect monocistronic and polycistronic functions (208). Recently it has been established that *Chironomus tentans* produces an approximately 70 S RNA that is a single polycistronic readout which presumably codes for proteins produced by the salivary glands. This long molecule which has a poly A terminus has been suggested to code for a giant protein precursor of the individual species of salivary gland proteins (78, 93a, 176a–d). When it was assumed that there was complete fidelity of transcription and that all the genome is transcribed, it seemed likely mRNA was "DNA-like." Since the $dA + dT/dC + dG$ ratio of mammalian DNA is 1.35, the corresponding $A + U/G + C$ ratio of the mRNA could be 1.35 (350). Some pools of RNA molecules have been found which have such a ratio. Many have a high A content which is now believed to reflect the added poly A on the 3′ end of the 8–18 S and 18 S RNA fractions (Table 5.2).

F. Isolation of Messenger RNA

The greatest contribution to studies on differentiating messenger RNA of cancer cells has been the continuing improvement of methods (Table 5.3) for the isolation and analysis of individual nuclear precursors or specific cytoplasmic mRNA molecules (52, 59, 316, 317). As yet, "messenger" functions have not been adequately demonstrated except in the very few instances shown in Table 5.1. Although the available methods (Table 5.3) have not yet discriminated between mRNA molecules of various cell types, intensive studies are being made to improve electrophoretic and other methods (77, 248, 249, 268).

Combinations of a number of centrifugation, chromatographic, and electrophoretic methods have provided for isolation of the cellular messenger RNA species isolated so far (Tables 5.1, 5.3). When combined with the isolation of cellular particles such as the polysomes, mitochondria, nuclei, and nucleoli or their subunits, improved opportunities will develop for purification of mRNA's since each of these cellular elements probably contains many fewer messenger RNA species than the total extractable from whole cells (see Chapters I and XIII).

G. Structure of mRNA

It is generally assumed from electron microscopic evidence as well as the logical basis for their operation that mRNA molecules are linear forms in their functional states (226, 350). However, it is clear that mRNA can assume a variety of conformations (117, 226); some of these may not be functional and accordingly factors that control its conformation could control mRNA translation into protein (105). The mRNA-associated proteins may also be responsible for maintenance of its structure in mammalian cells (33, 235); presumably they do not interfere with translation.* In the case of the polycistronic messenger RNA molecules of either RNA phages or viruses, the packing structure may vary markedly from that of the operational structure of these molecules. For

---

* In some instances, even DNA-RNA hybrids have been found to be translated (16).

TABLE 5.2

BASE COMPOSITION OF RNA FRACTIONS ISOLATED BY HOT PHENOL FRACTIONATION FROM EHRLICH CARCINOMA CELLS[a]

RNA Fraction	Extraction temperature (°C)	Newly synthesized RNA molar percent of					Total RNA molar percent of				
		A	U	G	C	A + U/G + C	A	U	G	C	G + C/A + U
Whole	0	—	—	—	—	—	19.3	19.6	31.8	29.2	0.64
	40	14.5	21.7	30.6	33.2	0.56	17.9	21.8	30.7	29.6	0.66
	55	17.6	25.2	28.2	29.0	0.75	21.7	23.7	28.0	26.6	0.83
	63	28.7	26.6	21.0	23.6	1.23	29.1	24.6	23.2	23.1	1.16
	85	28.4	28.1	21.5	21.8	1.30	27.0	28.7	24.3	20.0	1.25
<18 S	63	34.1	23.9	19.8	22.2	1.37	—	—	—	—	—
18 S	63	31.3	23.8	19.3	25.6	1.23	28.6	24.4	23.3	23.7	1.12
23 S	63	27.7	25.7	21.8	24.8	1.15	—	—	—	—	—
28 S	63	28.0	26.3	22.2	23.5	1.20	—	—	—	—	—
32 S	63	27.4	27.1	22.1	23.4	1.20	—	—	—	—	—
45 S	63	26.3	28.6	21.8	23.3	1.25	—	—	—	—	—
>45 S	63	26.2	27.9	21.6	24.3	1.18	—	—	—	—	—
18 S	85	26.1	26.4	22.3	25.2	1.11	—	—	—	—	—
28–45 S	85	26.4	27.9	21.5	24.2	1.19	—	—	—	—	—
45 S	85	26.4	29.1	21.3	23.2	1.25	—	—	—	—	—
>45 S	85	28.0	28.0	21.0	23.0	1.28	—	—	—	—	—

[a] From Georgiev (109a).

TABLE 5.3

METHODS FOR SEPARATION OF RNA SPECIES INTO GC-RICH AND AU-RICH GROUPS

Procedure	Detail	Ref.
Extraction procedures		
Thermal fractionation and phenol fractionation	Heating phenol-aqueous phase mixture at varying temperatures	110, 111, 166, 209, 210, 288, 301, 302, 316, 317
Salt extraction of nuclei or whole cells	Initial extraction with 0.15 M NaCl followed by extraction with 2 M NaCl; various treatments of the residue	53, 296, 316
Fractionation of nuclei or cells with pH changes	Initial extraction at pH 7.6 (Tris) followed by extraction at pH 9 (Tris)	39, 40, 180
Fractionation of chromatin	Heating, centrifugation	36, 37, 370
Fractionation of isolated RNA		
Sucrose density gradient centrifugation	Separations in the 7–28 S regions with intensive purification of the 8 S, 9 S, and associated bands	178, 216, 285, 338–340
Countercurrent fractionation of RNA species	2-Phase systems with equilibration	162–164, 245, 358, 359
Electrophoresis	Varying gel concentrations, pH	216, 248, 249, 268
Chromatography on substituted cellulose or Sephadex columns	Gradient elution with varying salt concentrations, pH	156, 210
Other types of columns, i.e., MAK columns, poly T and poly U columns	Salt gradients or pH gradients; added components such as SDS	112, 241, 325, 366, 367
Hybridization methods	Use of cellulose acetate, Millipore or other membranes; use of similar columns	22, 113, 114, 243, 271
Selective inhibition		
Treatment of cells with		
(a) Actinomycin D	(a) Low to high doses of actinomycin D	129, 266, 347
(b) 5-Fluoroorotic acid	(b) 5-FO also blocks rRNA synthesis	360

transport of RNA of phage or virus particles, it has been suggested that much of the RNA is internally hydrogen bonded to ensure minimal volume and maximum stability. When viral or phage RNA is functional intracellularly, it is mainly or completely single stranded (2, 3, 26, 27, 115, 157, 224, 318).

AU-RICH RNA

Although the general problem of isolation of specific mRNA has been resolved only in a few circumstances (Table 5.1), for separation of the GC-rich ribosomal

RNA and the AU-rich RNA of the cell, many procedures have been successfully employed (Table 5.3).

It was demonstrated early (110, 111, 120) that the initially synthesized RNA's differed in their aqueous extractability after phenol treatment of samples at varying temperatures (Tables 5.2, 5.3). Below 50°C, phenol extracted RNA with a nucleotide ratio $(A + U/G + C)$ of approximately 0.6 in both Ehrlich ascites cells and normal liver. The RNA extracted above 50°C ("D-RNA") had an $A + U/G + C$ ratio of approximately 1.25, more like that of DNA. Although it was suggested that this second type of RNA contained "informational" or "messenger RNA," it now appears that only a small portion of it has that function. After pulse labeling, the specific activity of the "informational" or mRNA was higher than that of the other RNA in normal liver but not in the tumors. In early studies, "D-RNA" or the AU-rich RNA was found to have a sedimentation coefficient of 8–28 S. RNA with similar characteristics with higher sedimentation coefficients (65 S and 85 S) has been referred to as "giant RNA" (14, 15, 204, 296) or HnRNA (cf. below).

III. Metabolism of mRNA

A. Synthesis

In mammalian cells there are multiple forms of RNA-synthesizing enzymes, the RNA polymerases; one is confined to the nucleolus and the others are localized to the nucleoplasm; these have different subunits and cofactor requirements (49, 50, 66, 356). The nucleoplasmic enzyme (RNA polymerase II) probably primarily serves for synthesis of mRNA (66, 351), but in isolated systems its activity persists far too short a time to demonstrate mRNA synthesis. The reactions involved in synthesis of the mRNA proceed from the 5' to the 3' end of the molecule (177, 274, 311) and probably only one strand of DNA is read at any given time, although it is not clear whether the complementary strand contains meaningful information (134, 135, 160, 311). It is presumed that most DNA-RNA hybrids that are necessarily formed have a short half-life; apparently they persist longer in some cells than in others. The RNA may be released by factors that are derived from the cytoplasm (19, 309, 312–314, 326). The initial synthetic products have high molecular weights and probably some defined secondary structures (111, 212, 279, 287).

The rates of mRNA synthesis in cells have not been adequately defined either in terms of total mass or molecular numbers. In general, cells undergoing rapid division and accordingly totally duplicating their mRNA content should have higher rates of synthesis of mRNA than nondividing cells or cells with longer cell cycles. However, the rate of synthesis of AU-rich nuclear RNA in many nontumor cells is equally as rapid as that of tumors (67, 87, 106, 122, 194, 214, 222, 335, 354). At present there is virtually no information available on rates of transfer of this rapidly synthesized RNA or its products to the cytoplasm;

the studies on the turnover of cytoplasmic mRNA of tumors and other tissues have not been clearly interpretable because of the technical problems encountered with RNases.

B. Heterogeneous RNA

After the initial studies on "D-RNA" in tumors (110, 111), others (15, 280–283, 349) reported that in the duck erythrocyte there was a rapidly sedimenting or "giant" RNA which had a high content of UMP and a low GC content. In duck erythrocytes, these initially synthesized RNA molecules were "metabolically unstable" and had a half-life of 30 minutes. The name "heterogeneous" RNA or HnRNA (308, 349) has stuck because this RNA sediments throughout the gradient from 8 S through the highest sedimentation regions. Much variability has been found with respect to the localization of this RNA in gradients and little real purification has been achieved. Its $A + U/G + C$ ratio was not so high, i.e., about 0.9–1.0 for this RNA, and it was lower than the 1.0–1.1 of the polysomal mRNA from these cells. Although it seems that the "heterogeneous nuclear RNA" or HnRNA in these cells is the precursor of the mRNA, hybridization studies indicate that large losses of nucleotide sequences must occur in processing of this RNA to mRNA. These early workers also suggested that the 9 S RNA in these cells might be the mRNA for hemoglobin synthesis (15, 280–283).

C. Processing of Newly Synthesized mRNA

There seems little question that the RNA first synthesized in the nucleus has properties different from subsequent products in that it is both more rapidly sedimenting in various types of sucrose gradients, binds tightly to columns such as MAK columns (28, 53, 94, 262), and also it has a higher turnover rate. Processing of ribosomal precursor RNA is understood very well at the present time (59) but processing of nonribosomal RNA is still only incompletely understood (8, 52, 59, 110, 111, 131, 132). The indications are that much of the newly synthesized RNA is destroyed in the nucleus (10, 30, 41, 79, 131, 132, Fig. 5.4), but clear-cut evidence for this has not been presented. Another possibility is that newly synthesized RNA is disaggregated (83, 197). Some regions of nuclear HnRNA have definitive secondary structures referred to as hairpins that may be lost during nuclear processing (4, 156a). Poly A residues are apparently added to the 3′ ends and protein ("informatin") is added for formation of the RNP particles (informofers) that transport the mRNA to the nuclear membranes (Fig. 5.5). Interestingly, in some human leukemic myeloblastic cells, the processing has been reported to be altered (336, 337) so that labeled high molecular weight RNA precursors accumulate. However, this is not a general phenomenon for leukemic cells inasmuch as chronic leukemic lymphocytes as well as a number of other leukemia cells do not accumulate highly labeled

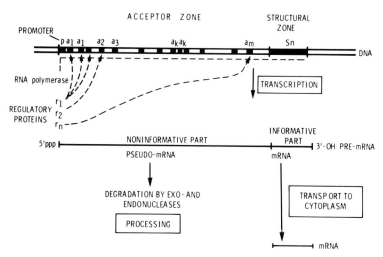

Fig. 5.4. Theoretical model of the transcriptional DNA units in eukaryotic cells (from 109a).

high molecular weight RNA, i.e., it is "unstable" like that of other cells (304, 342).

While most of the rapidly labeled, rapidly sedimenting RNA of tumor cells is a nucleolar precursor of ribosomal RNA of the cytoplasm (13, 50, 279, 315, 373), the membrane-associated "heterogeneous" RNA has been reported to arise from the mitochondria (14).

D. Poly A Terminal Sequences of mRNA

One aspect of the differing $A + U/G + C$ ratios of mRNA and HnRNA that has been clarified is the high content of adenylic acid in mRNA as compared to the nuclear HnRNA. For a number of years, reports appeared on the presence of segments of high molecular weight RNA rich in purine residues (88, 93, 123, 124, 270). Recent evidence indicated that a poly A segment was localized to the 3' terminus of high molecular weight RNA (80, 81, 93, 100, 180, 206, 251). Further, it is added to the RNA after the initial synthesis on the DNA templates. Although the synthetic process is certainly an enzymic one, perhaps of the "slippage" type described years ago for RNA polymerase, the synthetic reaction does not involve DNA templates for high molecular weight RNA (80, 81, 93, 180, 206, 251). Interestingly, these poly A residues are also added to RNA of tumor and other viruses prior to their transcription or replication (158, 175, 252, 299, 348a).

The function of this RNA segment is not known at present. Of the theories for its potential function, one is that poly A residues are involved in the transport of mRNA. Another, referred to as "ticketing," suggests that each time the mRNA is used for synthesis of a protein, one of the A residues is removed (323). Accordingly, in the cytoplasm there should be a variety of different degrees

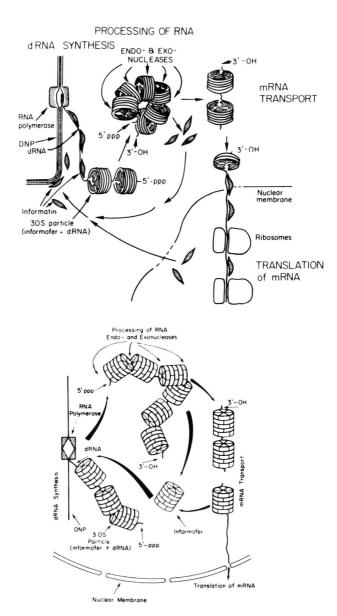

Fig. 5.5. Theoretical model of processing of "informofer-bound" RNA in the informofer cycle (from 109a).

of A contents for a given molecular species and this has been found for hemoglobin mRNA (17, 51, 181).

Another interesting use of the poly A terminals is for the binding of the mRNA species to poly T or poly U columns (112). This technique permits the isolation of many types of mRNA (17) but not all since some mRNA, e.g., histone mRNA, does not contain poly A residues (4).

E. Relationship of mRNA and HnRNA

Many subsequent studies on mRNA and HnRNA have still not completely answered the question of the chemical relationship betwen mRNA of mammalian cells and the nuclar heterogeneous RNA (109a, 308). Among the questions that persist are (1) is all the nuclear heterogeneous RNA the precursor of the mRNA which then undergoes modification by the addition of 200 nucleotide polyadenylic (poly A) sequences to the molecule (Fig. 5.4) and (2) is some heterogeneous mRNA of the nucleus a significantly different type of RNA or an aggregate that may need little further modification to exert its function. The model developed in Fig. 5.3 is based on the data of Table 5.4 which indicates that mRNA competes in hybridization with the 3′ end of HnRNA but not the 5′ end.

A continuing uncertainty relates to the "nativeness" of the nuclear heterogeneous RNA. In the presence of formaldehyde (197), thermal denaturation disaggregated the nuclear heterogeneous RNA to species of much smaller size with molecular weights from 100,000 to 1.4 million as compared to the size estimates of greater than 2 million for the aggregated RNA. As shown in Fig. 5.6, the RNA obtained from Ehrlich ascites cells no longer appeared as a radioactive sweep all over the gradient but rather as a peak in the 8–18 S region. This effect was noted in actinomycin-treated cells, which is important because under the conditions which inhibit synthesis of ribosomal RNA (59) there was a very sharp peak produced in the 10–12 S region which had a spread from the 4 S

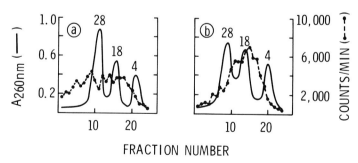

Fig. 5.6a. Effect of thermal denaturation in the presence of formaldehyde on giant heterogeneous nRNA of Ehrlich ascites cells. Cells were pulse labeled for 2 hours with [³H] adenine and heterogeneous nRNA was extracted with phenol at 65°C. (a) Before formaldehyde treatment, centrifuged for 12 hours at 35,000 revolutions/minute. (b) After formaldehyde treatment, centrifuged for 16 hours at 38,000 revolutions/minute (from 197).

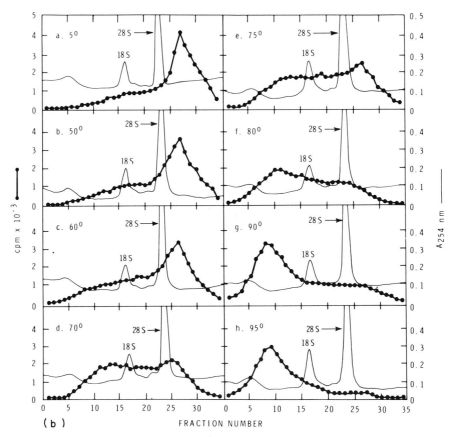

Fig. 5.6b. Aliquots of HnRNA (>28 S) were dissolved in water and heated at the temperature (°C) shown. The marker RNA was added after cooling. The shift of the sedimentation to low molecular weight regions after heating suggests this RNA is aggregated or that its conformational state is markedly altered.

to the 28 S region. Such studies (38a, 59) require demonstration that the RNA species in the aggregated and disaggregated forms were similar in chain length or chemically identical as defined either by nucleotide composition, terminal analysis, or nucleotide sequence.

In view of the high labeling of HnRNA and its likely role as a precursor of mRNA (see above), it seems essential that it be isolated in a satisfactory manner and subjected to fractionation procedures designed to demonstrate its identity or difference in tumors and other tissues. The lack of adequate methods for such studies represents a serious problem for further progress in this field. Since many workers have studied "messenger" activity of various fractions of RNA, it is clearly critical to ascertain whether they are studying meaningful fractions or simply the HnRNA that may be randomly distributed throughout the gradients (5, 154). Relative activities of various fractions may simply represent the degree of dilution of the HnRNA or the mRNA with the nonmessenger types of RNA. In such studies, there must be certainty of the "nativeness" (deg-

TABLE 5.4

HYBRIDIZATION AND COMPETITION PROPERTIES OF 5′ AND 3′ ENDS OF GIANT
PRE-mRNA FROM EHRLICH ASCITES CARCINOMA CELLS[a]

	RNA nonhybridized[b] cpm	RNA hybridized[c]		RNA hybridized in the presence of polysomal RNA as competitor		
		cpm	Hybridization (%)	cpm	Hybridization (%)	Competition (%)
5′-End analysis						
32P in pppNp	370	200	35	230	40	0
32P in Np	1,380,000	110,000	7.4	95,000	6.4	−14
pppNp/Np × 10^{-2}	0.027	0.18	—	0.24	—	—
3′-End analysis						
3H-end nucleoside	2200	494	18.3	155	5.7	−69
14C-internal nucleotides	3940	212	5.2	194	4.7	−10
3H/14C	0.56	2.3	—	1.25	—	—

[a] Figure of two typical experiments at intermediate Cot values (109a). These results support the concept that the polysomal RNA composes the 3′ end of the giant pre-mRNA of these cells.
[b] Original RNA sample.
[c] Hybridization in the absence of competitor.

radation and aggregation) of the RNA molecules isolated from various types of cells. In part, the problem has been resolved by the use of tumors that have low RNase activity although not all tumors share this important property (65). In addition, methods that limit RNase activity are also very helpful (58, 59).

F. Timing of mRNA Synthesis

The synthesis of gene products occurs in ordered time sequences ("the biological clock") in bacterial and viral systems to insure the production of products in an orderly manner for interaction with host factors and ultimate synthesis of new viruses or cells (35, 107, 169, 230, 246, 307, 328). Although aging and maturation processes must involve gene function, there is little evidence for such organized readouts in mammalian cells. Moreover, even in simple systems it is not known why one gene may be read many times while others may be read only once.

The timing of mRNA synthesis was investigated in HeLa cells to determine whether mRNA molecules produced are the same at all times in the cell cycle (242). Unfortunately, the limited sensitivity of the DNA-RNA hybridization method employed did not permit precise conclusions about differences in various phases of the cell cycle (202).

IV. Specific mRNA

A. Hemoglobin mRNA

The prototype of a messenger RNA in mammalian cells is the hemoglobin messenger RNA (Table 5.5). Sufficiently large amounts of this 9 S RNA have been isolated to demonstrate its definitive effect on stimulation of the labeling of specific peptides in hemoglobin and that the distribution of labeled amino acids conformed to the relative amounts of these in the peptides in the molecule. This RNA has subsequently been utilized to serve as a source of messenger for studies with oocytes in vivo (121, 205) which showed the RNA of mouse reticulocytes induced the formation of hemoglobin in amounts proportional to the amount of mRNA added.

The problem of hemoglobin mRNA has been complicated because of the similarity of the mRNA species for both α- and β-globin chains and the difficulty in separating these two species of RNA. Definitive isolation of single hemoglobin mRNA's is under study in several laboratories and with the availability of purer mRNA, it should soon be possible to characterize purer products.

As Table 5.5 indicates, many characteristics of this RNA have been defined and it has been isolated from enough sources to insure the validity of the claims made for its role as a messenger.

TABLE 5.5
HEMOGLOBIN MESSENGER RNA

Origin	Characteristics	Ref.
Rabbit reticulocyte	Nucleotide composition	189
	binding to protein	33
	Poly A sequences	17, 51
	Polysome source	89–91, 99, 146, 149, 150, 215, 234, 257, 330
	Electrophoretic characteristics	174
	Globin product	179, 183, 295
Duck erythrocytes	Giant size precursors, AU-rich	15, 281–283
Turtle, chicken erythrocytes	Stable mRNA	290
Liver nuclei[a]	Liver source	170–172
Fetal mouse yolk sac	Yolk sac synthesis	331

[a] Possibly from residual hematopoietic tissues in liver.

B. Other Types of Messenger RNA

Although the studies on hemoglobin messenger RNA have been preeiminent in the field of messenger RNA of mammalian cells, other systems have been developed or are being developed for studies on mRNA molecules (Table 5.1). At present, mRNA has been isolated from tissues producing myosin, immunoglobulins, and oviduct proteins. Thus far, no reports have appeared on specific "cancer mRNA" but histone mRNA has been isolated from HeLa cells, a tissue culture line derived from a human cervical cancer (38, 156, 161).

C. Hormone-Related mRNA

Among the systems most studied for the effects of cell responses on mRNA formation are those affected by hormones. Early studies in this field lacked specificity because of the problems in both the isolation and analytical methods. Many reports indicate that in response to estrogens (127, 128, 346), thyroid hormones (61–64), cortisol (294), aldosterone (92, 256), hydrocortisone (103), and growth hormone (273), there are changes in both the rate and type of RNA produced in the affected cells (119, 162, 329). These effects occur after binding of the hormone to cytoplasmic protein receptors, transport of the protein-bound hormones to the nucleus, and subsequent gene derepression (86a, 193). Not all of the effects of the hormones are stimulatory, i.e., there are examples of inhibition such as the inhibition of prostatic tumors by estrogens or diethylstilbesterol and inhibition of leukemic cells by cortisone or prednisone. Although these hormones also inhibit RNA synthesis (1), this inhibition is probably a secondary event.

Currently, much more sophisticated approaches to the isolation and definition of function of the products of hormone action have become possible, particularly the mechanisms of action of hormones on production of oviduct proteins (236–239). Specific mRNA's have been purified and their special roles have been shown in the specific synthesis of ovalbumin and other egg proteins (239). Also, inroads have been made into the mechanisms of action of prolactin and insulin on breast tissue (344). Synthesis of new proteins and RNA products have been demonstrated following administration of these hormones.

Although the response of many target cells to hormones includes increased production of both mRNA and rRNA, estradiol inhibits RNA polymerase activity in normal ovaries (48). In ovarian tumors in which the RNA polymerase activity is frequently 2–3 times greater than in the normal ovaries, no inhibition of RNA polymerase activity was produced by estradiol (48).

D. mRNA of Cancer Cells

Some early studies on D-RNA (110, 111) suggested the presence of distinct species of RNA in tumor cells (166, 240, 302). The methods based on the phenol fractionation procedure (316, 317) did not involve heat extraction but instead utilized differential salt concentrations in the aqueous extraction systems. One "heavy" RNA fraction extracted from mouse ascites tumor cells contained an "AU-rich" RNA $(A + U/G + C = 0.82)$ that was "DNA-like" (130).* An RNA bound to DNA had a nucleotide composition of A, 28%; U, 26%; G, 23%; and C, 23% $(A + U/G + C = 1.15)$. However, studies in this laboratory showed that the overall ^{32}P nucleotide compositions of nuclear RNA in a variety of tumors including a series of Morris hepatomas were quite similar; the $A + U/G + C$ ratio was found to be 0.74–0.78 by ^{32}P-nucleotide composition (56); all the tumor RNA had a lower AMP content (20–24%) than normal liver (30%) but most had a higher UMP content than the normal liver. In general, the UV nucleotide composition was different only in the higher GC (GMP + CMP) content of the tumor, i.e., 60% compared to 52% for liver (56, 296).

These initial results on D-RNA of tumors and the lack of clear differences on the basis of nucleotide compositions indicated that much more refined probes were necessary to differentiate RNA readouts in tumors and other tissues.

1. HYBRIDIZATION

The initiation of the hybridization method (190) which was followed by the development of the commonly used Millipore or filter paper method (113, 114) led to the development of more modern, yet still nondefinitive approaches to mRNA of tumor cells. In competition studies, one type of RNA competes with another for binding sites on DNA. If the unlabeled RNA competes well

---

* Reports that the kidney and the thymus contained "DNA-like" RNA, i.e., with an $A + U/G + C$ ratio of approximately 1.33 (129), suggested that the whole DNA is read in these cells. This idea is at variance with data on hybridization of RNA in a number of tissues which suggested that only a portion of the genome was read and that different cistrons were read in different tissues such as thymus and the kidney.

with labeled RNA, it is assumed to be the same or very similar but if it does not, it is different. Using this method, it was found that the RNA produced in normal liver did not completely compete with the RNA produced in the Morris or Yoshida hepatomas (68) and conversely, the RNA produced in these tumors did not completely compete with the RNA of normal liver. These and other hybridization studies suggested that different RNA molecules are produced in these types of tissues (162–164, 195). In other hybridization studies, similar differences were found in the RNA produced in mouse tumors, i.e., the products obtained differed in their competition capacity with that of nontumor tissues (69, 162–164).

Although some have concluded that there are marked differences in readouts from tissue to tissue (47, 198) and in tumor readouts from those of other tissues (68, 69, 168, 195), others (297, 298) report that there are no significant differences in the readouts of tumors and other tissues. It is generally conceded that tumors have a different distribution of RNA readouts than control tissues (111, 275), but it has not been possible to demonstrate a specific difference to this time. Such distribution differences may well relate to the significantly greater nucleolar activity and size of many tumors as compared to other tissues.

These important studies on hybridization should be carried forward, but they are hampered by the lack of methods for purification of the very small quantities of individual RNA molecules of tumors. Some successes are now being reported in studies on viral RNA (see p. 211) but at present there are serious difficulties in drawing any general conclusions about tumors inasmuch as they vary markedly from one another in gene readouts (254, 261, 300) (see Chapter XIII). The most important question is whether there is one general type of "cancer mRNA."

COT* VALUES AND REPETITIVE DNA SEQUENCES. Among the complexities (31) with respect to the hybridization of various types of RNA to DNA are those of the numbers of DNA sequences to which the RNA can bind and the stability of the hybrids that are formed. The idea is that the greater the number of places on the genome on which a given type of RNA molecule might fit, the more likely they are to find their proper complementary DNA (low Cot values). On the other hand, if the number of sites on which the given RNA might fit is relatively small, it would take longer for a given number of such RNA molecules to align themselves on the complementary DNA sites (high Cot value). Since some sequences are highly repetitive in DNA such as those for synthesis of rRNA, satisfactory hybridization comparisons are readily made for these. For some of the crucial messenger RNA molecules, only a few template sites may be present in the genome (31, 79).

Although there is no information available at present on the number of copies that exist for any cistron, it may be presumed that some are present in large

---

* Cot was originally defined as the product of the initial concentration of DNA (c_0) and the time required for DNA renaturation, and is defined for a given temperature, salt concentration, and DNA fragment size. The lower the Cot values, the larger the number of DNA binding sites. The same principles have now been applied to RNA hybridization to DNA.

numbers, i.e., several hundreds of copies, and others may be present in as small a number as only one copy. With this problem in mind, experiments on hybridization have now been extended markedly in time. For some studies on messenger RNA, periods of hybridization of 3 weeks or longer are being attempted. Even under the optimal conditions, complete saturation of DNA by RNA has not been shown. Moreover, the nonrepetitive portion of the genome (44, 45) was found to vary 20–60% (Table 5.6). This problem as well as some nonspecificity of hybridization (44, 45) limits interpretations of the earlier studies on tumor RNA hybridization (68, 69). There is some uncertainty about the value of such methods to establish differences in tumors and other tissues, although improved conclusions may be drawn with increased purity of the RNA being hybridized.

An interesting approach to separation of RNA species with different Cot values was tested by hybridizations that were interrupted at 3, 6, and 9 hours (243). After the initial "burst" of hybridization, each of the hybridizations at later time points resulted in a plateau of hybrid formation. For the "reiterated" segments of the genome, hybridization proceeded rapidly. For the less reiterated or nonreiterated portions of the genome, the hybridizations proceed much more slowly.

In another approach to the problem, efforts have been made to isolate individual or groups of chromosomes. Unfortunately, in the development of metaphase plate, even in the most "synchronized" cells, there is only limited synchrony of chromosome formation or condensation. Thus, while some chromosomes are just being formed, others are well into metaphase. Since chromosomes in metaphase continue to condense, or shrink in size, and some of the larger ones become smaller than the smaller chromosomes just entering metaphase, sucrose density gradient centrifugation was unable to separate clearly these into type specific or size specific groups. The separation of "big" and "small" chromosomes has not provided definitive results with respect to chromosomal hybridization (242). Hopefully isolation of specific chromosomes will permit more definitive studies in the near future.

TABLE 5.6
COMPLEXITY OF SOME GENOMES[a]

| Organisms | Genome size | | Percentage of genome which is nonrepetitive | Complexity in number of nucleotides |
	Picograms (pg)/ haploid genome	Number of nucleotides		
Scaphiopus	1.2	1.1×10^9	60	0.7×10^9
Engystomops	2.7	2.5×10^9	50	1.2×10^9
Xenopus (toad)	3.0	2.7×10^9	55	1.3×10^9
Bufo (frog)	5.0	4.6×10^9	20	0.9×10^9
Rana (frog)	8.0	7.3×10^9	22	1.6×10^9
Ambystoma	42.0	3.8×10^{10}	20	7.6×10^9
Bos (cow)	3.5	3.2×10^9	55	1.6×10^9

[a] From Britten and Davidson (45).

Since the critical task is the demonstration and isolation of the mRNA of the tumors that specify cancer, if such really exist, it seems unfortunate that thus far, only one messenger (presumptive) RNA, namely that of the histones has been reported to be isolated from cancer cells (38, 156, 161). Otherwise, all of the isolated messengers have been obtained from cells with highly specialized functions (Table 5.1). Attempts to isolate tumor-specific messenger RNA molecules have all suffered from the inherent biochemical problems of dealing with many molecular species; clearly by the very nature of the tumor cell, most of its life processes must be very similar to those of other tissues.

An early suggestion of differences in the RNA of tumors and liver was the report (75) that Novikoff hepatoma tumors contained less RNP and that major components in tumor RNA found by ECTEOLA chromatography were absent in similar liver preparations. The obverse was also true, i.e., major liver components were absent from the tumors. However, no subsequent reports have confirmed these differences.

2. Viral Genome Incorporation

One of the very informative results of studies on the incorporation of the viral genome into mammalian cells is that relatively few molecules are required for transformation of the mammalian cells. Although early reports (353) indicated 5–60 genome equivalents of SV40 DNA were present in transformed cells, as few as 1 to 5 such molecules may be sufficient to redirect the synthetic activity of the host genome and in oncogenesis to create those conditions necessary for neoplastic transformation (278, 284, 289). DNA reassociation kinetics on hydroxylapatite showed that 1 genome equivalent of SV40 DNA was present in 4 of 5 transformed lines and the other had 3 genome equivalents (108). Values of 0.45 to 0.5 were background values in these studies. The 0.5 copies per normal Green African monkey kidneys may either be integration sites or actually reflect the presence of such genomes in normal cells.* While it is not yet clear whether the DNA is integrated as a single genome at one site or whether there are many genome fragments distributed throughout the genome, it seems likely that integration occurs at one site, since reconstitution of the intact virus is possible.

Such results do not precisely define the response of the neoplastic cells to the presence of viral genes. It is necessary to define the number and type of viral RNA molecules produced in each affected cell (246). It is possible that there is a reading of one copy of mRNA from the integrated viral genome, or there may be many. If the number is small, i.e., 1 to 3 RNA molecules per cell, there are key technical problems in isolating such a few gene readouts. Moreover, it is not known whether such molecules are RNA species of the "heterogeneous" variety or are discrete entities that are readily separable on polyacrylamide gels (55, 268). Introduction of oncogenic virus such as polyoma

---

* To localize adenovirus DNA, *in situ* hybridization was carried out with adenovirus RNA (199), but no precise localization was found.

virus into cells produced a change in the gene readouts as shown by the rapid production of 20 S and 10 S RNA species (18). In addition, new 4 S RNA species were produced. The RNA from avian myeloblastosis virus exhibited template activity suggesting that the RNA from these species could be effective as an intracellular messenger (104, 263). In mouse and human mammary carcinomas, it has been found that 70 S RNA-directed DNA synthesis occurs. Both the polymerase and its 70 S RNA are found in oncornavirus particles (120a).

The presence of RNP particles in human tumor viruses, like those of animal tumor virus, has been more extensively studied (17a,b,c, 120a, 133a, 137a, 159a, 173a, 283a, 311a,b). These particles contain 70 S RNA which hybridizes well with DNA produced by reverse transcription of the viral RNA. In addition, these particles contain a reverse transcriptase. It seems possible that the RNA of these virus particles is the product of viral DNA produced in the infected cells by reverse transcription and then incorporated into the mammalian genome. Another possibility is that partial viral infections continue in the tumor cells during their growth and development. It is critical that "passenger viruses" be eliminated as the source of such particles.

3. Nucleotide Composition

Studies on nucleotide compositions of tumor and other RNA's have suffered from two major difficulties, (a) those arising from homogenization (255) and (b) pools of RNA precursors in tumors and other tissues (251, 298, 365). Some of the problems of homogenization relate to RNases, the relative amounts of RNA in the cytoplasm, and also the total number of polysomes in the cytoplasm (255).

In studies on high molecular weight nuclear RNA of tumors and other tissues, differences were found in ^{32}P-nucleotide compositions (Table 5.7). Such data indicate that tumors produce more GC-rich ribosomal precursor RNA than the normal liver which produces more AU-rich RNA (Table 5.7) (53, 110, 296). Such results would be anticipated from the types and sizes of nucleoli present in these tumors and normal liver (55, 56, 59, 204, 233).

TABLE 5.7

Distribution of ^{32}P in Nucleotides of Early-Labeled Nuclear RNA[a]

	Liver		Walker tumor	
	45 S	55 S	45 S	55 S
Adenylic acid (A)	24.9	26.1	15.3	17.6
Uridylic acid (U)	21.2	22.6	22.7	24.0
Guanylic acid (G)	29.5	26.5	32.3	30.0
Cytidylic acid (C)	24.4	24.8	29.7	28.5
A + U/G + C	0.86	0.95	0.61	0.71

[a] From Okamura and Busch (233).

The data of Table 5.7 (233) require consideration of the following possibilities:

1. The higher A + U/G + C ratio in liver results from the production of different types of messenger RNA in the liver than in the tumor.
2. The higher A + U/G + C ratio in the liver results from the production of more messenger RNA and less preribosomal RNA.
3. The result reflects artifactual differences that may arise from differences in *in vivo* labeling because of pools or differences in types of components in the system.

When the methods for isolation of nucleoli became routine (59), it was found that the marked differences in the labeling pattern of the whole nuclear high molecular weight RNA was reflected in the nucleolar RNA (Table 5.8). In a series of studies of the labeling of whole nuclear RNA in a variety of tumors of the Morris hepatoma series, some, like the hepatoma 7787, 7800 and the R3b tumors, had nucleotide compositions similar to those of the regenerating liver, particularly when the results were corrected for the ^{32}P-nucleotide compositions of the nucleolar RNA (Table 5.9).*

* For the residue ("nucleolochromosomal") fractions there were no significant differences by UV nucleotide analysis although the liver had a characteristic higher AMP content by ^{32}P analysis. The uncertainties resulting from this crude data (55, 56, 204, 233) were such that it was not possible to be certain of definitive differences between the RNA readouts of tumor and liver cells.

TABLE 5.8
^{32}P-NUCLEOTIDE COMPOSITION OF 45 S NUCLEOLAR RNA[a]

Source	AMP	UMP	GMP	CMP	r
Hepatomas					
Morris hepatoma					
9618A	14.7	19.5	34.4	31.4	0.52
9618B	14.4	20.4	34.4	30.8	0.53
9121	14.0	18.6	35.4	32.0	0.48
9098	13.1	20.7	34.0	32.1	0.49
7787	15.7	20.2	35.5	28.7	0.56
Novikoff hepatoma	12.1	21.3	33.5	33.1	0.50
Other tumors					
HeLa cells	13.1	17.2	36.6	33.2	0.44
H-50 cells-SV40 transformed	13.4	22.4	35.4	28.8	0.56
Walker tumor	13.2	20.6	34.4	31.7	0.51
Ehrlich ascites	12.6	22.1	33.2	32.0	0.53
Normal liver	19.3	16.6	39.4	24.7	0.56
Regenerating liver	19.3	17.9	38.8	24.0	0.59
Thioacetamide-treated liver (9 days)	18.5	16.4	37.6	26.1	0.55

[a] ^{32}P-nucleotide composition of 45 S nucleolar RNA after pulse labeling with [^{32}P] orthophosphate. The values are percentages of the total ^{32}P in each of the four nucleotides. The values for each of the tumors are averages of two to four determinations on individual samples. r, ratio of AMP + UMP/GMP + CMP.

TABLE 5.9
^{32}P-NUCLEOTIDE COMPOSITION OF 45 S NUCLEAR RNA[a]

	AMP	UMP	GMP	CMP	r
Hepatoma					
9618A	16.9	21.1	31.7	30.4	0.61
9121	16.8	20.6	33.5	29.0	0.60
9108	17.4	21.7	31.1	29.0	0.66
9098	15.8	22.6	31.5	30.1	0.61
8995	16.0	21.3	31.9	30.8	0.59
7800	21.6	25.3	29.8	23.5	0.88
7787	20.0	22.4	30.2	27.4	0.74
3924A	18.3	22.2	31.5	28.0	0.68
R7	17.0	21.7	31.9	29.1	0.63
R3B	19.5	24.6	30.8	25.1	0.79
Walker tumor	15.3	22.7	32.3	29.7	0.61
Normal liver	26.6	23.0	25.8	24.3	1.00
Regenerating liver	21.8	18.5	34.7	24.9	0.68
Thioacetamide-treated liver	25.6	23.0	26.2	25.1	0.95

[a] ^{32}P-nucleotide composition of 45 S nuclear RNA after pulse labeling with [^{32}P] orthophosphate. The values are percentages of the total ^{32}P in each of the four nucleotides. The
values for each of the tumors are averages of two to four determinations on individual samples.
r, ratio of AMP + UMP/GMP + CMP.

4. CHROMOSOMAL RNA

When successive salt extractions were made to separate nuclear high molecular
weight RNA into fractions soluble in 0.15 M NaCl (the "nuclear sap" fraction),
2 M NaCl (the "chromatin fraction"), and the insoluble residue (the "residue"
or "nucleolochromosomal fraction"), high molecular weight RNA was found
in each fraction. In the 2 M NaCl extract, the RNA was rich in uridylic acid
both by ^{32}P and UV nucleotide analysis, i.e., 31 and 27%, respectively. The
A + U/G + C ratio was approximately 1.1. This RNA was separable into sedimentation classes (Fig. 5.7) which had very similar nucleotide compositions.
Accordingly, it may be part of the "aggregated" HnRNA (see p. 203). This
RNA differs markedly from that of the "residue fraction" with the corresponding
sedimentation coefficients which have A + U/G + C ratios of 0.60–0.68. Further
studies are necessary to determine whether there are differences in individual
RNA species or hybridization characteristics of these RNA fractions in tumors
and other tissues. As yet, on the basis of nucleotide composition, clear-cut distinc-
tions have not been shown between the extranucleolar RNA of the tumors and
other tissues.

"Chromosomal RNA" has also been used to identify a type of low molecular
weight RNA extracted from a residue fraction of nuclei previously treated with
dilute saline solutions. This "cRNA" was said to have unusual properties (36,
37, 196): (1) a content of 30% dihydrouridylic acid; (2) a content of 10% dihy-
droribothymidylic acid; (3) a high content of adenylic and uridylic acids; (4)

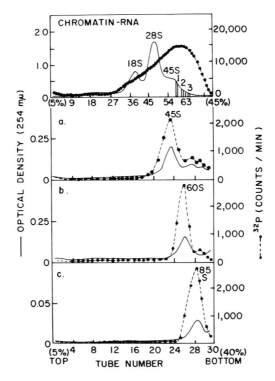

Fig. 5.7. (Top) Zonal ultracentrifugation pattern of RNA of the chromatin fraction. Samples containing 100 mg of RNA were centrifuged through a 5–45% linear sucrose gradient at 35,000 rpm for 15 hours at 4°C. Figure 5.7a, b, and c: RNA from the rapidly sedimenting fractions 1, 2, and 3 obtained by zonal ultracentrifugation (top) was precipitated and rerun on 5–40% sucrose gradients in a SB 110 rotor of International B-35 centrifuge at 25,000 rpm for 15 hours at 4°C: a, b, and c are the analytical patterns for fractions 1, 2, and 3, respectively. ——O.D.; --- ● --- ● --- radioactivity (from 296).

hybridization to 10% of the total DNA; (5) a low molecular weight and sedimentation coefficient of 3 S or less; and (6) function as gene repressors and activators. Some hybridization differences of this RNA have been reported for tumors, regenerating liver and other tissues (195, 196), but cRNA has been the subject of controversy. Several studies have suggested that cRNA is a degradation product (12). When tRNA was added to such chromatin preparations (140a), it was degraded to products similar to those noted above (36, 37, 197). Since dihydrouridylic acid and ribothymidylic acid have only been found in tRNA, degradation of such molecules could result in the formation of these products. Moreover, under the conditions for extraction of the chromosomal RNA, there was adherence of almost any type of added RNA in the medium to the "chromatin" (12). With citric acid nuclei and treatment with CsCl or 5 M urea, the "chromosomal RNA" fraction or "skin" fraction was not found. Although it was concluded (12) that the cRNA was an artifact, this has been debated recently (147a) on the grounds that tRNA was not degraded in its preparation.

5. Stimulatory Activity of Tumor RNA for Amino Acid Uptake

Demonstration of messenger activity by increased uptake of labeled amino acids into proteins (192, 227) has served to establish that tumor cells contain RNA with stimulatory activity. The RNA of the nuclear sap of the AH-130 hepatoma had high activity in stimulation of amino acid uptake in such systems. The RNA's that had the highest activity had sedimentation coefficients of 18 S and greater than 45 S. Similar results for stimulation of amino acid uptake were reported for whole liver nuclear RNA (154). The activity of the nucleolar RNA was less than that of the nuclear sap but higher than that of chromosomal RNA. The HnRNA is present throughout the sedimentation gradients, but some have reported its localization particularly in the 8–18 S region. It is possible that such RNA species account for the stimulatory activity in the systems employed (5, 154). Accordingly, the activity of the fractions studied may simply reflect the relative amounts of the heterogeneous RNA and the nonheterogeneous RNA (212).

6. Stability and Degradation of mRNA in Tumors

Degradation of mRNA is orderly in bacterial systems (20, 107, 303), but in mammalian cells studies on RNA degradation are complicated by enzymes that may not be normally involved in degradation of cellular RNA such as lysosomal RNases and latent or "masked" RNases (59). The release of these enzymes by procedures normally employed for disruption of cells has led to the extensive precautions necessary in studies on RNA of tumors and other tissues (Section II).

Nonetheless, many workers have dealt with the stability of mRNA, both membrane bound and in free polysomes (176). Turnover of this RNA probably reflects degradative processes but clear-cut evidence has not been unequivocally obtained for turnover that is not related to new cell synthesis. Indeed, recent studies indicate mRNA of tumors has a half-life similar to that of the cell (41, 118a).

The "DNA-like RNA" associated with the rough endoplasmic reticulum and polysomes of both the Morris hepatomas and the normal liver may be the mRNA or its precursor in liver and tumor cells (see Chapter XIII). Much of the data dealing with its stability (188, 305) has been criticized on the grounds that it is not possible to show that actinomycin D totally blocks new synthesis of mRNA (96, 319), that turnover rates based on enzyme activity may reflect protein turnover rather than mRNA turnover, and that convincing evidence for turnover of mammalian cell RNA has not been presented.

If any RNA turnover exists, the catabolic reactions must be mediated by specific enzymes. RNases of tumors and other tissues are both endo- and exonucleases. The content of RNases is lower in some tumors than in growing or nongrowing nontumor tissues, suggesting the possibility that RNA degradation is less in such cells. Some rapidly growing nontumor tissues have much larger contents of RNases than resting tissues (59, 65, 316); RNases may account for the half-life of rRNA of 5.5 days in normal liver and a reported half-life of mRNA as short as 3 hours up to the half-life of the cell (118a, 138–140).* Perhaps some "RNases" are processing or "trimming" enzymes but at this point it is not possible to distinguish these in the usual assays for RNase.

E. Transport

mRNA-Containing RNP Particles

Considerable evidence has accumulated that the transport of mRNA of the nucleus to the cytoplasm (Fig. 5.5) occurs in the form of RNP particles (138–140, 153, 167, 225, 275–277, 287) which have been called "informosomes" (207, 312–314). Conceptually, these particles may migrate to the nuclear membrane where polysome formation may occur. These RNP particles are both dissociable and reconstitutable under appropriate conditions (138–140, 211, 217–220). There is specific binding of the mRNA primarily with one protein (referred to as "informatin") and possibly with others (275–277, 355). Residues of associated RNP particles combined with mRNA, particularly 8–18 S nuclear RNA (200, 355). Protein binding is characteristic of mRNA even in the cytoplasm (32, 33, 217–220, 235).

Since the functioning element in protein synthesis in the cytoplasm is the polysome, its origin and transport have been of special interest, particularly whether polysomes are transported from the nucleus intact or whether the mRNA is transported alone (52, 59, 143, 148). It has been suggested that there is an altered transport of RNA to the cytoplasm in tumor cells (297, 298), but there is no certainty on this point possibly because of the difficulty of evaluating which of the molecules in the cytoplasm are representative of the newly synthesized RNA. Turnover of the protein associated with mRNA (33, 235, 275, 276) is not defined adequately either in tumors or other tissues.

F. mRNA and Polysomes

mRNA functions in association with ribosomes (133, 136, 192, 208, 213, 227, 250, 264, 277, 303, 349, 349a). Although methods have been sought for quantitatively releasing intact messenger RNA from polysomes (32, 34), there are only a few reports for isolation of purified messengers from tumor cells (38, 156, 161). There is clearly a great need for improved methods for such studies.

G. mRNA and Mitosis

Daughter cells may contain maternal specialized readouts that influence their functions both during and after mitosis. Protein synthesis decreases in mammalian cells and polysomes disaggregate during metaphase (145). However, even

---

* RNase activity may have accounted for the differences reported in polyribosome:ribosome ratios of hepatomas and normal liver (352).

when actinomycin D is added to the medium, polysomes are observed to reform within 30 minutes after metaphase, and within 45 minutes after metaphase there is an increase in protein synthesis. Selected proteins are synthesized as shown by some of the peptides formed. This finding is of considerable consequence with respect to persistent gene function inasmuch as it demonstrates that there is an important possibility that specific functions are transmitted to daughter cells by the mRNA left in the cells. It is possible that such RNA produces gene derepressors or inducers that are specific for one or more specialized genes. For example, if the gene derepressors for liver functions persist in the dividing cells of regenerating liver, the maintenance of the liver readout will continue in the daughter cells. This result also has important implications for the continuity of neoplastic traits in daughter cells of cancer cells and for paramutations as well (Chapter I).

V. Utilization of Informational RNA

One of the persistent questions in modern pharmacology is whether "genetic engineering" can take advantage of any specific gene information (54, 60) as an approach to cancer chemotherapy (57) or other disease states (118). One key question is whether some types of informational or structural RNA may be involved in "memory," control of specifying cellular gene readouts, or some other functional control that may be meaningful. For example, an RNA-rich extract was recently found (187) to be effective in increasing the avoidance responses of rats when the RNA was obtained from the brains of trained rats, particularly cerebral RNA. The RNA from the brains of untrained rats and other control RNA was less effective or ineffective. The conditions utilized for the extraction of the RNA should, in effect, only have released mainly ribosomal RNA and accordingly it is a question as to whether this is (a) a valid and specific result or (b) some sort of blocking of degradation of functional intracellular RNA. To understand the mechanisms, studies are required on the sites at which the RNA is localized and its function at these specific sites of action.

Another similar example is endometrial RNA (364) which was injected into regressed uteri; this was followed by increased production of alkaline phosphatase in the uterine epithelium. The injected controls i.e., with 0.15 M NaCl, liver RNA, and RNase-treated endometrial RNA, produced no similar effect. This system may also be useful for studies on mRNA utilization.

Studies of this type have endured much skepticism since it was reported (229) that RNA of normal liver converted hepatoma cells to normal liver cells, particularly since others were unable to repeat the work. Similarly, rat liver RNA was reported to inhibit growth of rat ascites hepatoma cells while ascites cell RNA, yeast RNA, and rabbit liver RNA were ineffective (11). Another approach to tumor inhibition has been the use of DNA which was shown to inhibit growth of Walker tumors (126). Calf spleen RNA was found to decrease malignancy and increase the oxygen consumption of leukemic cells (98).

Recently, increased immune responses to tumors have been reported (253, 333) after administration of "programmed" RNA to tumor-bearing animals. Moreover, injections of hemoglobin mRNA into oocytes was followed by hemoglobin production in these cells (121, 205). Clearly the controls in these studies must be very rigorous since cells contain surface nucleases and other protective mechanisms against extrinsic nucleic acids (76, 231, 232).

From the point of view of cancer chemotherapy, the results of current studies on mRNA of tumor cells have not provided targets or defined utilizable products (57). The former objective would be ideal for chemists interested in modifying RNA or synthesizing analog oligonucleotides that could be of chemotherapeutic value if definitive "cancer specific sequences" could be identified. Approaches to this type of "genetic engineering" have been suggested (54, 73, 112, 185, 341, 343, 362), but the lack of defined chemical targets and the problems of developing procedures for cellular transmembrane transport of oligonucleotides are the key limitations to developments in this field (54, 76, 231, 232).

If there were ways to define the critical limitations of cancer cells with respect to cellular controls, such as a mechanism that restrains growth of normal cells but not of cancer cells, it would be possible that mRNA with the appropriate codes for such controls could be extracted from nontumor cells and taken up into tumor cells in appropriately protected form (109). Possibly the growth patterns of tumors might be blocked or such RNA might be "reversely transcribed" into a DNA that would perpetuate the inhibition of the tumor cells (47a, 289). Alternatively, specific antinucleic acid antibodies might be utilized (97). Such intriguing possibilities await critical research developments in the field of mRNA to make them feasible.

VI. High Molecular Weight RNA of the Nucleolus

A. Controls of Synthesis of Ribosomal RNA

Although the mechanisms of control of rRNA synthesis are not yet defined, they appear to provide for a precise correlation with growth rates and protein synthesis of tissues (9, 59). As examples, in contact inhibited cells and mature lymphocytes, the synthesis of rRNA is markedly inhibited (95) while in regenerating liver cells there is a tenfold increase in rRNA synthesis. Among the mechanisms available for increasing rates of rRNA synthesis are increased availability of active RNA polymerase I, increased reading rates of rDNA (71, 137, 327), and, recently, amplification of rDNA genes that has been found to be important in amphibian oocytes (59). Involvement of reverse transcriptase in the amplification process has been suggested (47a, 101).

The morphological demonstrations of the relative increase in nuclear and nucleolar sizes in tumor cells (Chapter II) and the pleomorphism of the nucleoli of the cancer cell have naturally led to the question of whether the RNP products of the nucleus and nucleolus differ from those of other cells. The difficult task of purification of individual high molecular weight RNA has been achieved for only a few mammalian RNA species including some transfer RNA, some low molecular weight nuclear RNA species (Chapter VI), rRNA, and nucleolar high molecular weight species. Sequencing the RNA species of tumor cells has only recently been successful, largely due to the evolution of the ^{32}P-labeling method (147, 278). Although it may seem that the rate of information accumulation should be extremely rapid in this field, in 1973 the sequences are defined for only a few transfer RNA molecules of mammalian origin, nuclear 4.5 S RNA$_I$, 5 S RNA, and U2 RNA (55, 58, 267, 268). Only regional information is available for any higher molecular weight RNA species (152, 221, 291–293).

B. Ribosomal and Preribosomal RNA

The elegant studies on ribosomal and nucleolar RNA have been amply summarized in recent years (7, 13, 59, 361). Ribosomal RNA consists of four major types, 28 S, 18 S, 5.5 S, and 5 S RNA, with approximate molecular weights of 1.7 million, 0.6 million, 50,000, and 40,000 respectively. Each ribosome contains one each of these molecules in its total structure which has a sedimentation coefficient of approximately 80 S. The 18 S and 28 S rRNA molecules are the backbones of the 40 S and 60 S subunits of the ribosomes (13, 59, 100). The 5 S RNA molecule is apparently part of a small ribonucleoprotein particle in the 60 S ribosomal subunit that is essential for the function of the ribosome but for which a definitive function has not yet been defined. Unequivocal evidence has now been provided that the source of ribosomal 18 S and 28 S RNA is the nucleolus, but the source of the 5 S RNA is extranucleolar; it is apparently synthesized on a one to one basis with the other ribosomal RNA species.

Information on the differences of ribosomal RNA of various species has been accumulating slowly (29, 186, 291–293). Although there have been suggestions by many laboratories that in both 18 S RNA and 28 S RNA there may be several types with differing structures (77) with either macro- or microheterogeneity, the chemical evidence indicates the rRNA in a single species is very constant. Quantitative analysis of molar yields of fragments of ribosomal RNA indicates that there is only 1 major species each of 18 S and 28 S rRNA.* While the possibility cannot be completely ruled out yet that there are minor components of these molecules, convincing evidence has not been presented that they are not artifacts resulting from nonspecific cleavage of higher molecular weight molecules or aggregation products of smaller molecules (144).

C. Nucleolar Precursors of Ribosomal RNA

Extensive studies have been devoted both to the machinery for the development and organization of the nucleolus itself and for the reading of the nucleolar rDNA templates for the synthesis of rRNA (59, 213). The nucleolar apparatus

---

* In *E. coli* where the structure of 16 S rRNA seems also to be consistent with a single species (371a), much of the topography of relationship of this RNA and its associated proteins has been defined.

TABLE 5.10
RATES OF SYNTHESIS OF NUCLEOLAR RNA[a]

Tissue	Nucleolar RNA (fg/min/nucleolus)
Normal liver	3
Regenerating liver (18 hr)	15
Thioacetamide-treated liver	35
Novikoff hepatoma	45

[a] From Busch and Smetana (59).

is of great interest (Chapter II), and its ribosomal products are essential to the protein synthesizing machinery and hence to the life of the cell. The nucleolar rRNA precursor is largely one RNA species of rather great length, ranging from 12,000 to 36,000 nucleotides. The sedimentation coefficients of these RNA molecules are 45 S RNA, the elementary unit, 65 S RNA, a dimer, and 85 S RNA, a trimer of the 45 S RNA (141a). The rates of synthesis have been defined for several tissues (Table 5.10).

Many data show that 45 S nRNA contains both 18 S and 28 S rRNA (59). After the initial suggestion that such RNA was the precursor of ribosomal RNA (279), subsequent experiments (45a) showed that in enucleolate mutants, neither 45 S nRNA nor 28 S rRNA was formed. Thus, when the genes for ribosomal precursor RNA synthesis were missing, the products could not be formed.

The presence of both rRNA species in 45 S nRNA was proved by hybridization competition studies (13, 258). Both 18 S rRNA and 28 S rRNA compete with the hybridization of 45 S RNA and, when combined they compete independently (Fig. 5.8). These data indicate that each 45 S nRNA molecule contains one molecule of the two rRNA species.

Much chemical evidence supports these hybridization studies. The highly hydrogen-bonded B3 fragment was found in 45 S nRNA, 35 S nRNA and 28 S

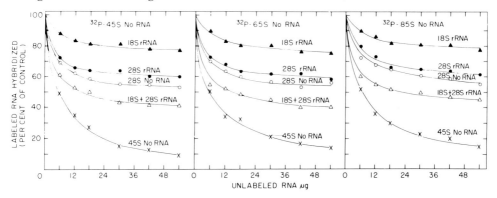

Fig. 5.8. Hybridization competition between ^{32}P-labeled 45 S, 65 S, and 85 S nucleolar RNA's and unlabeled 18 S rRNA, 28 S rRNA, 18 S + 28 S rRNA, 28 S nucleolar RNA (nRNA), and 45 S nucleolar RNA. Six micrograms of labeled nucleolar RNA were used for each point (from 258).

rRNA (365a). The octa-, nona-, deca-, undeca-, and dodecanucleotides produced by pancreatic RNase digestion of 28 S, 35 S, and 45 S were identical
for normal liver and Novikoff hepatoma (291). A tetradecanucleotide marker
of 18 S rRNA produced by pancreatic digestion was also found in 45 S nRNA.
Combined digestion with U2 RNase and T1 RNase produced common marker
polypyrimidine oligonucleotides from both 28 S and 18 S rRNA that are also
found in 45 S nRNA (Table 5.11). In another approach to this problem, marker-
methylated oligonucleotides and other oligonucleotides were found in 18 S and
28 S rRNA and also in 45 S nRNA (29, 186).

The scheme presented (Fig. 5.9) agrees with that of other workers (352a,
373) in most respects. Critical differences are the detection of a variety of subspecies of RNA including 41 S, 32 S, 24 S, and 20 S RNA, which have not

TABLE 5.11A

OLIGONUCLEOTIDE SEQUENCES COMMON TO 45 S nRNA AND 28 S rRNA

Fragment[a]	Sequence
	Longer sequences of 28 S rRNA
Partial T1 RNase digestion	
B3-9 Fragment (99)	ACCCCCUCUCCUUUCCGCCCGGGCCCGCCCCUCCUCU-CCCGCGGGGCCCCGCCGUCCCCGCGUCGUCGCCGU-GGUUCCCCCCUCUCCUCUUCCCGUCCGp.
β Fragment (20)	AAAUACCACmUACUUCCAUCGp
Δ Fragment (28)	AACCUAUCUUCAUCUCAAACUUUAAAUGp
GmU Fragment (15)	CUCCGmUAUUCAAUUAGp
UmGmU Fragment (23)	UmGmUUUCACCCAUAUCAAUACCAG
Combined U2 and T1 RNase digestion	
Octanucleotides (8)	CCCCCCCGp; CCUCUCCCAp; CUCUCUCGp; CUUUCCCGp; UCUCUUCGp
Nonanucleotides (9)	CUUCUCCCGp; CUCCUCUCGp
Decanucleotides (10)	CUUUCCUCCGp; UUUUCCUCCGp
Undecanucleotides (11)	CCCCCCUCCCAp; CUCUCCCCCCGp
Dodecanucleotides (12)	CCUCUCCCUCCGp
Tridecanucleotides (13)	CCCCCCCUUUCCGp; CCCUCCCUUUCCGp
Tetradecanucleotides (14)	CCCCUCCUCUCCCGp
Pentadecanucleotides (15)	(CCCCCUC)UCCUUCCGp; (CCCCCUU)CCUUCCCCGp
Hexadecanucleotide (16)	CCCCCUCUCCUUUCCGp
Unicosanucleotide (21)	(UUCCCCCUC)UCCUCUUCCCGp
	Shorter sequences of 28 S rRNA
Pancreatic RNase digestion	
Tetradecanucleotide (14)	(AAAAGp)(A-Gp)(Gp)(Gp)(Gp)AAACp
Undecanucleotides (11)	(AAGp)(A-Gp)(C-Gp)(Gp)(Gp)(Gp)Up
Decanucleotides (10)	(A-Gp)(Gp)(Gp)(Gp)AAGGUp; (AAAGp)(A-Gp)(Gp)(Gp)(Gp)Up
Nonanucleotides (9)	AAAAGGAACp; AGAGGAAACp; GGGAAGAGUp; (Gp)(Gp)(A-Gp)(A-Gp)AACp; (AAAAGp)(A-Gp)(Gp)Up
Octanucleotides (8)	GAAAAGACp; GAAGAAGCp; GAGGAAGCp; GAAAGAGUp
Heptanucleotides (7)	AAGAAGCp; GGGGGGUp
Hexanucleotides (6)	GGGGGUp; AAAAGCp; AAGAACp

[a] The numbers in parentheses are chain lengths.

TABLE 5.11B

OLIGONUCLEOTIDE SEQUENCES COMMON TO 18 S rRNA AND 45 S nRNA

Fragment	Sequence
18 S RNA	
Pancreatic RNase digestion	
Tridecanucleotide (13)[a]	$(C_3UGp)(AGp)(CGp)(Gp)(Gp)(Gp)Cp$
Combined U2 and T1 RNase digestion	
Pentanucleotides (5)	UmCCCAp; UUUUGp
Hexanucleotide (6)	UUUUCGp
Heptanucleotide (7)	UCCCCCAp
Octanucleotides (8)	$CUUCUCUGp$; $AmUC_2U_2Ap$
Decanucleotide (10)	CCCUUUUCUGp
Undecanucleotide (11)	CCCUUCUUCCAp
Dodecanucleotide (12)	CCCCCCUUCCCGp

[a] The numbers in parentheses are chain lengths.

CLEAVAGE REACTIONS
OF NUCLEOLAR 45S RNA

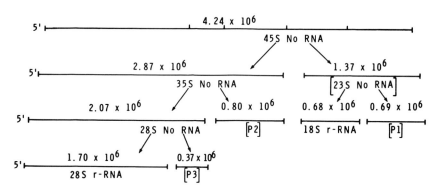

Fig. 5.9. No = nucleolar; r = ribosomal; P1, P2, and P3 = postulated polynucleotide intermediates that have not yet been identified (from 59).

been studied in this laboratory. Also, it was suggested that 5.5 S rRNA is a product of degradation of the high molecular weight nucleolar RNA that emerges from the conversion of 32 S RNA to 28 S RNA.*

* Although it is a small point in the context of the cancer problem, it seems clear that 18 S rRNA emerges from 45 S nRNA as part of a larger segment that was referred to as 23 S nRNA (59, 93b). This segment is approximately twice as long as 18 S rRNA, has the same 5′ terminal as 18 S rRNA and all of the same methylated dinucleotides, and hybridized with nucleolar DNA to approximately twice the extent as 18 S rRNA. Accordingly, there is little doubt that the 3′ end of the 45 S RNA contains the 18 S rRNA which is apparently the 5′ end of the 23 S fragment. Little more is known about this end of the molecule since virtually no sequence work has been done on this fraction of the 45 S RNA molecule. In one sense, the origin of the 18 S rRNA is still not completely resolved. Tiollais et al. (334) have found that high molecular weight RNA can be readily resolved into three bands referred to as 47, 46, and 45 S RNA, although these values are not verified. They suggested that one of these may be the precursor of 28 S rRNA and any other the precursor of 18 S rRNA.

TABLE 5.12

UV Nucleotide Compositions of Nucleolar RNA[a]

	Adenylic acid (A)	Uridylic acid (U)	Guanylic acid (G)	Cytidylic acid (C)	$\dfrac{A + U}{G + C}$
Normal rat liver					
45 S RNA	14.5	20.8	35.3	29.4	0.55
35 S RNA	14.3	19.8	35.1	30.8	0.52
28 S RNA	15.0	19.9	34.9	30.2	0.54
Walker tumor					
55 S RNA	15.3	19.2	36.7	28.8	0.53
45 S RNA	14.6	20.5	35.1	29.7	0.54
35 S RNA	15.4	19.0	35.0	30.6	0.52
28 S RNA	16.0	19.0	35.3	29.6	0.54

[a] Ultraviolet nucleotide composition of nucleolar RNA components. Each puri-fied RNA fraction was subjected to alkaline hydrolysis followed by chromatog-raphy on Dowex-1 column. The values for each purine or pyrimidine nucleotide are averages of the percentage of total purine and pyrimidine bases in the RNA frac-tion determined by ultraviolet absorption at the specific wavelength for each nucleotide. The nucleotide compositions are percentages of the total nucleotides. From Busch and Smetana (59).

D. Analytical Comparisons of the Nucleolar RNA of Tumors and Normal Liver

Initial studies on the various RNA species of the normal liver and the Walker tumor nucleoli indicated that there were no significant differences in the UV nucleotide compositions (221, 291–293) (Table 5.12). When similar studies were carried out using ^{32}P-labeling method, there were marked differences in the ^{32}P-nucleotide composition of 45 S nRNA of tumors and other tissues (Table 5.8). One possibility was that while the UV nucleotide compositions reflected marked similarities of the nucleolar RNA species in the bulk of the nucleolar RNA, the differences in the various isotope distributions might reflect differences in the newly synthesized products.*

* When these studies were made (365), it was already clear that pool factors were involved in the interpretation of such analytical data, i.e., disparate results could emerge if the labeling pools of nucleotide precursors were markedly different (255, 363) in tumors and other tissues. To eliminate such problems, the alkaline hydrolysis procedure was used for production of the 3′-terminal nucleotides from the RNA rather than the 5′-terminal nucleotides. In this way, the nucleotide entering the RNA would not account for the labeling (the 5′ nucleotide is incorporated) but rather the phosphate would be on the adjacent nucleotide. Thus, the ^{32}P-composition of the "newly synthesized" RNA might differ from the nucleotide composition of the unlabeled RNA present in the cell, and indeed this would be a virtue since most (approximately 90%) cellular RNA is ribosomal or transfer RNA. Other approaches to minimization of the pools emerged in later studies on oligonucleotides in the Rushizky-Knight method (265, 272, 365); however, there are still possibilities that the labeling procedure exhibits pool effects.

In recent studies in this laboratory (304a,b) it was shown that there were significant pool differences of labeled nucleotides in normal liver and Novikoff hepatoma. Although the

TABLE 5.13

RADIOACTIVITY DISTRIBUTION IN MONO- AND OLIGONUCLEOTIDES IN NUCLEOLAR
RNA AFTER 6-HOUR LABELING WITH ^{32}P-ORTHOPHOSPHATE[a,b]

Oligo-nucleotides	Normal liver			Morris hepatoma 9618A			Novikoff hepatoma		
	28 S	35 S	45 S	28 S	35 S	45 S	28 S	35 S	45 S
C	26.7	27.8	27.7	28.8	28.6	28.0	28.7	29.0	27.7
U	13.4	13.1	12.6	14.7	14.2	14.5	13.6	13.2	13.7
Pseudo-U	1.0	0.6	1.3	0.8	0.6	0.6	0.8	0.7	0.8
Total mono	41.1	41.5	41.7	44.2	43.4	43.1	43.1	42.9	42.2
AC	4.3	4.3	4.6	5.2	5.3	5.1	4.2	3.9	4.4
GC	13.2	14.0	13.5	18.3	18.5	19.9	14.4	14.6	15.0
AU	2.5	2.5	3.1	1.9	1.9	1.8	2.9	2.7	2.9
GU	5.8	5.9	5.8	6.3	6.4	6.4	9.3	9.4	9.8
Total di	25.8	26.7	27.0	31.7	32.1	32.4	30.8	30.6	32.1
AAC	2.1	2.5	2.8	2.0	2.0	1.8	1.8	1.7	1.7
(AG)C	6.5	6.5	5.6	7.5	7.2	7.3	5.0	5.5	4.9
GGC/A$_3$U	5.2	5.0	4.6	2.5	2.2	2.4	3.4	3.7	4.4
AAU	1.8	2.1	1.5	1.5	1.7	1.5	1.4	1.5	1.3
(AG)U	3.8	3.0	3.6	2.2	2.7	2.5	2.7	3.4	3.6
GGU	2.6	2.1	2.7	1.0	1.0	0.9	3.1	2.7	2.6
Total tri	22.0	21.2	20.8	16.7	16.9	16.4	17.4	19.5	18.5
A$_3$C	1.3	1.5	1.5	1.1	1.4	1.1	1.4	1.3	0.9
(AAG)C	2.8	2.9	2.9	2.6	2.6	3.0	2.4	2.6	1.7
(AGG)C	3.1	2.6	2.0	1.4	1.1	1.1	1.4	1.6	1.5
(AAG)U	2.7	2.2	2.8	1.4	1.5	2.3	1.6	1.4	1.6
(AGG)U	1.2	1.3	1.7	0.6	0.8	0.6	1.4	1.0	1.0
Total tetra	11.2	10.5	10.9	7.1	7.4	8.1	8.2	7.9	6.7

[a] From Yazdi et al. (365).

[b] The values for each sequence are the percentages of the total radioactivity from each RNA found in a given sequence. The abbreviations are those used by Roberts and D'Ari (265).

When the "oligonucleotide frequency method" (272) became available, it was employed to test these possibilities. Table 5.13 shows the results of these studies. Interestingly, the isotope content of the dinucleotide series was greater in the tumors than in the liver. The isotope content of the dinucleotides GC and GU was higher in the tumors than in the liver. On the other hand, the isotope contents of the dinucleotides AC and AU were not significantly different

specific activities were essentially the same for the nucleotides in the Novikoff hepatoma, the specific activity of AMP was approximately 1.5 times that of CMP, UMP, and GMP in normal liver. It is thus possible that the higher values for adenylic acid in the liver samples reflect primarily a difference in this specific activity rather than a difference in the sequences of the RNA molecules. Along with the data on hybridization indicated (see below) it would appear that some of the earlier differences found reflected pool differences rather than sequence differences in these RNA's.

in the tumors and the liver. Since the same precursor pools would be primarily responsible for labeling GU and AU or GC and AC in the liver in both cases, the pool contribution appears to be limited (365). However, the higher frequencies of the GU dinucleotide of the Novikoff hepatoma were not found for the Morris hepatoma 9618A and similarly the Morris hepatoma 9618A had a high GC content which was not found for the Novikoff hepatoma as compared to the normal liver. On the other hand, statistically meaningful differences were not found for the other oligonucleotides studied.

In extensions of these studies to partial hydrolysates produced by partial T1 RNase digestion of high molecular weight RNA from Novikoff hepatoma and normal liver nucleoli (357), it was found that there was a marked difference in the frequency of the dinucleotide UG in the tumors, i.e., some 7–10 UG dinucleotides more were present in the tumor than in normal liver (Table 5.14). Along with the higher GU dinucleotide frequency, it was concluded that there was probably a larger number of GUGU tetranucleotides in the nucleolar rRNA precursors of the Novikoff hepatoma than in the normal liver. However, it seemed possible that this result reflected either pool differences or terminal differences in view of the lack of differences found in the sequence studies (221, 291).

Recently it was reported (133a) that there are oligonucleotide differences between 18 S rRNA of mouse liver and mouse hepatoma. Further analysis will be required to determine whether this in fact represents a sequence or pool or terminal difference in this RNA.

E. Hybridization

In early studies on competitive hybridization of 18 S rRNA of liver ribosomes with that of tumor ribosomes, no significant differences were found and accord-

TABLE 5.14

COMPARISON OF DINUCLEOTIDES OF 28 S rRNA OF NORMAL LIVER
AND NOVIKOFF HEPATOMA PARTIALLY DIGESTED WITH T1 RNASE

	No. of dinucleotides			
	CG	AG	UG	GG
Ionophoresis[a]				
Normal liver	14	14	5	14
Novikoff hepatoma	8	15	12	14
Column chromatography[b]				
Normal liver	15	15	5	14
Novikoff hepatoma	8	14	12	15

[a] Number of dinucleotides is based on the total recovery of isotope from the identified spots and total subjected to electrophoresis (357).

[b] Number of dinucleotides is based on recovery of isotope from identified peaks (357).

ingly it was concluded that there were no marked dissimilarities. When similar studies were carried out with 28 S rRNA, no marked differences were found (357).

Recent studies have been carried out on the competitive hybridization of liver nucleolar 45 S RNA with that of Novikoff hepatoma nucleoli (Fig. 5.10). Although this method would not rule out minor differences such as a few GUGU or other tetranucleotides, no marked differences were found for competition with either liver or tumor nucleolar 45 S RNA. The suggestion that there were as much as 25% differences in the nucleotides of these RNA's (based on ^{32}P-nucleotide compositions) thus appears to mirror pool differences rather than sequence differences in these RNA species. Such data indicates that the high molecular weight nucleolar RNA is essentially the same in tumors and other tissues.

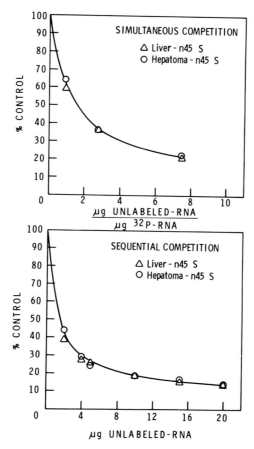

Fig. 5.10. (Upper) Simultaneous competition of liver or tumor unlabeled nucleolar 45 S RNA with labeled tumor nuclear 45 S RNA. No significant differences were found. (Lower) Two-step, presaturation competition for hybridization of Novikoff hepatoma nucleolar 45 S RNA with tumor nucleolar DNA. No significant difference was found in competition by unlabeled liver or tumor nucleolar 45 S RNA (304b).

F. "Fetal rRNA?"

Based on ^{32}P-nucleotide data, the intriguing suggestion was made that in the tumor cells there is activation of "fetal rRNA templates" (142). Since the same types of nucleotide composition and oligonucleotide frequencies were demonstrated in tumors and embryonic liver tissues, it was suggested that fetal gene activation may have occurred in the tumors (142). This idea needs to be supported by additional evidence such as hybridization data in view of the likely pool contributions to the results of labeling studies.

In summary of this work on the distribution of oligonucleotides and the ^{32}P-labeling method in preribosomal and ribosomal RNA, the general conclusion is that differences exist in the distribution of the isotope in the chains of newly synthesized nucleolar RNA of tumors and normal liver. However, studies on sequences of nucleotides of nucleolar precursors and 18 S rRNA and 28 S rRNA and hybridization-competition analysis have not revealed major differences between these species. Preliminary studies have suggested that the tetranucleotide GUGU and the dinucleotide GC are in higher concentration in tumor nucleolar and 28 S rRNA. However, such possible differences await unequivocal evidence, particularly in view of the very similar hybridization characteristics of nucleolar 45 S RNA of liver and tumor cells.

VII. Summary

Although the enormous expansion of information on high molecular weight RNA has been of great value in providing concepts relevant to protein synthesis, information transfer from genes to cell function, and understanding of potential mechanisms for gene regulation, it is clear that definitive information differentiating cancer cells from other cells has still not emerged.* As noted earlier, the methods are presently inadequate to isolate pure species of messenger RNA from cancer cells that are tumor specific. In a sense, this would be expected to be a most difficult problem in view of the fact that there are so many messengers for cell functions and the methods for their individual isolation are as yet unavailable except for a very few species. On the other hand, it may be hoped that within a relatively short time much new information will be obtained in this field.

For characterization of their structures as well as their effects, hopefully "cancer-specific messenger RNA's" may soon be isolated. In addition, analysis of the kinetics of their turnover will define whether such molecules turn over once

* It is of interest, for example, that no definitive differences have been reported for mRNA of regenerating and normal liver (212) or even fetal liver (42). Although morphological and quantitative changes in RNA occur in carcinogenesis (43, 317), no specific alterations have been reported.

or a few times in the life-time of the cell. If their labeling rates are slow, it may be a problem of extraordinary difficulty to carry out hybridization studies or to identify such molecular species by the usual labeling methods. Happily, in the last few years, new methods have been developed to attack such problems. It is now possible (151, 306) to label the N-7 position of guanine selectively with radioactive dimethyl sulfate and thereby obtain RNA molecules of sufficiently high specific activity for studies on hybridization with DNA. This procedure offers an alternative to the *in vivo* or biological labeling of the RNA, at least for studies on hybridization.

Although it was initially hoped that the task of isolating, purifying, and analyzing rRNA species (and other RNA species) would be readily accomplished and would lead to specific information about the cancer problem, this has not turned out to be the case. At present there is considerable uncertainty about the differences in these RNA species in tumors and other cells. In a sense, this might have been expected from the efficiency of cancer cells in protein synthesis, both for growth and specific protein products. On the other hand, it is still possible that there are regions of microheterogeneity in these molecules that may be critical in control of cell function. Accordingly, it is necessary that continuing studies be made on their sequences and structures.

The development of concepts of viral oncogenesis has also led to a search for viral RNA in tumor cells. However, it does not appear that this problem is any simpler than the general problem of specifying special RNA's of cancer cells, although methods being developed are currently relevant to both fields of endeavor. As in many areas, it is apparent that an enormous effort is required to clearly characterize the viral and other products of cancer cells and to differentiate them specifically from those of nontumor cells (see Chapter XI).

Acknowledgment

The original studies in this chapter were supported by the Cancer Center Grants, CA-10893 P. 1 and CA-10893 P. 7.

References

1. Abraham, A. D., and Sekeris, C. E. (1971). *Biochim. Biophys. Acta* **247**, 562–569.
2. Adams, J. M., Jeppesen, P. G. N., Sanger, F., and Barrell, B. G. (1969). *Nature (London)* **223**, 1009–1014.
3. Adams, J. M., Spahr, P.-F., and Cory, S. (1972). *Biochemistry* **11**, 976–988.
4. Adesnik, M., and Darnell, J. E. (1972). *J. Mol. Biol.* **67**, 397–406.
5. Akino, T., and Amano, M. (1970). *J. Biochem.* **67**, 533–539.
6. Alberts, B. M., and Frey, L. (1970). *Nature (London)* **227**, 1313–1318.
7. Amaldi, F. (1969). *Nature (London)* **221**, 95–96.
8. Arion, V. J., Mantieva, V. L., and Georgiev, G. P. (1967). *Biochim. Biophys. Acta* **138**, 436–438.
9. Arnaud, M., Beziat, Y., Borgna, J. L., Guilleux, J. C., and Mousseron-Canet, M. (1971). *Biochim. Biophys. Acta* **254**, 241–254.

10. Aronson, A. I. (1972). *Nature New Biol.* **235**, 40–44.

11. Artamonova, V. A., Tikhonenko, T. I., and Morgunova, T. D. (1964). *Voprosy Onkologii* **10**, T706–T708.

12. Artman, M., and Roth, J. S. (1971). *J. Mol. Biol.* **60**, 291–301.

13. Attardi, G., and Amaldi, F. (1970). *Ann. Rev. Biochem.* **39**, 183–226.

14. Attardi, G., and Attardi, B. (1968). *Proc. Nat. Acad. Sci. U.S.* **61**, 261–268.

15. Attardi, G., Parnas, H., Huang, M.-I. H., and Attardi, B. (1966). *J. Mol. Biol.* **20**, 145–182.

16. Avadhani, N. G., and Beutow, D. E. (1970). *Nature (London)* **228**, 242–245.

17. Aviv, H., and Leder, P. (1972). *Proc. Nat. Acad. Sci. U.S.* **69**, 1408–1412.

17a. Axel, R., Gulati, S. C., and Spiegelman, S. (1972). *Proc. Nat. Acad. Sci. U.S.* **69**. 3133–3137.

17b. Axel, R., Schlom, J., and Spiegelman, S. (1972). *Nature (London)* **235**, 32–36.

17c. Axel, R., Schlom, J., and Spiegelman, S. (1972). *Proc. Nat. Acad. Sci. U.S.* **69**, 535–538.

18. Azuma, M., Hodgson, J. R., Aizawa, C., and Fisher, H. W. (1969). *J. Virol.* **3**, 275–277.

19. Bagshaw, J. C., and Malt, R. A. (1971). *Biochem. Biophys. Res. Commun.* **42**, 1207–1213.

20. Baker, R. F., and Yanofsky, C. (1968). *Nature (London)* **219**, 26–29.

21. Bank, A., Terada, M., Metafora, S., Dow, L., and Marks, P. A. (1972). *Nature New Biol.* **235**, 167–169.

21a. Baserga, R., and Stein, G. (1971). *Fed. Proc.* **30**, 1752–1759.

22. Bautz, E. K. F., and Reilly, E. (1966). *Science* **151**, 328–330.

23. Bekhor, I., and Bavetta, L. A. (1971). *Biochem. Biophys. Res. Commun.* **42**, 615–620.

24. Ben-Hamida, F., and Schlessinger, D. (1965). *J. Bacteriol.* **90**, 1611–1616.

25. Berke, G., Sarid, S., and Feldman, M. (1971). *Biochim. Biophys. Acta* **254**, 440–446.

26. Billeter, M. A., Dahlberg, J. E., Goodman, H. M., Hindley, J., and Weissmann, C. (1969). *J. Cell. Physiol.* **74**, 197–204.

27. Billeter, M. A., Dahlberg, J. E., Goodman, H. M., Hindley, J., and Weissmann, C. (1969). *Nature (London)* **224**, 1083–1086.

28. Billing, R. J., Inglis, A. M., and Smellie, R. M. S. (1969). *Biochem. J.* **113**, 571–572.

29. Birnboim, H. C., and Coakley, B. V. (1971). *Biochem. Biophys. Res. Commun.* **42**, 1169–1175.

30. Birnboim, H. C., Pene, J. J., and Darnell, J. E. (1967). *Proc. Nat. Acad. Sci.* **58**, 320–327.

31. Birnstiel, M. L., Sells, B. H., and Purdom, I. F. (1972). *J. Mol. Biol.* **63**, 21–39.

32. Blobel, G. (1971). *Proc. Nat. Acad. Sci. U.S.* **68**, 832–835.

33. Blobel, G. (1972). *Biochem. Biophys. Res. Commun.* **47**, 88–95.

34. Blobel, G., and Sabatini, D. (1971). *Proc. Nat. Acad. Sci. U.S.* **68**, 390–394.

35. Bolle, A., Epstein, R. H., Salser, W., and Geiduschek, E. P. (1968). *J. Mol. Biol.* **31**, 325–348.

36. Bonner, J., and Huang, R. E. (1963). *Proc. Nat. Acad. Sci. U.S.* **50**, 169, 893–900.

37. Bonner, J., and Widholm, J. (1967). *Proc. Nat. Acad. Sci. U.S.* **57**, 1379–1385.

38. Borun, T. W., Scharff, M. D., and Robbins, E. (1967). *Proc. Nat. Acad. Sci. U.S.* **58**, 1977–1983.

38a. Bramwell, M. E. (1972). *Biochim. Biophys. Acta* **281**, 329–337.

39. Brawerman, G., Biezunski, N., and Eisenstadt, J. (1965). *Biochim. Biophys. Acta* **103**, 201–210.

40. Brawerman, G., Mendecki, J., and Lee, S. Y. (1972). *Biochemistry* **11**, 637–641.

41. Bresnick, E., and Burleson, S. S. (1970). *Cancer Res.* **30**, 1060–1063.

42. Bresnick, E., Eckles, S. G., and Lanclos, K. D. (1967). *Biochemistry* **6**, 2481–2488.

43. Briere, N. (1970). *J. Histochem. Cytochem.* **18**, 498–503.

44. Britten, R. J., and Kohne, D. E. (1968). *Science* **161**, 529–540.

45. Britten, R. J., and Davidson, E. H. (1971). *Quart. Rev. Biol.* **46**, 111–138.

45a. Brown, D. D., and Gurdon, J. B. (1964). *Proc. Nat. Acad. Sci. U.S.* **51**, 139–146.

46. Brown, D. D., and Littna, E. (1964). *J. Mol. Biol.* **8**, 669–687.

47. Brown, I. R., and Church, R. B. (1971). *Biochem. Biophys. Res. Commun.* **42**, 850–856.

47a. Brown, R. D., and Tocchini-Valentini, G. P. (1972). *Proc. Nat. Sci. U.S.* **69**, 1746–1748.
48. Bruzzone, S. (1971). *Brit. J. Cancer* **25**, 158–165.
49. Burgess, R. R. (1969). *J. Biol. Chem.* **244**, 6160–6167.
50. Burgess, R. R. (1969). *J. Biol. Chem.* **244**, 6168–6176.
51. Burr, H., and Lingrel, J. B. (1971). *Nature New Biol.* **233**, 41–43.
52. Busch, H. (1962). *In* "Biochemistry of the Cancer Cell," p. 356. Academic Press, New York.
53. Busch, H., Arendell, J. P., Morris, H. P., Neogy, R. K., and Schwartz, S. M. (1968). *Cancer Res.* **28**, 280–285.
54. Busch, H., Choi, Y. C., Crooke, S. T., and Okada, S. (1972). *Oncology* **26**, 152–179.
55. Busch, H., Choi, Y. C., Daskal, I., Inagaki, A., Olson, M., Reddy, R., Ro-Choi, T. S., Shibata, H., and Yeoman, L. (1972). *Karolinska Symp. Methods Reproductive Endocrinol.* **5**, 35–66.
56. Busch, H., Hodnett, J. L., Morris, H. P., Neogy, R., Smetana, K., and Unuma, T. (1968). *Cancer Res.* **28**, 672–683.
57. Busch, H., and Lane, M. (1967). "Chemotherapy." Year Book Publ., Chicago, Illinois.
58. Busch, H., Ro-Choi, T. S., Prestayko, A. W., Shibata, H., Crooke, S. T., El-Khatib, S. M., Choi, Y. C., and Mauritzen, C. M. (1971). *Persp. Biol. Med.* **15**, 117–139.
59. Busch, H., and Smetana, K. (1970). "The Nucleolus." Academic Press, New York.
60. Busch, H., and Starbuck, W. C. (1969). *Cancer Res.* **29**, 2454–2456.
61. Cartouzou, G., Aquaron, R., Mante, S., and Lissitzky, S. (1968). *Eur. J. Biochem.* **4**, 55–67.
62. Cartouzou, G., Attali, J.-C., and Lissitzky, S. (1968). *Eur. J. Biochem.* **4**, 41–54.
63. Cartouzou, G., Mante, S., and Lissitzky, S. (1965). *Biochem. Biophys. Res. Commun.* **20**, 212–217.
64. Cartouzou, G., Poiree, J. C., and Lissitzky, S. (1969). *Eur. J. Biochem.* **8**, 357–369.
65. Chakravorty, A. K., and Busch, H. (1967). *Cancer Res.* **27**, 780.
66. Chambon, P., Gissinger, F., Kedinger, C., Mandel, J. L., Meilhac, M., and Nutet, P. (1972). *Karolinska Symp. Methods Reproductive Endocrinol.* **5**, 222–246.
67. Cheevers, W. P., and Sheinin, R. (1970). *Biochim. Biophys. Acta* **204**, 449–461.
68. Chiarugi, V. P. (1969). *Biochim. Biophys. Acta* **179**, 129–135.
69. Church, R. B., Luther, S. W., and McCarthy, B. J. (1969). *Biochim. Biophys. Acta* **190**, 30–37.
70. Cohen, E. P. (1967). *Proc. Nat. Acad. Sci. U.S.* **57**, 673–680.
71. Colli, W., and Oishi, M. (1970). *J. Mol. Biol.* **51**, 657–669.
72. Comstock, J. P., O'Malley, B. W., and Means, A. R. (1972). *Biochemistry* **11**, 646–652.
73. Cowling, G. J., Jones, A. S., and Walker, R. T. (1971). *Biochim. Biophys. Acta* **254**, 452–456.
74. Cozzone, A., and Marchis-Mouren, G. (1967). *Biochemistry* **6**, 3911–3917.
75. Creaser, E. H., and Spencer, J. H. (1960). *Biochem. J.* **76**, 171–178.
76. Crooke, S. T., Okada, S., and Busch, H. (1972). *Cancer Res.* **32**, 1745–1752.
77. Dahlberg, J. E., and Peacock, A. C. (1971). *J. Mol. Biol.* **55**, 61–74.
77a. Daneholt, B. (1972). *Nature New Biol.* **240**, 229–232.
78. Daneholt, B., and Svedhem, L. (1971). *Exp. Cell Res.* **67**, 263–272.
79. Darnell, J. E., and Balint, R. (1970). *J. Cell Physiol.* **76**, 349–356.
80. Darnell, J. E., Philipson, L., Wall, R., and Adesnik, M. (1971). *Science* **174**, 507–510.
81. Darnell, J. E., Wall, R., and Tushinski, R. J. (1971). *Proc. Nat. Acad. Sci. U.S.* **68**, 1321–1325.
82. Davidson, E. H., and Hough, B. R. (1971). *J. Mol. Biol.* **56**, 491–506.
83. DeKloet, S. R., and Andrean, B. A. G. (1971). *Biochim. Biophys. Acta* **247**, 519–527.
84. Delovitch, T. L., Davis, B. K., Holme, G., and Sehon, A. H. (1972). *J. Mol. Biol.* **69**, 373–386.
85. DeWachter, R., and Fiers, W. (1967). *J. Mol. Biol.* **30**, 507–527.
86. DeWachter, R., Vandenberghe, A., Merregaert, J., Contreras, R., and Fiers, W. (1971). *Proc. Nat. Acad. Sci. U.S.* **68**, 585–589.

86a. Diczfalusy, E. (ed.) (1972). "Gene Transcription in Reproductive Tissue." Karolinska Inst., Stockholm.

87. DiGirolamo, A., DiGirolamo, M., Gaetani, S., and Spadoni, M. A. (1966). *Biochim. Biophys. Acta* **114**, 195–198.

88. Doi, R. H. (1965). *Nature (London)* **208**, 552–554.

89. Drach, J. C., and Lingrel, J. B. (1964). *Biochim. Biophys. Acta* **91**, 680–683.

90. Drach, J. C., and Lingrel, J. B. (1966). *Biochim. Biophys. Acta* **123**, 345–355.

91. Drach, J. C., and Lingrel, J. B. (1966). *Biochim. Biophys. Acta* **129**, 178–185.

92. Drews, J., and Brawerman, G. (1966). IEG 37 Memo #684.

93. Edmonds, M., Vaughan, M. H., Jr., and Nakazato, H. (1971). *Proc. Nat. Acad. Sci. U.S.* **68**, 1336–1340.

93a. Edstrom, J.-E. (1974). *In* "The Cell Nucleus" (H. Busch, ed.), Vol. II. Academic Press, New York.

93b. Egawa, K., Choi, Y. C., and Busch, H. (1971). *J. Mol. Biol.* **56**, 565–577.

94. Ellem, K. A. O. (1966). *J. Mol. Biol.* **20**, 283–305.

95. Emerson, C. P. (1971). *Nature New Biol.* **232**, 101–106.

96. Endo, Y., Tominaga, H., and Natori, Y. (1971). *Biochim. Biophys. Acta* **240**, 215–217.

97. Epstein, W. V., Tan, M., and Easterbrook, M. (1971). *New England J. Med.* **285**, 1502–1506.

98. Esposito, S. (1964). *Nature (London)* **203**, 1078–1081.

99. Evans, M. J., and Lingrel, J. B. (1969). *Biochemistry* **8**, 3000–3005.

100. Falvey, A. K., and Staehelin, T. (1970). *J. Mol. Biol.* **53**, 1–19.

101. Ficq, A., and Brachet, J. (1971). *Proc. Nat. Acad. Sci. U.S.* **68**, 2774–2776.

102. Fiers, W., Contreras, R., DeWachter, R., Haegeman, G., Merregaert, J., Min Jou, W., and Vandenberghe, A. (1971). *Biochimie* **53**, 495–506.

103. Finkel, R., Henshaw, E., and Hiatt, H. (1966). IEG 37, Memo #231.

104. Fridlender, B., Fry, M., Bolden, A., and Weissbach, A. (1972). *Proc. Nat. Acad. Sci. U.S.* **69**, 452–455.

105. Fukami, H., and Imahori, K. (1971). *Proc. Nat. Acad. Sci. U.S.* **68**, 570–573.

106. Fukuda, T., Akino, T., Amano, M., and Izawa, M. (1970). *Cancer Res.* **30**, 1–10.

107. Geiduschek, E. P., and Haselkorn, R. (1969). *Ann. Rev. Biochem.* **38**, 647–676.

108. Gelb, L. D., Kohne, D. E., and Martin, M. A. (1971). *J. Mol. Biol.* **57**, 129–145.

109. Georgatsos, J. G. (1972). *Proc. Soc. Exp. Biol. Med.* **139**, 667–669.

109a. Georgiev, G. P. (1973). *In* "The Cell Nucleus" (H. Busch, ed.). Academic Press, New York.

110. Georgiev, G. P., and Mantieva, V. L. (1962). *Biochim. Biophys. Acta* **61**, 153–154.

111. Georgiev, G. P., Samarina, O. P., Lerman, M. I., Smirnov, M. N., and Severtzov, A. N. (1963). *Nature (London)* **200**, 1391–1394.

112. Gilham, P. T. (1970). *Ann. Rev. Biochem.* **39**, 227–250.

113. Gillespie, S., and Gillespie, D. (1971). *Biochem. J.* **125**, 481–487.

114. Gillespie, S., and Spiegelman, S. (1965). *Proc. Nat. Acad. Sci. U.S.* **12**, 829–842.

115. Goodman, H. M., Billeter, M. A., Hindley, J., and Weissman, C. (1970). *Proc. Nat. Acad. Sci. U.S.* **67**, 921–928.

116. Gottlieb, A. A., and Tenney, D. N. (1972). *J. Nat. Cancer Inst.* **48**, 1457–1462.

117. Granboulan, N., and Scherrer, K. (1969). *Eur. J. Biochem.* **9**, 1–20.

118. Green, M. (1972). *Proc. Nat. Acad. Sci. U.S.* **69**, 1036–1041.

118a. Greenberg, J. R. (1972). *Nature (London)* **240**, 102–104.

119. Greenman, D. L., Wicks, W. D., and Kenney, F. T. (1965). *J. Biol. Chem.* **240**, 4420–4426.

120. Gros, F., Hiatt, H., Gilbert, W., Kurland, C. G., Riseborough, R. N., and Watson, J. D. (1961). *Nature (London)* **190**, 581–585.

120a. Gulati, S. R., Axel, R., and Spiegelman, S. (1972). *Proc. Nat. Acad. Sci. U.S.* **69**, 2020–2024.

121. Gurdon, J. B., Lane, C. D., Woodland, H. R., and Marbaix, G. (1971). *Nature (London)* **233**, 177–182.

122. Hadjiolov, A. A. (1966). *Biochim. Biophys. Acta* 119, 547–556.
123. Hadjivassiliou, A., and Brawerman, G. (1965). *Biochim. Biophys. Acta* 103, 211–218.
124. Hadjivassiliou, A., and Brawerman, G. (1966). *J. Mol. Biol.* 20, 1–7.
125. Haegeman, G., Min Jou, W., and Fiers, W. (1971). *J. Mol. Biol.* 57, 597–613.
126. Halpern, B. C., Halpern, R. M., Chaney, S. Q., and Smith, R. A. (1970). *Proc. Nat. Acad. Sci. U.S.* 67, 1827–1833.
127. Hamilton, T. H. (1963). *Proc. Nat. Acad. Sci. U.S.* 49, 373–379.
128. Hamilton, T. H. (1964). *Proc. Nat. Acad. Sci. U.S.* 51, 83–89.
129. Hanania, N., and Harel, J. (1968). *Bull. Soc. Chim. Biol.* 50, 693–707.
130. Harel, J., Harel, L., Lacour, F., Boer, A., and Imbenotte, J. (1963). *J. Mol. Biol.* 7, 645–651.
131. Harris, H. (1963). *Nature (London)* 198, 184–185.
132. Harris, H. (1964). *Nature (London)* 201, 863–867.
133. Haschemeyer, A. E. V., and Rich, A. (1962). *Biochim. Biophys. Acta* 55, 994–997.
133a. Hashimoto, S., and Muramatsu, M. (1973). *Eur. J. Biochem.* 33, 446–458.
134. Hayashi, M., Hayashi, M. N., and Spiegelman, S. (1963). *Proc. Nat. Acad. Sci. U.S.* 50, 664–672.
135. Hayashi, M., Hayashi, M. N., and Spiegelman, S. (1964). *Proc. Nat. Acad. Sci. U.S.* 51, 351–359.
136. Hayes, D. H., Hayes, F., and Guerin, M. F. (1966). *J. Mol. Biol.* 18, 499–515.
137. Haywood, A. M. (1971). *Proc. Nat. Acad. Sci. U.S.* 68, 435–439.
137a. Hehlmann, R., Kufe, D., and Spiegelman, S. (1972). *Proc. Nat. Acad. Sci. U.S.* 69, 1727–1731.
138. Henshaw, E. C. (1968). *J. Mol. Biol.* 36, 401–411.
139. Henshaw, E. C., and Loebenstein, J. (1970). *Biochim. Biophys. Acta* 199, 405–420.
140. Henshaw, E. C., Revel, M., and Hiatt, H. H. (1965). *J. Mol. Biol.* 14, 241–256.
140a. Heyden, H. W. von, and Zachau, H. G. (1971). *Biochim. Biophys. Acta* 232, 651–660.
141. Heywood, S. M., and Nwagwu, M. (1969). *Biochemistry* 8, 3839–3845.
141a. Hidvegi, E., Prestayko, A. W., and Busch, H. (1971). *Physiol. Chem. Phys.* 3, 17–35.
142. Higashi, K., Matsuhisa, T., Gotoh, S., Nishinaga, K., and Yukiya, S. (1971). *Biochim. Biophys. Acta* 232, 352–358.
143. Hill, M., Miller-Faures, A., and Errera, M. (1964). *Biochim. Biophys. Acta* 80, 39–51.
144. Hill, W. E., Rossetti, G. P., and Van Holde, K. E. (1968). *Biochem. Biophys. Res. Commun.* 33, 151–155.
145. Hodge, L. D., Robbins, E., and Scharff, M. D. (1969). *J. Cell Biol.* 40, 497–507.
146. Holland, J. J., Buck, C. A., and McCarthy, B. J. (1966). *Biochemistry* 5, 358–365.
147. Holley, R. W., Apgar, J., Everett, G. A., Madison, J. T., Marquisee, M., Merrill, S. H., Penswick, J. R., and Zamir, A. (1965). *Science* 147, 1462–1465.
147a. Holmes, D., Mayfield, J. E., Sander, G., and Bonner, J. (1972). *Science* 177, 72–74.
148. Houssais, J-F., and Attardi, G. (1966). *Proc. Nat. Acad. Sci. U.S.* 56, 616–623.
149. Huez, G., Burny, A., Marbaix, G., and Lebleu, B. (1967). *Biochim. Biophys. Acta* 145, 629–636.
150. Hunt, J. A., and Wilkinson, B. R. (1967). *Biochemistry* 6, 1688–1693.
151. Hynes, R. O., and Gross, P. R. (1972). *Biochim. Biophys. Acta* 259, 104–111.
152. Inagaki, A., and Busch, H. (1972). *J. Biol. Chem.* 247, 3327–3335.
153. Ishikawa, K., Ueki, M., Nagai, K., and Ogata, K. (1972). *Biochim. Biophys. Acta* 259, 138–154.
154. Jacob, S. T., and Busch, H. (1967). *Biochim. Biophys. Acta* 138, 249–257.
155. Jacob, F., and Monod, J. (1961). *J. Mol. Biol.* 3, 318–356.
156. Jacobs-Lorena, M., Baglioni, C., and Borun, T. W. (1972). *Proc. Nat. Acad. Sci. U.S.* 69, 2095–2099.
156a. Jelinek, W., and Darnell, J. E. (1972). *Proc. Nat. Acad. Sci. U.S.* 69, 2537–2541.
157. Jeppesen, P. G. N., Steitz, J. A., Gesteland, R. F., and Spahr, P. F. (1970). *Nature (London)* 226, 230–237.
158. Johnston, R. E., and Bose, H. R. (1972). *Proc. Nat. Acad. Sci. U.S.* 69, 1514–1516.

159. Jones, K. W. (1970). *Nature* (*London*) **225**, 912–915.
159a. Kacian, D. L., Mills, D. R., Kramer, F. R., and Spiegelman, S. (1972). *Proc. Nat. Acad. Sci. U.S.* **69**, 3038–3042.
160. Kano-Sueoka, T., and Spiegelman, S. (1962). *Proc. Nat. Acad. Sci.* **48**, 1942–1949.
161. Kedes, L. H., and Birnstiel, M. L. (1971). *Nature New Biol.* **230**, 165–169.
162. Kidson, C., and Kirby, K. S. (1964). *Nature* (*London*) **203**, 599–603.
163. Kidson, C., and Kirby, K. S. (1964). *Cancer Res.* **24**, 1604–1609.
164. Kidson, C., and Kirby, K. S. (1964). *J. Mol. Biol.* **10**, 187–198.
165. Kiho, Y., and Rich, A. (1965). *Proc. Nat. Acad. Sci. U.S.* **54**, 1751–1758.
166. Kimura, K., Tomoda, J., and Sibatani, A. (1965). *Biochim. Biophys. Acta* **108**, 540–550.
167. Knochel, W., Tiedemann, H., and Fellmann, I. (1972). *Biochim. Biophys. Acta* **269**. 104–117.
168. Kostraba, N. C., and Wang, T. Y. (1971). *Cancer Res.* **31**, 1663–1668.
169. Kozak, M., and Nathans, D. (1972). *Bacterial. Rev.* **36**, 109–134.
170. Kruh, J., Dreyfus, J. C., and Schapira, G. (1964).`Biochim. Bipophys. Acta* **91**, 494–505.
171. Kruh, J., Dreyfus, J. C., and Schapira, G. (1965). *Bull. Soc. Chim. Biol.* **47**, 1691–1696.
172. Kruh, J., Dreyfus, J. C., and Schapira, G. (1966). *Biochim. Biophys. Acta* **114**, 371–384.
173. Kuechler, E., and Rich, A. (1969). *Nature* (*London*) **222**, 544–547.
173a. Kufe, D., Magrath, I. T., Ziegler, J. L., and Spiegelman, S. (1973). *Proc. Nat. Acad. Sci. U.S.* **70**, 737–741. ·
174. Labrie, F. (1969). *Nature* (*London*) **221**, 1217–1222.
175. Lai, M. M. C., and Duesberg, P. H. (1972). *Nature* (*London*) **235**, 383–386.
176. Lamar, Jr., C., Prival, M., and Pitot, H. (1966). *Cancer Res.* **26**, 1909–1914.
176a. Lambert, B. (1972). *J. Mol. Biol.* **72**, 65–76.
176b. Lambert, B., Daneholt, B., Edstrom, J.-E., Egyhazi, E., and Ringborg, U. (1973). *Exp. Cell Res.* **76**, 381–389.
176c. Lambert, B., Egyhazi, E., Daneholt, B., and Ringborg, U. (1973). *Exp. Cell Res.* **76**, 369–380.
176d. Lambert, B., Wieslander, L., Daneholt, B., Egyhazi, E., and Ringborg, U. (1972). *J. Cell Biol.* **53**, 407–418.
177. Lamfrom, H., McLaughlin, C. S., and Araabhai, A. (1966). *J. Mol. Biol.* **22**, 355–358.
178. Lang, N., and Sekeris, C. E. (1964). *Life Sci.* **3**, 161–167.
179. Laycock, D. G., and Hunt, J. A. (1969). *Nature* (*London*) **221**, 1118–1122.
180. Lee, S. Y., Mendecki, J., and Brawerman, G. (1971). *Proc. Nat. Acad. Sci. U.S.* **68**, 1331–1335.
181. Lim, L., and Canellakis, E. S. (1970). *Nature* (*London*) **227**, 710–712.
182. Lingrel, J. B., Lockard, R. E., Jones, R. F., Burr, H. E., and Holder, J. W. (1971). *Ser. Haemat.* **4**, 37–69.
183. Lockard, R. E., and Lingrel, J. B. (1971). *Nature New Biol.* **233**, 204–206.
184. Mach, B., and Vassali, P. (1965). *Science* **150**, 622–626.
185. Mackey, J. K., and Gilham, P. T. (1971). *Nature* (*London*) **233**, 551–552.
186. Maden, B. E. H., Salim, M., and Summers, D. F. (1972). *Nature* (*London*) **237**, 5–9.
187. Malin, D. H., Golub, A. M., and McConnell, J. V. (1971). *Nature* (*London*) **233**, 211–212.
188. Mansbridge, J. N., and Korner, A. (1966). *Biochim. Biophys. Acta* **119**, 92–98.
189. Marbaix, G., Burney, A., Huez, G., and Chantrenne, H. (1966). *Biochim. Biophys. Acta* **114**, 404–406.
190. Marmur, J., and Lane, D. (1960). *Proc. Nat. Acad. Sci. U.S.* **46**, 453–461.
191. Marsh, J. B., and Drabkin, D. L. (1965). *Biochim. Biophys. Acta* **95**, 173–176.
191a. Mathews, M. B., Osborn, M., Berns, A. J. M., and Bloemendal, H. (1972). *Nature New Biol.* **236**, 5–7.
192. Matthaei, J. H., and Nirenberg, M. N. (1961). *Proc. Nat. Acad. Sci. U.S.* **47**, 1580–1588.
193. Matthysse, A. G., and Phillips, C. (1969). *Proc. Nat. Acad. Sci. U.S.* **63**, 897–902.
194. Mauritzen, C. M., Choi, Y. C., and Busch, H. (1971). In "Methods in Cancer Research" (H. Busch, ed.), Vol. VI, p. 253–282. Academic Press, New York.

195. Mayfield, J. E., and Bonner, J. (1971). *Proc. Nat. Acad. Sci. U.S.* **68**, 2652–2655.
196. Mayfield, J. E., and Bonner, J. (1972). *Proc. Nat. Acad. Sci. U.S.* **69**, 7–10.
197. Mayo, V. S., and De Kloet, S. R. (1971). *Biochim. Biophys. Acta* **247**, 74–79.
198. McCarthy, B. J., and Hoyer, B. H. (1964). *Proc. Nat. Acad. Sci. U.S.* **52**, 915–922.
199. McDougall, J. K., Dunn, A. R., and Jones, K. W. (1972). *Nature (London)* **236**, 346–348.
200. McParland, R., Crooke, S. T., and Busch, H. (1972). *Biochim. Biophys. Acta* **209**, 78–89.
201. Means, A. R., Comstock, J. P., Rosenfeld, G. C., and O'Malley, B. W. (1972). *Proc. Nat. Acad. Sci. U.S.* **69**, 1146–1150.
202. Miller, A. O. A. (1967). *Arch. Biochem. Biophys.* **122**, 270–279.
203. Min Jou, W., Haegeman, G., Ysebaert, M., and Fiers, W. (1972). *Nature (London)* **237**, 82–88.
204. Mizuno, N. S., Hof, H., and Collin, M. V. (1968). *Biochim. Biophys. acta* **166**, 656–662.
205. Moar, V. A., Gurdon, J. B., and Lane, C. D. (1971). *J. Mol. Biol.* **61**, 93–103.
206. Molloy, G. R., Sporn, M. B., Kelley, D. E., and Perry, R. E. (1972). *Biochemistry* **11**, 3256–3260.
207. Molnar, J., Samarina, O. P., and Georgiev, G. P. (1968). *Mol. Biol.* **2**, 627–636.
208. Monneron, A., Liew, C. C., and Allfrey, V. G. (1971). *J. Mol. Biol.* **57**, 335–350.
209. Morimoto, T., Yamamoto, O., Yamamoto, S., and Sibatani, A. (1965). *Biochim. Biophys. Acta* **108**, 152–155.
210. Moriyama, Y., Hodnett, J. L., Prestayko, A. W., and Busch, H. (1969). *J. Mol. Biol.* **39**, 335–349.
211. Moulé, Y., Andrieu, A., and Sarasin, A. (1969). *Bull. Soc. Chim. Biol.* **51**, 1139–1156.
212. Muramatsu, M., and Busch, H. (1965). *J. Biol. Chem.* **240**, 3960–3966.
213. Muramatsu, M., and Fujisawa, T. (1968). *Biochim. Biophys. Acta* **157**, 476–492.
214. Murthy, M. R. V. (1968). *Biochim. Biophys. Acta* **166**, 115–123.
215. Nair, K. G., and Arnstein, H. R. V. (1965). *Biochem. J.* **97**, 595–606.
216. Nakamura, T., Prestayko, A., and Busch, H. (1968). *J. Biol. Chem.* **243**, 1368–1375.
217. Naora, H., and Kodaira, K. (1969). *Biochim. Biophys. Acta* **182**, 469–480.
218. Naora, H., and Kodaira, K. (1970). *Biochim. Biophys. Acta* **224**, 498–506.
219. Naora, H., Kodaira, K., and Pritchard, M. J. (1971). *Biochim. Biophys. Acta* **246**, 280–290.
220. Naora, H., and Pritchard, M. J. (1971). *Biochim. Biophys. Acta* **246**, 269–279.
221. Nazar, R. N., and Busch, H. (1972). *Cancer Res.* **32**: 2322–2331.
222. Neiman, P. E., and Henry, P. H. (1971). *Biochemistry* **10**, 1733–1740.
223. Nemer, M., and Infante, A. A. (1965). *Science* **150**, 217–221.
224. Nichols, J. L. (1970). *Nature (London)* **225**, 147–151.
225. Niessing, J., and Sekeris, C. E. (1971). *Biochim. Biophys. Acta* **247**, 391–403.
226. Ninio, J. (1971). *Biochimie* **53**, 485–494.
227. Nirenberg, M. W., and Matthaei, J. H. (1961). *Proc. Nat. Acad. Sci.* **47**, 1588–1602.
228. Nishimura, S., Jacob, T. M., and Khorana, H. G. (1964). *Proc. Nat. Acad. Sci. U.S.* **52**, 1494–1501.
229. Niu, M. C., Cordova, C. C., and Lau, K. C. (1961). *Proc. N.Y. Acad. Sci.* **47**, 1689–1700.
230. Oda, K-I., and Joklik, W. K. (1967). *J. Mol. Biol.* **27**, 395–419.
231. Okada, S., and Busch, H. (1972). *Cancer Res.* **32**, 1737–1744.
232. Okada, S., and Busch, H. (1972). *Physiol. Chem. Phys.* **4**, 209–233.
233. Okamura, N., and Busch, H. (1965). *Cancer Res.* **25**, 693–697.
234. Olsen, G. D., Gaskill, P., and Kabat, D. (1972). *Biochim. Biophys. Acta* **272**, 297–304.
235. Olsnes, S. (1971). *Eur. J. Biochem.* **23**, 557–563.
236. O'Malley, B. W. (1971). *Metabolism* **20**, 981–988.
237. O'Malley, B. W., and McGuire, W. L. (1968). *Biochem. Biophys. Res. Commun.* **32**, 595–598.
238. O'Malley, B. W., and McGuire, W. L. (1968). *Proc. Nat. Acad. Sci. U.S.* **60**, 1527–1534.
239. O'Malley, B. W., Rosenfeld, G. C., Comstock, J. P., and Means, A. R. (1972). *Karolinska Symp. Methods Reproductive Endocrinol.* **5**, 381–395.

240. Ono, H., and Terayama, H. (1965). *Gann* **56**, 477–483.
241. Oravec, M., and Korner, A. (1971). *Biochim. Biophys. Acta* **247**, 404–407.
242. Pagoulatos, G. N., and Darnell, J. E., Jr. (1970). *J. Cell Biol.* **44**, 476–483.
243. Pagoulatos, G. N., and Darnell, J. E., Jr. (1970). *J. Mol. Biol.* **54**, 517–535.
244. Palacious, R., Palmiter, R. D., and Schimke, R. T. (1972). *J. Biol. Chem.* **247**, 2316–2321.
245. Parish, J. H., and Kirby, K. S. (1966). *Biochim. Biophys. Acta* **114**, 198–200.
246. Parsons, J. T., Gardner, J., and Green, M. (1971). *Proc. Nat. Acad. Sci. U.S.* **68**, 557–560.
247. Paul, J., Carroll, D., Gilmour, R. S., More, J. A. R., Threlfall, G., Wilkie, M., and Wilson, S. (1972). *Karolinska Symp. Methods in Reproductive Endocrinol.* **5**, 277–297.
248. Peacock, A. C., and Dingman, C. W. (1967). *Biochemistry* **6**, 1818–1827.
249. Peacock, A. C., and Dingman, C. W. (1968). *Biochemistry* **7**, 668.
250. Pedersen, S., and Hultin, T. (1963). *Biochim. Biophys. Acta* **68**, 328–330.
251. Perry, R. P., La Torre, J., Kelley, D. E., and Greenberg, J. R. (1972). *Biochim. Biophys. Acta* **262**, 220–226.
252. Philipson, L., Wall, R., Glickman, G., and Darnell, J. E., Jr. (1971). *Proc. Nat. Acad. Sci. U.S.* **68**, 2806–2809.
253. Pilch, Y. H., Ramming, K. P., and Deckers, P. J. (1973). *In* "Methods in Cancer Research" (H. Busch, ed.), Vol. IX. Academic Press, New York.
254. Pitot, H. C., and Jost, J.-P. (1967). *Nat. Cancer Inst. Mono.* **26**, 145–166.
255. Plaegeman, P. G. W. (1971). *J. Cell. Physiol.* **77**, 213–240, 241–258.
256. Porter, G. A., Bogoroch, R., and Edelman, I. S. (1964). *Proc. Nat. Acad. Sci. U.S.* **52**, 1326–1333.
257. Prichard, P. M., Piciano, D. J., Laycock, D. G., and Anderson, W. F. (1971). *Proc. Nat. Acad. Sci. U.S.* **68**, 2752–2756.
258. Quagliarotti, G., Hidvegi, E., Wikman, J., and Busch, H. (1970). *J. Biol. Chem.* **245**, 1962–1969.
259. Raff, R. A., Colot, H. V., Selvig, S. E., and Gross, P. R. (1972). *Nature (London)* **235**, 211–214.
260. Ralph, P., and Rich, A. (1971). *Biochemistry* **10**, 4717–4725.
261. Reid, E., and Morris, H. P. (1963). *Biochim. Biophys. Acta* **68**, 647–650.
262. Revel, M., Delemen, M., and Mandel, P. (1963). *Biochim. Biophys. Acta* **68**, 547–553.
263. Riman, J., Travnicek, M., and Veprek, L. (1967). *Biochim. Biophys. Acta* **138**, 204–207.
264. Ristow, H., and Kohler, K. (1967). *Biochim. Biophys. Acta* **142**, 65–74.
265. Roberts, W. K., and D'Ari, L. (1968). *Biochemistry* **7**, 592–600.
266. Roberts, W. K., and Newman, J. F. E. (1966). *J. Mol. Biol.* **20**, 63–73.
267. Ro-Choi, T. S., Moriyama, Y., Choi, Y. C., and Busch, H. (1970). *J. Biol. Chem.* **245**, 1970–1977.
268. Ro-Choi, T. S., Choi, Y. C., Savage, H. E., and Busch, H. (1973). *In* "Methods in Cancer Research" (H. Busch, ed.), Vol. IX. Academic Press, New York.
269. Rosenfeld, G. C., Comstock, J. P., Means, A. R., and O'Malley, B. W. (1972). *Biochem. Biophys. Res. Commun.* **46**, 1695–1703.
270. Rosenfeld, M. G., Abrass, I. B., Mendelsohn, J., Roos, B. A., Boone, R. F., and Garren, L. D. (1972). *Proc. Nat. Acad. Sci. U.S.* **69**, 2306–2311.
271. Rüger, W., and Bautz, E. K. F. (1968). *J. Mol. Biol.* **31**, 83–90.
272. Rushizky, G. W., and Knight, C. T. (1960). *Virology* **11**, 236–249.
273. Salaman, D. F., Betteridge, S., and Korner, A. (1972). *Biochim. Biophys. Acta* **272**, 382–395.
274. Salas, M., Smith, M. A., Stanley, Jr., W. M., Wahba, A. J., and Ochoa, S. (1965). *J. Biol. Chem.* **240**, 3988–3995.
275. Samarina, O. P. (1964). *Biochim. Biophys. Acta* **91**, 688–691.
276. Samarina, O., Krichevskaya, A., Molnar, J., Bruskov, V., and Georgiev, G. (1966). IEG #7, Memo #639.
277. Samec, J., Jacob, M., and Mandel, P. (1968). *Biochim. Biophys. Acta* **161**, 377–385.
278. Sanger, F. (1971). *Biochem. J.* **124**, 833–843.
279. Scherrer, K., and Darnell, J. E., Jr. (1962). *Biochem. Biophys. Res. Commun.* **7**, 486–489.

280. Scherrer, K., and Marcaud, L. (1965). *Bull Soc. Chim. Biol.* **47**, 1697–1713.
281. Scherrer, K., Marcaud, L., Zajdela, F., Breckenridge, B., and Gros, F. (1966). IEG #7, Memo #560.
282. Scherrer, K., Marcaud, L., Zajdela, F., London, I., and Gros, F. (1966). IEG #37, Memo #561.
283. Scherrer, K., Marcaud, L., Zajdela, F., Breckenridge, B., and Gros, F. (1968). *Bull. Soc. Chim. Biol.* **48**, 1037–1075.
283a. Schlom, J., Colcher, D., Spiegelman, S., Gillespie, S., and Gillespie, D. (1973). *Science* **179**, 696–698.
284. Schlom, J., Spiegelman, S., and Moore, D. (1971). *Nature (London)* **231**, 97–100.
285. Schochetman, G., and Perry, R. P. (1972). *J. Mol. Biol.* **63**, 577–590.
286. Schultz, G. A., Chen, D., and Katchalski, E. (1972). *J. Mol. Biol.* **66**, 379–390.
287. Schultz, G., Gallwitz, D., and Sekeris, C. E. (1968). *Eur. J. Biochem.* **4**, 149–156.
288. Schweet, R., and Heintz, R. (1966). *Ann. Rev. Biochem.* **35**, 723.
289. Scolnick, E. M., Aaronson, S. A., Todaro, G. J., and Parks, W. P. (1971). *Nature (London)* **235**, 318–321.
290. Scott, R. B., and Malt, R. A. (1965). *Nature (London)* **208**, 487–498.
291. Seeber, S., and Busch, H. (1971). *Cancer Res.* **31**, 1888–1894.
292. Seeber, S., and Busch, H. (1971). *J. Biol. Chem.* **246**, 7144–7150.
293. Seeber, S., and Busch, H. (1971). *J. Biol. Chem.* **246**, 7151–7158.
294. Sekeris, C. E., and Lang, N. (1964). *Life Sci.* **3**, 169–173.
295. Shaeffer, J., Favelukes, G., and Schweet, R. (1964). *Biochim. Biophys. Acta* **80**, 247–255.
296. Sharma, O. K., Hidvegi, E. J., Marks, F., Prestayko, A. W., Smetana, K., and Busch, H. (1969). *Phys. Chem. Phys.* **1**, 185–209.
297. Shearer, R. W., and Smuckler, E. A. (1971). *Cancer Res.* **31**, 2104–2109.
298. Shearer, R. W., and Smuckler, E. A. (1972). *Cancer Res.* **32**, 339–342.
299. Sheldon, R., Jurale, C., and Kates, J. (1972). *Proc. Nat. Acad. Sci. U.S.* **69**, 417–421.
300. Shonk, C. E., and Boxer, G. E. (1967). *In* "Methods in Cancer Research" (H. Busch, ed.), Vol. II, pp. 579–661. Academic Press, New York.
301. Sibatani, A., deKloet, S.-R., Allfrey, V. G., and Mirsky, A. E. (1962). *Proc. Nat. Acad. Sci. U.S.* **48**, 471–477.
302. Sibatani, A., Yamana, K., Kimura, K., and Takahashi, T. (1960). *Nature (London)* **186**, 215–217.
303. Singer, M., and Leder, P. (1966). *Ann. Rev. Biochem.* **35**, 195–230.
303a. Singer, R. H., and Penman, S. (1972). *Nature (London)* **240**, 100–102.
304. Sinks, L. F., and Hayhoe, F. G. J. (1967). *Nature (London)* **213**, 1140–1142.
304a. Sitz, T. O., Spohn, W., and Busch, H. (1973). *Proc. Amer. Ass. Cancer Res.* **14**, 55.
304b. Sitz, T. O., Nazar, R. N., Spohn, W. H., and Busch, H. *Cancer Res.* (in press).
305. Sladek, N. E., and Pitot, H. C. (1970). *Cancer Res.* **30**, 1598–1604.
306. Smith, K. D., Armstrong, J. L., and McCarthy, B. J. (1967). *Biochim. Biophys. Acta* **142**, 323–330.
307. Snyder, L., and Geiduschek, E. P. (1968). *Proc. Nat. Acad. Sci. U.S.* **59**, 459–466.
308. Soeiro, R., and Darnell, Jr., J. E., (1970). *J. Cell Biol.* **44**, 467–475.
309. Sonneborn, T. M. (1970). *Proc. Roy. Soc. B* **176**, 347–366.
310. Spelsberg, T. C., Steggles, A. W., and O'Malley, B. W. (1971). *Biochim. Biophys. Acta* **254**, 129–134.
311. Spiegelman, S. (1963). *Fed. Proc.* **22**, 36–54.
311a. Spiegelman, S., Axel, R., Baxt, W., Gulati, S. C., Hehlmann, R., Kufe, D., and Schlom, J. (1972). "RNA Viruses/Ribosomes," Vol. 27, 73–99. 8th Meeting, Federation of European Biochemical Societies, Amsterdam, North Holland.
311b. Spiegelman, S., Axel, R., and Schlom, J. (1972). *J. Nat. Cancer Inst.* **48**, 1205–1211.
312. Spirin, A. S. (1966). IEG #7, Memo #228.
313. Spirin, A. S., Belitsina, N. V., and Lerman, M. I. (1965). *J. Mol. Biol.* **14**, 611–615.
314. Spirin, A. S., and Nemer, M. (1965). *Science* **150**, 214–217.

315. Srinivasan, P. R., Miller-Faures, A., Brunfaut, M., and Errera, M. (1963). *Biochim. Biophys. Acta* **72**, 209–216.

316. Steele, W. J., and Busch, H. (1967). *In* "Methods in Cancer Research (H. Busch, ed.), Vol. III, pp. 61–152. Academic Press, New York.

317. Steele, W. J., Okamura, N., and Busch, H. (1965). *J. Biol. Chem.* **240**, 1742–1749.

318. Steitz, J. A. (1969). *Nature (London)* **224**, 957–964.

319. Stern, R., and Friedman, R. M. (1971). *Biochemistry* **10**, 3635–3645.

320. Stevenin, J., Samec, J., Jacob, M., and Mandel, P. (1968). *J. Mol. Biol.* **33**, 777–793.

321. Stewart, J. A., and Papaconstantinou, J. (1967). *Proc. Nat. Acad. Sci. U.S.* **58**, 95–102.

322. Stewart, J. A., and Papaconstantinou, J. (1967). *J. Mol. Biol.* **29**, 357–370.

323. Sussman, M. (1970). *Nature (London)* **225**, 1245–1246.

324. Suzuki, Y., and Brown, D. D. (1972). *J. Mol. Biol.* **63**, 409–429.

325. Swan, D., Aviv, H., and Leder, P. (1972). *Proc. Nat. Acad. Sci. U.S.* **69**, 1967–1971.

326. Szeszak, F., and Pihl, A. (1971). *Biochim. Biophys. Acta* **247**, 363–367.

327. Takahashi, H. (1969). *Biochim. Biophys. Acta* **190**, 214–216.

328. Takanami, M., Okamoto, T., and Sugiura, M. (1971). *J. Mol. Biol.* **62**, 81–88.

329. Tata, J. R. (1965). *Proc. Biochem. Soc., 453rd Meeting* Middlesix Hospital Medical School.

330. Temmerman, J., and Lebleu, B. (1969). *Biochim. Biophys. Acta* **174**, 544–550.

331. 'Terada, M., Banks, J., and Marks, P. A. (1971). *J. Mol. Biol.* **62**, 347–360.

332. Thach, R. E., Dewey, K. F., Brown, J. C., and Doty, P. (1966). *Science* **153**, 416–418.

333. Thor, D. E. (1968). *Fed. Proc.* **27**, 16–20.

334. Tiollais, P., Galibert, F., and Boivin, M. (1971). *Proc. Nat. Sci. U.S.* **68**, 1117–1120.

335. Tominaga, H., Ali, J., and Natori, Y. (1971). *Biochim. Biophys. Acta* **228**, 183–192.

336. Torelli, U. L., Torelli, G. M., Andreoli, A., and Mauri, C. (1970). *Nature (London)* **226**, 1163–1165.

337. Torelli, U. L., Torelli, G. M., Andreoli, A., and Mauri, C. (1971). *Acta Haematol.* **45**, 201–208.

338. Trakatellis, A. C., Axelrod, A. E., and Montjar, M. (1964). *Nature (London)* **203**, 1134–1136.

339. Trakatellis, A. C., Axelrod, A. E., and Montjar, M. (1964). *J. Biol. Chem.* **239**, 4237–4244.

340. Trakatellis, A. C., Montjar, M., and Axelrod, A. E. (1965). *Biochemistry* **4**, 1678–1686.

341. Tryfiates, G. P., and Krause, R. F. (1971). *Life Sci.* **10**, 1097–1103.

342. Tryfiates, G. P., and Laszlo, J. (1967). *Nature (London)* **213**, 1025–1027.

343. Tsugita, A., Fraenkel-Conrat, H., Nirenberg, M. W., and Matthaei, J. H. (1962). *Proc. Nat. Acad. Sci. U.S.* **48**, 846–853.

344. Turkington, R., and Kadohama, N. (1972). *Karolinska Symp. Methods Reproductive Endocrinol.* **5**, 346–368.

345. Uenoyama, K., and Ono, T. (1972). *J. Mol. Biol.* **65**, 75–89.

346. Ui, H., and Mueller, G. C. (1963). *Proc. Nat. Acad. Sci. U.S.* **50**, 256–260.

347. Unuma, T., Arendell, J. P., and Busch, H. (1968). *Exp. Cell Res.* **52**, 429–438.

348. Verma, I. M., Meuth, N. L., Bromfeld, E., Manly, K. F., and Baltimore, D. (1971). *Nature New Biol.* **233**, 131–134.

348a. Wall, R., and Darnell, J. E. (1971). *Nature New Biol.* **232**, 73–76.

349. Warner, J. R., Soeiro, R., Birnboim, C., Girard, M., and Darnell, J. E. (1966). *J. Mol. Biol.* **19**, 349–361.

350. Watson, J. D. (1965). "Molecular Biology of the Gene," 2nd ed. Benjamin, New York.

351. Weaver, R. F., Blatti, S. P., and Rutter, W. J. (1971). *Proc. Nat. Acad. Sci. U.S.* **68**, 2994–2999.

352. Webb, T. E., Blobel, G., and Potter, V. R. (1964). *Cancer Res.* **24**, 1229–1237.

352a. Weinberg, R. A., Loening, U., Willems, M., and Penman, S. (1967). *Proc. Nat. Acad. Sci. U.S.* **58**, 1088–1095.

353. Westphal, H., and Dulbecco, R. (1968). *Proc. Nat. Acad. Sci.* **59**, 1158–1165.

354. Whitcutt, J. M., and Roth, J. S. (1964). *Biochim. Biophys. Acta* **87**, 380–387.

355. Whitelam, J. M., and Naora, H. (1972). *Biochim. Biophys. Acta* **272**, 425–434.
356. Widnell, C. C., and Tata, J. R. (1966). *Biochim. Biophys. Acta* **123**, 478–492.
356a. Wikman, J., Howard, E., and Busch, H. (1969). *J. Biol. Chem.* **244**, 5471–5480.
357. Wikman, J., Quagliarotti, G., Howard, E., Choi, Y. C., and Busch, H. (1970). *Cancer Res.* **30**, 2749–2759.
358. Wilkinson, B. R., and Kirby, K. S. (1966). *Biochem. J.* **99**, 780–785.
359. Wilkinson, B. R., and Kirby, K. S. (1966). *Biochem. J.* **99**, 786–792.
360. Wilkinson, D. S., Cihak, A., and Pitot, H. C. (1971). *J. Biol. Chem.* **246**, 6418–6427.
361. Willems, M., Musilova, H. A., and Malt, R. A. (1969). *Proc. Nat. Acad. Sci. U.S.* **62**, 1189–1194.
362. Willis, D. B., and Starr, J. L. (1972). *Biochim. Biophys. Acta* **262**, 181–188.
363. Wu, R. S., and Soeiro, R. (1971). *J. Mol. Biol.* **58**, 481–487.
364. Yang, S.-F., and Hsu, C.-Y. (1970). *Proc. Soc. Exp. Biol. Med.* **133**, 485–489.
365. Yazdi, E., Ro-Choi, T. S., Wikman, J., Choi, Y. C., and Busch, H. (1969). *Cancer Res.* **29**, 1755–1762.
366. Yoshikawa, M., Fukada, T., and Kawade, Y. (1964). *Biochem. Biophys. Res. Commun.* **15**, 22–26.
367. Yoshikawa-Fukada, M. (1966). *Biochim. Biophys. Acta* **123**, 91–101.
368. Yot, P., Pinck, M., Haenni, A.-L., Duranton, H. M., and Chapeville, F. (1970). *Proc. Nat. Acad. Sci. U.S.* **67**, 1345–1352.
369. Yourno, J. (1971). *J. Mol. Biol.* **62**, 223–231.
370. Yu, V. I., Yu, V. K., Limborskaya, S. A., and Georgiev, G. P. (1972). *Stud. Biophys.* (in press).
371. Yudkin, M. (1966). IEG #7.
371a. Zimmerman, R. A., Muto, A., Fellner, P., Ehresmann, C., and Branlant, C. (1972). *Proc. Nat. Acad. Sci. U.S.* **69**, 1282–1286.
372. Zomzely-Neurath, C., York, C., and Moore, B. W. (1972). *Proc. Nat. Acad. Sci. U.S.* **69**, 2326–2330.
373. Zylber, E. A., and Penman, S. (1971). *Proc. Nat. Acad. Sci. U.S.* **68**, 2861–2865.

CHAPTER VI

Low Molecular Weight Nuclear RNA

TAE SUK RO-CHOI AND HARRIS BUSCH

I. Introduction*

All mammalian cells contain many types of transfer RNA, messenger RNA, and four types of ribosomal RNA (Chapter V). The main function of these various forms of RNA's is to provide links between genetic information contained in DNA sequences and the primary structures of proteins. Most RNA's are syn-

* Abbreviations: LMWN-RNA, low molecular weight nuclear ribonucleic acid; LMW-RNA, low molecular weight ribonucleic acid; Nu, nuclei; No, nucleoli; Rib, ribosome; $m^{2,2,7}G$, N^2,N^2-dimethyl 7-methylguanosine; Gly, glycerol; A', ^3H derivative of adenosine; the ribose moiety of the nucleoside was oxidized with sodium periodate and reduced with KB^3H_1; U', ^3H derivative of uridine; G', ^3H derivative of guanosine; C', ^3H derivative of cytosine; ψ', ^3H derivative of pseudouridine; m^6A', ^3H derivative of N^6-methyladenosine; m^2G', ^3H derivative of N^2-methylguanosine; B, background; A, adenosine; U, uridine; G, guanosine; C, cytidine; ψ, pseudouridine; T, ribothymidine; DhU, dihydrouridine.

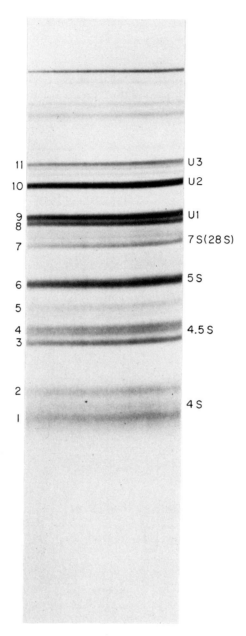

Fig. 6.1. Polyacrylamide gel (12%) electrophoresis of LMWN-RNA from Novikoff hepatoma cell nuclei. Electrophoresis was carried out for 50 hours with a current of 40 mA at a voltage of 300 V in a buffer containing 0.02 M Tris-HCl (pH 7.2), 0.02 M NaCl, and 0.04 M EDTA.

thesized in the nucleus on the DNA templates by various forms of DNA-dependent RNA polymerases (28, 132, 137) and transferred to the cytoplasm where they serve their specific functions.

Following the discovery of 5 S RNA in the ribosomes (138), other types of low molecular weight RNA have been found. With the aid of polyacrylamide gel electrophoresis methods (Fig. 6.1) (66, 84, 90, 115, 130, 157) and high level labeling, some low molecular weight RNA's were found to be specifically localized to the nucleus of tumor cells and other cells (40, 43, 65, 66, 70, 84, 85, 106, 108, 120, 130, 134, 157, 167). Although the cytoplasm contains low molecular weight RNA's other than transfer RNA, they are mainly found in the ribosomes where 5 S and 5.5 S RNA are present in a 1:1 molar ratio with 18 S and 28 S rRNA.

Although at the present time, the sequences of only a relatively small number of RNA species, isolated mostly from nonmammalian organisms, have been established, such studies have already uncovered important structure–function relationships. For example, the location of the anticodon triplet to tRNA and details of its interaction with messenger RNA code "letters" have provided the basis for understanding mechanisms of protein synthesis (Chapter IX). Some progress has been made in studies on specificity of amino acyl tRNA synthetase and structural differences in natural and suppressor tRNA.

More recently, ribosomal RNA and its precursors have been subjected to analysis of their primary sequences with particular respect to the relationship of their structures to the orientation of their accompanying proteins which provide the functional mosaics for protein synthesis (49, 58, 139). However, sequences of only four RNA's from mammalian cells have been determined, (a) 5 S rRNA from KB cells (46, 47); (b) 4.5 S RNA_I and U2 RNA from Novikoff hepatoma cell nuclei (136, 148a); (c) $tRNA^{ser}$ from rat liver (56); and (d) one viral RNA of mammalian cell origin, 6 S VA-RNA (113, 114). Among these RNA's, 4.5 S RNA_I and U2 are the only RNA's localized to the cell nucleus that have been sequenced. Although the functions of most of these LMWN

TABLE 6.1

GENERAL CHARACTERISTICS OF LMWN-RNA

1. Size ranges; 100–300 nucleotides: total number per cell; $1-2 \times 10^6$ molecules (157)
2. Stable half-lives of up to one cell cycle (158)
3. Specific localization; i.e.,
   (a) Nucleolus-associated RNA
       U3 RNA
   (b) Nucleoplasmic RNA
       4.5 S $RNA_{I, II, and III}$
       5 S RNA_{III}, U1 RNA
       U2 RNA
   (c) Cytoplasm: absent
4. Cell distribution: present in all eukaryotic cells studied; including human cells (Hela cells, KB cells, lymphocytes, fibroblast), rat cells (liver cells, Novikoff hepatoma cells), hamster cells (Chinese hamster ovary cells), mouse cells (3T3 cells, Yoshida ascites cells, Ehrlich ascites cells, L cells), *Xenopus laevis* cells, sea urchin eggs, and *Tetrahymena pyriformis*
5. Some exist in ribonucleoprotein complexes (43, 129)
6. Exhibit specificity of hybridization with nuclear and nucleolar DNA (149)
7. Specific sequences; some have an unusual distribution and content of modified nucleosides (128)

RNA's are not defined, they are a unique class of RNA species with specific characteristics (Table 6.1).

II. Classification and Number of Low Molecular Weight RNA

One of the criteria of classification of these RNA molecules is by size. Figure 6.2 is a representative gel pattern of low molecular weight nuclear and nucleolar RNA on 8% polyacrylamide gels. There are six major groups of LMWN RNA's which include 4 S RNA (tRNA), 5 S RNA, U1 RNA, U2 RNA, and U3 RNA. A comparison of nomenclature of these RNA's from several laboratories is presented in Table 6.2.

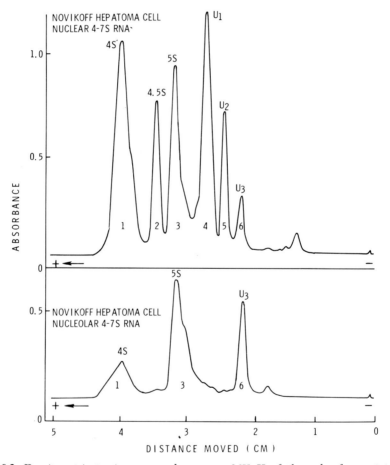

Fig. 6.2. Densitometric tracings on a chromoscan MK II of the gels after staining with methylene blue. Electrophoresis of the RNA was carried out on 8% polyacrylamide gels at pH 7.2. The arabic numbers are arranged from the fastest moving band 1 to the slowest moving band 6. The ordinate is band absorbance compared with a methylene blue standard (25 mg per liter).

TABLE 6.2

SPECIES OF LOW MOLECULAR WEIGHT NUCLEAR RNA OF MAMMALIAN CELLS

	Band number						Ref.
	1–2	3–4	5–6	7–8	9–10	11	
Species	4 S RNA	4.5 S RNA I, II, and III	5 S RNA I, II, and III	U1 RNA 5.5 S (28 S) U1a and U1b	U2 RNA	U3 RNA	24, 25, 135
Approximate chain length	I 78 80 (a)	H 97 100 96 (b)	G and G' 121 121 120 (c)	F and D 138–150 125–150	C 180 165 196 (d)	A 185 180	157 84 157 (a) 166; (b) 136, (c) 47; (d) 148a 157
Estimated number of molecules/nucleus	5×10^5	3×10^5	6×10^5	1×10^6	5×10^5	2×10^5	

TABLE 6.3

EVIDENCE THAT NUCLEAR LOW MOLECULAR WEIGHT RNA's
ARE NATIVE MOLECULAR SPECIES[a]

1. The polyacrylamide gel patterns of nuclear low molecular weight RNA's are reproducible for individual cell types and are similar from cell type to cell type including liver, spleen, fibroblasts, ovary, kidney, and tumors (65, 106, 130)
2. The nucleotide compositions of specific RNA fractions are constant and differ from those of high molecular weight RNA
3. The RNase content of Novikoff hepatoma nuclear preparations is low, and the residual RNase activity is inhibited at the low pH of citric acid used for these nuclear isolations
4. When labeled 18 S and 28 S rRNA were added to the preparations, no degradation was observed during isolation of nuclear RNA either with hot or cold phenol extractions
5. The nuclear RNA bands are found in preparations of RNA obtained from whole cells so they cannot be artifacts of nuclear isolation techniques
6. The special nuclear RNA bands are equally well extracted with either hot or cold phenol
7. The labeling patterns of the nuclear RNA with either [14C]sodium formate or [14C]methyl methionine differ from those of tRNA, 5 S RNA, or high molecular weight RNA
8. Unique and specific linear sequences of nucleotides have been demonstrated for 4.5 S RNA$_I$, U1, and U2 RNA

[a] From references 24, 70, and 106.

The complexity of LMWN-RNA was substantiated by 3'-terminal analysis which showed that A', U',U', and G' are, respectively, predominant 3' terminals of 4 S RNA, 4.5 S RNA, 5 S RNA, and U1 RNA. Both U2 and U3 RNA had more complex terminals (134). Some of these six groups of RNA's have been subfractionated into several subspecies by chromatography on DEAE-Sephadex columns. Although it is possible that these molecules exhibit internal microheterogeneity as in the case of tRNA, good evidence that this is the case has not been obtained. The possibility has been ruled out that these RNA species result from artifactual breakdown of high molecular weight RNA (Table 6.3).

III. Localization of Low Molecular Weight RNA in the Cell

Analysis of the low molecular weight RNA from fractionated subcellular organelles showed these RNA's have specific localizations. Figure 6.3 shows the sucrose density gradients of the RNA extracted from nucleoli, nuclei, and ribosomes of the Novikoff hepatoma cells. The shaded areas designated as 4–8 S RNA were reprecipitated and electrophoresed on 8% analytical polyacrylamide gels (Figs. 6.2 and 6.4). Whole nuclear RNA contains the greatest variety of LMWN-RNA's, and the cytoplasmic sap is largely composed of transfer or amino acid acceptor RNA which has the highest mobility of any of the types of LMW-RNA in these groups. The LMW-RNA of the ribosomal fraction contains at least two bands in the 4 S region, a dark band of 5 S RNA that has a slower migration rate and another dark band (5.5 S RNA) that follows the 5 S RNA, (Fig. 6.4). Only three main types of low molecular weight RNA are in the ribosomes; (a) 4 S transfer RNA, (b) 5 S RNA, and (c) 5.5 S (28 S) RNA (116, 122).

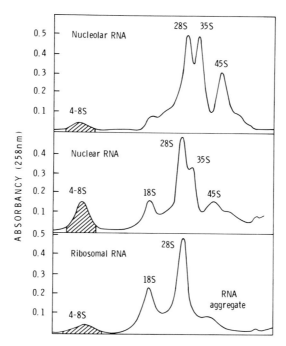

Fig. 6.3. Sucrose density gradient centrifugation profiles of Novikoff hepatoma nucleolar, nuclear, and ribosomal RNA. RNA was extracted with SDS-phenol at 65°C from each organelle. The 4–8 S RNA (shaded) was used for further studies.

In the whole nuclear RNA, obtained either from Novikoff hepatoma, normal liver, or other tissues, there is a dense band of 4.5 S RNA between the 4 S and 5 S bands, and a distinct region containing two dense bands referred to as U1a and U1b (Fig. 6.4). These two closely approximated bands are followed by a single dense band referred to as U2 RNA. The smaller U3 band which follows the U2 band is concentrated in the nucleolus (Fig. 6.2).

Nucleolar LMW-RNA is like the ribosomal RNA in that it contains only three major electrophoretic components (Fig. 6.2). The nucleolus also contains 4 S RNA, 5 S RNA, and the slower moving U3 RNA. Of six classes of low molecular weight RNA (4 S, 4.5 S, 5 S, U1, U2, and U3 RNA), 4 S RNA is present in all of the subcellular fractions. Although more than 99% is in the cytoplasm, some is present in nucleoplasm and nucleolus (Table 6.4).

The 4.5 S RNA is localized exclusively in the extranucleolar portion of the nucleus in the liver and Novikoff hepatoma cells (121, 134). However, approximately 30% of 4.5 S RNA was found in the nucleolar fraction of HeLa cells, KB cells, and Ehrlich ascites cells* (65, 157) (Table 6.4).

---

* For Novikoff cells, the sonication method (23) was used for the isolation of nucleoli, whereas for the other cells, an extraction method (117) was used to fractionate nuclei. When Novikoff hepatoma cell nuclei and rat liver nuclei were extracted with 0.14 M NaCl followed by 2 M NaCl extraction, part of the 4.5 S RNA remained in the residue fraction (120). This residue fraction contains the nuclear RNP network (109) and nuclear membrane in addition to nucleolar fraction.

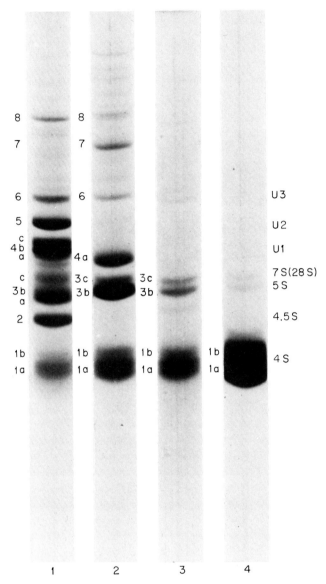

Fig. 6.4. Polyacrylamide gel (8% gel, pH 7.2., and 0.5×7 cm) electrophoresis patterns of 4 to 8 S RNA from different fractions of rat liver cells. Slot 1: nuclear 4 to 8 S RNA; slot 2: ribosomal 4 to 8 S RNA; slot 3: crude mitochondrial 4 to 8 S RNA; and slot 4: soluble cytoplasmic sap 4 to 8 S RNA. The patterns from the same fractions of the Novikoff hepatoma were virtually the same.

The U1 RNA and U2 RNA are exclusively localized to the nucleoplasm. Salt fractionation of the liver nuclei indicates that 65 to 75% of the total LMWN-RNA is associated with the chromatin fraction. The U2 RNA is exclusively in the chromatin fraction in the nucleus (120).

TABLE 6.4

ESTIMATED NUMBERS OF MOLECULES OF VARIOUS TYPES
OF RNA IN NUCLEI, THE NUCLEOPLASM,
AND THE CYTOPLASM[a]

Species of RNA	Estimated no. of molecules/cell		
	Cytoplasm	Nucleoplasm	Nucleolus
U3	—	—	2×10^5
U2	—	4×10^5	1×10^5
U1	—	1×10^6	7×10^4
5.5 S (28 S)	5×10^6	5×10^4	1×10^4
5 S	5×10^6	3×10^5	3×10^5
4.5 S	—	2×10^5	1×10^5
4 S tRNA	1×10^8	2×10^5	—
18 S	5×10^6	6×10^4	
28 S	5×10^6	7×10^4	
35 S	—	—	4×10^4
45 S	—	—	1×10^4

[a] Modified from Weinberg and Penman (157).

The U3 and 8 S nucleolar RNA are associated with preribosomal RNP particles of the nucleolus (24). Some U3 RNA is hydrogen bonded to the 28 S nucleolar RNA. Because it is only transitionally associated with the 28 S RNA molecule in the nucleolus, it may be part of the system that transports nucleolar products to the nucleoplasm (24).

The saturation values for several LMWN-RNA's have been reported to be $0.2–1 \times 10^{-4}$ for approximately 2000 cistrons per genome in the baby hamster kidney (BHK) cells (42a). The number of cistrons for U3 RNA in the Novikoff hepatoma cells was found to be approximately 3000 in nucleolar DNA (149).

IV. Presence of Low Molecular Weight RNA in Various Tissues

At least seven nucleus-specific LMWN-RNA have been found in Novikoff hepatoma cells in addition to tRNA and 5 S RNA. Some are predominantly located in the nucleolus and others are in the nucleoplasmic fraction (134). LMWN-RNA has been found in various tissues including human cells (HeLa cells, KB cells, lymphocytes), Chinese hamster cells, 3T3 cells, rat liver, Yoshida and Ehrlich ascites cells, L cells, sea urchin eggs, *Tetrahymena pyriformis*, and *Xenopus laevis* (41, 65, 66, 130, 157).

The gel electrophoretic patterns of LMWN-RNA components from mammalian cells (HeLa cells, Novikoff hepatoma cells, KB cells, Chinese hamster cells, Ehrlich and Yoshida ascites cells, and human lymphocytes) appear to be nearly identical, although minor differences have been reported between some species. Using a double-labeling method prior to electrophoresis of LMWN-RNA, it

TABLE 6.5

Existence of Low Molecular Weight RNA Other than tRNA

Species	Nuclei	Ribosomes	Soluble sap	Ref.
E. coli	—	5 S RNA	4.5 S RNA	67
			6 S RNA	18, 138
Tetrahymena pyriformis	5 S RNA	4.9 S RNA	5 S RNA	66
	T1, T2, T3 and T4 RNA	6 S RNA (To)		
Xenopus laevis	H, 5 S RNA, (G + G')	5 S RNA	5 S RNA	130
	D, C, B, and A[a]	5.5 S RNA		
Mammalian cells		See Table 6.2		
Viruses				
Adenovirus 2 (KB cell); VA-RNA (6 S RNA)				113, 114
λ Phage (*E. coli*); 6 S RNA				88
λ Phage (*E. coli*); 4 S oop RNA				34a
CEV (exocortis disease virus); 7–10 S RNA				144
PSTV (potato spindle tuber viroid); 4–6 S RNA				35
Visna virus; 5–7 S RNA				62
Qβ RNA; 6 S RNA				77
Avian leukosis virus (9 S RNA)				111
Rous sarcoma virus (7 S RNA)				9
φ 80 (*E. coli*) smaller than 4 S RNA				119a

[a] For nomenclature, see Table 6.2.

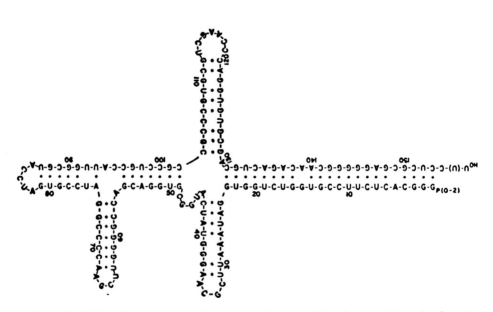

Fig. 6.5. Nucleotide sequence and one possible model for base pairing of adenovirus VA-RNA. Watson-Crick base pairs (G to C and A to U) as well as G to U base pairs are indicated by solid dots (113).

was found that the electrophoretic mobilities of three of the species, U1(D), U2(C), and U3(A), are different in mouse cells (3T3 and L cells) and human cells (HeLa cells and WI-38 cells) (130).

The gel electrophoretic patterns of LMWN-RNA of Ehrlich, Yoshida, and L5178Y ascites cells were identical although there were differences in the components of U3(A) and 4.5 S (H) RNA between HeLa cells and Ehrlich ascites cells. Three components were found in 4.5 S RNA of the Novikoff hepatoma cells and Ehrlich ascites cells, but in HeLa cells there was only one component (65, 130, 134). Thus, it appeared that the mobility of the respective RNA species was determined by the tissue of origin and not by the cell type, karyotype, or tumorigenicity of the cells (130). These LMW-RNA have also been found in other than mammalian cells (Table 6.5).

Low molecular weight RNA's associated with various viruses were also reported (79, 87, 88, 95, 144). One associated with adenovirus 2-infected KB cells (VA-RNA) has been sequenced (Fig. 6.5). Although the functions of these viral low molecular weight RNA's are not completely understood, some plant low molecular weight RNA (144) have been shown to be infectious.

V. Specific Classes of Low Molecular Weight RNA

A. 4 S RNA

The 4 S RNA which mainly contains transfer RNA is found in all types of cells and in several viruses. It is understandable that much of the older research on nucleic acid structure has centered on tRNA, because the tRNA molecule is relatively small and many individual molecular species have been isolated. The tRNA is very diverse in terms of the microheterogeneity and the variety and complexity of the chemical reactions in which it participates. Each tRNA molecule has specificity for a particular amino acid, is "recognized" by the corresponding aminoacyl tRNA synthetase, and "recognizes" a specific codon on mRNA. Since there is more than one triplet code for each amino acid and each tRNA molecule is capable of reading more than one codon *in vitro*, multiple species of each tRNA exist in cells.

Since the first sequence analysis of alanine tRNA (71), some 40 tRNA's have been sequenced. However, the only mammalian cell tRNA sequenced is tRNA[ser] from rat liver (56) (Chapter IX). The function of tRNA is to transfer amino acid from the free to the protein bound state. Studies on structure and function of tRNA (71, 166) have shown a number of universal characteristics of tRNA structure; particularly, the "clover-leaf" structure (Table 6.6).

1. PARTIAL CLEAVAGE AND FUNCTION OF tRNA

tRNA has been dissected by specific cleavage reactions; the isolated large fragments were reconstituted to regain a totally or partially biologically active

TABLE 6.6
UNIVERSAL CHARACTERISTICS OF tRNA

1. Chain length of the molecule: 80 ± 5 nucleotides
2. Loops:

	Dihydrouridine	Anticodon	ψ
Size	Variable	17 Nucleotides	17 Nucleotides
Stem	3–4 Base pairs	5 Base pairs $A \cdot \psi$ pair	5 Base pairs Rich in G:C pair
Loop	8–12 Nucleotides	7 Nucleotides	7 Nucleotides
Modified nucleotides	DhU	Hypermodified nucleotides	Universal pentanucleotide G-T-ψ-C-G (A)
Function	Aminoacyl-tRNA synthetase recognition site?	Binding site in the presence of triplet codons	Ribosome binding site? 5 S RNA binding site?

3. Amino acid acceptor stem and extra arm
   Amino acid acceptor stem:
   (a) 7 Base pairs at —C—C—A stem
   (b) —C—C—A is added post transcriptially
   (c) Similar in various tRNA species
   Extra arm: Variable in base compositions as well as in length.
4. The position of first anticodon nucleotide is at the 35 ± 1 from 5′ end of the molecule
5. Thymidine of the universal pentanucleotide is at 23 ± 1 from the 3′ end of the molecule
6. The length from 5′ end to anticodon is approximately 80 Å
7. The number of nucleotides between m^5C to T, m^2G to 5′ end, and m_2^2G to first anticodon are 5–6, 9–10, and 9, respectively

molecule (73, 103, 112, 146).[*] Such studies have been used to define the specifying parts of the molecule (31, 98, 104, 100, 146). Heterologous fragments of tRNA's from different species can be hybridized (101, 103, 154), and the hybrids retain part of the biological function. Amino acid acceptor activity was studied for fragments or various combinations of partial molecules in an attempt to find recognition sites for amino acyl tRNA synthetases. In yeast tRNA[ala], an isolated amino acid-accepting stem fragment retains some specificity for the amino acid accepting activity (72, 73, 99, 100). Although certain parts of the dihydrouridine loop and arm can be removed without loss of amino acid acceptor activity in *E. coli* tRNA[met], the removal of eight nucleotides in this region renders the molecule inactive (148).

2. SPECIFICITY OF AMINOACYL tRNA SYNTHETASES

Since each tRNA has a specific anticodon for a specific amino acid, it seemed possible that the anticodon might specify which amino acid should be accepted. However, single breaks at the anticodon produced no change in amino acid acceptor activity. The tRNA$_1$[tyr] of yeast and tRNA$_1$[tyr] and tRNA$_2$[tyr] of *E. coli* have the same anticodon (GUA), but they can be aminoacylated only by the

[*] Cleavage into two halves and reconstitution was also done for the ribosomal 5 S RNA from *E. coli* (76). The reconstituted 5 S RNA from two fragments, I (nucleotide number 42 to 120) and II (nucleotide number 1 to 41) has been shown to have identical fingerprints and conformation to that of native 5 S RNA. Moveover, this reconstituted 5 S RNA bound to reconstituted 50 S ribosomal subunits with essentially the same efficiency as native 5 S RNA.

homologous aminoacyl tRNA synthetase. Also, tRNA^{tyr} from *E. coli* Su_{III^+} has the anticodon CUA; this tRNA can be aminoacylated by same tyrosyl tRNA synthetase as the wild type tRNA^{tyr} which has GUA as anticodon. From these studies, the anticodon was eliminated as a recognition site. The fact that the sequences of tRNA^{phe} from yeast tRNA^{phe} from wheat and tRNA^{val} from *E. coli,* all of which are phenylalanylated by yeast phenyalanyl tRNA synthetase, have the highest sequence homology in the dihydro U loop and its stem (37) suggested that this area contained recognition sites. However, at present, several lines of evidence suggest that this may not be true for all of the tRNA studied.

The amino acid acceptor region is another site which has been proposed to contain tRNA synthetase recognition sites. In yeast tRNA^{ala}, after UV irradiation, the acceptor activity was decreased markedly, the UV target was found to be the 5th, 6th, and 7th nucleotide from 3′ end of the molecule. In addition, fragments including the acceptor stem can distinguish the appropriate synthetase and amino acid (27, 143) and thus may be considered the recognition site. However, at present, it seems that the amino acyl tRNA synthetase may recognize the appropriate tRNA molecule by its exterior shape.

3. Mutant tRNA

The relationship of the nucleotide sequence, structure, and function of tRNA has been studied for a number of mutants. These include the mutants that read the UAG terminator codon as an amino acid; the amber (UAG) suppressor of Su_{I^+} serine tRNA, Su_{II^+} glutamine tRNA and Su_{III^+} tyrosine tRNA and the suppressor of the UGA nonsense codon which is a tryptophan tRNA (68, 69). The wild type of Su_{III} gene (Su_0^-) is the structural gene for one of the tyrosine tRNA's of *E. coli* which recognizes the codon UAU and UAC. The Su_{III^+} tRNA recognizes only the amber codon UAG. The mutation to Su^- can occur not only by reversion to Su_0^- but also by changes in the tRNA sequence which produces a defective tRNA.[*]

Suppressor tRNA^{trp} for the nonsense codon UGA was unchanged in the anticodon CCA which is complementary to the tryptophan codon, UGG. This RNA had changes in the dihydrouracil arm where A was substituted for G

[*] Some mutants of the Su_{III} tyrosine suppressor transfer RNA, (1, 150), differ from the wild type Su_{III}^+ tRNA molecule by a single base change. Three mutant tRNA's^{tyr} have G → A substitutions at positions 15, 17, and 31, respectively. A mutant tRNA containing an A residue in place of G in the "dihydrouracil loop" appears to be defective in a step after the acylated tRNA is bound to the ribosome. There was no change in kinetics of aminoacylation or the ribosome binding of the tRNA. Another mutant tRNA having an A residue in place of a G in the "anticodon" stem has been shown to be defective in its apparent affinity for the tyrosyl tRNA synthetase. In two temperature-sensitive mutants, single base substitutions at the amino acid acceptor stem and dihydrouracil arm were observed which produced mispaired bases from a GC to an AC pair. These do not have suppressor activity *in vivo*. However, second site revertants of these mutant to wild type suppressors produce a tRNA with an AU pair at this position. These changes from GC to AU pairs do not alter the K_m of aminoacylation of tRNA with tyrosine tRNA synthetase which suggests these regions are not involved in recognition by the synthetase.

to make an AU pair. Tryptophan tRNA from several related *Su⁻* strains denatured on isolation but that from the suppressor strain is stable.

Although mutant tRNA's have not yet been found in neoplastic cells, it seems important that they be searched for as a possible mechanism for altered growth controls.

4. NUCLEOLAR 4 S RNA

Fractionation of nucleolar 4–8 S RNA by polacrylamide gel electrophoresis or gel filtration separated three major components, 4 S, 5 S, and U3 RNA and two minor components, 5.5 S (28 S) and 8 S RNA. The nucleolar 4 S RNA is unique in its minor nucleoside content and amino acid acceptor activities.

The major and minor nucleoside content of the 4 S RNA, (126) is the same for the nucleus, ribosomes, and cell sap, i.e., 11.5% are modified (Table 6.7). On the other hand, the nucleolar 4 S RNA differed markedly from these RNA's in its higher content of U and A and lower content (9.5%) of modified nucleosides. There was significantly less dihydro-U and N²-methyl-G. Although the reason for these differences is not clear, it is possible that the 4 S RNA from nucleoli contains RNA other than tRNA since nucleolar 4 S RNA had only 60% of the amino acid acceptor activity of nuclear or cytoplasmic 4 S RNA, (Table 6.8; 25, 108, 131). Modification of precursor nucleosides to dihydro-U

TABLE 6.7

NUCLEOSIDE COMPOSITION OF 4 S RNA's FROM NUCLEOLI,
NUCLEI, RIBOSOMES, AND CELL SAP

	% Total nucleosides			
	Nucleoli	Nuclei	Ribosomes	Cell sap
Major nucleosides				
U	19	17	17	17
A	20	19	19	19
C	24	26	26	26
G	27	27	27	27
	91	89	89	89
Modified nucleosides				
m^1A	0.7	0.9	0.9	0.9
m^6A	0.2	0.2	0.2	0.2
m^3C	0.2	0.2	0.2	0.2
m^5C	1.2	1.2	1.3	1.3
m^1G	0.6	0.7	0.6	0.7
m^2G	0.6	1.2	1.1	1.2
m_2^2G	0.4	0.5	0.5	0.5
m^7G	0.6	0.6	0.5	0.6
T	0.4	0.5	0.4	0.5
ψ	2.8	2.9	2.9	3.0
DhU	1.6	2.3	2.5	2.5
	9.5	11.1	11.2	11.6

TABLE 6.8
AMINO ACID ACCEPTOR CAPACITIES OF 4 S RNA's

tRNA	Valine acceptance (% cytoplasm)	Leucine ($\mu\mu$moles/A_{260})
Novikoff cytoplasmic	100	85
Novikoff nuclear	71	42
Novikoff nucleolar	37	28
Rat liver cytoplasmic	63	31

and N^2-methyl-G in nucleoli may be a slower process compared to other modifications so that nucleolar 4 S RNA may contain a greater proportion of "immature" tRNA.

The low content of dihydro-U and N^2-methylguanosine in nucleolar 4 S RNA may be related to its low amino acid acceptor activity. As noted above, the recognition site of aminoacyl tRNA synthetase may reside in the dihydro-U loop and its stem (37–39, 148). The N^2-methyl G appears to be specifically localized to the dihydro-U stem in several tRNA's (59, 91). The lower rates of synthesis as determined by kinetics of labeling with ^{32}P and the different compositions have appeared to rule out a role for the nucleolar 4 S RNA as a precursor of nuclear and cytoplasmic tRNA. In summary, nucleolar 4 S RNA is different from the 4 S RNA of the remainder of the cell with respect to amino acid acceptor activity and content of modified nucleosides.

5. NUCLEAR 4 S RNA

The 4 S RNA of the nucleus is primarily amino acid acceptor or tRNA and has activity like that of cytoplasmic tRNA. Whether nuclear 4 S RNA participates in protein synthesizing machinery (which has not been found in the nucleus) is doubtful; whether nuclear 4 S RNA can act as an amino acyl transfer RNA *in vivo* is unknown at present. Since the amino acid accepting activity of nuclear 4 S RNA is essentially similar to that of the cytoplasmic tRNA, it appears that the newly synthesized tRNA is converted to an active form as soon as it is formed or in close proximity to the site of its formation. A close proximity of methylation and modification reactions to biosynthetic sites has also been found for high molecular weight nucleolar precursors of ribosomal RNA (29, 107), but not yet for tRNA.

6. CYTOPLASMIC 4 S RNA

Cytoplasmic 4 S RNA's are essentially all transfer RNA's. The amino acid acceptor activity and content of modified nucleosides of Novikoff hepatoma were essentially the same as reported values for tRNA from human tissues and tRNA from rat liver and brain (125, 127). Some evidence exists for differences of 4 S RNA of mitochondria and the cytoplasmic sap and there are differences in the major and minor nucleoside compositions of these 4 S RNA's (124).

Although their amino acid acceptor activities are not known, mitochondrial tRNA's have high $A + U/G + C$ ratios with an unusually high A content and fewer modified nucleosides (hypomethylation). Whether tRNA is involved in regulatory processes in the cytoplasm is not clear at the present time (152).

Some special functions have been suggested for specific tRNA molecules. The tRNA that inserts serine into position 3 of the α-chain of hemoglobin is not the same molecule involved in insertion of serine into either position 49 or 52 of the chain (57). Similarly, the tRNA$_I^{Arg}$ and tRNA$_{II}^{Arg}$, purified from yeast tRNA, inserted arginine residues into different positions of the α-chain of hemoglobin (160). Two species of E. coli tRNA^{leu} distributed leucine differently into various peptides of the α-chain of rabbit hemoglobin (161). These results suggest that a relatively rare molecular species of tRNA, responsible for inserting amino acid into one location of a given protein molecule, could become the rate-limiting factor in the synthesis of this molecule. This form of control could occur even though an excess of other tRNA molecules capable of transferring amino acid was available. Recently, 4 S RNA associated with 10–30 S particulate material from postribosomal fraction has been isolated from Chinese hamster cells (60, 142). Lysyl tRNA$_{II}$ disappears from the soluble fraction and appears in particulate fractions after fertilization of sea urchin systems suggesting that this particle-associated tRNA may play a role in cell regulation (165). tRNA has also been a subject of intensive study in relation to neoplasia (11).

a. STUDIES ON tRNA METHYLASE. High levels of methylated purines in whole RNA of S180 ascites cells and C3H mammary adenocarcinoma (7) and high levels of 7-methyl G in tRNA of rats treated with dimethylnitrosamine (92) have been reported. These results led to the proposal that alterations in tRNA methylase might be involved in carcinogenesis. Since then, numerous reports have indicated that increases occur in tRNA methylase activity as well as an increase in specific purine methylation in tRNA of various human and other mammalian tumor cells (Table 6.9).[*]

Using BHK 21 cells, the methylating activity was studied before and after transformation by Rous sarcoma virus or polyoma virus and no difference was found in the extent of methylation. However, a threefold increase was found in methylated A in Rous sarcoma virus transformed cells and an unidentified methyl A was found in polyoma-transformed cells. In a comparison of the specificity and extent of methylase activity from normal and neoplastic cells, the guanylate residue-specific tRNA methylase from tumors and normal rat liver were found to be the same in specificity for guanine residues in tRNA^{fmet} (G_{27}) and tRNA^{val} (G_{10}) (82). Using a mixture of enzyme extracts from mouse liver and plasmocytoma, some differences were found in "populations" of tRNA methylases in these two tissues (110). Quantitative increases in methylases were also found.

On the other hand, analysis of the modified base content of Morris hepatoma

---

[*] The rates, extent, and pattern of methylation largely depend on the ionic environment of the *in vitro* assay system and a precise relationship of increased methylase activity with carcinogenesis has not been established (80).

TABLE 6.9
INCREASED tRNA METHYLASE ACTIVITY IN NEOPLASTIC TISSUE[a]

Neoplastic tissue	Control tissue used
Human tissue	
Leukocytes from leukemic patients	Leukocytes from normal subjects
Mammary carcinoma	Adjacent normal tissue
Carcinoma of colon and rectum	Adjacent normal tissue
Medulloblastoma	Normal brain frontal lobe
Spongioblastoma	Normal brain frontal lobe
Astrocytoma	Normal brain frontal lobe
Oligodendroglioma	Normal brain frontal lobe
Glioblastoma	Normal brain frontal lobe
Neurinoma	Normal brain frontal lobe
Hamster tissue	
SV40-induced tumor (undifferentiated sarcomas)	Connective tissue, liver, thymus, and skeletal muscle
Adenovirus-12 induced tumor	Liver, lung, kidney, spleen, skin, and muscle
Chicks	
Liver tumor with Marek's disease	Uninfected liver
Rat	
Novikoff hepatoma	Liver
Morris hepatoma 5123C	Liver
Mammary carcinoma	Lactational mammary gland
Ethionine-induced tumor of the liver	Normal liver
Spleen with the Dunning leukemia	Liver and spleen of normal rat
Polyoma-transformed rat embryo cells	Normal embryo cells
Diethylnitrosamine-induced tumors	Muscle, kidney, and liver
Mouse	
Glioma	Normal brain
Mammary carcinoma	Liver and lactational mammary gland
Melanoma	Liver
Ehrlich ascites cells	Liver
Hepatoma BW 7756	Liver
Spleen infected with murine leukemia RNA virus	Normal spleen
SV40-transformed kidney cells	Normal kidney cells
Neoplastic line of mouse embryo *in vitro* culture	Nonneoplastic line of mouse embryo *in vitro* culture
Myeloma	Liver

[a] From Borek and Kerr, 11.

5123D showed that this tumor had a lower content of methylated nucleosides (Table 6.10) than normal liver.

b. CHROMATOGRAPHIC DIFFERENCES AND ISOACCEPTING tRNA. A search for different tRNA's in tissues was also carried out using different column chromatographic techniques. The most commonly used methods are MAK(94), BD cellulose (56), and reversed phase (162) column chromatographic methods.

The population of tRNA's extracted from different tumors and nontumor tissues was charged with same amino acids carrying different isotopes and cochro-

TABLE 6.10

Total and Modified Base Composition of 4 S RNA Extracted from 15,000 × g Pellets of Tissue Homogenates of Liver and Morris 5123D Hepatoma[a]

	Total base composition		Modified base composition	
	Host liver	Hepatoma 5123D	Host liver	Hepatoma 5123D
Nucleosides				
U	14.91	15.62	—	—
A	18.73	19.74	—	—
C	25.34	25.58	—	—
G	26.63	26.40	—	—
m^5U	0.51	0.41	3.56	3.29
hU	2.49	2.05	17.36	16.25
ψ	3.78	3.30	26.29	26.10
m^1A	1.32	1.21	9.19	9.57
I	0.29	0.28	2.06	2.26
X	0.41	0.41	2.88	3.26
m^3C	0.28	0.23	1.96	1.86
m^5C	1.87	1.62	13.02	12.82
m_2^2G	0.55	0.54	3.84	4.30
m^2G	1.33	1.23	9.31	9.77
m^1G	0.77	0.68	5.37	5.42
m^7G	0.73	0.63	5.11	5.06
Total	100.00	100.00	100.00	100.00
Modified nucleosides				
Major nucleosides	0.168	0.145		

[a] K. Randerath, E. Randerath, and L. S. Y. Chia, unpublished data. Values are averages of 4 analyses. Note that the modified base content of the hepatoma RNA is lower than that of the liver RNA. Similar modified base composition differences between liver and Morris 5123D hepatoma 4 S RNA were found following isolation of the RNA from 15,000 × g supernatant solutions of tissue homogenates. The differences in total base composition for U, A, C, G, m^5U, ψ, hU, m^1A, m^3C, m^5C, m^2G, m^1G, and m^7G and in modified base composition for m^5U, hU, m^1A, m^3C, m_2^2G, and m^2G are statistically significant (p < 0.05, Student's t-Test), as is the difference in the total modified base content (p = 0.001). X = trialcohol of an unidentified nucleoside.

matographed to assess identity or nonidentity. Table 6.11 summarizes the reports of altered tRNA species in neoplastic tissues (11). Since such experiments do not discriminate between changes in the primary sequence of nucleotides in the transfer RNA and changes in modification, such as methylation, their interpretation will depend on more extensive studies on isolated tRNA species.

Although the exact role of methylated nucleotides in tRNA species is still unknown, it is evident from the studies on several suppressor mutant tRNA species that subtle changes in primary sequences may alter tRNA functions.[*]

[*] For example, it was reported that in *Staphylococcus aureus* the development of resistance to erythromycin is accompanied by the appearance of N^6-dimethyladenine in the 23 S RNA (83). In addition, there is some correlation between methylation of preribosomal 45 S RNA and its processing in the blast cells of acute leukemia (155, see also Chapter V).

TABLE 6.11
ALTERED tRNA SPECIES IN NEOPLASTIC TISSUES[a]

Neoplastic tissues	Altered tRNA's	Control tissues used
Human		
Spleen with malignant lymphoma, chronic leukemia, myelogenous leukemia	Phe	Normal spleen
HeLa cells	Tyr	Human liver
Leukemic lymphoblast	Leu, Ser, Thr, Pro, Tyr, Gln	Normal lymphoblast
Hamster cells		
Adenovirus-31 transformed cells	Asp, Tyr	Reticulocytes and liver
Rous-transformed BHK 21	Tyr	Normal kidney
SV40-transformed cells	Tyr	Hamster liver
Adenovirus-7 transformed cells	Tyr	Hamster liver
Chicken		
Fibroblast	Tyr	Chicken liver
Rat		
Reuber hepatoma	Asp, Tyr	Reticulocytes and liver
HTC hepatoma	Asp, Tyr	Reticulocytes and liver
Morris hepatoma 5123d	Ser, Phe, His	Rat liver
Morris hepatoma 9618A	Lys, Phe	Rat liver
Morris hepatoma 5123 and 5123C	Asn, Gln, Phe	Rat liver
Novikoff hepatoma	His, Tyr, Asn, Phe, Val, Ser, Arg, Leu, Lys, Meth, Ser, Ala, Tryp, Asp	Rat liver
Mouse		
Fibrosarcoma	Tyr, Asp	Liver
Reticulum cell sarcoma	Tyr, Asp	Liver
L-M cell tumors	Asp, Tyr, Phe, His	L-M cells, reticulocytes, and liver cells
Plasma cell tumor (MOPC 31C)	Asp, Tyr	Regressing plasma cells tumor
Ehrlich ascites	Phe, Ser, Tyr	Mouse embryo
Tumor cells	Gly	Mouse liver
Mouse sarcoma-1 cells (Sa-1 cells)	Phe	Kidney
Mouse L cells	Tyr	Liver
P-388 Lymphocytic leukemia	His, Lys, Ser	Rat liver
Leukemia	Val	Rat liver
Mouse plasma cell tumor (K-type immunoblobulin light chain producer)	Leu	Mouse liver

[a] From Borek and Kerr, (11).

c. EFFECTS OF CARCINOGENS ON tRNA. Several investigators (45) have reported that ethionine interacts with liver tRNA's. The reaction is mostly through ethylation of one or more of the bases and ribose. Since ethionine is converted to S-adenosyl-ethionine, it is possible that the ethionine ethyl group participates in alkylation of the RNA's. Moreover, it was also reported (5) that ethionine-fed rats have a loss of leucyl-tRNA which codes for UUG. Increased ethylating activity was also found in embryonic and neoplastic liver by comparison to normal liver (61). Guanylic acid has been shown to be the nucleotide which is most extensively ethylated.

Several aminoazo carcinogens are N-hydroxylated and then can react with protein, RNA, and DNA (97). Acetylaminofluorene (AAF) has been shown to react with tRNA, and an AAF-tRNA complex can be separated from other tRNA by BD-cellulose column chromatography (159, see also Chapter X).

N-acetoxy AAF-treated E. coli tRNA has been shown to be different from untreated tRNA in that most of the tRNA's examined had reduced activities while valine and alanine acceptance was increased (159). Another aminoazo carcinogen, 3′-methyl-4-dimethylaminoazobenzene, fed to male albino rats produced different chromatographic patterns of lysyl, leucyl, phenylalanyl, and tyrosyl tRNA's and slight distortions of arginyl, glutamyl, seryl, and isoleucyl tRNA's on reversed-phase columns. Changes have been found in the chromatographic behavior of phenylalanine tRNA and tyrosine tRNA after direct methylation with diazomethane or dimethyl sulfoxide. Alterations in tRNA structure and function were also observed after UV irradiation of purified tRNA (yeast alanyl tRNA). At present, the precise effects of these alterations in tRNA induced by carcinogenic agents (chemical, viral, and physical) are still unknown.

B. 4.5 S RNA

Almost all studies on LMWN-RNA molecules (24, 25, 65, 66, 70, 84–87, 108, 167) have shown the existence of nucleus-specific 4.5 S RNA's (Fig. 6.1, 6.6). Although the functions of these RNA's are not known, their localization differs from that of some other nuclear RNA's since they are not found in the nucleolus and thus are limited in location to the chromatin or nucleoplasm (Fig. 6.2, 6.4). This RNA was not found in any of the cytoplasmic fractions (Fig. 6.4). The purified 4.5 S RNA from Novikoff hepatoma cell nuclei was separated into three molecular species using DEAE-Sephadex column chromatography (134). The same results were obtained with Ehrlich ascites tumor cells in which the 4.5 S RNA region was also separated into three bands on 13%

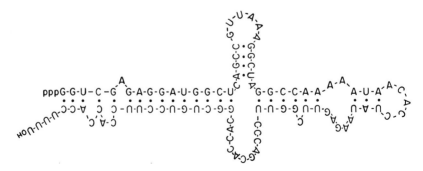

Fig. 6.6. One of the possible secondary structures of 4.5 S RNA$_I$ of Novikoff hepatoma cell nuclei. The secondary structure was constructed to have maximal base pairing with high stability numbers and to fit partial hydrolytic products of this RNA molecule with limited enzyme digestions with pancreatic RNase or T1 RNase (136).

gel (66). However, in KB cells (86), HeLa cells (157, 158), and CHO cells, this region was only a single monodisperse peak even on 15% gels. The low molecular weight RNA from 3T3 (130) also showed heterogeneity in this region. The significance of these differences is not known at the present time. The three fractions obtained from DEAE-Sephadex column chromatography also migrated as single bands with the same mobilities as the original 4.5 S RNA on 8% analytical gels.

The complete sequence of 4.5 S RNA$_I$ has been determined (Fig. 6.6). This RNA contains 96 nucleotides and no modified nucleotides. A striking feature of this molecule is the regional difference in the content of purines and pyrimidines. The 5′ end is rich in purines and the 3′ end is rich in pyrimidines. The center of the molecule has a high content of AMP residues since half of the total adenylic acid residues are clustered in the center between residue 37 and 55. The 5′ terminus was found to be pGp when the RNA was labeled *in vivo*, whereas mixtures of pGp, ppGp, and pppGp were found when the RNA was labeled *in vitro*. Like a number of other RNA species, there was some heterogeneity of the 3′ terminal of 4.5 S RNA$_I$. Two 3′-terminal fragments were found which differed in their content of UMP, i.e., —U—U—U—U$_{OH}$ and —U—U—U—U—U$_{OH}$ (136). The former accounted for two-thirds of the terminals and the lat-

TABLE 6.12

NUCLEOSIDE COMPOSITION OF LOW MOLECULAR WEIGHT RNA'S FROM NUCLEI, NUCLEOLI, AND RIBOSOMES[a]

	U	A	C	G	ψ	m⁶A	m²G	m²,²,⁷G	Alkali-stable oligonucleotides
Nuclei									
4.5 S$_I$	24	25	25	26	0.1				
4.5 S$_{II}$	26	25	25	24					
4.5 S$_{III}$	23	25	21	26	2.9	0.8	0.8		AmpAp GmpAp GmpGp
5 S$_I$	24	19	25	31	0.4				
5 S$_{II}$	24	20	26	30					
5 S$_{III}$	31	24	20	23	1.7				UmpUp,GmpCp
U1a	25	19	27	30					
U2	26	22	24	23	5.5			0.5	CmpUp,Cmpψp A′mpGp,G′mpGp UmpAp,m²GmpAp GmpGmpCp (AmpUmp)m²,²,⁷Gp
U3	25	20	25	29	0.9			0.4	
Nucleoli									
5 S	24	20	27	30					
5.5 S	23	21	27	30	0.4				
U3	24	20	25	29	1.1			0.4	
Ribosomes									
5 S	24	20	27	30					
5.5 S	23	20	27	30	0.4				

[a] From Reddy *et al.*, (128).

ter accounted for one-third. This type of heterogeneity has been previously found in KB cell and mouse cell 5 S rRNA (46, 164) and adenovirus VA-RNA (114).

The 4.5 S RNA_{III} is a unique RNA species with pAp as the 5′ terminal and 2′-O-methyl uridine as the 3′-terminal nucleoside. It has a very low T_m of 37.5°C compared to 65°C for the 4.5 S RNA_I. As shown in Table 6.12 this RNA has a higher ψ and a lower C content than 4.5 S RNA_I. Analysis of the alkali-resistant dinucleotides showed that 4.5 S RNA_{III} contains four alkali resistant dinucleotides, i.e., AmpAp, GmpAp, and 2 GmpGp residues. Analysis of base-modified nucleosides of 4.5 S RNA_{III} (Fig. 6.7, Table 6.12) has indi-

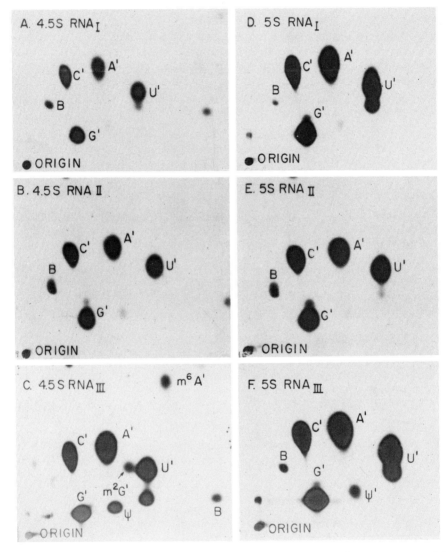

Fig. 6.7. Fluorographs of two-dimensional thin layer chromatography. Separation of ^{3}H-nucleoside derivatives from nuclear low molecular weight RNA's (128). A, 4.5 S RNA_I; B, 4.5 S RNA_{II}; C, 4.5 S RNA_{III}; D, 5 S RNA_I, E, 5 S RNA_{II}; and F, 5 S RNA_{III}.

cated that this RNA contains ψ, N^2-methyl-G, and N^6-methyl-A which accounted for 2.9%, 0.8%, and 0.8% of the total nucleosides, respectively. Since the approximate chain length of this RNA is 93 (41), the number of ψ, N^2-methylguanosine, and N^6-methyladenosine residues is 3, 1, and 1, respectively. The presence of N^6-methyladenosine is unique to this RNA since no other RNA of mammalian origin, including tRNA (125, 128), contains this N^6-methyladenosine. In addition, this is the only RNA known to have a 2'-O-methylated 3' end. As in the case of 4.5 S RNA$_I$, its function is unknown.

C. Ribosome-Associated LMW-RNA

1. 5 S RNA

5 S ribosomal RNA has been shown to be associated with large ribosomal subunits from all bacterial (34, 42, 52, 138, 141), animal (6, 15, 33, 34, 50–52, 81, 156), plant (26, 89), and lower eukaryotic cells (34, 96) thus far examined. The 5 S rRNA from three cell types, E. coli (20), P. fluorescens (36), and KB cells (46), have been completely sequenced (Fig. 6.8). E. coli 5 S RNA was found to be 120 nucleotides long while the KB cell 5 S RNA exists in two forms, 120 and 121 nucleotides long, respectively. In E. coli 5 S RNA various sequences are repeated twice in the molecule and the whole molecule can be divided into two halves which display a considerable similarity. On the other hand, the KB cell 5 S RNA which has a base composition very similar to that of E. coli 5 S RNA has a different nucleotide sequence with only a limited amount of homology to its E. coli counterpart. However, both nucleotide

A.
```
                 10                    20                   30
pU-G-C-C-U-G-G-C-G-G-C-C-G-U-A-G-C-G-C-G-G-U-G-G-U-C-C-C-A-C-C-U-G-A-C-C-C-
   40                   50                   60                   70
A-U-G-C-C-G-A-A-C-U-C-A-G-A-A-G-U-G-A-A-A-C-G-C-C-G-U-A-G-C-G-C-C-G-A-U-G-G-U-
   80                   90                  100                  110                  120
A-G-U-G-U-G-G-G-G-U-C-U-C-C-C-C-A-U-G-C-G-A-G-A-G-U-A-G-G-G-A-A-C-U-G-C-C-A-G-G-C-A-U_OH
```

B.
```
                 10                    20                   30
pU-G-U-U-C-U-G-U-G-G-U-G-A-C-G-A-G-U-A-G-U-G-G-C-A-U-U-G-G-A-A-C-A-C-C-U-G-A-U-U-C-C-C-
   40                   50                   60                   70
A-U-C-C-C-G-A-A-C-U-C-A-G-A-G-G-U-G-A-A-A-A-C-G-A-U-G-C-A-U-C-G-C-C-G-A-U-G-G-U-
   80                   90                  100                  110                  120
A-G-U-G-U-G-G-G-G-U-U-U-C-C-C-C-A-U-G-U-C-A-A-G-A-U-C-U-C-G-A-C-C-A-U-A-G-A-G-C-A-U_OH
```

C.
```
                 10                    20                   30
Gp-U-C-U-A-C-G-G-C-C-A-U-A-C-C-A-C-C-C-U-G-A-A-C-G-C-G-C-C-C-G-A-U-C-U-C-G-U-
   40                   50                   60                   70
C-U-G-A-U-C-U-C-G-G-A-A-G-C-U-A-A-G-C-A-G-G-G-U-C-G-G-G-C-C-U-G-G-U-U-A-G-U-A-C-U-
   80                   90                  100                  110                  120
U-G-G-A-U-G-G-G-A-G-A-C-C-G-C-C-U-G-G-G-A-A-U-A-C-C-G-G-G-U-G-C-U-G-U-A-G-G-C-U-U_OH
```

Fig. 6.8. Primary sequences of ribosomal 5 S RNA's. A, E. coli 5 S rRNA; B, P. fluorescens 5 S rRNA; and C, KB cell 5 S rRNA.

sequences permitted extensive base pairing between the 5′ and 3′ ends of the molecule and permitted more than one possible arrangement of base-paired regions among the internal nucleotide sequences. The 5′-terminal nucleotide is uridylic acid and the 3′-terminal nucleoside is uridine in both *E. coli* and *P. fluorescens* 5 S RNA. Although these two sequences show marked similarities in their primary sequences, they do not fit exactly to any of the proposed models for the secondary structure of other 5 S RNA's.

There is some microheterogeneity in internal sequences differing by one nucleotide in only one position which has been found in an *E. coli* strain as well as *P. fluorescens* (20, 36). The 5 S RNA precursor in exponentially growing *E. coli* cells contains the 5′-terminal sequences of pAUUUG, pUUUG, and pUUG in addition to pUG which is found in mature 5 S RNA (19, 75). These precursor molecules were also found when maturation of 5 S RNA had been arrested by antibiotics or amino acid starvation. These findings suggest that processing or maturation takes place from the 5′ end. In this case, the final cleavage (pUUG → pUG . . .) may be prevented by the secondary structure of the precursor 5 S RNA molecule. The fact that the larger precursor form has an adenine nucleotide at its 5′ end can be correlated with the known transcription initiating preference of RNA polymerases (93).*

Although the function of 5 S RNA remains unknown, its release results in loss of biological activity (3). Three possible functions have been postulated, (a) formation of peptidyl 5 S RNA in the peptide elongation reaction in protein synthesis, suggested by model building studies (123); (b) tRNA binding sites on ribosomes (20), based on the presence of sequences complementary to the universal pentanucleotide of tRNA,

$$G—T—\psi—C—G(A)—$$

which has been considered as a possible ribosome binding site (74, 80); and (c) an essential structural component which provides crucial protein binding sites. Reconstitution of 50 S subunits in the absence of 5 S RNA resulted in greatly reduced activity, presumably because of four of the ribosomal proteins containing 5 S RNA (44). Recently, a single 5 S RNA-binding protein was isolated from rat liver and rabbit reticulocyte ribosomes (10); this protein has a molecular weight of about 35,000.

Although it is clear that 5 S RNA is a component of ribosomal RNA and synthesis of this RNA is coordinated with 18 S and 28 S rRNA, it has been shown that 5 S RNA cistrons are located at different sites from 18 S and 28 S rRNA cistrons. In anucleolate *Xenopus laevis* embryos which do have 5 S RNA genes (16), there is no 5 S RNA synthesis and there is coordinated acceler-

---

* It is interesting that in mammalian cell ribosomal 5 S RNA (KB cell, mouse liver cell, and Novikoff hepatoma cell), microheterogeneity was found at the 3′ end, i.e., a one-nucleotide difference is found. All of these 5 S RNA's from mammalian cells appear to have identical sequences which have pGp as the 5′ terminal and uridine as the 3′ terminal. Mixtures of pppGp, ppGp, and pGp as the 5′ terminal were found in HeLa cells as well as in Novikoff hepatoma cells (64, 136). It is possible that in mammalian cells processing of ribosomal 5 S RNA takes place from the 3′ end as is the case for preribosomal RNA (118).

TABLE 6.13

GENOME REDUNDANCY FOR RIBOSOMAL RNA COMPONENTS AND 4 S RNA[a,b]

Organism	18 S + 28 S RNA	5 S rRNA	tRNA
HeLa cells	280	2000	1260
Rabbit	250	—	—
Chick	100	—	—
Rat liver	300	—	—
Novikoff hepatoma cell	300	—	—
Xenopus laevis	450–610	9000–24,000	6500–1150
Drosophila melanogaster	130	—	860
Tobacco	cyt 3450	—	—
Pea	cyt 4500	—	—
Neurospora crassa	125	—	—
B. subtilis	8–9	4–5	42
E. coli	5–6	11	50–60

[a] From Attardi and Amaldi (2).

[b] The values are the number of cistrons per genome.

ated synthesis of all three RNA species in amphibian oocytes,* in which no amplification of the 5 S genes is detectable (14). In addition, by RNA-DNA hybridization experiments along with labeling kinetics, it has been estimated that an equal number of 5 S, 16 S, and 23 S RNA molecules are synthesized in *E. coli* in a given period of time. The observation that there are different numbers of cistrons for 5 S RNA compared to those of high molecular weight rRNA (Table 6.13) also speaks against the existence of a common precursor of high molecular weight rRNA and 5 S RNA as does the presence of pools of 5 S RNA (105). Recently, the 5 S DNA purified from *Xenopus laevis* was shown to have a very low GC (33–35%) content and each repeat has a molecular weight of 500,000 daltons; large "spacers" must be present.

2. 5.5 S RNA

In animal cells a low molecular weight RNA is found associated with 28 S rRNA. This component which has been designated as 7 S RNA (81) or 5.5 S RNA (157) has not been found in *E. coli*. However, the postribosomal supernatant of *E. coli* contains a 6 S RNA (18), which recently has been sequenced (Fig. 6.9). No function has been suggested for the 5.5 S RNA and the 6 S RNA. The 5.5 S RNA (7 S RNA) in mammalian cells was found to be associated with 28 S rRNA by hydrogen-bonding. RNA with the same mobility was also found in nuclear and nucleolar low molecular weight RNA from Novikoff hepatoma cells (121) and HeLa cells (157). Moreover, it was associated with nucleolar 28 S RNA when RNA was extracted at room temperature and was released by heating. However, 5.5 S RNA was not released from 35 S and 45 S RNA by heating. The precise role of this RNA in maturation of ribosomes is uncertain at the present time.

* These oocytes exhibit rDNA gene amplification (14, 25).

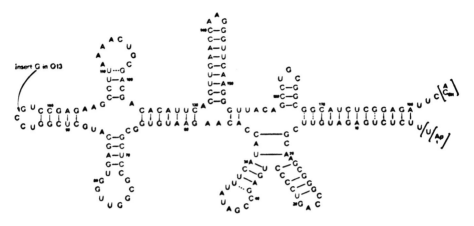

Fig. 6.9. A possible secondary structure model of 6 S RNA of *E. coli* (MRE 600). Possible base pairs are indicated as follows: G–C, A–U, and G–U. Square brackets are drawn around the terminal nucleotides which are absent in a fraction of the normal population of 6 S RNA molecules. Q13 is another strain of *E. coli* which has a G inserted as shown in a fraction of the population of 6 S RNA molecules (18).

D. Nuclear 5 S RNA$_{III}$

When the nuclear 5 S RNA was analyzed by chromatography on DEAE-Sephadex, a new species of 5 S RNA was discovered; it is referred to as 5 S RNA$_{III}$ (135). The three nuclear 5 S RNA's include two ribosomal types, 5 S RNA$_I$, and 5 S RNA$_{II}$, which are conformational isomers (Table 6.12, Fig. 6.10, 158) and a nucleus-specific species, 5 S RNA$_{III}$, which has been isolated best by chromatography of whole nuclear 5 S RNA on DEAE-Sephadex columns (135). By all the criteria used, 5 S RNA$_I$ and 5 S RNA$_{II}$ are the same. The nucleotide compositions of nuclear 5 S RNA$_I$ and 5 S RNA$_{II}$, as well as 5 S rRNA and nucleolar 5 S RNA, are virtually identical (Table 6.12).[*]

The composition of nuclear 5 S RNA$_{III}$ differs in its higher AMP and UMP content and lower CMP content. The AMP + UMP/GMP + CMP ratio for the ribosomal type 5 S RNA's are 0.74–0.80, but that of 5 S RNA$_{III}$ is 1.24. Its 3′ terminals are cytidine and uridine as compared with uridine alone for ribosomal 5 S RNA (134). A precursor of bacterial 5 S RNA described earlier has been shown to be different at the 5′ end by 2–3 nucleotides. However, its characteristics differ significantly from those of the 5 S RNA$_{III}$ of mammalian cells. The 5 S RNA$_I$ and 5 S RNA$_{II}$ do not contain any modified nucleotides which is in agreement with those reported for KB cell ribosomal 5 S RNA

---

[*] Although 5 S RNA has been reported to exist in two conformational states that are interconvertible by heat (4), the finding of only one 5 S peak in the nucleolar and ribosomal RNA fractions suggests that there may be other restrictions on conformation in these molecules in these sites. Whether this is related to the maturation process of ribosomes is unclear at the present time.

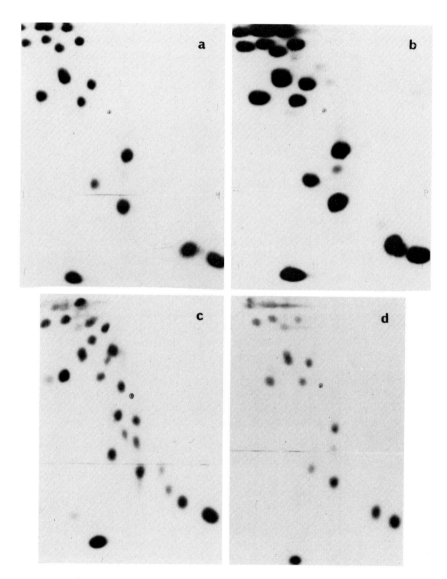

Fig. 6.10. Autoradiograph of two-dimensional electrophoretic patterns of P-RNase digestion products of 5 S RNA's. (a) Nuclear 5 S RNA$_I$; (b) nuclear 5 S RNA$_{II}$; (c) nuclear 5 S RNA$_{III}$; and (d) nucleolar 5 S RNA.

(46). Moreover, 5 S RNA$_{III}$ contains the two alkali-stable dinucleotides, UmpUp and GmpCp, and two ψ residues. As shown by the absence of 5 S RNA$_{III}$ in the nucleolus and cytoplasm, this is also a unique nucleoplasmic RNA. The function of this RNA is also unknown.

Recently, a 5 S RNA was found to be associated with chick liver chromatin; this RNA contains 28% uridylic acid. This RNA is stimulatory to RNA synthesis when chick liver chromatin is used as template with *E. coli* RNA polymerase (78).

E. U1 RNA

Among the earliest findings in studies on the LMWN-RNA's was the presence of a dense double-banded zone, referred to as the U1 RNA, that has a lower electrophoretic mobility than that of 5 S RNA (Fig. 6.1). The two bands in the U1 RNA were not adequately separated by gel electrophoresis or chromatography on DEAE-Sephadex. Recently it was found that these bands are also conformational isomers. U1 RNA has a 3'-terminal guanosine and apparently lacks a 5'-terminal phosphate. Although it seems probable that there is a minimum number of four bands in the U1 region (Fig. 6.1), two are minor bands. The U1 RNA is also a nucleoplasmic RNA, i.e., it is not found either in the nucleolus or cytoplasm. U1 RNA appears to have two alkali-stable dinucleotides but no base-modified nucleotides (Table 6.12).*

F. U2 RNA

The U2 RNA fraction was the first LMWN-RNA that was obtained in a high state of purity by preparative gel electrophoresis (70). Like U1 RNA, the U2 RNA is localized to the extranucleolar portions of the nucleus and although its function is uncertain, its linear sequence of nucleotides is almost completely defined (Fig. 6.11). It is probably only synthesized once during the cell cycle and hence may serve as a structural or initiating element in gene readouts. The nucleotide compositions of this RNA in the liver and tumor are very similar.

A most unique feature of the U2 RNA is its remarkable polarity (Fig. 6.11). Its 5' end contains many modified nucleotides including the unusual base $N^{2,2}$-7-trimethylguanosine (Fig. 6.12). The modified nucleotides are clustered in the 5' half of the molecule but the 3' half of the molecule does not have any modified nucleotides and is rich in pyrimidines. The fact that all the modified nucleotides are clustered at the 5' end of the molecule suggests that this RNA

---

* This RNA is part of a small RNP particle (20–30 S) (Hermolin et al., unpublished).

Nm–(Am, Um)–$m_3^{2,2,7}$G–C–G–C–Gm–Gm–C–(U–C)–(C, ψ–ψ)–C–ψ–U–U–U–Gm–G–C–

U–A–A–G'm–A–U–C–A–A'm–G–U–G–ψ–A–G–ψ–A–ψ–Cm–ψ–G–ψ–ψ–U–C–Um–A–U–C–A–

G–U–ψ–U–U–A–A–ψ–A–U–Cm–U–U–C–G–A–U–A–C–G–U–C–C–U–C–U–A–U–C–C–G–A–

G–G–A–C–A–A–U–A–ψ–U–A–ψ–U–A–A–A–U–G–G–A–U–U–U–U–G–G–A–A–C–U–A–G–

G–A–G–U–U–G–G–A–A–U–A–G–G–A–G–C–U–U–G–C–U–C–C–G–U–C–C–A–C–C–U–C–A–

C–G–C–A–U–C–G–A–C–C–U–G–G–U–A–U–U–G–C–G–C–A–G–U–A–C–C–U–C–A–G–G·

A–A–C–G–G–U–G–C–A–C–C–A$_{OH}$

Fig. 6.11. Nucleotide sequence of the U2 RNA of Novikoff hepatoma cell nuclei.

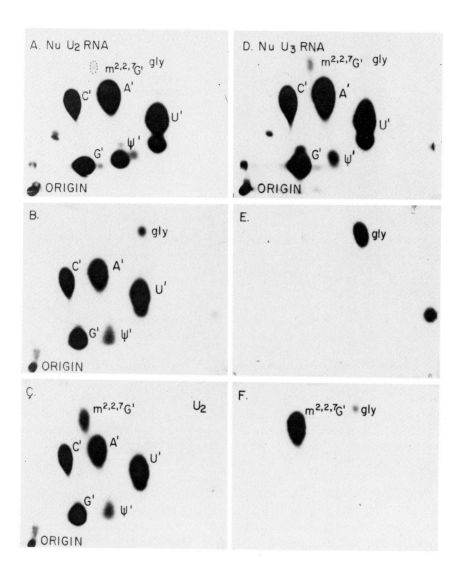

Fig. 6.12. Fluorographs of two-dimensional thin layer chromatography. Separation of ³H-nucleoside derivatives from nuclear U2 RNA and nucleolar U3 RNA. A, Nuclear U2 RNA; B, sample A heated at 95°C for 2 hours in 10% piperidine; C, sample A cochromatographed with [³H]trialcohol derivative of N^2,N^2-dimethyl 7-methylguanosine; D, nucleolar U3 RNA; E, ³H-derivative of N^2,N^2-dimethyl 7-methylguanosine heated at 95°C for 2 hours in 10% piperidine; and F, ³H-derivative of N^2,N^2-dimethyl 7-methylguanosine.

Trimethylguanosine first found in low molecular weight RNA from Chinese hamster ovary cells (140) was synthesized according to the method described (155) which defined the structure of this nucleoside; it was labeled with ³H (136). Figure 6.11F shows the fluorograph of the position of this labeled trimethyl-G derivative as well as its purity. After heating this derivative in 10% piperidine, all of the compound was degraded and glycerol was produced as shown in Fig. 6.11E. When labeled nucleoside derivatives from U2 RNA were heated in piperidine, the unusual spot disappeared and a dark glycerol spot appeared. Chromatography of a mixture of nucleoside derivatives of U2 RNA and trimethylguanosine (Fig. 6.11C) shows the comigration of the derivative of synthesized trimethylguanosine and the unusual nucleoside of the U2 RNA. From these experiments, it was concluded that U2 and U3 RNA contain this unusual nucleoside N^2,N^2-dimethyl 7-methylguanosine in the amount of 1 residue each.

might form specific complexes with other macromolecules or have a specific conformation for its function.*

G. U3 RNA

The U3 RNA along with the 8 S (28 S) RNA is of special interest because of its specific localization to the nucleolus. Both the U3 RNA and 8 S RNA are associated with nucleolar 28 S RNA as is 5.5 S (28 S) RNA. Several molecular species may be present in the U3 and 8 S (28 S) RNA's since the major 3'-terminal nucleosides of U3 RNA are adenosine and uridine and the major 3'-terminal nucleosides of 8 S (28 S) RNA are cytidine and uridine. The U3 RNA is a sharp single band on 8–10% gel and can be resolved into three to four closely moving bands on 16% polyacrylamide gel electrophoresis. The U3 RNA from Novikoff hepatoma cell nuclei and Walker 256 carcinosarcoma cell nuclei was separated into four bands; that of normal and thioacetamide-treated liver separated into three bands (122). The fastest moving band which was absent in normal cells and present in tumor cells had a different nucleotide composition. Preliminary sequence analysis of U3 RNA shows there is one main chain of U3 RNA with possible microheterogeneity at the 3' end of the molecule.

Neither nucleolar 45 S RNA nor 35 S RNA contain the U3 or 8 S RNA components present in nucleolar 28 S RNA. However, these RNA species (U3 and 8 S RNA) do not appear to be precursors of cytoplasmic RNA's and therefore their function must be restricted to the nucleus and, more specifically, to the nucleolus. The finding that 5.5 S (28 S) RNA is present in the molar ratio of approximately 1:1 to nucleolar 28 S RNA suggests that it binds to nucleolar 28 S RNA in a relatively specific site. On the other hand, the molar ratio of 8 S (28 S) and U3 (28 S) RNA to nucleolar 28 S RNA is only approximately 1:2, suggesting that only some of the nucleolar 28 S RNA's are bound to these molecules. These results suggest that these small molecules may serve a role in processing of nucleolar 28 S RNA and hence are associated with it only for a limited time. Since the nucleolar 35 S and 45 S RNA's are not bound to any of these molecular species, it seems probable that in the course of processing of nucleolar 35 S RNA to nucleolar 28 S RNA, the 5.5 S (28 S), U3 (28 S), and 8 S (28 S) RNA's are added from preexisting pools.

It is noteworthy that species differences in LMWN-RNA mobilities on gel electrophoresis were most significant in the region of U3 RNA. The U3(A) RNA, from different sources, migrated differently, i.e., that from 3T3 cells and Ehrlich ascites cells migrated faster than that of HeLa cells (65, 130).

VI. Functions of Low Molecular Weight RNA

A number of species of low molecular weight RNA are present in many types of cells. The major known function of the low molecular weight RNA

---

* By sequence analysis (Fig. 6.11), it was found that the U2 RNA has only one 5' end but has two types of 3' ends (C and A) which differ by one nucleotide.

is the amino acid acceptor and transfer activity of tRNA. The possible involvement of low molecular weight RNA in gene regulatory functions proposed (13, 54) are (1) gene activation, (2) primers for nucleic acid synthesis, and (3) structural components of chromatin.

A. Gene Activator RNA

Some models for gene regulation in higher organisms include RNA (13, 54). Recently, a stimulatory activity was found for certain species of low molecular weight chromatin RNA in *in vitro* RNA synthesizing systems (78). These results suggest that these RNA's might function as specific or nonspecific "depressors" for gene activity.

B. Primer for Nucleic Acid Synthesis

Another possibility is that these RNA's may function as primer molecules for DNA (21, 153, 163) or RNA synthesis. The existence of pppGp as a 5′ end of 4.5 S RNA_I (136) suggests that this RNA could be an initiation site for nucleic acid synthesis. The lack of a 5′ phosphate and the hypermodified nature of 5′ end of U2 RNA suggests that this RNA may be part of some processing or binding particle. The unusual modification of the 5′ end of U2 RNA including $N^{2,2}$-7-trimethyl-G might serve as a recognition site for specific processing enzyme(s). These RNA's in complexes with specific protein(s) may localize at the initiation or termination site(s) of gene transcriptional unit(s) and direct the RNA polymerase activity. Recently, an RNA composed of 81 nucleotides, referred to as the oop RNA, was found in λ phage infected *E. coli* to be a primer for DNA synthesis (34a, 64a). Sequence similarities of 4.5 S RNA_I and the oop RNA suggest that 4.5 S RNA_I might have an analogous function.

C. Structural Elements

The 5 S RNA of three different species has been sequenced. This RNA is essential for function of the 50 S ribosomal subunit. It may be a critical site for binding important proteins. A similar function was proposed for the nucleolar U3 RNA for binding structural or processing protein(s) for the immature ribosomal particles (121).

Acknowledgments

The original studies in this chapter were supported by the Cancer Center Grant, CA-10893 P. 4.

References

1. Abelson, J. N., Gefter, M. L., Barnett, L., Landy, A., Russell, R. L., and Smith, J. D. (1970). *J. Mol. Biol.* **47**, 15–28.

2. Attardi, G., and Amaldi, F. (1970). *Ann Rev. Biochem.* **39**, 183–226.
3. Aubert, M., Monier, R., Reynier, M., and Scott, J. F. (1967). *Proc. FEBS Meeting, 4th* **3**, 151–168.
4. Aubert, M., Scott, J. F., Reynier, M., and Monier, R. (1968). *Proc. Nat. Acad. Sci. (Wash.)* **61**, 292–299.
5. Axel, R., Weinstein, I. B., and Farber, E. (1967). *Proc. Nat. Acad. Sci. U.S.* **58**, 1255–1260.
6. Bachvaroff, R. J., and Tongur, V. (1966). *Nature (London)* **211**, 248–250.
7. Bergquist, P. L., and Matthews, R. E. F. (1962). *Biochem. J.* **85**, 305–313.
8. Bernhardt, D., and Darnell, Jr., J. (1969). *J. Mol. Biol.* **42**, 43–56.
9. Bishop, J. M., Levinson, W. E., Sullivan, D., Fanshier, L., Quintrell, N., and Jackson, J. (1970). *Virology* **42**, 927–937.
10. Blobel, G. (1971). *Proc. Nat. Acad. Sci. U.S.* **68**, 1881–1885.
11. Borek, E., and Kerr, S. J. (1972). *Advan. Cancer Res.* **15**, 163–190.
12. Briscoe, W. T., Taylor, W., Griffin, A. C., Duff, R., and Rapp, F. (1972). *Cancer Res.* **32**, 1753–1755.
13. Britten, R. J., and Davidson, E. H. (1969). *Science* **165**, 349–357.
14. Brown, D. D., and Dawid, I. B. (1968). *Science* **160**, 272–280.
15. Brown, D. D., and Littna, E. (1966). *J. Mol. Biol.* **20**, 95–112.
16. Brown, D. D., and Weber, C. S. (1968). *J. Mol. Biol.* **34**, 681–697.
17. Brown, D. D., Wensink, P. C., and Jordan, E. (1971). *Proc. Nat. Acad. Sci. U.S.* **68**, 3175–3179.
18. Brownlee, G. G. (1971). *Nature New Biol.* **229**, 147–149.
19. Brownlee, G. G., and Cartwright, E. (1971). *Nature New Biol.* **232**, 50–52.
20. Brownlee, G. G., Sanger, F., and Barrell, B. G. (1968). *J. Mol. Biol.* **34**, 379–412.
21. Brutlag, D., Schekman, R., and Kornberg, A. (1971). *Proc. Nat. Acad. Sci. U.S.* **68**, 2826–2829.
22. Burdon, R. H. (1971). *Progr. Nucleic Acid Res. Mol. Biol.* **11**, 33–79.
23. Busch, H. (1967). *In* "Methods in Enzymology" (L. Grossman and K. Moldave, eds.), Vol. 12. pp. 421–448. Academic Press, New York.
24. Busch, H., Ro-Choi, T. S., Prestayko, A. W., Shibata, H., Crooke, S. T., El-Khatib, S. M., Choi, Y. C., and Mauritzen, C. M. (1971). *Persp. Biol. Med.* **15**, 117–139.
25. Busch, H., and Smetana, K. (1970). "The Nucleolus." pp. 285–317. Academic Press, New York.
26. Chakravorty, A. K. (1969). *Biochim. Biophys. Acta* **179**, 67–82.
27. Chambers, R. W. (1969). *J. Cell Physiol. Suppl. 1* **74**, 179.
28. Chambon, P., Gissinger, F., Mandel, Jr., J. L., Kedinger, C., Gniazdowski, M., and Meilhac, M. (1970). *Cold Spring Harbor Symp.* XXXV, 693–707.
29. Choi, Y. C., and Busch, H. (1970). *J. Biol. Chem.* **245**, 1954–1961.
30. Chugnev, I. I., Axelrod, V. D., and Bayev, A. A. (1969). *Biochem. Biophys. Res. Commun.* **34**, 348–353.
31. Clark, B. F. C., Dube, S. K., and Marcker, K. A. (1968). *Nature (London)* **219**, 484–485.
32. Clason, A. E., and Burdon, R. H. (1969). *Nature (London)* **223**, 1063–1064.
33. Comb, D. G., and Katz, S. (1964). *J. Mol. Biol.* **8**, 790–800.
34. Comb, D. G., Sarkar, N., DeVallet, J., and Pinzino, C. J. (1965). *J. Mol. Biol.* **12**, 509–513.
34a. Dahlberg, J. E., and Blattner, F. R. (1973). *Fed. Proc.* **32**: 664 Abs.
35. Diener, T. O., and Smith, D. R. (1971). *Virology* **46**, 498–499.
36. DuBuy, B., and Weissman, S. M. (1971). *J. Biol. Chem.* **246**, 747–761.
37. Dudock, B. S., Diperi, C., and Michael, M. S. (1970). *J. Biol. Chem.* **245**, 2465–2468.
38. Dudock, B. S., Diperi, C., Scileppi, K., and Reszelbach, R. (1971). *Proc. Nat. Acad. Sci. U.S.* **68**, 681–684.
39. Dudock, B. S., Katz, G., Taylor, E., and Holley, R. W. (1969). *Proc. Nat. Acad. Sci. U.S.* **62**, 941–945.

40. Egyhazi, E., Daneholt, B., Edstrom, J. E., Lambert, B., and Ringborg, U. (1969). *J. Mol. Biol.* **44**, 517–532.
41. El-Khatib, S. M., Ro-Choi, T. S., Choi, Y. C., and Busch, H. (1970). *J. Biol. Chem.* **245**, 3416–3421.
42. Elson, D. (1961). *Biochim. Biophys. Acta* **53**, 232–234.
42a. Engberg, J., Hellung-Larsen, P., and Frederiksen, S. (1973). Ninth International Congress of Biochemistry, Stockholm, p. 161.
43. Enger, M. D., and Walters, R. A. (1970). *Biochemistry* **9**, 3551–3562.
44. Erdman, V. A., Fahnestock, S., Higo, H., and Nomura, M. (1971). *Proc. Nat. Acad. Sci. U.S.* **68**, 2932–2936.
45. Farber, E., McConomy, J., Franzen, B., Marroquin, F., Stewart, G. A., and Magee, P. N. (1967). *Cancer Res.* **27**, 1761–1772.
46. Forget, B., and Weissman, S. M. (1968). *J. Biol. Chem.* **243**, 5709–5723.
47. Forget, B. G., and Weissman, S. M. (1969). *J. Biol. Chem.* **244**, 3148–3165.
48. Fresco, J. R., Adams, A., Ascione, R., Henley, D., and Lindahl, T. (1966). *Cold Spring Harbor Symp. Quant. Biol.* **31**, 527–537.
49. Fuller, W., and Hodgson, A. (1967). *Nature (London)* **215**, 817–821.
50. Galibert, F., Larsen, C. J., Lelong, J. C., and Boiron, M. (1965). *Nature (London)* **207**, 1039–1041.
51. Galibert, F., Larsen, C. J., Lelong, J. C., and Boiron, M. (1966). *Bull. Soc. Chem. Biol.* **48**, 21–36.
52. Galibert, F., Lelong, J. C., Larsen, C. J., and Boiron, M. (1966). *J. Mol. Biol.* **21**, 385–390.
53. Gartland, W. J., and Sueoka, N. (1966). *Proc. Nat. Acad. Sci. U.S.* **55**, 948–956.
54. Georgiev, G. P. (1972). *Current Topics Develop Biol.* **7**, 1–60.
55. Gillam, I., Millward, S., Blew, D., von Tigerstrom, M., Wimmer, E., and Tener, G. M. (1967). *Biochemistry* **6**, 3043–3056.
56. Ginsberg, T., Rogg, H., and Staehelin, M. (1971). *Eur. J. Biochem.* **21**, 249–257.
57. Gonano, F. (1967). *Biochemistry* **6**, 977–983.
58. Gould, H. J. (1967). *J. Mol. Biol.* **29**, 307–313.
59. Griffin, A. C., and Black, D. D. (1971). In "Methods in Cancer Research" (H. Busch, ed.), Vol. VI, p. 189–251. Academic Press, New York.
60. Hampel, A. E., Saponara, A. G., Walters, R. A., and Enger, M. D. (1972). *Biochim. Biophys. Acta* **269**, 428–440.
61. Hancock, R. L. (1968). *Cancer Res.* **28**, 1223–1230.
62. Harter, D. H., Schlom, J., and Spiegelman, S. (1971). *Biochim. Biophys. Acta* **240**, 435–441.
63. Hashimoto, S., Kawata, M., and Takemura, S. (1969). *Biochem. Biophys. Res. Commun.* **37**, 777–784.
64. Hatlen, L. E., Amaldi, F., and Attardi, G. (1969). *Biochemistry* **8**, 4989–5005.
64a. Hayes, S., and Szybalski, W. (1973). *Fed. Proc.* **32:** 529 Abs.
65. Hellung-Larsen, P., Frederiksen, S., and Plesner, P. (1971). *Biochim. Biophys. Acta* **254**, 78–90.
66. Hellung-Larsen, P., and Frederiksen, S. (1972). *Biochim. Biophys. Acta* **262**, 290–307.
67. Hindley, J. (1967). *J. Mol. Biol.* **30**, 125–136.
68. Hirsh, D. (1971). *J. Mol. Biol.* **58**, 439–458.
69. Hirsh, D., and Gold, L. (1971). *J. Mol. Biol.* **58**, 459–468.
70. Hodnett, J. L., and Busch, H. (1968). *J. Biol. Chem.* **243**, 6336–6342.
71. Holley, R. W., Apgar, J., Everett, G. A., Marquisee, M., Merrill, S. H., Penswick, J. R., and Zamir, A. (1965). *Science* **147**, 1462–1465.
72. Imura, N., Schwam, H., and Chambers, R. W. (1969). *Proc. Nat. Acad. Sci. U.S.* **62**, 1203–1209.
73. Imura, N., Weiss, G. B., and Chambers, R. W. (1969). *Nature (London)* **222**, 1147–1148.
74. Jordan, B. R. (1971). *J. Mol. Biol.* **55**, 423–439.
75. Jordan, B. R., Feunteun, J., and Monier, R. (1970). *J. Mol. Biol.* **50**, 605–615.

76. Jordan, B. R., and Monier, R. (1971). *J. Mol. Biol.* **59**, 219–222.
77. Kacian, D. L., Mills, D. R., and Spiegelman, S. (1971). *Biochem. Biophys. Acta* **238**, 212–223.
78. Kanehisa, T., Tanaka, T., and Kano, Y. (1972). *Biochim. Biophys. Acta* **277**, 584–589.
79. Kaper, J. M., and West, C. K. (1972). *Prep. Biochem.* **2**(3), 251–263.
80. Kaye, A. M., and Leboy, P. S. (1968). *Biochim. Biophys. Acta* **157**, 289–302.
81. Knight, E., and Darnell, J. E. (1967). *J. Mol. Biol.* **28**, 491–502.
82. Kuchino, Y., Endo, H., and Nishimura, S. (1972). *Cancer Res.* **32**, 1243–1250.
83. Lai, C. J., and Weisblum, B. (1971). *Proc. Nat. Acad. Sci. U.S.* **68**, 856–860.
84. Larsen, C. J., Galibert, F., Hampe, A., and Boiron, M. (1969). *Bull. Soc. Chim. Biol.* (*Paris*) **51**, 649–668.
85. Larsen, C. J., Galibert, F., Lelong, J. C., and Boiron, M. (1967). *C. R. Acad. Sci. Paris* **D264**, 1523–1526.
86. Larsen, C. J., Lebowitz, P., Weissman, S. M. and Dubuy, B. (1970). *Cold Spring Harbor Symp. Quant. Biol.* **XXXV**, 35–46.
87. Larsen, C. J., Ravicovitch, R. E., Bazilier, M., Mauchauffe, M., Robin, J., and Boiron, M. (1972). *C. R. Acad. Sci. Paris* **274**, 1396–1398.
88. Lebowitz, P., Weissman, S. M., and Radding, C. M. (1971). *J. Biol. Chem.* **246**, 5120–5139.
89. Li, P. H., and Fox, R. H. (1969). *Biochim. Biophys. Acta* **182**, 255–258.
90. Loening, U. E. (1967). *Biochem. J.* **102**, 251–257.
91. Madison, J. T. (1968). *Ann. Rev. Biochem.* **37**, 131–148.
92. Magee, P. N., and Farber, E. (1962). *Biochem. J.* **83**, 114–124.
93. Maitra, U., and Hurwitz, J. (1965). *Proc. Nat. Acad. Sci. U.S.* **54**, 815–822.
94. Mandelt, J. D., and Hershey, A. D. (1960). *Anal. Biochem.* **1**, 66–77.
95. Marcaud, L., Portier, M. M., Kourilsky, P., Barrell, B. G., and Gros, F. (1971). *J. Mol. Biol.* **57**, 247–261.
96. Marcot-Queiroz, J., Julien, J., Rosset, R., and Monier, R. (1965). *Bull. Soc. Chim. Biol.* **47**, 183–194.
97. Miller, J. A., and Miller, E. C. (1967). *In* "Carcinogenesis: A Broad Critique," pp. 387–420. Williams and Wilkins, Baltimore, Maryland.
98. Mirzabekov, A. D., Grünberger, D., and Bayev, A. A. (1968). *Biochim. Biophys. Acta* **166**, 68–74.
99. Mirzabekov, A. D., Kazarinova, L., Ya., Lastity, D., and Bayev, A. A. (1969). *FEBS Lett.* **3**, 268–270.
100. Mirzabekov, A. D., Kazarinova, L. Ya., and Bayev, A. A. (1969). *Mol. Biol.* **3**, 879–892.
101. Mirzabekov, A. D., Kazarinova, L. Ya., Lastity, D., and Bayev, A. A. (1969). *Mol. Biol.* **3**, 909–919.
102. Mirzabekov, A. D., Lastity, D., and Bayev, A. A. (1969). *FEBS Lett.* **4**, 281–284.
103. Mirzabekov, A. D., Levina, E. S., and Bayev, A. A. (1969). *FEBS Lett.* **5**, 218–220.
104. Mirzabekov, A. D., Lastity, D., Levina, E. S., and Bayev, A. A. (1970). *FEBS Lett.* **7**, 95–98.
105. Morell, P., and Marmur, J. (1968). *Biochemistry* **7**, 1141–1152.
106. Moriyama, Y., Hodnett, J. L., Prestayko, A. W., and Busch, H. (1969). *J. Mol. Biol.* **39**, 335–349.
107. Muramatsu, M., and Fujisawa, T. (1968). *Biochim. Biophys. Acta* **157**, 476–492.
108. Nakamura, T., Prestayko, A. W., and Busch, H. (1968). *J. Biol. Chem.* **243**, 1368–1375.
109. Narayan, K. S., Smetana, K., Steele, W. J., and Busch, H. (1966). *Proc. Amer. Ass. Cancer Res.* **7**, 52.
110. Nau, F., Garbit, F., and Dubert, J-M. (1972). *Biochim. Biophys. Acta* **277**, 80–86.
111. Obara, T., Bolognesi, D. P., and Bauer, H. (1971). *Int. J. Cancer* **7**, 535–546.
112. Oda, K., Kimura, F., Harada, F., and Nishimura, S. (1969). *Biochim. Biophys. Acta* **179**, 97–105.
113. Ohe, K., and Weissman, S. M. (1970). *Science* **167**, 879–881.
114. Ohe, K., and Weissman, S. M. (1971). *J. Biol. Chem.* **246**, 6991–7009.

115. Peacock, A. C., and Dingman, C. W. (1967). *Biochemistry* 6, 1818–1827.
116. Pene, J. J., Knight, E., and Darnell, J. E. (1968). *J. Mol. Biol.* 33, 609–623.
117. Penman, S., Smith, I., and Holtzman, E. (1966). *Science* 154, 786–789.
118. Perry, R. P., and Kelley, D. E. (1972). *J. Mol. Biol.* 70, 265–279.
119. Philippsen, P., Thiebe, R., Wintermeyer, W., and Zachau, H. G. (1968). *Biochem. Biophys. Res. Commun.* 33, 922–928.
119a. Pieczenik, G., Barrell, B. G., and Gefter, M. L. (1972). *Arch. Biochem. Biophys.* 152, 152.
120. Prestayko, A. W., and Busch, H. (1968). *Biochim. Biophys. Acta* 169, 327–337.
121. Prestayko, A. W., Tonato, M., and Busch, H. (1970). *J. Mol. Biol.* 47, 505–515.
122. Prestayko, A. W., Tonato, M., Lewis, B. C., and Busch, H. (1971). *J. Biol. Chem.* 246, 182–187.
123. Raacke, I. D. (1971). *Proc. Nat. Acad. Sci. U.S.* 68, 2357–2360.
124. Randerath, K. Personal communication.
125. Randerath, K. (1971). *Cancer Res.* 31, 658–661.
126. Randerath, K., and Randerath, E. (1971). *In* "Procedures in Nucleic Acid Research" (G. L. Cantoni and D. R. Davies, eds.), Vol. 2, p. 796. Harper, New York.
127. Randerath, E., Yu, C. T., and Randerath, K. (1971). *Anal. Biochem.* 48, 172–198.
128. Reddy, R., Ro-Choi, T. S., Henning, D., Shibata, H., Choi, Y. C., and Busch, H. (1972). *J. Biol. Chem.* 247, 7245–7250.
129. Rein, A. (1971). *Biochim. Biophys. Acta* 232, 306–313.
130. Rein, A., and Penman, S. (1969). *Biochim. Biophys. Acta* 190, 1–9.
131. Ritter, P. O., and Busch, H. (1971). *Physiol. Chem. Phys.* 3, 411–425.
132. Ro, T. S., and Busch, H. (1964). *Cancer Res.* 24, 1630–1633.
133. Ro-Choi, T. S., Choi, Y. C., Savage, H., and Busch, H. (1973). *In* "Methods in Cancer Research" (H. Busch, ed.), Vol. IX, pp. 71–153. Academic Press, New York.
134. Ro-Choi, T. S., Moriyama, Y., Choi, Y. C., and Busch, H. (1970). *J. Biol. Chem.* 245, 1970–1977.
135. Ro-Choi, T. S., Reddy, R., Henning, D., and Busch, H. (1971). *Biochem. Biophys. Res. Commun.* 44, 963–972.
136. Ro-Choi, T. S., Reddy, R., Henning, D., Takano, T., Taylor, C. W., and Busch, H. (1972). *J. Biol. Chem.* 247, 3205–3222.
137. Roeder, R. G., and Rutter, W. J. (1969). *Nature (London)* 224, 234–237.
138. Rosset, R., and Monier, R. (1963). *Biochim. Biophys. Acta* 68, 653–656.
139. Sanger, F. (1971). *Biochem. J.* 124, 833–843.
140. Saponara, A. G., and Enger, M. D. (1969). *Nature (London)* 223, 1365–1366.
141. Schleich, T., and Goldstein, J. (1966). *J. Mol. Biol.* 15, 136–146.
142. Schlimme, E., von der Haar, F., and Cramer, F. (1968). *Z. Naturforsch.* 24b, 631–637.
143. Schulman, L. H., and Chambers, R. W. (1968). *Proc. Nat. Acad. Sci. U.S.* 61, 308–315.
144. Semancik, J. S., and Weathers, L. G. (1972). *Nature New Biol.* 237, 242–244.
145. Seno, T., Kobayashi, M., and Nishimura, S. (1969). *Biochim. Biophys. Acta* 174, 408–411.
146. Seno, T., Kobayashi, M., and Nishimura, S. (1969). *Biochim. Biophys. Acta* 182, 280–283.
147. Seno, T., Kobayashi, M., and Nishimura, S. (1969). *Biochim. Biophys. Acta* 190, 285–303.
148. Seno, T., Kobayashi, I., Fukuhara, M., and Nishimura, S. (1971). *Fed. Eur. Biochem. Soc. Lett.* 7, 343–346.
148a. Shibata, H., Reddy, R., Ro-Choi, T. S., Henning, D., and Busch, H. *Mol. Cell. Biochem.* (In press).
149. Sitz, T., Spohn, W., and Busch, H. (1973). *Proc. Amer. Ass. Cancer Res.* 14, 55.
150. Smith, J. D., Barnett, L., Brenner, S., and Russell, R. L. (1970). *J. Mol. Biol.* 54, 1–14.
151. Smith, J. D., Anderson, K., Cashmore, A., Hooper, M. L., and Russell, R. C. (1970). *Cold Spring Harbor Symp. Quant. Biol.* XXXV, 21–27.
152. Strehler, B. L., Hendley, D. D., and Hirsch, G. P. (1967). *Proc. Nat. Acad. Sci. U.S.* 57, 1751–1758.
153. Sugino, A., Hirose, S., and Okazaki, R. (1972). *Proc. Nat. Acad. Sci. U.S.* 69, 1863–1867.

154. Thiebe, R., and Zachau, H. G. (1969). *Biochem. Biophys. Res. Commun.* **36,** 1024–1031.
155. Torelli, U. L., Torelli, G. M., Andreoli, A., and Mauri, C. (1970). *Nature (London)* **226,** 1163–1165.
156. Watson, J. D., and Ralph, R. K. (1967). *J. Mol. Biol.* **26,** 541–544.
157. Weinberg, R. A., and Penman, S. (1968). *J. Mol. Biol.* **38,** 289–304.
158. Weinberg, R. A., and Penman, S. (1969). *Biochim. Biophys. Acta* **190,** 10–29.
159. Weinstein, I. B. (1970). *In* "Genetic Concepts and Neoplasia." Williams and Wilkins, Baltimore, Maryland.
160. Weisblum, B., Cherayil, J. D., Bock, R. M., and Söll, D. (1967). *J. Mol. Biol.* **28,** 275–280.
161. Weisblum, B., Gonano, F., Von Ehrenstein, G., and Benzer, S. (1965). *Proc. Nat. Acad. Sci. U.S.* **53,** 328–334.
162. Weiss, J. F., and Kelmers, A. D. (1967). *Biochemistry* **6,** 2507–2513.
163. Wickner, W., Brutlag, D., Schekman, R., and Kornberg, A. (1972). *Proc. Nat. Acad. Sci. U.S.* **69,** 965–969.
164. Williamson, R., and Brownlee, G. G. (1969). *FEBS Lett.* **3,** 306–308.
165. Yang, S. S., and Comb, D. G. (1968). *J. Mol. Biol.* **31,** 138–142.
166. Zachau, H. G. (1967). *FEBS Symp. 4th,* p. 169–174.
167. Zapisek, W. F., Saponara, A. G., and Enger, M. D. (1969). *Biochemistry* **8,** 1170–1181.

CHAPTER VII

Nucleotides: Biosynthesis, Inhibition of Synthesis, and Development of Resistance to Inhibitors

EDWARD BRESNICK

I. Introduction*

The development of chemotherapeutic approaches to the treatment of cancer is fraught with difficulties. It is generally based upon two tactics: (a) a blockade of a process or pathway which appears unique to the particular neoplasm, i.e., selective toxicity, and (b) an inhibition of the growth of the neoplastic tissue by taking advantage of the relative difference in its proliferation, i.e., differential toxicity. The former approach has not been successfully utilized to date primarily because of the paucity of information on the biochemistry of the cancer cell. The latter technique, since it involves growth, generally is aimed at blockade of either nucleic acid or protein synthesis.

Fortunately, many types of neoplasms possess elevated levels of enzymes which operate in the nucleic acid pathway and consequently, the armamentarium of the oncologist includes a large number of antimetabolites which affect the latter, i.e., purine and pyrimidine analogs. However, since nucleic acid synthesis is also required for growth and division of normal cells, antimetabolite therapy often leads to toxicity (103).

At present, the use of antimetabolites results in significant prolongation of life of cancer patients and in some select cases, in cures. The mechanism of action of many of these agents is interwoven with nucleotide biosynthesis. Unfortunately, even effective cancer chemotherapy is more often than not accompanied by the development of resistance to the antimetabolite and this chapter presents some of the mechanisms by which the neoplastic cells develop resistance to the purine and pyrimidine antimetabolites.

II. Pyrimidine Biosynthesis

A. De Novo Pathway

Our knowledge of the synthesis of the pyrimidine moiety comes largely from investigations (85) with both bacterial and mammalian systems. The precursors

* Abbreviations: The following abbreviations are employed in this chapter: CP, carbamyl phosphate; AG, N-acetylglutamate; DON, 6-diazo-5-oxo-L-norleucine; ATC'ase, aspartate transcarbamylase; UMP, UDP, and UTP, 5'-mono, di-, and triphosphates of uridine; CDP, CTP, 5'-di- and triphosphates of cytidine; ADP, ATP, 5'-di- and triphosphates of adenosine; OMP, orotidine-5'-monophosphate; UDP-G.A., UDP-glucuronic acid; UDPG, UDP-glucose; NADP, nicotinamide-adenine dinucleotide; NADPH, reduced nicotinamide-adenine dinucleotide phosphate; XDP, dXDP, 5'-diphosphates of purine or pyrimidine ribonucleosides and deoxyribonucleosides, respectively; dAMP, dADP, dATP, 5'-mono-, di-, triphosphates of deoxyadenosine; dGMP, dGTP, 5'-mono-, triphosphates of deoxyguanosine; dUMP, dUTP, 5'-mono-, triphosphates of deoxyuridine; dTMP, dTTP, 5'-mono-, triphosphates of deoxythymidine; araC, 1β-D-arabinosylcytosine; $N^{5,10}$-CH$_2$-THFA, $N^{5,10}$-methylenetetrahydrofolic acid; FUdR, 5-fluoro-2'-deoxyuridine; TdR, deoxythymidine; UdR, deoxyuridine; CdR, deoxycytidine; BUdR, IUdR, CF$_3$UdR, 5'-bromo-, iodo-, or trifluoromethyl deoxyuridine; IdUTP, 5'-iodo-deoxyuridine triphosphate; PRPP, phosphoribosyl pyrophosphate; PRA, phosphoribosylamine; THFA, tetrahydrofolate; HX, hypoxanthine; X, xanthine; G, guanine; 6MP, 6 mercaptopurine.

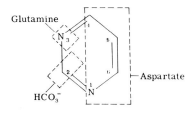

Fig. 7.1. Precursors for pyrimidine moiety.

for the atoms which constitute the pyrimidine structure are summarized in Fig. 7.1. In eukaryotes, nitrogens 1 and 3 stem from aspartic acid and the amide of glutamine, respectively. The details of these reactions are discussed later in this chapter. Carbon 2 originates from bicarbonate (or carbon dioxide) and carbons 4, 5, and 6 derive from aspartic acid. Orotic acid, a pyrimidine occurring naturally in milk, is the first pyrimidine moiety synthesized in the *de novo* pathway (85, Fig. 7.2.)

1. CARBAMYLPHOSPHATE (CP) SYNTHETASE

In mammalian systems, 2 enzymes are responsible for the synthesis of carbamyl phosphate: (a) an NH_3-requiring enzyme, dependent upon N-acetylglutamate (AG) as cofactor, present mostly in liver, and localized mainly in mitochondria (69). The reaction catalyzed by this liver enzyme is shown in Eq. (7.1).

$$NH_3 + CO_2 + ATP \xrightarrow{AG} CP + 2\,ADP + PO_4^{3-} \tag{7.1}$$

(b) The second is a glutamine-dependent enzyme, found more frequently in mitotically active tissues and present in the cytosol, i.e., particulate-free supernatant fraction (48). The reaction catalyzed by this enzyme is shown in Eq. (7.2).

$$Glutamine + CO_2 + 2\,ATP \rightarrow CP + Glutamate + 2\,ADP + PO_4^{3-} \tag{7.2}$$

For a number of years, the NH_3-requiring enzyme was the only one known which was capable of catalyzing CP formation. Most of pyrimidine biosynthesis was assumed to occur in the cytosol yet enzyme activity was only demonstrable

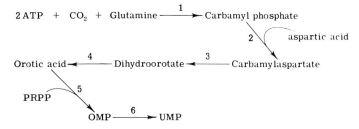

Fig. 7.2. *De novo* synthesis of pyrimidines. (1) Carbamylphosphate synthetase; (2) aspartate transcarbamylase; (3) dihydroorotase; (4) dihydroorotic acid dehydrogenase; (5) orotidine monophosphate (OMP) pyrophosphorylase; and (6) OMP decarboxylase.

in the mitochondria. The biosynthesis of pyrimidines should be extremely active in rapidly proliferating tissues, yet the activity of the NH_3-requiring enzyme was not readily demonstrable in tissues other than liver. Although NH_3 should supply nitrogen 3 of the pyrimidine moiety, ^{15}N studies indicated the amide nitrogen of glutamine to be an efficient precursor of uracil (90). Finally, although uracil biosynthesis *de novo* was inhibited by the glutamine antagonists, azaserine (*O*-diazoacetyl-L-serine) and 6-diazo-5-oxo-L-norleucine (DON), no step in the then accepted pathway appeared to require glutamine.

This apparent dilemma was settled by the findings of a number of investigators (49, 68) who succeeded in demonstrating that pyrimidine formation required the action of a labile glutamine-dependent enzyme. Thus, the blockade of pyrimidine biosynthesis by glutamine antagonists noted earlier was explainable by an inhibition at the first stage in the *de novo* pathway.

The NH_3-requiring mitochondrial enzyme is probably involved exclusively in the formation of arginine via the urea cycle. Thus, two highly compartmentalized systems exist in nature which are required for the synthesis of 2 different but important molecules, arginine and uracil, from a common intermediate, carbamyl phosphate, for the elaboration of the macromolecules, protein and nucleic acid, respectively. Apparently, pyrimidine biosynthesis is regulated at least in part at the carbamylphosphate synthetase step (98). Pyrimidine nucleotides, particularly UMP, are potent inhibitors of the activity of the glutamine-dependent enzyme. On the other hand, these nucleotides exhibit no such inhibitory effect on the other enzyme responsible for carbamyl phosphate formation.

2. Aspartate Transcarbamylase (ATC'ase)

ATC'ase catalyzes the carbamylation of the amine group of aspartic acid with carbamyl phosphate as the donor to yield carbamylaspartate [see Fig. 7.2 and Eq. (7.3)].

$$NH_2\text{—}\overset{\overset{\text{O}}{\|}}{C}\text{—O—PO}_3H_2 + H_2N\text{—}\overset{\overset{\text{COOH}}{|}}{\underset{\underset{\text{COOH}}{|}}{\underset{CH_2}{|}}}{C}\text{—H} \rightarrow NH_2\text{—}\overset{\overset{\text{O}}{\|}}{C}\text{—NH—}\overset{\overset{\text{COOH}}{|}}{\underset{\underset{\text{COOH}}{|}}{\underset{CH_2}{|}}}{CH} + P_i \qquad (7.3)$$

The regulatory subunit serves as the attachment site for the allosteric inhibitor, CTP, and activator, ATP, while the substrates bind to the catalytic subunit.

Attempts to demonstrate a similar regulatory mechanism at the activity level with mammalian systems have not been successful (11). Control at this step is exerted at the level of synthesis, i.e., enzyme concentration increases in response to increased cellular activity.

3. Other Enzymes in the *de novo* Pathway

Dihydroorotase catalyzes the intramolecular cyclization of carbamylaspartate to form dihydroorotate (Fig. 7.2). Although little is known of its action in mammalian systems, it is inhibited by a number of preformed pyrimidines and consequently, may serve as a locus of control in these higher organisms.

The sequence of reactions leading to the formation of UMP from orotic acid, catalyzed by OMP pyrophosphorylase and OMP decarboxylase, is also subject to modulation, as determined by the state of proliferation of a tissue (9); it is end product inhibited by UDP (4).

B. Salvage Pathway for UMP Formation

Most eukaryotic organisms possess salvage mechanisms for the reutilization of pyrimidines and their nucleosides that arise from the catabolism of nucleic acids or of nucleoside di- and triphosphates. These salvage pathways are indicated in Fig. 7.3. Uracil is ultimately converted into its nucleotide via the intermediate, uridine. The latter sequence is of particular importance because (a) uridine kinase activity is a positive indicator of the degree of proliferation of a tissue, (b) uridine kinase is inhibited by its end product, UTP, and in an analogous manner, CTP can inhibit cytidine kinase, (c) the pathway serves as the mechanism for activation of many pyrimidine analogs to their inhibitory forms, i.e., lethal synthesis, and (d) resistance to the pyrimidine analogs is often effected by an alteration of this pathway.

C. Anabolism of Nucleoside Monophosphates

Prior to utilization by the organism, UMP must be phosphorylated to di- and triphosphates and a fraction of the latter is aminated to CTP. These reactions are indicated in Eq. (7.4) and (7.5).

$$\text{UMP} \xrightarrow{\text{ATP}} \text{UDP} \xrightarrow{\text{ATP}} \text{UTP} \tag{7.4}$$

$$\text{UTP} + \text{glutamine} + \text{ATP} + H_2O \rightarrow \text{CTP} + \text{glutamate} + P_i + \text{ADP} \tag{7.5}$$

The phosphorylation reactions are accomplished by a kinase which is present in most mammalian tissues in excess of its need thus ensuring that most of the UMP formed will be elevated to the higher nucleotide levels.

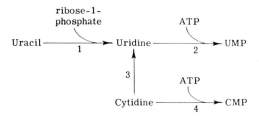

Fig. 7.3. Salvage mechanism for UMP formation. (1) Uridine phosphorylase; (2) uridine kinase; (3) cytidine deaminase; and (4) cytidine kinase.

The formation of CTP is effected by a glutamine-requiring enzyme, CTP synthetase, and consequently is azaserine and DON sensitive (59). CTP synthetase is also under allosteric control with GTP serving as a positive effector. CTP may also be formed from the monophosphate by a series of phosphorylations involving kinases.

Pyrimidine nucleoside triphosphates may be utilized in the synthesis of vital cofactors which are employed in biotransformation, i.e., preparation of metabolites or drugs for transport or excretion from the host, and in the formation of glycoproteins. The cofactors, UDP-glucuronic acid (UDP G.A.) and UDP glucose (UDPG), which can transfer glucuronic acid and glucose, respectively, to appropriate acceptors, are produced according to Eq. (7.6) and (7.7):

$$\text{UTP} + \text{glucose-1-phosphate} \xrightarrow{\text{UDPG pyrophosphorylase}} \text{UDPG} + \text{pyrophosphate} \quad (7.6)$$

$$\text{UDPG} + \text{NADP} \rightarrow \text{UDP-G.A.} + \text{NADPH} \quad (7.7)$$

These nucleoside diphosphate sugars react in the following manner (Eq. 7.8):

$$\begin{matrix} \text{UDPG} \\ \text{or} \\ \text{UDP-G.A.} \end{matrix} + \text{acceptor} \rightarrow \begin{matrix} \text{acceptor-glucoside} \\ \text{or} \\ \text{acceptor-glucuronide} \end{matrix} + \text{UDP} \quad (7.8)$$

D. Inhibitors of de Novo Synthesis of Pyrimidines

Antimetabolites which affect the *de novo* pathway for pyrimidine synthesis are generally of little value clinically because of their very low efficacy, although in their favor they exhibit little toxicity. The most widely known in this category belongs to the class of azapyrimidines with 6-azauracil or its nucleoside as representative members (Fig. 7.4). 6-Azauracil is formed by substitution of the carbon in the 6 position by a nitrogen atom (51, 94, 97). The azapyrimidine is anabolized by the identical pathway as is uracil to produce 6-azauridine-5'-monophosphate (6-aza-UMP). These reactions are shown in Fig. 7.5.

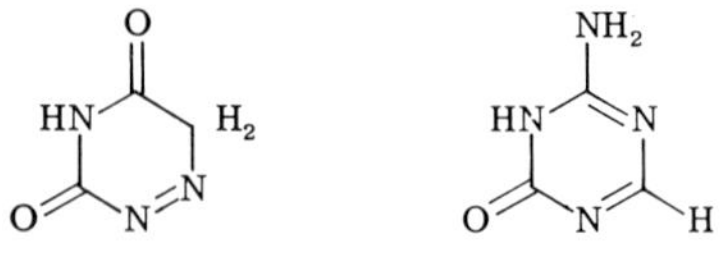

Fig. 7.4. Azapyrimidines. (A) 6-azauracil; (B) 5-azacytosine.

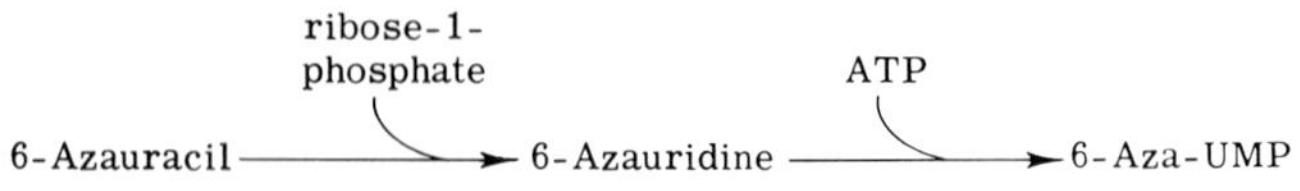

Fig. 7.5. Anabolism of 6-azauracil.

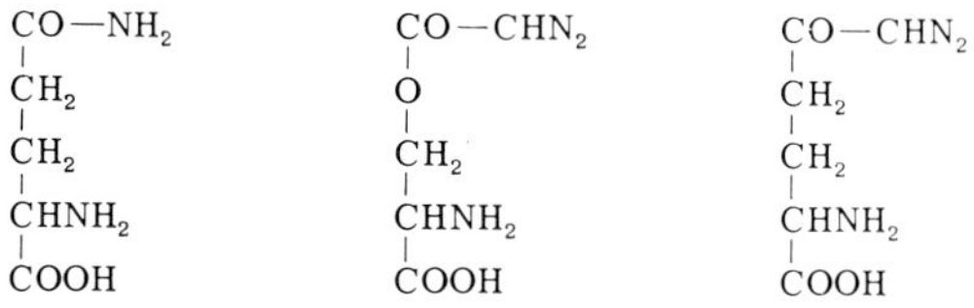

$$
\begin{array}{ccc}
\text{CO}-\text{NH}_2 & \text{CO}-\text{CHN}_2 & \text{CO}-\text{CHN}_2 \\
| & | & | \\
\text{CH}_2 & \text{O} & \text{CH}_2 \\
| & | & | \\
\text{CH}_2 & \text{CH}_2 & \text{CH}_2 \\
| & | & | \\
\text{CHNH}_2 & \text{CHNH}_2 & \text{CHNH}_2 \\
| & | & | \\
\text{COOH} & \text{COOH} & \text{COOH} \\
\\
A & B & C
\end{array}
$$

Fig. 7.6. Glutamine, azaserine, and DON. (A) Glutamine; (B) azaserine; and (C) DON.

The formation of 6-aza-UMP is absolutely required for chemotherapeutic efficacy with the site of action being OMP decarboxylase (51). Thus in inhibited systems, there is an increase in the amounts of orotic acid, orotidine, and other precursors. Considerable attention has recently been devoted to exploiting the use of the ribonucleoside, 6-azauridine, in the treatment of psoriasis.

Resistance to these derivatives develops rapidly by the loss of uridine kinase activity, the latter enzyme being required for the formation of the nucleotide, the "true" inhibitor (51).

5-Azacytidine has also been reported to possess tumor-inhibitory properties (96). This analog, which must also be anabolized to the nucleotide, blocks the *de novo* synthesis at the OMP decarboxylase step but in addition is incorporated into RNA and DNA, which could lead to genetic damage to the cell. The analog must be converted to di- and triphosphorylated derivatives and these reactions do not readily occur with 6-azauracil. Resistance to 5-azacytidine also occurs with a loss in kinase activity.

Azaserine and DON, antibiotics originally isolated from culture filtrates of streptomyces, are potent inhibitors of tumors in laboratory animals (see review 51). However, these agents appear too toxic for general usage in cancer patients. The antibiotics are glutamine antagonists (Fig. 7.6) which primarily affect purine biosynthesis. Since glutamine is needed for carbamyl phosphate and CTP synthesis, the analogs also decrease pyrimidine formation *de novo;* the exact role of this blockade in the mechanism of action of these glutamine antagonists has not been clarified.

E. Enzyme Levels in Neoplastic Tissues

Many of the enzymes involved in the *de novo* synthesis of pyrimidines are markedly elevated in neoplastic tissues. In this regard, ATC'ase activity was increased in a series of Morris rat hepatomas (6), in a series of mouse hepatomas (17), in kidney adenocarcinomas (15), and in human gastrointestinal tumors (95). Furthermore, the increase in many of the neoplasms was directly related to the rapidity of tumor growth.

The formation of UMP from orotic acid, via OMP pyrophosphorylase and decarboxylase, is also elevated in rapidly proliferating systems (9). Uridine kinase is another enzyme whose activity can serve as a marker for the relative degree of proliferation of the cell (for example, see 15).

F. Synthesis of Pyrimidine Deoxyribonucleotides

As early as 1953, it was suggested (87) that deoxyribonucleotides arose through the reduction of the corresponding ribonucleotides. However, the prevailing opinion favored deoxyribose-5-phosphate aldolase (84), which catalyzes the reversible reaction shown in Eq. (7.9) as the means for formation of the deoxyribonucleotides [Eq. (7.10)].

$$\text{Acetaldehyde} + \text{glyceraldehyde-3-phosphate} \rightleftarrows \text{deoxyribose-5-phosphate} \qquad (7.9)$$

$$\text{Deoxyribose-5-phosphate} \xrightleftharpoons{\text{mutase}} \text{deoxyribose-1-phosphate} \qquad (7.10)$$

$$\text{Base} + \text{deoxyribose-1-phosphate} \xrightarrow{\text{phosphorylase}} \text{deoxyribonucleoside} + \text{P}_i$$

$$\text{Deoxyribonucleoside} + \text{ATP} \xrightarrow{\text{kinase}} \text{deoxyribonucleotide} + \text{ADP}$$

The deoxyribose-5-phosphate generated from carbohydrate precursors undergoes a conversion to the 1-phosphate, which in the presence of the base and pyrimidine deoxyribonucleoside phosphorylase forms the deoxyribonucleoside. The latter may be phosphorylated in the presence of a kinase and ATP to yield the deoxyribonucleotide.

In support of this mechanism, diphenylsuccinate, a "selective" inhibitor of the aldolase enzyme, blocked deoxyribonucleotide formation in regenerating liver (47). However, in studies with double isotopes it was concluded (65) that deoxyribonucleotides could only arise by the direct reduction of the corresponding ribonucleotides. Subsequent investigations (100) clarified this controversy by showing that diphenylsuccinate was not a selective inhibitor; it inhibited the reductive pathway as well. At present, the mechanism originally proposed by Rose and Schweigert (87) is accepted. The aldolase pathway, in contrast, would predominantly function in mammalian cells in the catabolism of the deoxy sugar.

RIBONUCLEOTIDE REDUCTASE

Our knowledge of the pathway by which ribonucleotides are reduced to deoxyribonucleotides without rupture of the glycosidic bond originates from the outstanding work of Reichard and his colleagues in Sweden using bacterial model systems (66). It was found that 4 proteins, divalent cations, ribonucleoside diphosphates, H⁺, and NADPH are required for fruition of the reductive process [Eq. (7.11) and (7.12)].

$$\text{XDP} + \text{thioredoxin (SH)}_2 \xrightarrow[\text{Mg}^{2+}]{\text{proteins B}_1 + \text{B}_2} \text{dXDP} + \text{thioredoxin} \underset{S}{\overset{S}{\diagdown|}} + \text{H}_2\text{O} \qquad (7.11)$$

$$\text{Thioredoxin} \underset{S}{\overset{S}{\diagdown|}} + \text{NADPH} + \text{H}^+ \xrightarrow[\text{reductase}]{\text{thioredoxin}} \text{thioredoxin (SH)}_2 + \text{NADP}^+ \qquad (7.12)$$

The complex sequence involves, first of all, the interaction of a sulfhydryl-containing protein, thioredoxin, and 2 other proteins, B_1 and B_2, with the pyrimidine ribonucleotide. The B_2 protein represents the catalytic subunit to which the ribonucleotide binds while the B_1 protein is the regulatory subunit. Unlike ATC'ase (Section II, A,2), no activity is demonstrable unless B_2 is bound to B_1. The end result of these interactions is the reduction of the nucleoside diphosphate, XDP, and the oxidation of thioredoxin. Reduced thioredoxin is regenerated by means of NADPH and the enzyme, thioredoxin reductase. Of particular interest with regard to this system is that a single enzyme is capable of reducing deoxyribonucleotides of all 4 bases.

Subsequent investigations (73) established a similar mechanism for the reductive process in mammalian tissues and, in particular, in the Novikoff hepatoma. In addition, the reductase is allosterically influenced by both negative and positive effectors. It was found that: (a) the reduction of CDP and UDP requires ATP as activator; the reduction of ADP requires dGTP as the activator; and the reduction of GDP requires dTTP as the activator while ATP stimulates the reaction further; (b) the reduction of UDP and CDP is inhibited by dATP, dGTP, and dTTP; the reduction of GDP is inhibited by dATP and dGTP; and the reduction of ADP is inhibited by dATP; and (c) the regulatory control of deoxyribonucleotide formation is similar in tumor and in rat embryonic tissue (73, 76).

The end result of this complex regulatory mechanism is a cascade effect in which dTTP activates dGDP formation for subsequent dGTP production; the latter then activates dADP synthesis required for dATP formation. If dATP cannot be used for DNA synthesis, the reduction of all the ribonucleotides is blocked.

A number of investigators have compared the activity of ribonucleotide reductase in normal and neoplastic tissues. A marked increase in enzyme activity was found in the spleens of mice infected with a murine leukemia virus as compared to normal spleen (42). No significant differences were observed in the relative inhibitory or activating effects of deoxyribonucleotides on the enzyme from either the normal or tumor-bearing host. Infection of kidney cells with an oncogenic polyoma virus also produced significant elevation in enzyme activity (60).

The relationship between enzyme activity and the rate of tumor growth was investigated in a series of rat hepatomas and compared to normal and host liver (31). Within the sensitivity of the assay, no enzyme activity was observed in liver while only marginal activity was noted in tumors with growth rates in excess of 3 months. The highest enzyme activity was found in fetal rat liver. In the series of hepatomas, a closer correlation of enzyme activity with growth rate was found than with a number of other enzymes involved in DNA synthesis.

INHIBITORS OF TUMOR GROWTH AND OF RIBONUCLEOTIDE REDUCTASE. Many studies have shown that hydroxyurea (Fig. 7.7A) and certain other hydroxamates can block DNA synthesis in mammalian cells in culture and in other rapidly proliferating systems (93, 106) in addition to causing profound inhibition of

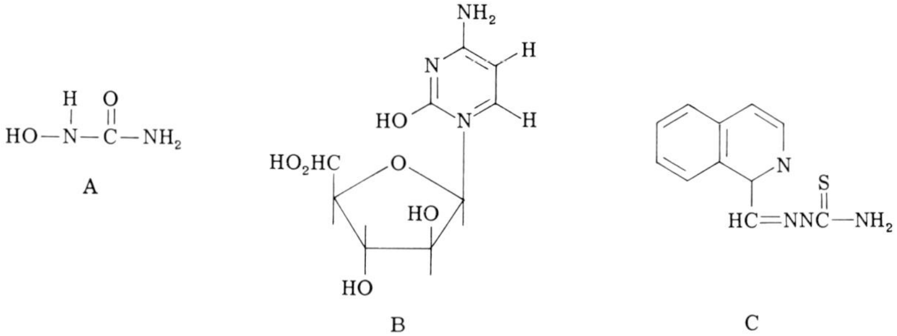

Fig. 7.7. Inhibitors of ribonucleotide reductase. (A) Hydroxyurea; (B) arabinosylcytosine; and (C) 1-formyl isoquinoline thiosemicarbazone.

tumor growth. The site of action of hydroxyurea is ribonucleotide reductase (37). Apparently, the antitumor agent interacts in some fashion with a nonheme iron of protein B_2 of the enzyme complex (62).

D-Arabinose analogs of some nucleotides, e.g., β-1-D-arabinosylcytosine (araC) (Fig. 7.7B), have demonstrated significant antitumor and antiviral activities (26, 83). In both bacterial and mammalian cells, the analog profoundly inhibits DNA synthesis after activation by lethal synthesis to the arabinosyl nucleotide (see Section II,G,4,b). Several investigators have suggested the action of this inhibitor is localized to ribonucleotide reductase and in particular is limited to the reduction of CDP to dCDP. Later studies have taken issue with this proposal (see 26) and instead have implicated the polymerization of deoxyribonucleoside triphosphates to DNA, i.e., DNA polymerase, as the major site of action of this analog. The *coup de grace* to the former theory came with the finding (74) that di- and triphosphates of araC inhibit the reduction of all 4 ribonucleoside diphosphates at high concentrations and only weakly and, consequently, this action could not play any role in the inhibition of DNA synthesis observed *in vivo*.

A number of α-(N)-heterocyclic carboxaldehyde thiosemicarbazones have been shown to be potent inhibitors of the growth of a variety of experimental neoplasms (91); the most potent in this series was 1-formyl isoquinoline thiosemicarbazone (Fig. 7.7C). Initial reports had implicated some step in DNA synthesis as the locus of action of this inhibitor. Subsequent work (75) more precisely established the inhibition to occur at ribonucleotide reductase. The heterocycle apparently binds to an iron-charged enzyme or the iron-chelate of the inhibitor may interact with the enzyme at a site occupied by reduced thioredoxin (or similar protein).

G. Deoxyribonucleotide Interconversions

The scheme depicting the formation of the deoxyribonucleotides and their interconversions is shown in Fig. 7.8. Following the reduction of UDP to dUDP, the latter is phosphorylated to dUTP or dephosphorylated to dUMP. With the

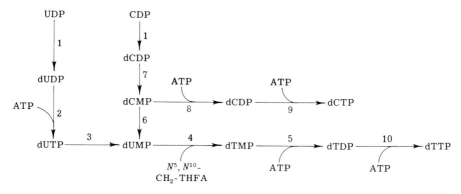

Fig. 7.8. Deoxyribonucleotide formation and interconversions. (1) Ribonucleotide reductase; (2) dUDP kinase; (3) dUTP pyrophosphatase; (4) dTMP synthetase; (5) dTMP kinase; (6) dCMP deaminase, (7) phosphatase; (8) dCMP kinase; (9) dCDP kinase; and (10) dTDP kinase.

observation that purified *E. coli* DNA polymerase can incorporate dUTP into DNA (3), it was difficult to explain the absence of the latter from the polydeoxyribonucleotide *in vivo*. However, with the finding that most mammalian cells contain a powerful dUTP pyrophosphatase (enzyme 3 of Fig. 7.8) which hydrolyzes dUTP to pyrophosphate and dUMP, the mechanism which excludes deoxyuridine from DNA consisted of lowering the concentration of dUTP far below that of dTTP by this enzyme.*

1. INHIBITORS OF dTMP SYNTHETASE

dTMP synthetase is an extemely important enzyme since it catalyzes a unique reaction leading to the synthesis of a deoxyribonucleotide which is required for the formation of DNA. Consequently, blockade of its activity is accompanied by profound effects upon the tissue or organism. Toward this end a number of substances have been designed which inhibit dTMP synthetase and which are therapeutically active. These analogs generally owe their differential toxicity in neoplastic tissues to the presence of higher concentrations of dTMP synthetase in rapidly proliferating systems. However, their use is often accompanied by profound toxicity to the gastrointestinal tract, hematopoietic tissues, and buccal mucosa, since rapid cell division occurs in the latter tissues as well.

FLUORINATED PYRIMIDINES. The development of pyrimidine analogs was initially based upon the observation (89) that uracil was utilized to a much greater extent for nucleic acid synthesis in a chemically induced rat hepatoma than in normal liver. This phenomenon was soon shown to reflect differences in the catabolism of pyrimidines by various tissues and in the level of enzymes which govern anabolism in neoplastic tissue. Subsequently, the synthesis of 5-fluoroura-

---

* dUMP undergoes a very interesting reaction involving an activated derivative of folic acid, $N^{5,10}$-methylenetetrahydrofolic acid ($N^{5,10}$-CH$_2$-THFA), and an enzyme (38), dTMP synthetase (enzyme 4 of Fig. 7.8). The activated folate derivatives are considered later in this chapter.

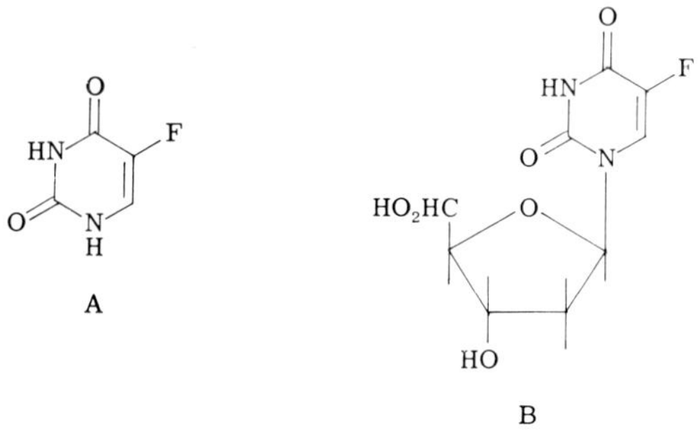

Fig. 7.9. Fluorinated pyrimidines. (A) 5-fluorouracil; (B) FUdR, (5-fluoro-2′-deoxyuridine).

cil was announced in 1957 (30). Its synthesis was based upon similarity in the relative van der Waals radii of the fluorine and hydrogen atoms, i.e., approximately 1.3 Å. It was soon found that the fluorinated analog exhibited profound antitumor activity and that 5-fluoro-2′-deoxyuridine (FUdR) (Fig. 7.9) was less toxic and more effective than the parent 5-fluorouracil (55). Subsequent studies have also demonstrated that FUdR is a potent inhibitor of DNA virus replication, e.g., vaccinia virus or herpesviruses (see 83).

In studies on its mechanism of action, FUdR inhibited the incorporation of most precursors into DNA after suitable activation to the monophosphate (5a). The latter presumably is formed via the action of deoxythymidine (TdR) kinase (10) as discussed below. 5-Fluoro-dUMP is a powerful inhibitor of dTMP synthetase (56); the inhibitor combines irreversibly and very tightly to the enzyme because of the structural resemblance to the natural substrate, dUMP (86). In this regard, the inhibition can more aptly be classified as of the pseudo-irreversible type. The size of the atom at the 5 position of the pyrimidine ring is critical in determining the efficacy of the resultant analog as an inhibitor of dTMP synthetase. For example, a pyrimidine substituted at this position with a larger halogen, Cl, Br, or I, has little action at this step, but is more of a structural analog of deoxythymidine (TdR) rather than deoxyuridine (UdR). The TdR analogs are considered in Section II,G,4,a.

dTMP synthetase is inhibited strongly by another group of antimetabolites, the antifols, e.g., amethopterin and aminopterin (39). These substances prevent the cyclic regeneration of tetrahydrofolic acid. A more detailed discussion of this group follows in Section II,G,3.

2. dCMP DEAMINASE

As noted earlier, the formation of the vitally important precursor for DNA synthesis, dTMP, requires the availability of sufficient amounts of dUMP. The latter may be generated ultimately from dUDP or through the action of dCMP deaminase [Eq. (7.13)].

$$\text{dCMP} \xrightarrow{\text{H}_2\text{O}} \text{dUMP} + \text{NH}_3 \tag{7.13}$$

This enzyme is specific for the deamination of dCMP, its 5-methyl, 5-hydroxy-methyl, and 5-halogeno compounds to the corresponding dUMP derivatives. There has been considerable work on the purification and properties of the enzyme (5). The enzyme is of particular interest since it is present in rate-limiting amounts in mammalian tissues and is subject to a complex pattern of allosteric activations and inhibitions in accordance with its key role in DNA synthesis.

dCMP deaminase is apparently composed of 4 subunits each of which has a catalytic site and one or more regulatory sites capable of complexing with effectors. dTTP is a potent and specific inhibitor and its interaction with the enzyme is accompanied by a conformational change leading to an alteration in sedimentation characteristics of the enzyme. The addition of the activator, dCTP, is accompanied by aggregation of the enzyme. Thus, a very delicate balance between activity and inactivity exists which is dependent on the intracellular concentrations of dTTP and dCTP.

3. NUCLEOTIDE KINASES

Little or no dTMP kinase activity is observed in nonproliferating tissues, e.g., liver, while in neoplastic, regenerating, or embryonic livers, dTMP is extensively phosphorylated (79). dTDP kinase, on the other hand, is present in normal and neoplastic tissues in exceedingly high levels suggesting that the phosphorylation of dTMP to dTDP is the rate-limiting step in supplying sufficient dTTP for DNA synthesis.

The enzymic phosphorylation of dCMP has been examined in normal rat liver and in hepatoma cells (79). dCMP kinase is very stable in normal liver and unstable in the tumor cells. In contrast to dTMP kinase, the level of enzyme activity appeared higher in control liver than in hepatoma. The presence of activators in the control tissue, i.e., thiols, was responsible for this apparent anomaly.

4. SALVAGE PATHWAY FOR DEOXYRIBONUCLEOTIDE FORMATION

In addition to the *de novo* pathway for synthesis, deoxyribonucleotides may be formed from preformed pyrimidines. The "salvage" enzymes involved are TdR kinase, deoxycytidine (CdR) kinase, and pyrimidine deoxyribosyltransferase. The enzymes catalyze the reactions in Eq. (7.14–16).

$$\text{TdR} + \text{ATP} \xrightarrow[\text{kinase}]{\text{TdR}} \text{dTMP} + \text{ADP} \qquad (7.14)$$

$$\text{CdR} + \text{ATP} \xrightarrow[\text{kinase}]{\text{CdR}} \text{dCMP} + \text{ADP} \qquad (7.15)$$

$$\text{TdR} + \text{Uracil} \underset{\text{transferase}}{\overset{\text{dR}}{\rightleftarrows}} \text{UdR} + \text{T} \qquad (7.16)$$

$$\text{T} + \text{Deoxyribose-1-phosphate} \longrightarrow \text{TdR} + \text{P}_i$$

a. TdR KINASE. The enzyme catalyzes the phosphorylation of TdR by ATP to yield dTMP and ADP [Eq. (7.14)]. The reaction is relatively specific for TdR, UdR, and some of the TdR analogs (10). The enzyme has proved an enigma to biochemists since no definitive information is available as to its role within the cell. In all probability, however, the enzyme functions to offset the balance between degradation of dTMP by phosphatases and the anabolism of deoxyribonucleotides. Rapidly proliferating systems, e.g., neoplastic cells, require large amounts of dTMP ultimately destined for DNA synthesis and cell division and hence, cannot "afford" to catabolize any of this deoxyribonucleotide. However, in the event of the occurrence of this degradation, the high intracellular concentration of TdR kinase would catalyze reformation of dTMP.

TdR kinase was initially purified from *E. coli* (81) and found to be allosterically influenced by the phosphorylating agent, ATP, and by dCDP, the latter serving as an activator. Furthermore, dTTP, the end product of TdR anabolism, proved a potent feedback inhibitor of the bacterial enzyme, acting as a simple competitive inhibitor with respect to TdR.

TdR kinase has also been partially purified from animal tumors (10). The enzyme also exhibited allosteric properties with regard to ATP and dTTP although no activation was apparent upon addition of dCDP. The inhibition by dTTP was markedly affected by the concentration of ATP; in the presence of low ATP, profound inhibition by dTTP was manifested. The end product inhibitory requirements were investigated in series of rat and mouse hepatomas as well as in embryonic liver; no significant difference was noted in the efficacy of dTTP in this regard (8).

TdR kinase is not only regulated by end product inhibition, but its actual intracellular level is modulated as well according to the cell division requirements. For example, TdR kinase is barely detectable in adult liver but is markedly elevated in neoplastic, embryonic, and regenerating livers (16). After partial hepatectomy the increase was prevented by inhibitors of protein or RNA synthesis and was not the result of any change in the rate of degradation of enzyme protein (13).

i. Inhibition by Halogenated Pyrimidines. A number of substances can serve as substrates for TdR kinase including TdR analogs in which the 5 position is substituted by a constituent possessing a similar van der Waals radius as the methyl moiety, i.e., approximately 2.00 Å. Thus, the 5-Cl, 5-Br, 5-I, and 5-CF$_3$ derivatives of UdR have K_m values which are similar to that of the natural substrate, TdR (10, 12). In contrast, UdR and 5-FUdR with an H and F in the 5 position, respectively, are only 10% as efficacious a substrate as TdR.

Not only can the 5-Br, 5-I, 5-Cl, or 5-CF$_3$ derivatives serve as substrates, but these analogs are potent inhibitors of TdR kinase with TdR as substrate (10, 12). Furthermore, the halogenated analogs can substitute at each of the anabolic steps for TdR phosphorylation and block the formation of the respective thymine deoxyribonucleotide (Fig. 7.10). A sequential blockade is established with these analogs which results in potent inhibition of DNA synthesis.

When halogenated derivatives are incorporated into DNA in lieu of TdR, there are profound effects upon the structure of the macromolecule. The electronic configuration of the pyrimidine ring is altered by the inductive effect of the halogen resulting in a more acidic dissociation constant (reviewed in 83). At pH 7, only 0.16% of TdR is in the anionic form, but 8% of BUdR is in this form.

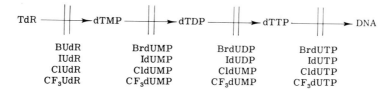

Fig. 7.10. Blockade of TdR anabolism by halogenated pyrimidines.

These changes may be in part responsible for the physical effects seen in substituted DNA molecules including (a) increased shearing of DNA during isolation, (b) increased melting temperature and buoyant density, (c) increased rate of mutation of organisms possessing substituted DNA, (d) inhibition of cell reproduction, and (e) increased sensitivity to both UV- and X-irradiation.

The halogenated derivatives exhibit another effect which may have biological import. The triphosphates, e.g., IdUTP, can act as pseudo-feedback inhibitors of TdR kinase and dCMP deaminase (83). The blockade of DNA synthesis, therefore, is compounded further by inhibition at the end product level.

The CF₃UdR analog has been shown (56) to inhibit dTMP synthetase after conversion to the deoxyribonucleotide, a reaction catalyzed by TdR kinase. The inhibition appears to be noncompetitive and possibly irreversible.

ii. Biological action of the halogenated pyrimidines. IUdR and BUdR exhibit potent antiviral activity, particularly against the DNA viruses (83). In the latter category, they have special utility in the treatment of infections caused by herpesviruses. CF₃UdR also is active against herpes simplex and apparently can effectively block the growth of the IUdR-resistant organism as well (61).

b. DEOXYCYTIDINE KINASE. CdR kinase, like TdR kinase, is found predominantly in rapidly proliferating tissues (46). The highest levels of the enzyme are noted in lymphatic organs and in tumors derived from them (28).

CdR kinase catalyzes the phosphorylation of CdR to yield dCMP. The enzyme is subject to allosteric modification with UDP, dCMP, dCDP, and dCTP serving as inhibitors and UTP, dUTP, and dTTP capable of reversing this inhibition (29).

i. Arabinosylcytosine and CdR kinase. AraC is phosphorylated by a lethal synthesis to its active form in the reaction catalyzed by CdR kinase (28, 70). Furthermore, the phosphorylation of araC can be blocked by cytosine deoxyribonucleotides thus explaining the reversal of toxicity of this analog in mammalian cells in culture (25).

AraC is rapidly deaminated to arabinosyluracil *in vivo* in the human (27) presumably through the action of cytosine nucleoside deaminase. The toxicity of the analog for a particular tissue is related in part to the level of this deaminase in that tissue and to the intracellular concentration of CdR kinase since araCMP is not a suitable substrate for the former. These facts explain the rather selective toxic action of araC on lymphatic tissues and their tumors since these have lower levels of deaminase.

In an analogous manner to the halogenated pyrimidines, araC after phosphorylation to araCTP, can pseudo-feedback inhibit its own phosphorylation by CdR kinase but apparently exerts little action on CdR phosphorylation (71). Therapy of experimental tumors with araC is accompanied by the development of resistance to the analog. The mechanism of resistance appears associated with the loss of the lethal synthesis mechanism, that is, in the ability of the resistant cells to phosphorylate (catalyzed by CdR kinase) araC as demonstrated in leukemic L1210 cells (92).

c. DEOXYRIBOSYL TRANSFER. The transfer of a deoxyribosyl moiety from pyrimidine deoxyribonucleosides [Eq. (7.16)] is catalyzed by TdR phosphorylase. The latter enzyme is also responsible for the reversible phosphorolysis of TdR [see Eq. (7.16)] (107). The transfer of the deoxyribosyl group was studied in detail with purified preparations from human leukocytes (43). The transfer reaction can be inhibited by various purines.

The relative activity of TdR phosphorylase (deoxyribosyltransferase) was investigated in control and leukemic leukocytes (44). Although the properties of the enzyme were similar in leukocytes from normals and from patients with chronic myelogenous leukemia, the activity was considerably lower in the latter. The lowered activity was not the result of an inhibitor but was due to a decreased number of enzyme molecules.

H. Catabolism of Pyrimidines

Within the liver, a delicate balance exists between the utilization of pyrimidine for nucleic acid synthesis and its catabolism for more usable materials. Preformed pyrimidines are largely degraded in adult liver tissue. The reactions by which this catabolism is accomplished (20) are depicted in Fig. 7.11. The initial step,

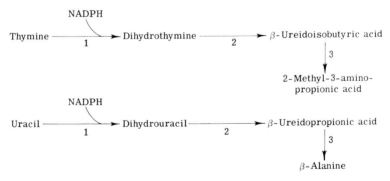

Fig. 7.11. Catabolism of pyrimidines. (1) Dihydrouracil (dihydrothymine) dehydrogenase; (2) dihydrouracil (dihydrothymine) hydrase; and (3) β-ureidopropionic (β-ureidoisobutyric) acid decarbamylase.

involving the reduction of either uracil or thymine, is the rate-limiting step in the catabolism of the pyrimidine. Although it was proposed (21) that a decrease in the uracil-degrading system represented an obligate part of any growth process in liver, more recent evidence (40) is not entirely in accord with this hypothesis.

The development of neoplasia is associated with a marked reduction and in many cases, a complete loss of the activity of these catabolic enzymes (17, 82). Furthermore, the administration of carcinogens, e.g., 2-acetylaminofluorene, was accompanied by a reduction in uracil catabolism in liver which was partially reversible upon cessation of carcinogen treatment (41).

Catabolism of a number of pyrimidine analogs, e.g., 5-halogenated pyrimidines and 6-azapyrimidines, also proceeds by means of this pathway (80). Thus, 5-fluorouracil is metabolically degraded to dihydrofluorouracil, α-fluoro-β-ureido-propionic acid, urea, carbon dioxide, and α-fluoro-β-alanine (24).

III. Purine Biosynthesis

A. De Novo Pathway

Although the reactions comprising the *de novo* pathway for purine biosynthesis are ubiquitous in nature, the classic work was conducted in the pigeon (5, 54). The major advantage of this species for these investigations is related to the elaboration of uric acid as the end product of purine metabolism. Uric acid is extremely insoluble and, hence, can be isolated in relatively pure form after administration of labeled isotopes *in vivo* or *in vitro* and degraded to its component parts. The structure and the source of the atoms of uric acid are depicted in Fig. 7.12.

Carbon dioxide supplies the carbon atom at position 2 while formate (or the 1-carbon pool) is responsible for positions 2 and 8. Glycine is incorporated into positions 4, 5, and 7 while the amide nitrogen of glutamine makes up the nitrogens at positions 3 and 9. The final nitrogen at position 1 is derived from aspartic acid.

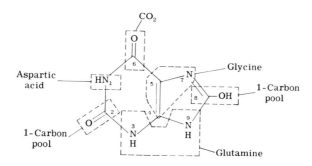

Fig. 7.12. Uric acid; source of its atoms.

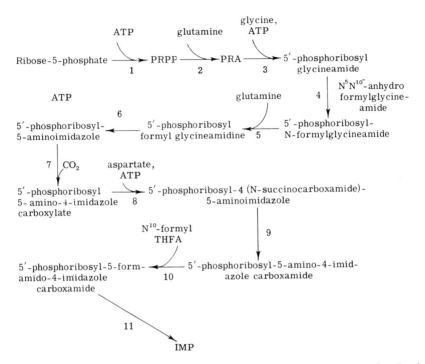

Fig. 7.13. Biosynthesis of IMP. PRPP, Phosphoribosyl pyrophosphate; PRA, phosphoribosyl-amine; (1) ribosephosphate pyrophosphokinase; (2) phosphoribosyl-pyrophosphate amido-transferase; (3) phosphoribosyl-glycineamide synthetase; (4) phosphoribosyl-glycineamide formyltransferase; (5) phosphoribosylformyl-glycineamidine synthetase; (6) aminoimidazole ribonucleotide synthetase; (7) phosphoribosyl-aminoimidazole carboxylase; (8) phosphoribosyl-aminoimidazolesuccinocarboxamide synthetase; (9) adenylosuccinate lyase; (10) phosphoribosyl-aminoimidazolecarboxamide formyltransferase; and (11) IMP cyclohydrolase.

The first purine moiety, inosine-5'-monophosphate (IMP), is formed through a complex series of reactions beginning with very simple materials. The reactions are shown in Fig. 7.13.

1. PRPP FORMATION

The formation of PRPP is an important process in the mammalian cell since this intermediate is required for the synthesis of pyrimidines, i.e., OMP, and of purines, i.e., by both the *de novo* and preformed pathways. Since PRPP formation ultimately derives from glucose via ribose-5-phosphate, it is conceivable that regulation could be effected by modulating the intracellular carbohydrate stores (57).

The PRPP which is normally utilized for purine synthesis can be depleted by diverting this supply to other fates. As noted in Section II, A, OMP pyrophosphorylase catalyzes the formation of OMP from orotic acid and PRPP.

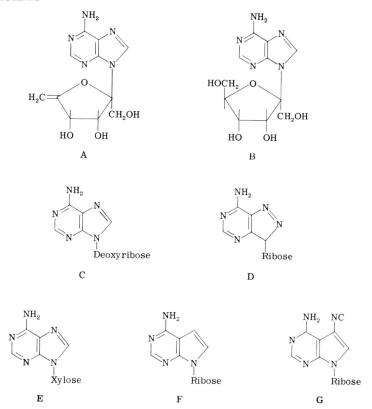

Fig. 7.14. Purine analogs which affect PRPP formation. (A) Decoyinine; (B) psicofuranine; (C) 3'-deoxyadenosine (cordycepin); (D) formycin; (E) 9β-D-xylofuranosyladenine; (F) tubicidin; and (G) toyocamycin.

The administration of large amounts of orotic acid to rats leads to the production of fatty livers which presumably is caused by an inhibition of purine synthesis *in vivo* as a result of the depletion of PRPP (14, 34, 50).

INHIBITION OF PRPP FORMATION. The synthesis of PRPP is subject to inhibition by a number of purine analogs which include decoyinine, psicofuranine, cordycepin (3'-deoxyadenosine), formycin, tubercidin, and 9β-D-xylofuranosyladenine (Fig. 7.14). These analogs all have the common feature of possessing a 6-amino group and apparently after suitable phosphorylations (if possible) they occupy the site on the PRPP kinase which is normally reserved for ATP (72).

2. AMIDOTRANSFERASE

The formation of phosphoribosylamine (PRA) from PRPP and glutamine may actually be regarded as the first step in the pathway which is unique to the synthesis of purine nucleotides. In this irreversible enzyme-catalyzed reaction, a Walden inversion takes place at position 1 of PRPP, i.e., the configuration which is α in PRPP at this point inverts to β in PRA.

The requirement of this enzyme for glutamine synthesis has been examined in tumor cells (36). The synthesis of glutamine in these tumor cells was operating at only a minimal level. Since purine biosynthesis includes 2 steps which require glutamine, the amidotransferase and phosphoribosyl-formyl-glycineamidine synthetase (Fig. 7.13), one might expect formation of this base to proceed extremely slowly. It was demonstrated that the neoplastic cells could replace glutamine by NH_4Cl or asparagine in the former reaction, but only at high concentrations. Consequently, in neoplastic tissues, the amidotransferase represents a very significant rate-limiting step in purine synthesis not only because of its presence in low amounts within the cell but additionally because a substrate, glutamine, is available only in minimal amounts.

The amidotransferase is also unique in exhibiting allosteric kinetics with PRPP as substrate (58) and is inhibited (end product) by a number of purine nucleotides (23, 53, 58). Consequently, the activity of this enzyme is a complex function of the amount of the enzyme, the concentration of the substrates, and the concentrations of adenine and guanine nucleotides. In this regard, the enzyme is inhibited only by purine 5'-ribonucleotides and not by 3'-nucleotides (104). Apparently, different and independent sites exist on the enzyme for attachment by adenine and guanine nucleotides (23). Therefore, under conditions of growth when the ribonucleotide concentration would be expected to be at a low level because of the demand for nucleic acid synthesis, the formation of purines would proceed at a maximum rate. However, in conditions of stasis when the purine nucleotide concentration within the cell would increase, further purine synthesis *de novo* would be minimal because of end product inhibition at the PRPP amidotransferase steps. Of particular interest in this regard is the pseudo-feedback inhibition of the enzyme by a number of purine analogs, e.g., 6-mercaptopurine ribonucleotide.

EFFECT OF GLUTAMINE ANTAGONISTS. The *de novo* synthesis of IMP utilizes 2 glutamine-requiring steps, PRPP amidotransferase and phosphoribosyl-formyl-glycineamidine synthetase (Fig. 7.13). Both steps are irreversibly inhibited by azaserine and DON. However for some reason, the more sensitive reaction is that catalyzed by the latter enzyme (54). The chemotherapeutic efficacy of these glutamine antagonists is due to the very potent blockade exerted on purine synthesis.

3. FOLATE-MEDIATED REACTIONS

Several reactions of purine biosynthesis require activated forms of folic acid (Fig. 7.13). These include phosphoribosyl-glycineamide formyltransferase and phosphoribosyl-aminoimidizolecarboxamide formyltransferase. Of interest is the fact that each of these enzymes utilizes a different form of THFA. The former requires N^5,N^{10}-anhydroformyl THFA for addition of a formyl group to the growing imidazole ring while the latter utilizes N^{10}-formyl THFA for insertion of a formyl moiety at position 2 of the purine ring. The structures of these

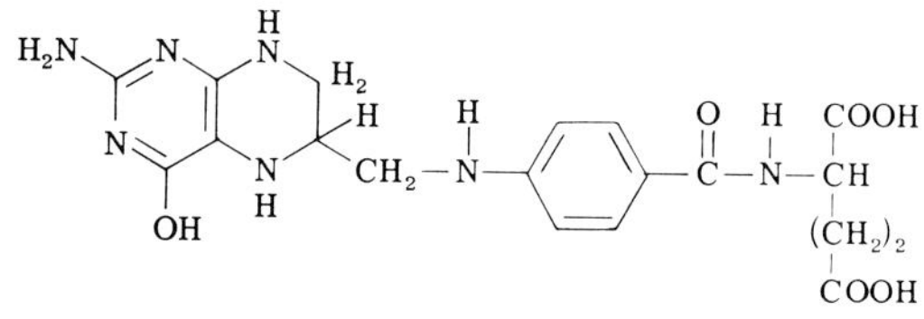

THFA

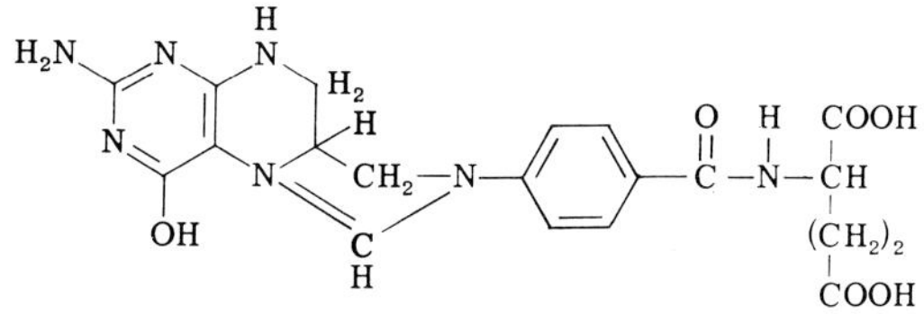

A

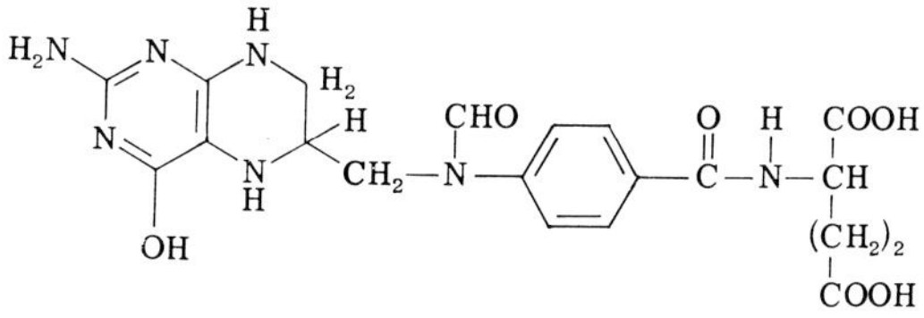

B

N¹⁰-formyl THFA.

Fig. 7.15. Activated forms of folic acid. (A) N^5,N^{10}-Anhydroformyl THFA; and (B) forms are shown in Fig. 7.15. These reactions are secondary sites of action of the antifolic acid drugs, e.g., amethopterin (Section IV).

4. UTILIZATION OF IMP

Inosine monophosphate is centrally located in the metabolism of purines; it serves as the bridge point to the synthesis of AMP and GMP (22, 67) (Fig. 7.16). In the formation of adenylosuccinate, aspartate is the donor of the amino

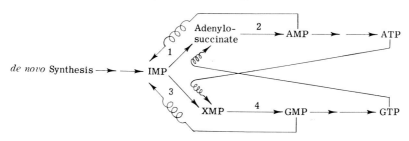

Fig. 7.16. Utilization of IMP and its regulation. (1) Adenylosuccinate synthetase; (2) adenylosuccinate lyase; (3) IMP dehydrogenase; and (4) XMP aminase. The regulatory mechanisms are indicated by the curling arrows. If in the direction of the reaction, then the nucleotide serves as an activator; if in the reverse direction, then as an inhibitor.

group and GTP serves as an activator. The reaction is inhibited (end product) by AMP. This particular reaction is the site of action of several antimetabolites, such as hadacidin (N-formyl-N-hydroxyaminoacetic acid), and 6-mercaptopurine ribonucleotide.

The formation of GMP proceeds via the intermediate XMP. The synthesis of the latter requires ATP as activator, and is inhibited by its end product, GMP. The series of activations and inhibitions presents an interesting picture where the levels of adenine and guanine nucleotides play an important role in controlling the balance between the two. Thus, if too much ATP accumulates within the cell, IMP dehydrogenase activity will be activated in an attempt to increase GTP and concomitantly, AMP formation will be inhibited at the adenylosuccinate synthetase step.

IMP dehydrogenase is also inhibited by 6-mercaptopurine ribonucleotide in a pseudo-feedback manner (54). XMP aminase, which catalyzes the formation of GMP, utilizes glutamine as the preferred nitrogen donor although high concentrations of NH_3 may substitute (64). Consequently, this reaction is blocked by azaserine and DON. Psicofuranine (Fig. 7.14) exerts profound inhibition at this step by complexing irreversibly with the aminase in the presence of XMP.

Although the routes from IMP to AMP or to GMP involve intermediate steps, the reverse pathways are executed in single steps. In this manner, AMP may be deaminated to IMP as catalyzed by AMP deaminase or GMP may be reductively deaminated to IMP as catalyzed by GMP reductase. Each of these pathways is also allosterically effected; AMP or ATP activates AMP deaminase, ATP inhibits GMP reductase, and GTP inhibits the deaminase. Once again, the powerful regulatory role of ATP is seen. The fine control of adenine nucleotides on the AMP deaminase step may play a key role in maintaining a constant level of intracellular purine. This is further balanced by the counter effect of guanine nucleotides.

B. Salvage Pathway or Synthesis from Preformed Purines

The first demonstration that exogenously administered adenine could participate in the anabolic pathway was the observation (18) that dietary adenine was incorporated into tissue nucleic acids in the rat. These studies were followed by the demonstration that AMP could be formed directly from the base in contrast to the pyrimidines [Eq. (7.17)].

$$\text{Adenine} + \text{PRPP} \rightarrow \text{AMP} + \text{pyrophosphate} \tag{7.17}$$

The enzyme which catalyzes this transformation, AMP pyrophosphorylase, can also use 2,6-diaminopurine and aminoimidazole carboxamide as substrates (2).

In addition, a different pyrophosphorylase has been isolated which is capable of utilizing hypoxanthine (HX), xanthine (X), guanine (G), and 6-mercaptopurine (6MP) [Eq. (7.18)]. This enzyme is of particular importance since it is responsible for the activation of 6-mercaptopurine, i.e., lethal synthesis.

$$\left.\begin{array}{c} \text{HX} \\ \text{G} \\ \text{X} \\ \text{6MP} \end{array}\right\} + \text{PRPP} \rightarrow \left.\begin{array}{c} \text{IMP} \\ \text{GMP} \\ \text{XMP} \\ \text{6MP-MP} \end{array}\right\} + \text{pyrophosphate} \qquad (7.18)$$

Recent work has implicated the purine nucleotide pyrophosphorylases in the activity of rapidly growing tissues (77, 78). The activity of both AMP and IMP pyrophosphorylases increases markedly in regenerating liver and during the rapid growth phase of Ehrlich ascites cells. Furthermore, both enzymes increase during the rapid growth phase in postnatal liver.

1. 6-MERCAPTOPURINE

This purine analog (Fig. 7.17) which was synthesized by Elion *et al.* (32) was designed as a specific inhibitor of the naturally occurring purines and soon shown to have significant antitumor activity; the agent has proved most effective in the treatment of acute lymphocytic leukemia in children. Although some question exists as to its exact mechanism of action, after conversion to the nucleotide this analog inhibits the following:

(a) *De novo* synthesis of purines by a pseudo-feedback inhibition of PRA formation
(b) AMP synthesis by blockade of adenylosuccinate formation
(c) GMP synthesis by blockade of IMP dehydrogenase
(d) Nucleic acid formation by virtue of the inhibition of purine synthesis
(e) Coenzyme synthesis which may require AMP or GMP formation

Furthermore, 6MP may be incorporated into RNA or coenzymes (in place of ATP) and exert effects upon their functions.

Resistance develops to 6MP both in bacterial and neoplastic cells, the mechanism of which appears related to the loss of the activating enzyme, IMP pyrophosphorylase [Eq. (7.19)].

2. ADENOSINE KINASE AND INHIBITORS OF PURINE SYNTHESIS

Under the action of purine nucleoside phosphorylase, adenine and other purines may be converted to ribonucleosides [Eq. (7.19)] and the latter phosphorylated to ribonucleotides in the presence of ATP and adenosine kinase [Eq. (7.20)].

$$\text{Purine} + \text{ribose-1-phosphate} \rightarrow \text{nucleoside} + \text{P}_i \qquad (7.19)$$

$$\text{Nucleoside} + \text{ATP} \rightarrow \text{nucleotide} + \text{ADP} \qquad (7.20)$$

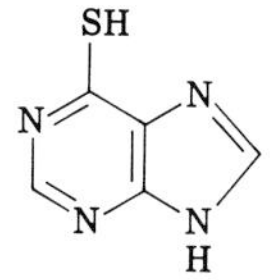

Fig. 7.17. 6-Mercaptopurine.

The latter reaction is activated by ATP but its importance in chemotherapy is due to its low substrate specificity. Consequently, it is able to form nucleotides from a variety of nucleosides of purine analogs (Fig. 7.14), including tubercidin, toyocamycin, formycin, psicofuranine, xylosyladenine, and arabinosyladenine. Resistance is accompanied by the loss in adenosine kinase activity such that no nucleotide, the active form of these analogs, can be formed.

3. OTHER ENZYMES

As mentioned earlier (Section II,G,4,b), the enzyme responsible for the phosphorylation of CdR also functions in the formation of dAMP and dGMP from deoxyadenosine and deoxyguanosine, respectively [Eq. (7.21)].

$$\begin{array}{ccc} \text{Deoxyadenosine} & \text{dAMP} & \\ \text{or} & + \text{ATP} \rightarrow & \text{or} & + \text{ADP} \\ \text{deoxyguanosine} & \text{dGMP} & \end{array} \qquad (7.21)$$

The deoxyadenosine kinase is markedly inhibited by nucleotides of cytosine; the deoxy derivatives are the most potent (63).

C. Catabolism of Purines

The catabolism of purine ribo- and deoxyribonucleotides yields the free purine bases, adenine, guanine, hypoxanthine, and xanthine, through the concerted action of a number of enzymes. As seen earlier (Section III, B), each of these bases can be returned to the ribonucleotide pool via the action of the pyrophosphorylases; the latter are generally more active in neoplastic tissue, hence favoring the anabolic pathway.

However, a substantial amount of purines is not recycled but instead is oxidized to uric acid for purposes of excretion. In most mammals, the filtered uric acid is reabsorbed by the kidney tubules and in the liver converted by uricase to the readily soluble allantoin which can be excreted in the urine. In man, however, this capability has been lost sometime during evolution and he must excrete the relatively insoluble uric acid. This can be of clinical significance since its limited solubility can lead to the deposition of crystals in various tissues. The mechanisms for uric acid production are shown in Fig. 7.18. Xanthine oxidase is the enzyme which catalyzes the oxidation of both hypoxanthine to xanthine and of xanthine to uric acid. The enzyme is also capable of catalyzing the oxidation of adenine (2,8-dihydroxyadenine is the agent responsible for adenine toxicity) and 6-mercaptopurine. The product of detoxification of the latter is 2,8-dihydroxy-6-mercaptopurine or 6-thiouric acid.

Since 6-thiouric acid has no chemotherapeutic efficacy, the thought was entertained that destruction of 6-mercaptopurine could be prevented by simultaneous administration of an agent which inhibited xanthine oxidase activity, thus allowing the use of smaller amounts of the antileukemic agent with the reduction of drug toxicity. The hypothesis was tested with 4-hydroxypyrazolo-(3,4-d)-pyrimi-

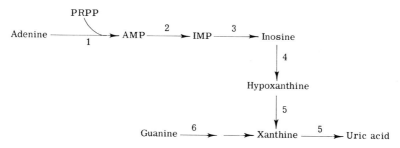

Fig. 7.18. Production of uric acid. (1) AMP pyrophosphorylase; (2) AMP deaminase; (3) phosphatase; (4) purine nucleoside phosphorylase; (5) xanthine oxidase; and (6) guanase.

dine (allopurinol) as the inhibitor (33) and although found partially correct, a more useful clinical observation was made. The excretion (and consequently the production) of uric acid in patients was markedly reduced. This observation has led to use of allopurinol in the treatment of gout. Hyperuricemia with uric acid nephropathy may be a life-threatening condition in patients with chronic myeloproliferative diseases, e.g., chronic myelocytic leukemia, with acute leukemias, or with any disease in which the turnover of cells is greatly accelerated (88). The rapid destruction of malignant cells by chemotherapeutic agents can augment this hyperuricemia which can be inhibited by allopurinol administration.

IV. Antifolic Acid Drugs

The discovery and subsequent elucidation of the functions of folic acid were quickly followed by the synthesis of a variety of antifolic acid drugs (Fig. 7.19). Two classes of antifols were readily identified: (a) those in which the pyrimidine (or triazine) moiety contained amino groups in both 2 and 4 positions—all these analogs possessed antitumor activity—and (b) those in which changes were made in other parts of the molecule, e.g., aspartic acid substituted for glutamic acid. These analogs had no substantial antitumor activity.

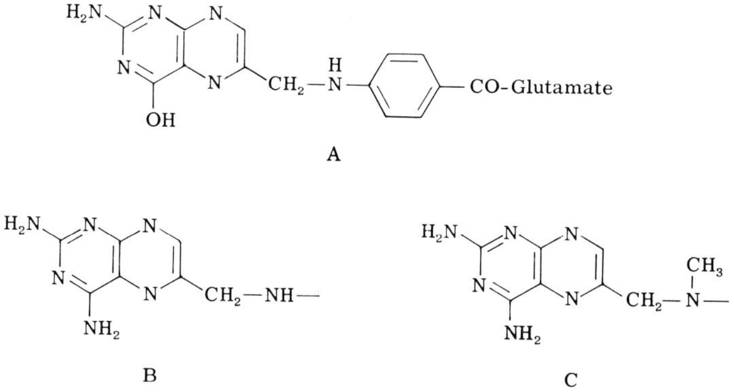

Fig. 7.19. Folic acid and its analogs. (A) Folic acid; (B) aminopterin; and (C) amethopterin.

For purposes of this discussion, only the analogs which fall into the first class will be considered. Two of the more important members in this class are aminopterin and amethopterin (Fig. 7.19). Interest in these analogs was spurred by the report that temporary remissions were observed upon treatment of children with acute leukemia with these drugs (35). Since that time, amethopterin has been employed in the treatment of other forms of neoplasia and sometimes with remarkable results, e.g., in choriocarcinoma.

A. Mechanism of Action of the Antifols

The antifols function by affecting the pathway for the activation of folic acid to its various forms. This pathway involves the reduction of folate to dihydrofolate and, subsequently, to tetrahydrofolate (THFA) (Fig. 7.20), a reduction which is markedly elevated in rapidly proliferating tissues such as in neoplastic cells. Apparently, amethopterin has profound affinity for the reductase and binds to the latter 10^5–10^6 times more tightly than the normal substrate, folic acid (102). The end result of this binding is a pseudo-irreversible inhibition with a prolonged drug retention.

Since the activated forms of THFA are required for 1-carbon transformations such as take place in purine and pyrimidine synthesis and some amino acid interconversions, the administration of the antifols exerts profound effects upon RNA, DNA, and protein synthesis. However, not all of the 1-carbon transformations are inhibited to the same degree. In this regard, dTMP synthesis is much more sensitive to their inhibitory action than purine synthesis (1, 99). This differential effect may be caused by the following: the formation of the purine skeleton results in the regeneration of THFA which can be recycled; the utilization in dTMP synthesis, however, involves the conversion of the activated folate to dihydrofolic acid which cannot recycle because of the blockade.

B. Resistance to the Antifols

That leukemic cells can become resistant to the antifols and other agents (Table 7.1) was first demonstrated in experimental animals (19). Since that time, the phenomenon of resistance has been demonstrated in many tumors in many species including man. The basis for the development of resistance is the tight almost irreversible complexation of drug to reductase. For all practical purposes, the enzyme has "titrated" out one molecule of inhibitor. The neo-

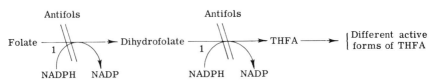

Fig. 7.20. Activation of folic acid and blockade by antifols. (1) Dihydrofolic acid reductase.

TABLE 7.1

DEVELOPMENT OF RESISTANCE TO CHEMOTHERAPEUTIC AGENTS

Mechanism	Examples
1. Loss of transport mechanisms responsible for permeability	Azaserine; 6-mercaptopurine
2. Loss of activation mechanism, i.e., inability to effect "lethal synthesis"	6-Mercaptopurine; 5-fluorouracil
3. Increased destruction (development of inactivating enzymes)	Arabinosylcytosine
4. Development of larger quantities of target enzyme, i.e., "titrating" out the inhibitor	Amethopterin
5. Alteration in target enzyme conformation such that inhibitor does not bind as tightly; k_i is increased	Amethopterin; 5-fluorouracil
6. Development of pathways circumventing blockade	L-Asparaginase (development of asparagine synthase); alkylating agents (development of repair mechanisms?)

plastic cell consequently responds by an enhanced elaboration of dihydrofolic reductase which may reach 1000-fold the intracellular concentration of enzyme present prior to administration of drug. At first blush, this would appear to be a very expensive method which the cell has adopted for the inactivation of a potent toxin, yet the end result is most effective, i.e., the removal of the inhibitor. A number of investigators have attempted to utilize the level of dihydrofolate reductase present in the neoplastic tissue as a means for determining either the susceptibility of that tumor to antifol therapy or as a means for determining the best timing for administration of antifol therapy (52).

V. Resistance

It is appropriate that this chapter be ended with a discussion of the mechanism by which resistance to purine and pyrimidine analogs develops in neoplastic cells. Generally, the application of a particular therapeutic regimen to a patient with a primarily responsive disease is sooner or later terminated by the onset of resistance. Although aspects of the resistance question have been covered in brief when the mechanism of action of an analog was under consideration, this particular section will be devoted to a general survey of types of mechanisms with examples cited for illustrative purposes (Table 7.1).

The phenomenon of resistance which was first clearly recognized by Paul Ehrlich in 1907 has for many years plagued clinical oncologists and individuals responsible for devising chemotherapeutic agents. A central question must be asked which relates to the origin of this phenomenon. How does resistance emerge? One might imagine that (a) resistance is the result of an induction by the particular drug being employed in therapy, *phenotypic adaptation,* or

(b) every population is composed of cells, which have varying susceptibilities to therapeutic agents, including small numbers of resistant organisms (genetically resistant) and therapy results in the subsequent selection of the latter. For a variety of reasons, the second hypothesis is generally favored.

The biochemical mechanisms by which neoplastic cells manifest resistance are many and include (Table 7.1):

1. Reduction in the transport of the chemotherapeutic agent across the plasma membrane, i.e., permeability is markedly impaired. The transport may be either passive or active, and resistance with the latter mechanism may be a reflection of an alteration of the transport protein. Resistance to the glutamine antagonists, azaserine and DON, is sometimes associated with this type of mechanism.

2. Decreased lethal synthesis. As we have seen previously, most of the purine and pyrimidine analogs require an activation reaction, e.g., the formation of ribonucleotide. In resistant cells, this mechanism has been markedly reduced. Leukemic cells which are resistant to 6-mercaptopurine generally cannot form the ribonucleotide.

3. Increased detoxification of the agent. Many agents are slowly metabolized to innocuous substances; this pathway may be significantly elevated in resistant organisms. Arabinosylcytosine may be deaminated to arabinosyluracil, an ineffective agent in tumor therapy, as catalyzed by deoxycytidine deaminase. In some resistant cells, this pathway is augmented.

4. Increased production of the target enzyme. Some antitumor agents bind almost irreversibly to the target enzyme. The resistant cells elaborate much more target enzyme to help in the elimination of the agent. This is the mechanism of resistance to amethopterin.

5. Decreased affinity of drug for target enzyme. In some resistant organisms, the target enzyme has been conformationally altered such that its specificity is exquisite. In this regard, cells resistant to 5-fluorodeoxyuridine elaborate a dTMP synthetase to which 5-FdUMP cannot bind, and hence cannot inhibit.

References

1. Balis, M. E., and Dancis, J. (1955). *Cancer Res.* **15**, 603–608.
2. Balis, M. E. (1968). "Antagonists and Nucleic Acids," pp. 5–37, North-Holland Publ., Amsterdam.
3. Bessman, M. J., Lehman, I. R., Adler, J., Zimmerman, S. B., Sims, E. S., and Kornberg, A. (1958). *Proc. Nat. Acad. Sci. U.S.* **44**, 633–640.
4. Blair, D. G. R., and Potter, V. R. (1961). *J. Biol. Chem.* **236**, 2503–2506.
5. Blakley, R. L., and Vitols, E. (1968). *Ann. Rev. Biochem.* **37**, 201–224.
5a. Bosch, L., Harbers, E., and Heidelberger, C. (1958). *Cancer Res.* **18**, 333.
6. Bresnick, E. (1964). *Advan. Enzyme Reg.* **2**, 213–236.
7. Bresnick, E., and Blatchford, K. (1964). *Biochim. Biophys. Acta* **81**, 150–157.
8. Bresnick, E., Thompson, U. B., Morris, H. P., and Liebelt, A. G. (1964). *Biochem. Biophys. Res. Commun.* **16**, 278–284.
9. Bresnick, E. (1965). *J. Biol. Chem.* **240**, 2550–2556.
10. Bresnick, E., and Thompson, U. B. (1965). *J. Biol. Chem.* **240**, 3967–3974.

11. Bresnick, E., and Mossé, H. (1966). *Biochem. J.* **101**, 63–69.
12. Bresnick, E., and Williams, S. S. (1967). *Biochem. Pharmacol.* **16**, 503–507.
13. Bresnick, E., Williams, S. S., and Mossé, H. (1967). *Cancer Res.* **27**, 469–475.
14. Bresnick, E., Mayfield, E. D., Jr., and Mossé, H. (1968). *Mol. Pharmacol.* **4**, 173–180.
15. Bresnick, E., Mainigi, K. D., Mayfield, E. D., Jr., and Morris, H. P. (1969). *Cancer Res.* **29**, 1932–1936.
16. Bresnick, E. (1971). *In* "Methods in Cancer Research" (H. Busch, ed.), Vol. VI, pp. 347–397. Academic Press, New York.
17. Bresnick, E., Mayfield, E. D., Jr., Liebelt, A. G., and Liebelt, R. A. (1971). *Cancer Res.* **31**, 743–751.
18. Brown, G. B., Roll, P. M., Plentyl, A. A., and Cavalieri, L. F. (1948). *J. Biol. Chem.* **172**, 469–484.
19. Burchenal, J. H., Robinson, E., Johnston, S. F., and Kushida, M. K. (1950). *Science* **111**, 116–117.
20. Canellakis, E. S. (1956). *J. Biol. Chem.* **221**, 315–322.
21. Canellakis, E. S., Jaffe, J. J., Mantsavinos, R., and Krakow, J. S. (1959). *J. Biol. Chem.* **234**, 2096–2099.
22. Carter, C. E., and Cohen, L. H. (1956). *J. Biol. Chem.* **222**, 17–30.
23. Caskey, C. T., Ashton, D. M., and Wyngaarden, J. B. (1964). *J. Biol. Chem.* **239**, 2570–2579.
24. Chaudhuri, N. K., Mukherjee, L. L., and Heidelberger, C. (1958). *Biochem. Pharmacol.* **1**, 328–341.
25. Chu, M. Y., and Fischer, G. A. (1962). *Biochem. Pharmacol.* **11**, 423–430.
26. Cohen, S. S. (1966). *Progr. Nucleic Acid Res.* **5**, 1–88.
27. Creasey, W. A., Papac, R. J., Markiw, M. E., Calabresi, P., and Welch, A. D. (1966). *Biochem. Pharmacol.* **15**, 1417–1428.
28. Durham, J. P., and Ives, D. H. (1969). *Mol. Pharmacol.* **5**, 358–375.
29. Durham, J. P., and Ives, D. H. (1970). *J. Biol. Chem.* **245**, 2276–2284.
30. Duschinsky, R., Pleven, E., and Heidelberger, C. (1957). *J. Amer. Chem. Soc.* **79**, 4559–4560.
31. Elford, H. L., Freese, M., Passamani, E., and Morris, H. P. (1970). *J. Biol. Chem.* **245**, 5228–5233.
32. Elion, G. B., Burgi, E., and Hitchings, G. H. (1952). *J. Amer. Chem. Soc.* **74**, 411–414.
33. Elion, G. B., Callahan, S., Nathan, H., Bieber, S., Rundles, R. W., and Hitchings, G. H. (1963). *Biochem. Pharmacol.* **12**, 85–93.
34. Euler, L. H. von, Rubin, R. J., and Handschumacher, R. E. (1963). *J. Biol. Chem.* **238**, 2171–2177.
35. Farber, S., Diamond, L. K., Mercer, R. D., Sylvester, R. F., and Wolfe, J. A. (1948). *New England J. Med.* **238**, 787–793.
36. Fontenelle, L. J., and Henderson, J. F. (1969). *Biochim. Biophys. Acta* **177**, 88–93.
37. Frenkel, E. P., Skinner, W. N., and Smiley, J. D. (1964). *Cancer Chemotherap. Rep.* **40**, 19–22.
38. Friedkin, M., and Kornberg, A. (1957). *In* "The Chemical Basis of Heredity" (W. D. McElroy and B. Glass, eds.), pp. 609–614. Johns Hopkins Press, Baltimore, Maryland.
39. Friedkin, M. (1963). *Ann Rev. Biochem.* **32**, 185–214.
40. Fritzson, P. (1964). *Biochim. Biophys. Acta* **91**, 374–379.
41. Fritzson, P., and Efskind, J. (1965). *Cancer Res.* **25**, 703–707.
42. Fujioka, S., and Silber, R. (1970). *J. Biol. Chem.* **245**, 1688–1693.
43. Gallo, R. C., and Breitman, T. (1968). *J. Biol. Chem.* **243**, 4936–4942, 4943–4951.
44. Gallo, R. C., and Perry, S. (1969). *J. Clin. Invest.* **48**, 105–116.
45. Gerhart, J. C., and Schachman, H. C. (1965). *Biochemistry* **4**, 1054–1062.
46. Grav, H. J. (1967). *In* "Methods in Cancer Research" (H. Busch, ed.), Vol. III, pp. 243–389. Academic Press, New York.

47. Groth, D. P., and Jiang, N. (1966). *Biochem. Biophys. Res. Commun.* **22**, 62–68.
48. Hager, S. E., and Jones, M. E. (1965). *J. Biol. Chem.* **240**, 4556–4563.
49. Hager, S. E., and Jones, M. E. (1967). *J. Biol. Chem.* **242**, 5667–5673, 5674–5680.
50. Handschumacher, R. E., Creasey, W. A., Jaffe, J. J., Pasternak, C. A., and Hankin, L. (1960). *Proc. Nat. Acad. Sci.* **46**, 178–186.
51. Handschumacher, R. E., and Welch, A. D (1960). *In* "The Nucleic Acids" (E. Chargaff and J. N. Davidson, eds.), Vol. III, pp. 453–526. Academic Press, New York.
52. Hardesty, C. T., Chen, D., and Mead, J. A. R. (1972). *Cancer Res.* **32**, 458–461.
53. Hartman, S. C. (1963). *J. Biol. Chem.* **238**, 3024–3035.
54. Hartman, S. C. (1970). *In* "Metabolic Pathways" (D. M. Greenberg, ed.), 3rd ed., Vol. IV, pp. 1–68. Academic Press, New York.
55. Heidelberger, C., Griesbach, L., Cruz, O., Schnitzer, R. J., and Grunberg, E. (1958). *Proc. Soc. Exp. Biol. Med.* **97**, 470–475.
56. Heidelberger, C. (1967). *Ann. Rev. Pharmacol.* **7**, 101–124.
57. Henderson, J. F., and Khoo, M. K. Y. (1965). *J. Biol. Chem.* **240**, 2349–2357, 2358–2362, 3104–3109.
58. Hill, D. L., and Bennett, L. L., Jr. (1969). *Biochemistry* **8**, 122–130.
59. Hurlbert, R. B., and Kammen, H. O. (1960). *J. Biol. Chem.* **235**, 443–449.
60. Kara, J., and Weil, R. (1967). *Proc. Nat. Acad. Sci. U.S.* **57**, 63–70.
61. Kaufman, H. E., and Heidelberger, C. (1964). *Science* **145**, 585–586.
62. Krakoff, I. H., Brown, N. C., and Reichard, P. (1968). *Cancer Res.* **28**, 1559–1565.
63. Krygier, V., and Momparler, R. L. (1971). *J. Biol. Chem.* **246**, 2752–2757.
64. Lagerkvist, U. (1958). *J. Biol. Chem.* **233**, 138–142, 143–149.
65. Larsson, A., and Nielands, J. B. (1966). *Biochem. Biophys. Res. Commun.* **25**, 222–226.
66. Larsson, A., and Reichard, P. (1967). *Progr. Nucleic Acid Res.* **7**, 303–348.
67. Lieberman, I. (1956). *J. Biol. Chem.* **223**, 327–339.
68. Mayfield, E. D., Jr., Lyman, K., and Bresnick, E. (1967). *Cancer Res.* **27**, 476–481.
69. Metzenberg, R. L., Hall, L. M., Marshall, M., and Cohen, P. P. (1957). *J. Biol. Chem.* **229**, 1019–1025.
70. Momparler, R. L., and Fischer, G. A. (1968). *J. Biol. Chem.* **243**, 4298–4304.
71. Momparler, R. L., Brent, T. P., Labitan, A., and Krygier, V. (1971). *Mol. Pharmacol.* **7**, 413–419.
72. Montgomery, J. A. (1971). *In* "Oncology 1970" (R. L. Clark, R. W. Crumley, J. A. McCoy, and M. M. Copeland, eds.), Vol. II, pp. 57–63. Yearbook Med. Publ., Chicago, Illinois.
73. Moore, E. C., and Hurlbert, R. B. (1966). *J. Biol. Chem.* **241**, 4802–4809.
74. Moore, E. C., and Cohen, S. S. (1967). *J. Biol. Chem.* **242**, 2116–2118.
75. Moore, E. C., Zedeck, M. S., Agrawal, K. C., and Sartorelli, A. C .(1970). *Biochemistry* **9**, 4492–4498.
76. Murphree, S., Moore, E. C., and Beall, P. T. (1968). *Cancer Res.* **28**, 860–863.
77. Murray, A. W. (1967). *Biochem. J.* **104**, 675–678.
78. Murray, A. W. (1966). *Biochem. J.* **100**, 664–670.
79. Nakamura, H., and Sugino, Y. (1966). *Cancer Res.* **26**, 1425–1429.
80. Newmark, P., Stephens, J. D., and Barrett, H. W. (1962). *Biochim. Biophys. Acta* **62**, 414–416.
81. Okazaki, R., and Kornberg, A. (1964). *J. Biol. Chem.* **239**, 275–284.
82. Potter, V. R., Pitot, H. C., Ono, T., and Morris, H. P. (1960). *Cancer Res.* **20**, 1255–1261.
83. Prusoff, W. H. (1967). *Pharmacol. Rev.* **19**, 209–250.
84. Racker, E. (1952). *J. Biol. Chem.* **196**, 347–365.
85. Reichard, P. (1959). *Advan. Enzymol.* **21**, 263–294.
86. Reyes, P., and Heidelberger, C. (1965). *Mol. Pharmacol.* **1**, 14–30.
87. Rose, I. A., and Schweigert, B. S. (1953). *J. Biol. Chem.* **202**, 635–645.
88. Rundles, R. W., Wyngaarden, J. B., Hitchings, G. H., and Elion, G. B. (1969). *Ann. Rev. Pharmacol.* **9**, 345–362.
89. Rutman, R. J., Canterow, A., and Paschkis, K. E. (1954). *Cancer Res.* **14**, 119–123.

90. Salzman, N. P., Eagle, H., and Sebring, E. D. (1958). *J. Biol. Chem.* **230**, 1001–1012.
91. Sartorelli, A. C., and Creasey, W. A. (1969). *Ann. Rev. Pharmacol.* **9**, 51–72.
92. Schrecker, A. W. (1970). *Cancer Res.* **30**, 632–641.
93. Schwartz, H. S., Garafolo, M., Sternberg, S. S., and Phillips, F. S. (1965). *Cancer Res.* **25**, 1867–1870.
94. Seibert, W. (1947). *Chem. Ber.* **80**, 494–502.
95. Smith, E. E., and Rutenberg, A. M. (1967). *Cancer Res.* **27**, 1470–1473.
96. Šorm, F., and Veselý, J. (1964). *Neoplasma* **11**, 123–130.
97. Šorm, F., and Škoda, J. (1956). *Coll. Czech. Chem. Commun.* **21**, 487–488.
98. Tatibana, M., and Ito, K. (1967). *Biochem. Biophys. Res. Commun.* **26**, 221–227.
99. Totter, J. R. (1955). *In* "Antimetabolites and Cancer" (C. P. Rhoads, eds.), pp. 153–162. Amer. Ass. Advan. Sci., Washington, D. C.
100. Turner, M. K., Abrams, R., and Lieberman, I. (1966). *J. Biol. Chem.* **241**, 5777–5780.
101. Weber, K. (1968). *Nature (London)* **218**, 1116–1119.
102. Werkheiser, W. C. (1961). *J. Biol. Chem.* **238**, 888–893.
103. Woglom, W. H. (1947). *In* "Approaches to Tumor Chemotherapy" (F. R. Moulton, ed.), pp. 1–10. Amer. Ass. Advan. Sci., Washington, D. C.
104. Wyngaarden, J. B., and Ashton, D. M. (1958). *J. Biol. Chem.* **234**, 1492–1496.
105. Yates, R. A., and Pardee, A. B. (1956). *J. Biol. Chem.* **221**, 757–770.
106. Young, C. W., and Hodes, S. (1964). *Science* **146**, 1172–1174.
107. Zimmerman, M. (1964). *J. Biol. Chem.* **239**, 2622–2627.

CHAPTER VIII

Nuclear Proteins*

MARK O. J. OLSON, WESLEY C. STARBUCK, AND HARRIS BUSCH

* The original studies in this chapter were supported by Cancer Center Grant, CA 10893
P. 3, Robert A. Welch Foundation, and National Science Foundation.

I. Introduction

Studies on nuclear proteins of cancer cells have been predicated on the concept that some aberrations of gene control mechanisms are responsible either for the initiation or continuation of tumor growth (44, 45). Although it has long been postulated that specific proteins are responsible for "gene control" in mammalian systems (40, 45, 118, 259), only recently has evidence been presented that supports this idea. In part, the experimental difficulties in testing this concept were related to the inadequacies of the methods available for definition of the number, types, and functions of nuclear proteins. Fortunately, these problems are now being rapidly overcome.

The nuclear proteins are divisible into two broad classes: (a) histones and (b) nonhistone proteins (NHP)* which include the nuclear enzymes. The histones are basic and tightly bound to DNA predominantly by multiple ionic bonds. Because of their small number, common features of structure, and relatively limited modifications, they are generally considered to be primarily structural proteins although special regulatory functions cannot be ruled out. Generally, it has been considered that if histones have a gene regulatory role, it involves the fixation of the specific phenotype of cells rather than their responses to various stimuli or environmental changes. On the other hand, cogent evidence has been provided that NHP are involved in gene derepression in eukaryotic cells.

Many of the nonhistone nuclear proteins are bound to RNA, either in particles (see Chapter II) or lengthy strands such as those of the granular and fibrillar elements of the nucleolus (Chapter II). In addition, many of the RNP particles of the nucleus are either completed ribosomes on the outer layer of the nuclear envelope or preribosomal particles which contain many of the ribosomal proteins. Thus in the definition of the NHP involved in gene control, it is essential to differentiate those that have structural functions as part of the nucleolar and other particulate elements from those that may be associated specifically with DNA. The nuclear enzymes involved in synthesis of DNA and RNA contain subunits that must also be distinguished from NHP that may have gene control functions.

In recent years, extensive progress has been made in nuclear protein chemistry, particularly of the histones, and this has served as a base for further consideration of their interrelationships with DNA. Moreover, vast improvements in methods for isolation, separation, and analysis of the nonhistone proteins (see p. 332) have given rise to the hope that further comprehension of their functions may be forthcoming. In view of this progress, it is the plan of this chapter to deal with the histones first and then with the NHP, about which less is understood and yet much is being learned at present. At least, at this point, with the aid of two-dimensional electrophoretic separation methods, it is possible

---

* The abbreviations used in this chapter are NHP, nonhistone protein(s); RNP, ribonucleoprotein; DNP, deoxyribonucleoprotein; BME, β-mercaptoethanol; SDS, sodium dodecyl sulfate.

to estimate the numbers and types of nuclear proteins (Fig. 8.1). Hopefully, gene control proteins may soon be identified and those involved in neoplasia may be differentiated from those that are not.

II. General Characteristics of Histones

Histones were first observed by Miescher (173) who found them associated with the DNA ("soluble nuclein") of unripe salmon testes. Kossel, whose primary interest was protamines, named them histones (145). Since the late 1940's when it was first proposed that histones might have a role in gene regulation (259), the histones of a number of species have been purified and chemically defined.

A. Definition of Histones

The histones are the basic proteins associated with DNA in the somatic cells of all eukaryotes but not in prokaryotes (34, 45, 130).* The histones have a number of common characteristics, including a content of more than 20% of basic amino acids, no tryptophan, and small amounts of cysteine or cystine (the arginine-rich histone, f3, is the only one which contains cysteine).

B. Number and Types of Histones

Although the actual number of unique species of histones was not clear until recently (40), the development of high resolution chromatographic and electrophoretic systems showed that in most tissues there are five classes of histones. By polyacrylamide gel electrophoresis (197), which is widely used as a tool for the analysis of histones (Fig. 8.2), the fastest moving band is the GAR (f2a1,IV) histone (Table 8.1) followed by the triplet of bands of the SLR (f2b,IIb2), AL (f2a2,IIb1), and AR (f3,III) histones. The slowest moving band is the VLR (f1,I) histone. Some properties of calf thymus histones, which are the most characterized, are shown in Table 8.1.

III. The Structures of Histones

The primary amino acid sequences of most of the histones have been defined (Figs. 8.3–8.7). The glycine- and arginine-rich histone (GAR,f2a2, histone IV) (Fig. 8.3), was the first to be sequenced (68, 182). When the sequence of the GAR histone from pea seedling was compared with that of calf thymus (69), only two conservative amino acid substitutions were found, an isoleucine substituted for a valine at position 60 and an arginine for a lysine at position 77. This finding shows that in the course of evolution, most of the histone sequence was conserved and most mutations were probably lethal.

---

* In some recent studies, small amounts of VLR (f1,I) histones have been found in cytoplasmic ribosomes (105a).

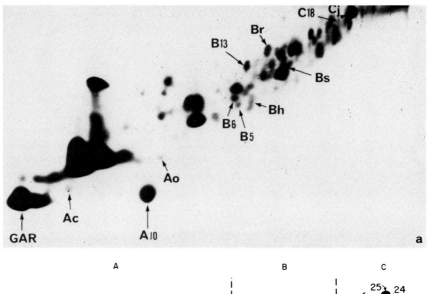

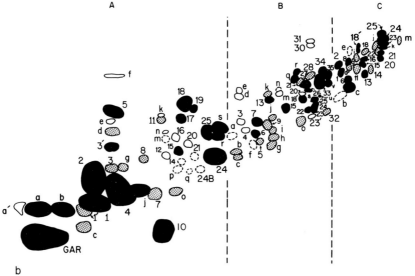

Fig. 8.1. Two-dimensional electrophoresis of 0.4 *N* H₂SO₄-extracted nuclear proteins of normal liver and Novikoff hepatoma. (a) Novikoff hepatoma nuclear proteins, (b) diagram of (a), (c) normal liver nuclear proteins, (d) diagram of (c) (from 296).

The SLR (f2b,IIb2) histone (Fig. 8.4) has little sequence homology to the GAR histone (125). However, in both sequences, there is clustering of basic residues (underlined) and the center of the molecule is largely hydrophobic.*

In the complete sequence of amino acids (70) of the AR (f3,III) histone, the distribution of the amino acids (Fig. 8.6) is similar to that of the GAR histone in that the center of the molecule is largely hydrophobic.

* Recently amino terminal sequences (Fig. 8.5) of several subfractions of the very lysine-rich histone, f1,I, from rabbit thymus were also determined (219).

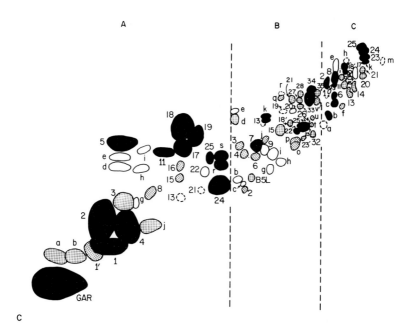

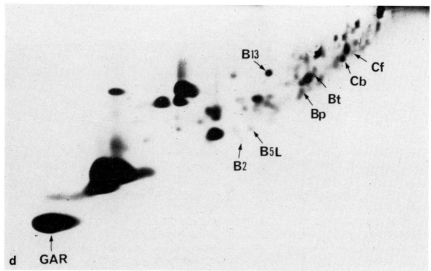

The most recently completed histone sequence (Fig. 8.7) is that of the AL (f2a1,IIb1) histone (183, 271, 295). Strikingly, the first nine residues of the AL and GAR histones are identical except for the glutamine at position 6:

	1	5	10
AL:	AcetylSer-Gly-Arg-Gly-Lys-Gln-Gly-Gly-Lys-Ala-Arg-Ala-Lys - -
GAR:	AcetylSer-Gly-Arg-Gly-Lys - Gly-Gly-Lys-Gly-Leu-Gly-Lys-Gly-Gly

	15	20	25
AL:	-Ala-Lys-Thr-Arg-Ser-Ser-Arg-Ala-Gly-Leu-Gln-Phe-Pro-Val-Gly-Arg-
GAR:	-Ala-Lys - Arg-His-Arg-Lys-Val-Leu-Arg-Asp-Asn-Ile-Gln-Gly-Ile-

TABLE 8.1

Major Histone Fractions from Calf Thymus

Class	Fraction	Number of sub-fractions	% Lys	% Arg	Total residues	Molecular weight	NH₂ terminal	COOH terminal
Lys rich	Very Lys rich VLR (f1,I)	3–4	26.8	1.8	212	19,500–21,000	AcetylSer	Lys
Intermediate	Slightly Lys rich SLR (f2b,IIb2)	1	16.0	6.4	125	13,800	Pro	Lys
	Arg, Lys rich AL (f2a2,IIb1)	1	10.8	9.3	129	14,000	AcetylSer	Lys
Arg rich	Arg rich AR (f3,III)	3	9.6	13.3	135	15,300	Ala	Ala
	Gly, Arg rich GAR (f2a1,IV)	2	9.8	13.7	102	11,300	AcetylSer	Gly

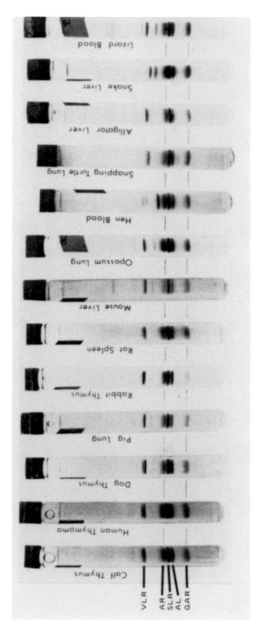

Fig. 8.2. Polyacrylamide gel electrophoresis patterns of vertebrate histones (from 197). The direction of migration is from top to bottom.

10
AcetylSer-Gly -Arg-Gly -Lys-Gly -Gly -Lys-Gly -Leu-Gly -Lys-Gly -Gly -Ala-

20
Lys (Ac)- Arg -His -Arg -Lys (Me) -Val -Leu-Arg-Asp-Asn - Ile -Gln -Gly - Ile -

30   40
Thr -Lys -Pro -Ala - Ile -Arg-Arg-Leu-Ala -Arg-Arg-Gly -Gly -Val -Lys-Arg-

50   60
Ile - Ser - Gly - Leu- Ile -Tyr-Glu -Glu -Thr-Arg-Gly -Val - Leu-Lys-Val -Phe-

70
Leu- Glu - Asn- Val - Ile -Arg-Asp-Ala -Val -Thr-Tyr-Thr-Glu -His -Ala -Lys-

80   90
Arg -Lys -Thr-Val -Thr-Ala -Met-Asp-Val -Val -Tyr-Ala -Leu-Lys-Arg-Gln -

100
Gly - Arg-Thr-Leu-Tyr-Gly -Phe-Gly -Gly-COOH.

Fig. 8.3. Sequence of the GAR(f2a1,IV) histone from calf thymus. Basic clusters are under-lined. (from 182).

5   10   15
H-Pro- Glu-Pro-Ala -Lys-Ser -Ala -Pro-Ala -Pro-Lys-Lys-Gly -Ser -Lys -Lys-Ala -Val -Thr-

20   25   30   35
Lys-Ala -Gln - Lys-Lys-Asp-Gly -Lys-Lys-Arg-Lys-Arg-Ser -Arg-Lys-Glu -Ser -Tyr-Ser -

40   45   50   55
Val -Tyr-Val -Tyr-Lys-Val -Leu-Lys-Gln -Val -His -Pro-Asp-Thr-Gly - Ile - Ser -Ser -Lys-

60   65   70   75
Ala -Met-Gly - Ile - Met-Asn-Ser -Phe-Val -Asn-Asp - Ile -Phe-Glu -Arg - Ile -Ala -Gly -Glu -

80   85   90   95
Ala -Ser -Arg-Leu-Ala -His -Tyr-Asn-Lys-Arg-Ser -Thr - Ile -Thr-Ser -Arg-Glu - Ile -Gln -

100   105   110
Thr-Ala -Val -Arg-Leu-Leu-Leu-Pro-Gly -Glu -Leu-Ala -Lys-His -Ala -Val -Ser -Glu -Gly -

115   120   125
Thr-Lys-Ala -Val -Thr-Lys-Tyr-Thr-Ser -Ser -Lys-OH.

Fig. 8.4. Sequence of the SLR (f2b, IIb2) histone from calf thymus (from 125).

10
Ac -Ser -Glu -Ala -Pro-Ala -Glu -Thr-Ala -Ala -Pro-Ala -Pro-Ala -Glu -Lys-Ser -Pro-Ala -

20   30
Lys-Lys-Lys-Lys-Ala -Ala -Lys-Lys-Pro-Gly -Ala -Gly -Ala -Ala -Lys-Arg-Lys-Ala -Ala -

40   50
Gly -Pro-Pro-Val -Ser -Glu -Leu - Ile -Thr-Lys-Ala -Val -Ala -Ala -Ser -Lys-Glu -Arg-Asn-

60   70
Gly -Leu-Ser -Leu-Ala -Ala -Leu-Lys-Lys-Ala -Leu-Ala -Ala -Gly -Gly -Tyr-

Fig. 8.5. The amino terminal amino acid sequence of VLR(f1,I) histone of rabbit thymus, fraction 3 (from 219).

$$\text{H}_2\text{N-Ala -Arg-Thr-Lys-Gln -Thr-Ala -}\underset{9}{\underline{\text{Arg- Lys}}}\,(\text{CH}_3)_{0-2}\text{-}\underset{10}{\text{Ser}}\text{- Thr-Gly -Gly -}\underset{14}{\text{Lys}}\,(\text{Ac})\text{-Ala -}$$

$$\text{Pro-}\underset{20}{\text{Arg}}\text{-Lys-Gln -Leu-Ala -Thr-}\underset{23}{\text{Lys}}\,(\text{Ac})\text{-Ala -Ala -}\underset{27}{\underline{\text{Arg- Lys}}}\,(\text{CH}_3)_{0-2}\text{-Ser -Ala -}\underset{30}{\text{Pro}}\text{-Ala -}$$

$$\text{Thr-Gly -Gly -Val -Lys-Lys-Pro-His -}\underset{40}{\text{Arg}}\text{-Tyr-Arg-Pro-Gly -Thr-Val -Ala -Leu-Arg-}\underset{50}{\text{Glu-}}$$

$$\text{Ile - Arg-Arg-Tyr-Gln -Lys-Ser -Thr-Glu -}\underset{60}{\text{Leu-}}\text{Leu - Ile -}\underline{\text{Arg- Lys}}\text{-Leu- Pro- Phe-Gln -Arg-}$$

$$\underset{70}{\text{Leu-}}\text{Val -Arg-Glu - Ile - Ala -Gln -Asp-Phe-Lys-}\underset{80}{\text{Thr-}}\text{Asp- Leu-Arg-Phe-Gln -Ser -Ser -Ala -}$$

$$\underset{90}{\text{Val}}\text{ -Met-Ala -Leu-Gln -Glu -Ala -Cys-Glu -Ala -}\underset{100}{\text{Tyr-}}\text{Leu-Val -Gly -Leu-Phe-Glu -Asp-Thr-}$$

$$\underset{110}{\text{Asn-}}\text{Leu-Cys-Ala - Ile - His -Ala -Lys-Arg-Val -Thr -}\underset{120}{\text{Ile}}\text{ -Met-Pro-Lys-Asp - Ile -Gln -Leu-}$$

$$\underset{130}{\text{Ala}}\text{ -}\underline{\text{Arg-Arg}}\text{ - Ile -Arg-Gly -Glu -Arg-Ala -COOH.}\quad\underset{135}{}$$

Fig. 8.6. The amino acid sequence of the AR (f3,III) histone from calf thymus (from **70**).

This finding suggests that these regions of the AL and GAR histones have similar functions (183). It is of interest that three histones have the same amino terminal, N-acetylserine, and three have a carboxyl-terminal lysine.

IV. Histones and Chromatin Structure

Chromatin is the functional form of the eukaryotic chromosome in which DNA is found in close association with various other macromolecules. The structure of chromatin is dependent on the cell type, its cycle stage, its age, and the method of extraction. Metaphase chromatin contains 13–20% DNA, 8–15% RNA, and 68–79% protein (63). Most studies were performed on interphase chromatin which represents chromatin fibers largely in an extended form. Interphase chromatin contains about 25% DNA, less RNA (3–5%), and about 70% protein. The histone to NHP ratio ranges from 0.25:1 to approximately 1:1 and varies from cell type to cell type (45, 51, 63, 77, 92, 118, 143, 164, 231). It has been suggested that some increases in RNA synthesis are associated with structural modifications in chromatin (28, 196, 284) that make new sites of DNA available for transcription (140, 282, 294a; also, see Chapter IV).

Although the structure of chromatin is not well defined, a number of recent studies have provided some insight into how histones fit into the chromatin matrix (Fig. 8.8) and how they interact with DNA (See Chapter IV). Whether histones bind to the large or small groove of the DNA double helix has been an open question. The elucidation of the amino acid sequence of the GAR (f2a1,IV) histone allowed construction of space-filling models in which the amino terminal region of the GAR histone (243, 272) was fitted as an α-helix in the large groove of the DNA double helix (Fig. 8.8). The α-amino groups

```
 1                            10                      15
AceylSer-Gly -Arg-Gly- Lys-Gln -Gly -Gly -Lys-Ala -Arg-Ala -Lys-Ala -Lys-Thr-Arg-Ser -

   20                  25                   30                   35
Ser -Arg -Ala -Gly -Leu-Gln -Phe-Pro-Val -Gly -Arg-Val -His -Arg-Leu-Leu-Arg-Lys-Gly -

         40                 45                    50                   55
Asn-Tyr-Ala -Glu -Arg-Val -Gly -Ala -Gly -Ala -Pro-Val -Tyr-Leu-Ala -Ala -Val -Leu-Glu -

           60                  65                   70                   75
Tyr-Leu-Thr-Ala -Glu - Ile - Leu-Glu -Leu-Ala -Gly -Asn-Ala -Ala -Arg-Asp-Asn-Lys-Lys-

             80                  85                   90
Thr-Arg - Ile - Ile - Pro-Arg-His -Leu-Gln -Leu-Ala - Ile - Arg-Asn-Asp-Glu -Glu -Leu-Asn-

 95                 100                   105                   110
Lys-Leu-Leu-Gly -Lys-Val -Thr - Ile -Ala -Gln -Gly -Gly -Val -Leu-Pro-Asn - Ile -Gln -Ala -

   115                120                   125                   130
Val -Leu-Leu-Pro-Lys-Lys-Thr-Glu -Ser -His -His -Lys-Ala -Lys-Gly -Lys-COOH.
```

A

Fig. 8.7A. Sequence of the AL (f2a2,II1) histone from calf thymus (from 295).

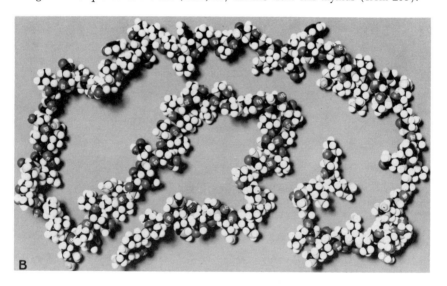

Fig. 8.7B. Molecular model of the AL histone.

of lysine residues in this model aligned to form salt bridges with the phosphate residues in DNA. A similar arrangement is possible with the AL (f2a2,IIb1) histone (183). Since histone I does not inhibit the binding of actinomycin D, it may also bind to the major groove of DNA (182a, 208a).

Numerous physical studies including circular dichroism studies showed that the GAR histone assumes a more α-helical structure when bound to DNA than when free in solution (245). Conversely, when the lysine-rich histone is bound to DNA, the physical behavior is that of a protein in the extended form (246). Proton magnetic resonance studies on the SLR (f2b,IIb2) histone support the idea that basic regions are the primary sites of interaction (43). Nonbasic regions

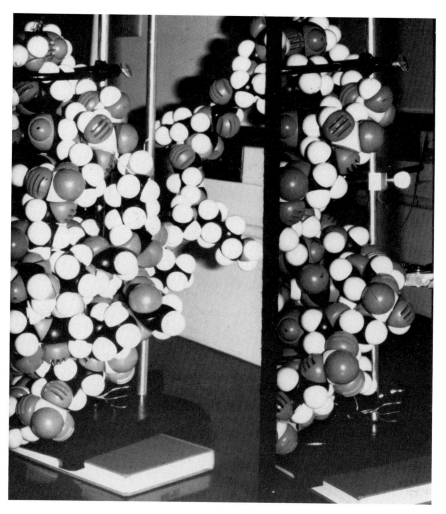

Fig. 8.8. DNA-histone molecular model showing dense packing of atoms in the complex. Left, GAR (f2a1,IV) histone in the large groove of DNA. Right, "naked" DNA double helix.

seem to have secondary structures that may be sites for histone—histone interactions. Thermal denaturation profiles of various DNA histone complexes indicate that the effects of each histone on DNA structure are quite specific (16). Similar studies on the interaction of half molecules of the SLR (f2b,IIb2) histone with DNA show that the amino terminal half of this molecule stabilizes the DNA against thermal denaturation better than the carboxyl terminal portion (155).

Various histones differ in their apparent manner of attachment to the chromatin matrix. The lysine-rich groups of histones (f1, f2b, and f2a2) are more easily extracted with NaCl than are the arginine-rich (f2a1 and f3) histones (38). If deoxycholate which apparently specifically binds to hydrophobic regions is used as a dissociating agent, the arginine-rich and slightly lysine-rich histones are selectively removed while the very lysine-rich histones are last to be extracted (106). In addition, histones appear to interact with DNA both by electrostatic and hydrophobic types of bonds (29).

Although the number of basic amino acids nearly equals the number of negatively charged nucleotides in chromatin (278), there is evidence to suggest that the proteins are unevenly distributed on the DNA. Titration of chromatin with polylysine, nuclease digestion, and exchange of protein between radioactively labeled and unlabeled DNA indicate that one third to one half of the DNA is "open" and not covered by protein (62, 124). Other studies have shown that the accessibility of DNA in chromatin was such that up to 71.5% of the DNA was digested (174).

The proteins associated with chromatin have basic regions, presumably contributed mostly by histones, which are exposed and not tightly bound to DNA. Modification of rabbit liver chromatin with acetic anhydride reached a limiting value of acetylation of 54 amino acid residues/100 DNA base pairs (242). A subsequent study employing limited digestion of chromatin with trypsin showed that 55 peptide bonds per 100 DNA base pairs were susceptible to cleavage (250). Tryptic digestion did not alter thermal denaturation profiles appreciably, indicating that sites of DNA–histone interaction were not altered. Moreover, other physical characteristics such as flow dichroism, specific viscosity, and circular dichroism of the modified chromatin appeared to be identical to those of free DNA. Among others, one idea is that chromatin has a supercoil conformation and that the histones act to promote supercoiling. The center regions of histones may interact with one another to produce this effect while the ends of the proteins bind to DNA. X-Ray diffraction studies also support a supercoil model for nucleohistones (200).

V. Modified Amino Acids in Histones

Figures 8.3–8.7 show that a number of amino acids in histones are modified by phosphorylation, acetylation, and methylation. The presence of these modifying groups introduces microheterogeneity into some of the histone fractions. The structures of the modified amino acids are shown in Table 8.2.

A. Phosphorylation of Histones

Phosphate is esterified to the hydroxyl of serine and possibly to a lesser extent to threonine; under various conditions, phosphate is found in all of the major histones. The placement of a negatively charged phosphate moiety on a positively charged protein might be expected to change the conformation of that protein or to lessen its binding affinity for DNA. Therefore, phosphorylation could act to (a) "uncover" specific genes which are repressed by histones, (b) modify the structure of chromatin in preparation for DNA synthesis and cell division, or (c) aid in the removal of the histones from DNA to facilitate replacement

TABLE 8.2
CHEMICAL MODIFICATIONS OF HISTONES

Modifying group	Structure of modified amino acid	Histones modified	References
Phosphoryl	Phosphoserine[a]	GAR (f2a1, IV)	169
		AL (f2a2, IIb1)	169, 272a
		AR (f3, III)	112, 169
		VLR (f1, I)	23, 112, 142, 150, 169, 241
		SLR (f2b, IIb2)	112, 169
		V (f2c)	2, 177
Acetyl[b]	α-N-Acetylserine	AL (f2a2, IIb1),	205, 206
		GAR (f2a1, V)	219
		VLR (f1, I)	
	ε-N-Acetyllysine	GAR (f2a, IV)	198, 211–213
		and AR (f3, III)	55, 57, 68, 70, 280, 280a
		(best acceptors)	55-57, 280-280a
		Other histones	
Methyl	ε-N-Mono- and dimethyllysine[c]	GAR (f2a1, IV),	68, 70, 114, 115, 182, 233
		AR (f3, III)	
		(major)	
	3-Methylhistidine	VLR (f1, I) and	94
		V (f2c)	

Structure of Phosphoserine:
$H_2N-\overset{H}{\underset{CH_2}{C}}-COOH$, $CH_2-O-P(=O)(OH)-O^-$

Structure of α-N-Acetylserine:
$CH_3\overset{O}{\overset{\|}{C}}-N-\overset{H}{\underset{CH_2}{C}}-COOH$, with OH

Structure of ε-N-Acetyllysine:
$H_2N-\overset{H}{\underset{(CH_2)_4}{C}}-COOH$, $HN-\overset{O}{\overset{\|}{C}}-CH_3$

Structure of ε-N-Mono- and dimethyllysine:
$H_2N-\overset{H}{\underset{(CH_2)_4}{C}}-COOH$, $N(CH_3)_{(1-2)}$, $H_{(0-1)}$

Structure of 3-Methylhistidine

TABLE 8.2 (*Continued*)

Modifying group	Structure of modified amino acid	Histones modified	References
	ω-N-methylarginine[d]	Crude histone	192

$$H_2N-C-COOH$$
$$(CH_2)_3$$
$$NH-C\overset{NH}{\underset{H}{\diagup}}N-CH_3$$

[a] Phosphothreonine has been reported to be present but was not observed in sequence studies (142, 189).

[b] The presence of O-acetyl groups has been noted in some instances (91a, 180, 180a, 212, 213).

[c] Trimethyllysine has been reported but not confirmed in peptides derived from histones (114, 115, 191).

[d] *In vitro* studies have shown that histones can be enzymically modified to contain 2-methyl-guanidinomethylarginine (135).

by another type of protein. Table 8.3 shows a number of correlations of histone phosphorylation with biological events.

A specific kinase of liver catalyzes the *in vitro* incorporation of phosphate into histones and this activity is stimulated by adenosine-3′, 5′-cyclic phosphate (cyclic AMP) (149). *In vivo* experiments demonstrated that a specific serine residue in a lysine-rich histone is phosphorylated in liver cells treated with dibutyryl cyclic AMP (150). Glucagon and, to a lesser extent, insulin stimulated this cyclic AMP-mediated phosphorylation of a lysine-rich histone in liver (151). At present, studies on other histone kinases are in progress.

TABLE 8.3
PHOSPHORYLATION OF HISTONES

Possible function of phosphorylation	Biological event or system	Site of phosphorylation	Ref.
Gene activation	Glucagon stimulation	VLR (f1,I) histones	149, 150, 151
Cell division	Regenerating liver	VLR (f1,I) histones	23, 43a, 189a, 270a
		AL (f2a2,IIb1) histone	272a
		All histone fractions	105b
	Morris hepatomas	VLR (f1,I) histones	21
	Cultured Ehrlich ascites and	VLR (f1,I) histones	241
	Morris hepatoma cells		22
	Cultured Chinese hamster ovary cells	VLR (f1,I) and SLR (f2b,IIb2)	237, 238
Replacement of histones	Spermiogenesis in trout testes	All major fractions	168

The level of glucagon-stimulated phosphorylation is on the order of 1% of the total lysine-rich histones (151). This is consistent with the activation of a small percentage of the genome of nondividing cells. However, this is the only well-defined instance which correlates histone phosphorylation with gene activation; the exact molecular events are still obscure.

A second type of phosphorylation has been observed which seems to be associated with cell division in regenerating liver and cell cultures (Table 8.3). With high resolution electrophoretic techniques for the study of lysine-rich histone phosphorylation (23, 241), one subfraction (the major one) of VLR (f1,I) histones reaches its maximum level of phosphorylation 29 hours after partial hepatectomy (23). The rapidly dividing Ehrlich ascites tumor cells (241) or Morris hepatoma cells in culture (22) have a much higher level of phosphorylation in the lysine-rich histones than normal tissues (23). When these studies were extended to a series of Morris hepatomas with varying growth rates (21), a positive correlation was found between growth rate and the degree of phosphorylation of one of the VLR (f1,I) histone subfractions (Fig. 8.9). Phosphorylation of the VLR (f1,I) histone may be an obligatory event in DNA synthesis or cell replication since the f1 histone is phosphorylated only during DNA syntheses (24). Since this type of phosphorylation is largely present in rapidly replicating tissues and essentially absent in stationary tissues, this modification is probably related more to cell division than gene expression.

A third type of histone phosphorylation occurs in the transformation of precursor cells to sperm cells (168). This process is accompanied by an increase in

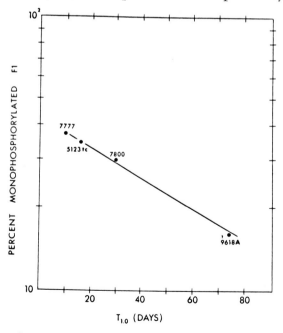

Fig. 8.9. Phosphorylation of VLR (f1,I) histone correlated with growth rate. $T_{1.0}$ is the time required for a transplanted tumor to grow to 1 gm. The numbers on the data points indicate the type of Morris hepatoma studied (from 22).

histone content and a decrease in nonhistone proteins of trout testis and later by a complete replacement of the histones by the highly basic protamines. A marked decrease in template activity of DNA results from this process. In this replacement process, preformed histones are phosphorylated (168). This phosphorylation may be related to the removal of histones from DNA in preparation for replacement by protamine or may serve as a signal for specific histone proteases (169). However, it is equally plausible that phosphorylation and subsequent dephosphorylation are important in the "annealing" of highly basic portions of histones onto the DNA double helix (160).

B. Acetylation of Histones

Two distinct types of acetylation are found in the histones, (a) acetylation of amino terminal moieties and (b) "internal" acetylation of the ϵ-amino groups of lysine. The amino terminal serine residues of the GAR (f2a1,IV), AL (f2a2,IIb1), and lysine-rich (f1,I) histones are N-acetylated (205, 206, 219). During the life-time of the histone, the α-NH$_2$-acetyl groups do not appear to turn over appreciably (95, 292). In the f2a (GAR and AL) histones, N-acetyl-seryl-tRNA has been reported to serve as the initiator complex for synthesis of these proteins (157). Chain initiation in these histones seems to be a unique case since N-formylmethionine or methionine has been found to be the initiator in other systems.

The acetyl groups of the ϵ-amines of lysine are metabolically active, turn over at varying rates in different tissues, and are found in fractional molar ratios at specific sites in histone molecules. These acetyl groups have been found in all histones except the VLR (f1,I) histones.

C. Physiological Significance of Histone Acetylation

The physiological significance of histone acetylation is uncertain. Acetylation of the free ϵ-amino groups of lysine eliminates the positive charge of this group. As with phosphorylation, this modification should be capable of changing the charge characteristics, the conformation, or the mode of binding of the histone to DNA.

Some examples of correlation of acetylation with events in cell cycle or gene expression have been reported (10). In various calf organs (198), the rapidly dividing tissues contain roughly equal amounts of the acetylated form of the GAR histone (f2a1,IV) and the nonacetylated parent histone. Slowly dividing tissues contain considerably more of the unmodified GAR histone. In regenerating liver, an increase in acetylation of arginine-rich histones was reported to precede the increase in RNA synthesis (212, 213). Similar changes occur in human lymphocytes stimulated with phytohemagglutinin (211). However, turnover rates of acetyl groups in arginine-rich histones do not vary appreciably with growth rate in a series of Morris hepatomas and liver (53). Moreover, in Novikoff hepatoma the acetyl groups of histones turn over much more slowly than in normal liver. Although this effect could be explained by the low level of histone deacetylase found in Novikoff hepatoma (156), it does not support the concept of an important control function for acetylation.

Although there are temporal relationships between histone acetylation and various events in the cell cycle or gene activation, no direct relationship has been proved. Acetylation may be one of several processes that must occur before a specific gene segment is selected for activation (12). Alternatively, partial acetylation of specific residues of histones may serve to neutralize the repulsive effects of closely spaced amino groups during histone binding to DNA (56, 57, 160). During the slow annealing of histones onto the DNA double helix, acetylases and deacetylases may serve to properly orient the amino groups of the histones.

D. Methylation of Histones

ε-Methylation of lysine (176) in histones is highly specific. The GAR (f2a1,IV) histone (calf thymus) is methylated at lysine 20 (68, 182); 75% of the molecules contained a dimethyl-and 25% a monomethyllysine (182). Pea seedlings do not contain methylated residues in the GAR histone (69).

In addition to methylated lysine, methylated histidine and arginine have been found (94). 3-Methylhistidine is present in duck erythrocyte histone fractions I and V. Calf thymus histones contain small amounts of methylarginine while rat liver histones contain significant amounts of this derivative (193).

In contrast to phosphorylation and acetylation reactions which occur in S phase or early in the cell cycle (238, 239), methylation of histones seems to occur late in the cell cycle (110, 231a, 275). In addition, the turnover rate of methyl groups seems to be similar to that of the parent histones, indicating that methylation is essentially an irreversible process (54).

E. Function of Methylation of Histones

Because of the small size of the methyl group and the relatively small change in the pK of the ε-amino group by introduction of the methyl moiety, any change in the general characteristics of the protein must be subtle. Changes in conformation or in susceptibility to specific proteolysis may result. Methylation may play a role in the condensation of chromatin late in the cell cycle prior to mitosis (94, 275).

VI. Histone Synthesis and Metabolism

A. Site of Histone Synthesis

Although it seemed possible that histone synthesis occurred in the nucleus (8, 9, 84, 220, 221), evidence for cytoplasmic synthesis of histones first emerged from cytochemical studies on developing grasshopper spermatids (34a). Later, HeLa cells synchronized by selective detachment of cells in mitosis were found to synthesize histones on isolated small polysomes during S phase. A rapidly labeled 7–9 S mRNA fraction (Chapter V) was associated with these polysomes (41).

Cytoplasmic histone synthesis was confirmed by studies on HeLa cell microsome preparations (89–91) and in sea urchin embryo polyribosomes (146, 179). Messenger RNA coding for histones has been isolated from HeLa cells and translated into protein by cell free extracts of mouse ascites tumor (see Chapter V).

Although there is now good evidence that histones are synthesized in the cytoplasm in several cell types, it is not yet clear whether all synthesis occurs in the cytoplasm. Since some cytoplasmic contamination of nuclear preparations may occur and vice versa, more definitive studies are needed to finally establish whether no histone synthesis occurs in the nucleus.

B. Time of Synthesis

The synthesis of DNA and histones generally appear to be closely coupled in the S phase. Early histochemical and autoradiographic studies indicated that histones and DNA were synthesized concurrently in several tissues including liver and mouse fibroblasts (35), in *Euplotes eurytomus* (216), and in HeLa cells and Chinese hamster cells in tissue culture (170b, 224). Histone synthesis stopped when DNA synthesis was inhibited by hydroxyurea in HeLa cell microsomal preparations (91). In some studies, only part of the histone synthesis in HeLa cells was parallel with DNA synthesis (228), and different histone fractions differed in the degrees of their association with DNA synthesis (58). The degree of concurrence of synthesis of DNA and histones may vary from cell to cell depending on the physiological or developmental state of each cell. Rapidly proliferating and relatively undifferentiated cell types seem to have less correlation between histone and DNA synthesis. Significant amounts of histone synthesis, however, have been reported during G_2, M, and G_1 phases in addition to the major amount of synthesis during S phase (105).

Thus, there is general agreement that the bulk of histone synthesis occurs concurrently with DNA synthesis; some histone synthesis and turnover may occur during other times of the cell cycle independent of DNA synthesis. Operationally, a small degree of asynchrony in cell populations could account for apparent independence from DNA synthesis.

C. Histone Turnover

The DNA-histone complex is metabolically stable as shown by the lack of significant differences in turnover rates of DNA and histones (52). In Chinese hamster cells in tissue culture, all histones except the lysine-rich group were metabolically stable. However, during inhibition of DNA synthesis, all the histones turned over slowly and the lysine-rich histones turned over faster than all other types of histones. In HeLa cells and mouse mastocytes there was essentially no turnover of histones unrelated to new DNA synthesis over eight generations (108).

In general, histone turnover appears to be very slow in the systems studied to date. Any observed turnover of histones may be attributed to cell death, cell replacement, or possibly gene regulation.

D. Differential Rates of Histone Synthesis

There are conflicting reports of differential rates of synthesis of various histone subfractions. Differences in rates of biosynthesis of histone fractions were found in liver and hepatoma (83, 120, 121). In Walker tumor, [^{14}C]lysine was incorporated faster in the arginine-rich histones than in the VLR histones. In other studies [^{14}C]leucine incorporation into lysine-rich histones was greatest in tissues undergoing cell division while incorporation was more active in the arginine-rich histones in cells not synthesizing DNA at a significant rate (59).

During pregnancy and lactation, the rates of synthesis for lysine-rich and arginine-rich histones were greater than for slightly lysine-rich fractions (270). In mouse mammary gland explants, a mixture of cortisol, prolactin, and insulin first depressed the incorporation of lysine into one of the lysine-rich subfractions and later elevated incorporation into another. There is need for care in interpretation of these results because of possible pool effects and possible contamination with rapidly labeled NHP (nonhistone proteins) in preparations used for these metabolic studies (118).

VII. Functions of Histones

The histones are found in the chromatin of all eukaryotic organisms but not in the prokaryotes. Along with the nuclear membrane, the presence of histones is a feature which distinguishes the eukaryotes from prokaryotes. Although the proposal that histones repress genome segments was supported by *in vitro* studies on transcription, neither the precise roles they play in specific genetic regulation nor their roles as structural elements of chromatin are well defined.

Histones in Genetic Restriction

Studies on pea seedlings first showed that histones added to DNA dramatically reduced its transcription by RNA polymerase (122). However, the insolubility of the DNA-histone complex is such that this addition of histones simply resulted in unavailability of DNA as a template. Subsequent studies have shown that stepwise removal of histones from chromatin increase its template activity (14, 19) possibly also because of its greater solubility (130b, 252a).

Since histone synthesis is closely coupled to DNA synthesis, it has been presumed that histones are either needed immediately to repress segments of newly synthesized DNA or that they are necessary for functional chromatin structure. Histones may also be required to suppress further synthesis of DNA (118, 287) or to prevent its cleavage by DNase (62).

Even if such evidence indicated participation of histones in gene repression, the problem of the specificity of histones for such repression is a difficult one. There are simply not enough unique species of histones to serve the function of specifically repressing the multitude of genes that need to be repressed in each cell type. Further, there is no evidence that specific histones combine with specific genes (244). Although the relative amounts of various histones vary somewhat from tissue to tissue, the histone electrophoretic patterns are generally very similar within a given organism (196).

A notable exception to the above general rule is seen in avian erythrocytes where there is a unique histone (V, f2c) which is rich in lysine and serine (116, 178). This histone replaces the lysine-rich histones during maturation of erythrocytes in birds, (71) and the nucleus becomes genetically inactive. The appearance of histone V is believed to be associated with the complete repression of the erythrocyte genome. Tissue specificity of histones has been reported for lung which has little cell replication; an extra histone (f1°) is present in lung that is absent in the rapidly dividing cells such as ascites tumors (199). However, its absence or reduction in amount does not seem to be universally related either to neoplasia or rapid growth (24a). This histone is similar to the lysine-rich histones but has a greater electrophoretic mobility.

Since mouse mamary gland explants in a medium containing insulin, cortisol, and prolactin first reduce the incorporation of lysine into one of the lysine-rich subfractions and then increase the synthesis of another subfraction (119), it was suggested that this restructuring of newly synthesized chromatin could alter the state of differentiation of cells.

Another instance of a relation between histones and gene regulation is the observation that one fraction of the VLR(f1,I) histones of rabbit thymus (fraction 3) is readily phosphorylated by a specific histone kinase whereas fraction 4 does not respond to the enzyme (152). The serine residue which is phosphorylated in fraction 4 is replaced by an alanine residue in fraction 3. It is conceivable that the chromatin of a cell type programmed to respond to phosphorylation could have a different distribution of the fractions 3 and 4 of the VLR histones in the chromatin matrix.

The above examples point to a special role which seems to be played by the VLR histones. Although the role played by most histones in gene expression appears to be somewhat limited, it has not been established whether they act alone or in concert with the nonhistone proteins. Because of the large amounts of histones present in the chromatin, their function would appear to be largely structural although a regulatory role cannot yet be excluded. Up to the present time, histones of cancer cells have not been found to have unique or differentiating features from histones of other cells (45).

VIII. Nonhistone Nuclear Proteins

In view of the uncertainties about the role of the histones as gene regulatory proteins, studies were initiated in our and other laboratories on the possible gene regulatory role of the NHP (nonhistone proteins) more than a decade ago (45).* One proposal for possible gene regulation by the NHP was that these proteins might be capable of forming complexes with histones and displacing them from DNA (Fig. 8.10), and another was that such proteins bind directly to DNA (45, 60, 164, 269, 277). Although early studies were made on turnover, composition, and terminals of these proteins in mammalian tissues (45), the initial studies of their roles as gene regulators were made with prokaryotic cells. Recently, it became possible to identify and characterize the "*lac* repressor" of *E. coli* (96), the lambda phage repressor (5, 27, 222), a repressor for the tryptophan operon (27, 301), and factors involved in control of the bacterial RNA polymerases (131).

The studies on bacterial systems had the remarkable advantages of the availability of mutants, including temperature-sensitive mutants that permitted very rapid advances in the isolation and structural analyses of the *lac* repressor (3) which have led to a partial sequence (Fig. 8.11) and some understanding

* There are now many reviews on the subject of nonhistone nuclear proteins (10–12, 30, 37–39, 44–51, 63, 72, 92, 113, 117, 118, 138, 143, 164–166, 170a, 258, 263, 266, 276).

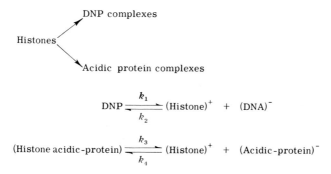

$$\text{Histones} \Big\langle \begin{array}{l} \text{DNP complexes} \\ \text{Acidic protein complexes} \end{array}$$

$$\text{DNP} \underset{k_2}{\overset{k_1}{\rightleftharpoons}} (\text{Histone})^+ + (\text{DNA})^-$$

$$(\text{Histone acidic-protein}) \underset{k_4}{\overset{k_3}{\rightleftharpoons}} (\text{Histone})^+ + (\text{Acidic-protein})^-$$

Fig. 8.10. A proposed scheme of gene regulation by NHP. NHP form complexes with histones thereby displacing them from DNA.

H₂N-Met-Lys-Pro-Val-Thr-Leu-Tyr-Asp-Val-Ala-Glu-Tyr-Ala-Gly-Val-Ser-Tyr-

Gln-Thr-Val-Ser-Arg-Val-Val-Asp-Gln-Ala-Ser-His-Val-Ser-Ala-Lys-Thr-

Arg-Glu-Lys-Val-Glu-Ala-Ala-Met-Ala-Glu-Leu-Asx-Tyr-Ile-Pro-Asx-

Fig. 8.11. The amino acid sequence of the *N*-terminal region of the *lac* repressor (from 3).

of its mechanism of binding to DNA. One of the most interesting features of the *lac* repressor is its very tight binding to its operator DNA; its dissociation constant is 10^{-12} M (129). Although DNA binding proteins have been found in a variety of mammalian cells and it is possible that they control growth and possibly other cellular activities such as rRNA synthesis (64), clear correlation of their binding, mRNA synthesis, and specific cell functions have not yet been provided despite some evidence that such controls exist in a number of endocrine glands (see Section VIII,H).

A. NHP and Chromatin

On the basis of evidence from bacterial systems, it is generally assumed that gene repressors have specific binding sites on DNA. However, unlike the bacterial systems where most of the DNA-binding proteins appear to have repressor function, in the mammalian cells it appears that the active chromatin has a higher content of NHP than inactive chromatin and that NHP involved in gene control generally have derepressor rather than repressor function. In current studies, the systems for binding analysis of the NHP are similar to those developed for the prokaryotes (104, 141, 158b, 282) and include affinity chromatography which has been useful for the steroid-binding proteins and other binding proteins (65, 66, 289a).

Nuclei and chromatin preparations of active tissues contain larger amounts of NHP than corresponding preparations of inactive tissues (266). However, it seems likely that many of these proteins are synthetic enzymes, proteins of nuclear ribonucleoprotein (RNP) complexes engaged in transport of preribosomal RNP particles, or proteins of preribosomal RNP particles. There appear to be much larger numbers of NHP with faster turnover rates than histones (260, 261, 264, 266) in nuclei and nucleoli (Fig. 8.1) which would be appropriate for regulator molecules. It seems likely that gene control proteins are present in very small numbers. Despite remarkable improvements in methods for identification and analysis of these proteins, significantly improved methods will be necessary to identify them satisfactorily. In studies on gene regulatory proteins, it is also important to note that some may not be "nucleus-specific" but may be "cytonucleoproteins" that travel to-and-fro from the nucleus to the cytoplasm and are only fleetingly chromatin bound (100–102, 194). Some of these proteins may be in the saline (0.15 M NaCl) extracts of cell nuclei (19, 20, 45).

B. Extrinsic Effects on NHP

Additional evidence for a role of the NHP in nuclear function is their change in various biological events. Recently, interactions have been reported for specific NHP and carcinogens, drugs, and plant and mammalian hormones (5, 6, 25, 81, 82, 107, 111, 126, 132, 146, 159, 185, 227, 263, 272a, 279). Moreover, the

NHP vary with different stages of the cell cycle (30, 165, 215, 266, 276) and with age (162, 208, 281, 299). Similarly, changes in enzymes have been related to specific NHP molecules (83a, 209, 214, 215). On the basis of evidence from prokaryotes, induced changes in biologically active tissues and their large number, the NHP apparently are important control molecules.

C. Sources of Nonhistone Proteins

The nonhistone nuclear proteins include the nuclear enzymes and other proteins of the nucleus except for the histones. Therefore, the source material for studies on these proteins may be the whole nucleus or parts of it such as chromatin, the nucleoplasm, or nucleoli. Many of the studies have been performed on isolated chromatin, because its nonhistone proteins are presumably closely associated with DNA and evidence for some functional specificity has been provided.

The nucleoprotein complex of chromatin may be isolated as a residue from whole cells after extraction with dilute saline followed by differential centrifugation through sucrose density gradients (38, 167) to remove cytoplasmic and soluble nuclear components. Alternatively, chromatin may be prepared similarly from isolated cellular components such as nuclei (195, 235) or nucleoli (290) to avoid contamination by cytoplasmic proteins which tend to adhere to chromatin strands (130a).

D. Isolation of Nonhistone Proteins

Because methods for isolation of NHP are relatively primitive (Table 8.4) by comparison to procedures for histones, many methods have been employed (33, 45, 51, 63, 74, 75, 81, 118, 143, 164, 166, 231, 234, 258, 270). In general, the nonhistone proteins may be dissociated from the nucleoprotein complex and solubilized by high concentrations of NaCl (2–3 M) and urea (5–7 M) (17, 31, 235, 298) or guanidine hydrochloride in concentrations up to 5 M (153). Separation of histones from nonhistones may be achieved by ion exchange chromatography (153, 163), selective precipitation of the DNA-histone complex by 0.15 M NaCl (201), or preextraction of the histones with dilute mineral acid (79). Proteins which are difficult to solubilize or to dissociate from DNA may be extracted with sodium dodecyl sulfate (SDS) from preextracted chromatin or nuclei (153, 286, 290). Phenol extraction has been used to obtain a class of residual proteins which contain covalently bound phosphate (85, 274).

E. Fractionation and General Characteristics of NHP

Because of the limited resolution and sensitivity of present methodology, the precise number of NHP species is not known in any tissue. In rat liver, the

TABLE 8.4

SUMMARY OF PRINCIPLE METHODS FOR OBTAINING NHP

Method[a,b]	Purpose of method	Reference
Bring to 1.5 M NaCl, ppt NHP with H$_2$SO$_4$	Solution and dissociation of DNP with high salt, ppt NHP from DNP	298
Suspension in large volumes of water, shear with Waring blender	Use of very dilute solutions for solubilization of DNP; NHP will ppt as gel	300
Bring to 1 M NaCl and disperse with Dounce homogenizer; dialyze against water	Dissociation with 1 M NaCl, removal of the DNA-histone complex after dialysis	286
Dissociated DNP, treat with Bio-Rex-70: discard resin	Bio-Rex-70 resin binds and removes histones	148
Apply solubilized NHP to column of DNA cellulose	Affinity chromatography removes specific DNA-binding proteins[c]	7
Wash nuclei with 0.35 M NaCl prior to extraction	Removes saline soluble NHP and cytoplasmic contamination	130a
Extract directly with 6 M urea, 0.4 M guanidine-HCl, 0.1% BME; remove nucleic acids by ultra-centrifugation; apply to Bio-Rex-70 column	Extraction and dissociation with high urea, separation of histones and NHP on column	153
Bring to 3 M NaCl and 7 M urea, DNA ppt	Avoidance of pH extremes by dissociation in high salt urea; a "mild" procedure	235
Bring to 3 M NaCl, separate DNA on Bio-gel A-50	Similar to above	235
Bring to 2 M NaCl and 0.05 M AlCl$_3$	AlCl$_3$ will ppt DNA + NHP; leaves histones in solution; a "mild" procedure	158a
Extract nuclei directly with 8 M urea, 0.05 M phosphate, pH 8.0.	One-step procedure to solubilize and extract NHP	103
Bring to 2 M NaCl with 5 M urea and then 0.0135 M LaCl$_3$	High salt solubilizes and dissociates DNP; LaCl$_3$ causes DNA to ppt leaving protein in solution	297
Extract nuclei directly with 0.1 M Salyrgan; sediment through sucrose	Salyrgan solubilizes chromatin including all NHP; a "mild" procedure	72a

[a] Starting material may be whole cells, nuclei, or chromatin. The treatment may dissociate and solubilize any one or combination of NHP, histones, and DNA.

[b] The starting material is usually in dilute or isotonic salt solutions at this point.

[c] Affinity chromatography can be used to isolate specific steroid-binding NHP proteins also (see text).

number of chromosomal NHP as observed after one-dimensional SDS gel electrophoresis is from 14 to 27 bands, with 70% of the protein found in 10–15 bands (80). Similar or greater numbers of proteins were found in the rabbit, spleen, kidney, and liver chromatin NHP fraction by SDS gels (153). In chromatin it appears that there is a limited number of the major NHP present. However, numerous minor protein bands not visible by staining techniques were detected by radioactive labeling (42, 154, 267). Recent studies on 0.4 N sulfuric acid extracts of nuclei and nucleoli of rat liver and Novikoff hepatoma have revealed the presence of 96 distinct protein spots on two-dimensional polyacrylamide gel electrophoresis as shown in Fig. 8.12 (190, 296). While 7–10 of these spots are histones, most of the proteins visualized are nonhistone proteins. This technique offers a vastly improved method for cataloging and surveying the NHP of various tissues.

The NHP of rat chromatin have been reported to range in molecular weight from about 5000 to 100,000 under dissociating conditions (79, 80) although many are probably larger in their undenatured state. In HeLa cells, chromosomal NHP had molecular weights from 15,000 to 180,000; 85% of the proteins had molecular weights greater than 40,000 (36).

Amino acid analyses carried out on various preparations have demonstrated that these mixtures are generally rich in glutamic and aspartic acids or their amides. Since the NHP are generally retained by anion exchange resins at approximately neutral pH, most are probably acidic. By isoelectric focusing, the isoelectric point of the rat liver chromatin NHP was reported to be 6–10 (17, 103).

Very little structural information is available on purified NHP. Recently, two nonhistone proteins θ and ϵ were isolated from rat liver chromatin (80). Protein ϵ had a single N-terminal glycine. A major protein of Novikoff hepatoma nucleoli has been isolated in a state of high purity (144); it has an amino terminal serine, a molecular weight of 60,000, and was found as a single band on one-dimensional gel electrophoresis. Comparison of the amino acid compositions of these proteins are shown in Table 8.5. Improved isolation and characterization of all the NHP is required.

F. Organ and Species Specificity

Unlike the histones which have similar electrophoretic profiles when obtained from various species and tissues, the nonhistone proteins have been found to vary from organ to organ and from species to species (67, 79, 80, 88, 142a, 152a, 236, 274, 288, 290). However, surveys of various tissues in the rat, chicken, and pea indicate that many of the nonhistone proteins are common to all organs of these species (79). Although very few tissue or species differences were found in comparing the NHP of several mouse and bovine tissues (163), the corresponding proteins from mouse brain had markedly different electrophoretic characteristics than other mouse tissues. As noted earlier, discrepancies in these reports may result from the presence of ribosomal and preribosomal proteins in the NHP as well as proteins of the informosomes (see Chapter V).

In particular, the nuclear phosphoproteins have been reported to have species specificity, both in their patterns of phosphorylation and electrophoretic mobilities (210, 274). Additional evidence of species specificity was obtained by an examination of their ability to form complexes with DNA of various species (161, 274). The greatest degree of binding of the nuclear phosphoproteins was found with the DNA from the same species. Rat phosphoproteins complexed best with rat DNA, to a lesser extent with mouse DNA, and not at all with

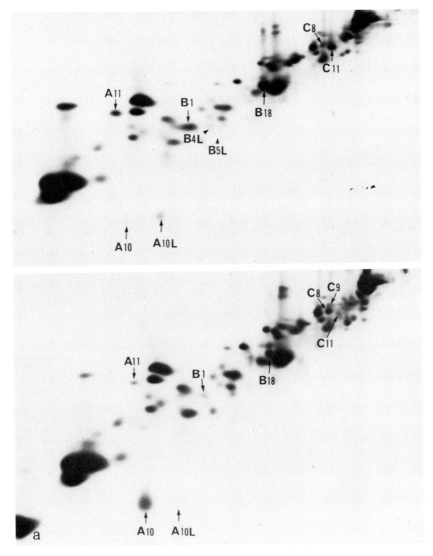

Fig. 8.12. Two-dimensional electrophoresis of nucleolar proteins. (a). Top, normal liver nucleolar proteins. Bottom, Novikoff hepatoma nucleolar proteins. (b) Diagrammatic representation of (a) (from 190).

calf, human, or dog DNA (274). The electrophoretic profiles of DNA-binding phosphoproteins from rat liver and rat kidney are shown in Fig. 8.13.

Immunochemical studies have demonstrated specificity of the antigenic properties of the nonhistone protein. NHP–DNA complexes from chick oviduct produced high levels of complement fixation with rabbit antisera prepared against chick oviduct chromatin by comparison to NHP–DNA complexes of both liver and spleen (61, 257). These antisera markedly decreased transcription of chick chro-

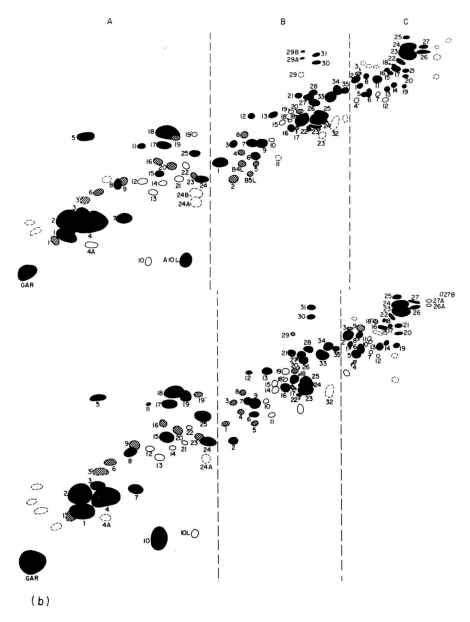

(b)

matin by *E. coli* RNA polymerase. The specificity resides in the nonhistone proteins since these differences in complement fixation were found for both the intact and dehistonized chromatins. Differences were also found in chromatin from different stages of development of chick oviduct (61, 257). Recently, similar antigenic differences were reported for NHP of rat thymus and liver, Novikoff hepatoma, Walker tumor, and rat 30 D hepatoma (285).

In summary, the NHP of chromatin contain a number of common proteins, probably including a number of enzymes. In addition, there appear to be some

TABLE 8.5

Amino Acid Compositions of NHP

	Nucleolar extract[a]	Nucleolar[a] band 15	Chromosomal[b] acidic proteins	NHP$_{\theta 1}$[c]	NHP$_\epsilon$[c]
Lysine	7.3	10.2	6.2	4.2	13.3
Histidine	2.4	1.0	2.2	1.3	1.3
Arginine	6.0	4.3	9.8	2.7	5.3
Aspartic acid	10.0	11.2	9.4	9.0	10.6
Threonine	5.1	5.3	4.9	5.5	3.7
Serine	7.6	6.2	5.2	13.3	9.1
Glutamic acid	13.8	15.9	13.6	12.8	17.2
Proline	5.3	4.7	4.4	6.1	4.8
Glycine	7.6	10.6	8.3	16.4	9.5
Alanine	7.0	9.8	8.4	9.0	8.2
Valine	6.0	5.6	6.4	4.2	2.5
Methionine	2.1	0.8	1.3	1.5	1.4
Isoleucine	4.1	3.3	4.9	2.7	2.8
Leucine	8.9	6.9	8.6	4.8	4.5
Tyrosine	2.4	1.2	1.8	2.6	2.8
Phenylalanine	3.6	3.1	3.2	3.9	2.9
Tryptophan	—	—	—	—	—
Total A	23.8	27.1	23.0	21.8	27.8
Total B	15.7	15.5	18.2	8.2	19.9
A/B	1.5	1.75	1.26	2.7	1.4
Molecular weight	—	66,000	—	49,000	31,000

[a] From 144.

[b] From 200a.

[c] From 80.

organ and species specific NHP. Although the functions of these proteins are largely unknown, some of these apparently have gene regulatory capacities.

G. Effects of NHP on Template Activities

The capacity of chromatin as a template for synthesis of RNA by DNA-dependent RNA polymerase is less than that of highly purified DNA (122). In early studies, histones were found to restrict RNA synthesis, particularly the amount of RNA synthesized (see p. 327). In more recent investigations, qualitatively different RNA produced from chromatins of various sources were analyzed by RNA–DNA hybridization (93, 203, 203a). In addition, the amount of RNA synthesized was also quantitated. The RNA transcribed *in vitro* from chromatin of mouse tissues competed with RNA from the corresponding tissue but not with *E. coli* RNA (204). Moreover, the RNA produced was reported to be specific for the tissue from which the chromatin was derived. Similar studies performed on dehistonized chromatin also indicated there was species specificity of the RNA produced (255, 256). Although evidence for specificity was obtained in these studies, the hybridization techniques used in these ex-

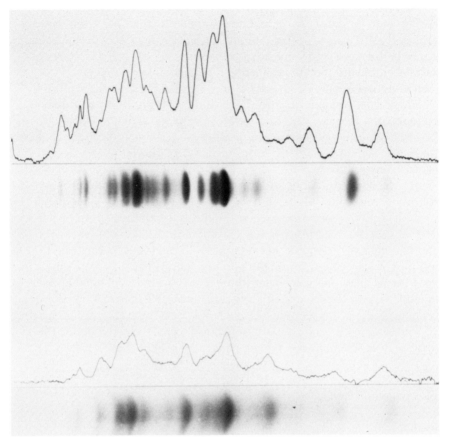

Fig. 8.13. Electrophoretic separation of phenol-soluble nuclear proteins. Top, rat liver; bottom, rat spleen (from 274).

periments would only detect RNA with relatively low Cot values, which indicates they originated from relatively highly reiterated DNA sequences (see Chapter V).

The logical extension of this work was to reconstitute chromatin with various types of proteins. Chromatin was shown to have essentially native properties after dissociation and reconstitution (31, 38, 123). The reconstitution was achieved after the chromatin was solubilized in 2 M NaCl and 5 M urea in the initial solvent with subsequent removal of the urea and salt by dialysis. The reconstituted chromatin possessed the ability to synthesize RNA that was indistinguishable from RNA derived from normal chromatin (97). Using the nonhistone proteins from a number of rabbit tissues for reconstitution experiments, it was found that the type of RNA produced was dependent on the source of the NHP (98). Thus, organ specificity seems to relate to the NHP of the chromatin.

Recently, similar studies have been applied to the comparison of tumor and normal tissues. When Walker tumor nonhistone proteins were used to activate the synthesis of RNA from normal rat liver chromatin, the RNA produced was similar to that produced by Walker tumor chromatin (147). In the converse experiment, activation of Walker tumor chromatin by rat liver nonhistone proteins resulted in production of RNA similar to rat liver RNA. Here, also, the nonhistone chromatin proteins seemed to dictate template specificity.

Nuclear phosphoproteins have been shown to stimulate transcription by RNA polymerase. The complex formed by addition of rat liver or kidney nuclear phosphoproteins to rat DNA had greater template activities than DNA alone (274). The phosphoproteins may constitute a positive control mechanism for transcription. As noted earlier, phosphorylation of the histones was also related to increased gene activity.

There is then, considerable evidence that the nonhistone proteins may enhance transcription reactions. Although their role in cancer cells is not understood, the loss of growth control may occur at the transcriptional level. That specific nonhistone chromosomal proteins may be important in this process was suggested by the finding that, in mouse fibroblasts, DNA synthesis is correlated with the appearance of a specific DNA-binding protein (229). The data available at present suggest there may be significant differences in the numbers and types of chromatin NHP of tumors and other tissues (147, 190, 289a, 296a). For example, one-dimensional polyacrylamide gel electrophoresis of NHP of normal lymphocytes, leukemic cells, and Burkitt lymphoma cells showed that in the tumors there was an increase in the higher molecular weight NHP (289a).

H. Nonhistone Proteins and Hormones

There is considerable evidence that protein receptors in the plasma membranes and in the cytoplasm (cytosol) of specific cells carry some hormones or activator substances into the nucleus where they localize at specific gene sites (15, 78, 109, 126, 170, 181, 183, 184, 185, 185a, 231, 252, 293). Furthermore, some steroid hormones increase the rates of synthesis of specific NHP fractions (26, 237, 273). The presence and functional activity of such receptors in endocrine tissues is being used clinically as a means for evaluation of prognosis and therapy of human breast and uterine cancer (294).

In chick oviducts, estrogen induces growth and differentiation as well as production of ovalbumin and other egg white proteins. Another protein, avidin, is synthesized in response to progesterone administration (187). When progesterone enters the cell, it forms a complex with a cytoplasmic receptor protein (240). This complex in turn migrates into the nucleus where it binds to chromatin (188). The cytosol receptor contained two types of subunits of which only one bound specifically to chromatin. Both of these, however, possessed equal progesterone-binding abilities.

There is specificity in this binding in that the natural target chromatin binds the steroid receptor complex much better than chromatins from other cell types (257, 262). The chromatin proteins associated with the steroid-receptor complex are acidic and exhibit tissue specificity (186). Studies with reconstituted chromatins indicate that receptor capacity is retained by the NHP and DNA from the oviduct. When reconstitution was carried out with histones from various sources, no evidence was found for tissue specificity of the histones. On the other hand, when the chromatin was reconstituted with NHP from sources other than the oviduct, the binding capacity was lost. The NHP fraction, then contains the specific binding elements for the cytosol receptor hormone complex.[*]

An analogous system is found in uteri of rats. Estradiol enters the cells of target tissue and forms a complex with a cytoplasmic receptor. This complex is transported into the nucleus where it associates with chromatin (127). The formation of the nuclear receptor is dependent on the prior presence of the cytosol receptor-estradiol complex in the cell (128, 247). The formation of a chromatin receptor for estradiol in the nonhistone chromatin fraction of calf endometrium does not require exposure of the cell to estradiol (5). A specific NHP is induced by estrogen in rat uterine chromatin (25); it is associated with the AR (f3,III) histone by disulfide linkages. Its relationship to other estrogen-induced proteins has not been established.

The above examples indicate the NHP have a role in the mechanism of action of some hormones. Certain NHP of target chromatins serve as acceptors for hormone-receptor complexes while others are synthesized in response to hormonal stimulation. Presumably, the NHP play a role in repression and derepression of the genome of hormonally sensitive tissues, but their exact functions remain to be determined.

I. NHP Biosynthesis and Turnover

Unlike the histones which are primarily synthesized during S phase in the cell cycle, the nonhistone proteins appear to turn over much faster than the histones throughout the cell cycle (45, 158, 260). Like the histones, the NHP of HeLa cells have been shown to be synthesized in the cytoplasm (134, 265). In synchronized HeLa cells the incorporation of [14C]leucine into tightly bound chromatin NHP increases after mitosis and reaches its maximum rate in late G_1 phase, just prior to the beginning of DNA synthesis (207, 264). During the S and G_2 phases there is a declining rate of NHP synthesis until it is the same as in G_1. By the use of inhibitors of DNA synthesis it was shown that unlike histone synthesis the NHP synthesis was not coupled to DNA replication. In addition, electrophoresis of the NHP produced at different stages of the cell cycle revealed the presence of phase-specific proteins. For example, one protein peak is present in much greater quantity in the G_2 phase than in the G_1 or S phase; another protein is present in the S and G_2 phases but absent in the G_1 phase. The turnover rate of individual proteins also varied greatly. In the G_2 phase, relatively high molecular weight proteins turned over rapidly, while lower molecular weight proteins seemed to be more metabolically stable (42). In the G_1 phase the opposite was found to be the case; the high molecular weight proteins generally turned over more slowly.

[*] The chromatin acceptor protein was dissociable from DNA by 2 M NaCl and 5 M urea (see Table 8.4).

One-dimensional polyacrylamide gel electrophoresis of NHP of normal lymphocytes, leukemic cells, and Burkitt lymphoma cells showed that in the tumors there was an increase in the higher molecular weight NHP (289a).

Increased rates of synthesis of NHP were observed in other systems where cell division is induced by a change in the environment of cells. Uptake of labeled amino acids into chromosomal NHP increased in mouse salivary glands stimulated with isoproterenol (264), in proliferating rat mammary gland explants (270), and in fibroblast cultures stimulated to divide by a change of medium (226).*

Such studies point to the complex chain of events involved in cell division. An initial stimulus causes activation or derepression of certain genes required for cell division (266). The macromolecules synthesized then participate in the biochemical events of cell division and cause further modifications in genetic expression throughout the cell cycle.

The above events should be distinguished from the nonreplicative genetic regulation of stationary cells. Early studies indicated that there were higher rates of labeled amino acid incorporation into the NHP of nondividing cells of kidney, pancreas, and liver than into their histones (13). In addition, active chromatin (euchromatin) had twice the amount of NHP as did inactive chromatin (heterochromatin) (86, 87, 158). In active chicken tissues there is a greater rate of synthesis of NHP than in inactive tissues (73). Increased NHP synthesis is also observed when rat mammary glands begin to lactate (270).

It is probable that there are two classes of regulatory chromosomal NHP: those concerned with cell division and those concerned with nonreplicative events in the life of the cell. The former are likely to be important in neoplasia and cell proliferation in general.

J. Nuclear Proteins and Carcinogens

Some carcinogens bind to proteins which are similar in some cases to the steroid binding proteins. The "h-protein" is a nonhistone saline soluble protein that can be isolated from both cytoplasm and nuclei and may function in a transport system similar to that for steroid hormones. The "h-protein" (19, 20, 139, 156, 175, 251, 253, 254) is known to bind dye carcinogens. It has been postulated (1) that the "h-protein" carries hydrocarbons including carcinogens from the cytoplasm to the nucleus.

The protein of liver cytosol that is designated as steroid binder 1 (251) also binds the carcinogen, 3-methylcholanthrene. This protein has been isolated and characterized (147a, 175) as a particle with a sedimentation coefficient of approximately 3.58 S and a molecular weight of 22,000. Another protein, ligandin, not only binds some carcinogen metabolites but also anionic steroid hormone metabolites with different degrees of affinity (241). Apparently, the receptors for 3-methylcholanthrene- and estrogen-binding are distinctly different.

* Guinea pig lymphoid cells stimulated by phytohemagglutinin (PHA) show a rapid increase in the synthesis of cell nonhistone proteins but not of histones (154). Several of the NHP were preferentially synthesized during PHA activation.

The chemical carcinogens N-hydroxy-N-2-fluorenylacetamide, *p*-dimethyl-aminoazobenzene, and 7,12-dimethylbenz(*a*)anthracene have been shown to bind *in vivo* to histones and nonhistone proteins of rat liver nuclei (133). The specificity of binding seemed to be greater for the histones than for nonhistone proteins, although no purified nonhistone fractions were tested. The carcinogen, 2-acetamidofluorene also binds to NHP when injected into rats (159).

Although it can be demonstrated that carcinogens bind to certain macromolecules, a direct link between the binding and carcinogenesis has not been established (see Chapter X). It is conceivable that carcinogen binding might alter the regulation by nuclear proteins of genes involved in growth control and thereby produce a loss of control of growth and cell division.

IX. The Nuclear Enzymes

Of the nuclear enzymes, most is known about the RNA polymerases, largely as the result of the extension of early findings of their presence (223) to their isolation (18, 18a, 59, 99, 136, 137, 171, 225, 232, 289) and separation into subunits (Fig. 8.14, Tables 8.6, 8.7). Major differences have been found in the RNA polymerases that transribe the nucleolar rDNA (and possibly other nucleolar genes) and those that transcribe the extranucleolar genes with respect to their

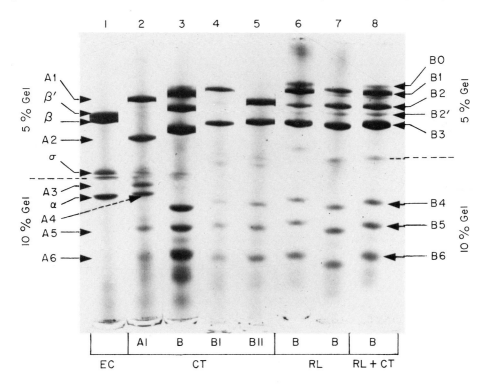

Fig. 8.14. Polyacrylamide gel electrophoresis showing the multiple subunits of RNA polymerase from various tissues. EC, *Escherichia coli;* CT, calf thymus; RL, rat liver (from 59).

TABLE 8.6

NOMENCLATURE AND LOCALIZATION OF ANIMAL DNA-DEPENDENT
RNA POLYMERASES[a]

Class of enzyme	Enzymes	Other terminology	Location
A	Enzyme AI	Enzyme I, enzyme IA	Nucleolar
(insensitive to amanitin)	Enzyme AII	Enzyme I, enzyme IB	Nucleolar
	Enzyme AIII	Enzyme III	Nucleoplasmic
	Enzyme AIV	Enzyme IV, pre-A,IA	Nucleolar
B	Enzyme BI	Enzyme II,IIA	Nucleoplasmic
(sensitive to low concentrations of amanitin, $10^{-9}-10^{-8}$ M)	Enzyme BII	Enzyme II,IIB	Nucleoplasmic
C	Enzyme C	—	Cytoplasmic
(sensitive to high concentrations of amanitin, $10^{-5}-10^{-4}$ M)			

[a] From 59.

physical characteristics, solubility, and sensitivity to inhibitors (Tables 8.6, 8.7). Virtually nothing is known with certainty regarding the initiation or termination factors in mammalian cells or plants (76, 110–111) that may be analogous to the sigma, rho, and other factors involved in bacterial RNA synthesis (230, 263–268, 274). It is possible that some ribonucleoprotein particles containing low molecular weight RNA may serve similar functions in mammalian cells (Chapter VI). Studies on these enzymes in cancer cells and carcinogenesis have thus far been only preliminary (4, 171, 172, 223, 290, 291).

After RNA molecules have been synthesized, many supplementary modifications and additions must be made; for example, in the case of nuclear U2 RNA (see Chapter VI), the 5′ portion of the molecule is subjected to 25 highly specific modifications of 69 nucleotides including formation of 11 pseudouridylic acid residues, 11 2′-O-methyl residues and three modified bases including the unique base $N^{2,2}$-7-trimethylguanine. In addition, the tRNA molecules undergo a variety of other modifications on specific nucleotides that can only occur as a result of activities of special enzymes that have definitive cellular localization.

Additional modifications of newly synthesized RNA molecules include the processing and/or "trimming" of newly synthesized high molecular weight RNA that is either preribosomal or premessenger HnRNA (Chapter V). The enzymatic reactions involved in these cleavages are specific and not random digestions of the precursor molecules (49, 217, 218).

In addition to the enzymes of RNA synthesis, modification, trimming, and other metabolism, the nucleus must contain at some point all of the enzymatic factors involved in the synthesis, repair, and modification of DNA (Table 8.8, also see Chapter IV). It is obvious that much needs to be learned about the similarities and differences of these molecules in cancer cells and other cells, but thus far, the problems involved in their isolation and characterization have been formidable (Chapter IV).

TABLE 8.7

CURRENT KNOWLEDGE CONCERNING THE SUBUNIT STRUCTURE OF MAMMALIAN RNA POLYMERASES[a]

	CT form BI			CT form BII			RL B mixture			CT form AI			RL form AII	
Sub-unit	MW	Molar ratio	Sub-unit	MW	Molar ratio	Sub-unit	MW	Molar ratio	Sub-unit	MW	Molar ratio	Sub-unit	MW	Molar ratio
—	—	—	—	—	—	B0	220,000	0.2	A1	197,000	1	A1	170,000	1
B1	214,000	1	—	—	—	B1	214,000	0.4	A2	126,000	1	A2	126,000	1
—	—	—	B2	180,000	1	B2	180,000	0.3	A3	51,000	1	A3	?	?
—	—	—	—	—	—	B2'	165,000	0.1	A4	44,000	1	A4	40,000	?
B3	140,000	1	B3	140,000	1	B3	140,000	1	A5	25,000	2	A5	?	?
B4	34,000	1	B4	34,000	1	B4	34,000	1	A6	16,500	2	A6	?	?
B5	25,000	1-2	B5	25,000	1-2	B5	25,000	2						
B6	16,500	3-4	B6	16,500	3-4	B6	16,500	3-4						

[a] From 59. For abbreviations see Fig. 8.14.

TABLE 8.8

NUCLEAR ENZYMES

---

1. RNA synthesis and processing
   a. RNA polymerases A, B, etc.
   b. RNA modification enzymes; methylases, formation of modified nucleosides
   c. RNA trimming or special cleavage enzymes
   d. RNases: exo- and endonucleolytic
2. DNA synthesis
   a. "True" synthetases
   b. Ligases
   c. Excision enzymes
   d. Terminal addition enzymes
   e. DNases
   f. Modification enzymes (methylases, etc.)
3. Other modification and synthetic enzymes
   a. Histone phosphokinases, methylases, acetylases, deacetylases, proteases
   b. NHP kinases and methylases
   c. Nucleoside kinases
   d. NAD pyrophosphorylase
4. Dehydrogenases
   a. Steroid dehydrogenase
   b. Cytochrome oxidase
   c. Glycerol-3-phosphate dehydrogenases
   d. Glyceraldehyde-3-phosphate dehydrogenase
   e. Succinate, malate, isocitrate, lactate, NADH, NADPH, glucose-6-phosphate, phospho-
      gluconate
5. Transferases—glycosyl for glycogen phosphorylases and branching enzymes
6. Enzymes of uncertain function
   a. ATPases
   b. Carboxylesterases
   c. Phosphatases
   d. 5'-Nucleotidases
   e. Phosphodiesterase

The only other enzyme for which unequivocal demonstration of nuclear localization has been effected is NAD synthetase or pyrophosphorylase which is localized to the nucleolus (49). There is no clear understanding at present for this localization and there has been some concern as to whether this enzyme may not be the "true" synthetic enzyme for NAD; needless to say, this question has been raised for many other enzymes, particularly for the cytoplasmic localization of enzymes that appear to be involved in DNA synthesis (45, 202). Enzymes that modify proteins, including the histones and the nuclear phosphoproteins are also found in the nucleus and although there is much interest in their functions, the factors controlling their activities are just now being studied. Recently, a histone-specific deacetylase for the GAR (f2a,IV) and AR (f3,III) histones was highly purified (280); this enzyme is a phosphorylated, acidic protein that binds to chromatin *in vitro*.

The nucleus has been studied extensively by cytochemists for many other enzymes including a variety of dehyrogenases, transferases, and hydrolyases (Table 8.8). Although there is convincing evidence for the presence of some

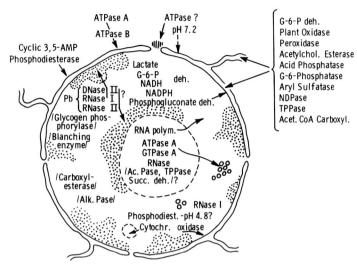

Fig. 8.15. Localization of various enzymes in the cell nucleus (from 283).

of these enzymes in the nucleus, its outer membrane, and the intermembrane space (Fig. 8.15; 32, 283), it is not clear what functional role these enzymes play. Within the limits of error in isolation of nuclei and nucleoli and the diffusion problems that attend cytochemical studies, it is somewhat uncertain whether these enzymes really have nuclear functions. In this connection, extensive discussions of enzyme and particle localization still absorb the attention of many cytologists and histochemists (217, 283) as well as biochemists (44, 45, 49, 248, 248a, 249).

In summary, significant progress has been made in the isolation, purification, and enzymatic characterization of nuclear and nucleolar RNA polymerases. Less meaningful progress has emerged from studies on DNA synthetases and there is little clear understanding yet of the roles of the multiple modification enzymes of the nucleus that affect specific bases of the nucleic acids or particular amino acids of the nuclear proteins. Although a variety of other enzymes have been localized to the nucleus which carry out oxidative, transfer, and hydrolytic reactions, their roles in nuclear function are as yet largely unexplored. The relationship of all of these enzymes to the proteins involved in gene control and the many nuclear proteins now readily visualized in two-dimensional gel systems are topics that require extensive study in the future, particularly with respect to the differences between cancer cells and other cells.

References

1. Abell, C. W., and Heidelberger, L. (1962). *Cancer Res.* **22**, 931–946.
2. Adams, G. H. M., Vidali, G., and Neelin, J. M. (1970). *Can. J. Biochem.* **48**, 33–37.
3. Adler, K., Beyreuther, K., Fanning, E., Geisler, N., Gronenborn, B., Klemm, A., Müller-Hill, B., Pfahl, M., and Schmitz, A. (1972) *Nature* (*London*) **237**, 322–327.

4. Akao, M., Kuroda, K., and Miyaki, K. (1972). *Gann* **63**, 1–10.
5. Alberga, A., Massol, N., Raynaud, J.-P., and Beulieu, E. (1971). *Biochemistry* **10**, 3835–3841.
6. Albert, A. E. (1972). *Chem. Biol. Interactions* **4**, 287–296.
7. Alberts, B. M., Amodio, F. J., Jenkins, M., Gutman, E. D., and Ferris, F. L. (1968). *Cold Spring Harbor Symp. Quant. Biol.* **33**, 289–306.
8. Allfrey, V. G. (1954). *Proc. Nat. Acad. Sci. U.S.* **40**, 881–885.
9. Allfrey, V. G., Faulkner, R., and Mirsky, A. E. (1964). *Proc. Nat. Acad. Sci. U.S.* **51**, 786–794.
10. Allfrey, V. G. (1969). *In* "Biochemistry of Cell Division" (R. Baserga, ed.), pp. 179–205. Thomas, Springfield, Illinois.
11. Allfrey, V. G. (1970). *In* "Aspects of Protein Synthesis" (C. B. Anfinsen, Jr., ed.), Part A, pp. 247–366. Academic Press, New York.
12. Allfrey, V. G. (1971). *In* "Histones and Nucleohistones" (D. M. P. Phillips, ed.), pp. 241–294. Plenum, New York.
13. Allfrey, V. G., Daly, M. M., and Mirsky, A. E. (1955). *J. Gen. Physiol.* **38**, 415–424.
14. Allfrey, V. G., Littau, V. C., and Mirsky, A. E. (1963). *Proc. Nat. Acad. Sci. U.S.* **49**, 414–421.
15. Anderson, J., Clark, J. H., and Peck, E. J., Jr. (1972). *Biochem. J.* **126**, 561–567.
16. Ansevin, A. T., and Brown, B. W. (1971). *Biochemistry* **10**, 1133.
17. Arnold, E. A., and Young, K. E. (1972). *Biochim. Biophys. Acta* **257**, 482–486.
18. Astier-Manifacier, S., and Cornuet, P. (1971). *Biochim. Biophys. Acta* **232**, 484–493.
18a. Austoker, J., Cox, D., and Mathias, A. P. (1972). *Biochem. J.* **129**, 1139–1156.
19. Bakey, B., and Sorof, S. (1969). *Cancer Res.* **29**, 22–27.
20. Bakey, B., Sorof, S., and Siebert, G. (1969). *Cancer Res.* **29**, 28–32.
21. Balhorn, R., Balhorn, M., Morris, H. P., and Chalkley, R. (1972). *Cancer Res.* **32**, 1775–1784.
22. Balhorn, R., Chalkley, R., and Granner, D. (1972). *Biochemistry* **11**, 1094–1098.
23. Balhorn, R., Rieke, W. O., and Chalkley, R. (1971). *Biochemistry* **10**, 3952–3958.
24. Balhorn, R., Oliver, D., Hohmann, P., Chalkley, R., and Granner, D. (1972). *Biochemistry* **11**, 3915–3921.
24a. Ballal, R., and Busch, H. *Cancer Res.* (In press).
25. Barker, K. L. (1971). *Biochemistry* **10**, 284–291.
26. Barnes, A. and Gorski, J. (1970). *Biochemistry* **9**, 1899.
27. Barret, A., and Dingle, J. (eds.) (1971). "Tissue Proteinases." North-Holland Publ., Amsterdam.
28. Bartley, J. A., and Chalkley, R. (1968). *Biochim. Biophys. Acta* **160**, 224–228.
29. Bartley, J. A., and Chalkley, R. (1972). *J. Biol. Chem.* **247**, 3647–3655.
30. Baserga, R., and Stein, G. (1971). *Fed. Proc.* **30**, 1752–1759.
31. Bekhor, I., Kung, G. M., and Bonner, J. (1969). *J. Mol. Biol.* **39**, 351–364.
32. Berezney, R., Macauley, L. K., and Crane, F. L. (1972). *J. Biol. Chem.* **247**, 5549–5561.
33. Birnie, G. D. (1972). "Subcellular Components; Preparation and Fractionation." Univ. Park Press, Baltimore, Maryland.
34. Bloch, D. P. (1969). *Genetics Suppl.* **61**(1), 93–111.
34a. Bloch, D. P., and Brack, S. D. (1964). *J. Cell Biol.* **22**, 327–340.
35. Bloch, D. P., and Godman, G. C. (1955). *J. Biophys. Biochem. Cytol.* **1**, 17–28.
36. Bhorjee, J. S., and Pederson, T. (1972). *Proc. Nat. Acad. Sci. U.S.* **69**, 3345–3349.
37. Bonner, J. (1965). "The Molecular Biology of Development." Oxford Univ. Press, London and New York.
38. Bonner, J., Chalkley, G. R., Dahmur, M., Fambrough, D., Fujimura, F., Huang, R. C., Huberman, J., Jensen, R., Marushige, K., Ohlenbusch, H., Olivera, B., and Widholm, J. (1968). *Methods in Enzymol.* **12**, Part B, 3–84.
39. Bonner, J., Dahmus, M., Fambrough, D., Huang, R., Marushige, K., and Tuan, D. (1968). *Science* **159**, 47–56.

40. Bonner, J., and Ts'o, P. O. P. (eds.) (1964). "The Nucleohistones." Holden-Day, San Francisco, California.
41. Borun, T. W., Scharff, M., and Robbins, E. (1967). Proc. Nat. Acad. Sci. U.S. 58, 1977–1983.
42. Borun, T. W., and Stein, G. S. (1972). J. Cell Biol. 52, 208–215.
43. Bradbury, E. M., Cary, P. D., Crane-Robinson, C., Riches, P. L., and Johns, E. W. (1971). Nature New Biol. 233, 265–267.
43a. Buckingham, R. H., and Stocken, L. A. (1970). Biochem. J. 117, 157–160.
44. Busch, H. (1962). "Biochemistry of the Cancer Cell." Academic Press, New York.
45. Busch, H. (1965). "Histones and Other Nuclear Proteins." Academic Press, New York.
46. Busch, H., Choi, Y. C., Daskal, I., Inagaki, A., Olson, M. O. J., Reddy, R., Ro-Choi, T. S., Shibata, H., and Yeoman, L. C. (1972). In Karolinska Symp. Res. Res. Methods Reproductive Tissue (E. Dizfaluzy, ed.). Bogtrykkeriet Forum, Copenhagen.
47. Busch, H., Choi, Y. C., Starbuck, W. C., Olson, M. O. J., and Wikman, J. (1971). In "Drugs and Cell Regulation" (E. Mihich, ed.), pp. 51–62. Academic Press, New York.
48. Busch, H., and Davis, J. R. (1958). Cancer Res. 18, 1241–1256.
49. Busch, H., and Smetana, K. (1970). "The Nucleolus." Academic Press, New York.
50. Busch, H. Starbuck, W. C., Singh, E. J., and Roe, T. S. (1964). Symp. Growth, Amherst pp. 51–71.
51. Busch, H., and Steele, W. J. (1964). Advan. Cancer Res. 8, 42–121.
52. Byvoet, P. (1966). J. Mol. Biol. 17, 311–318.
53. Byvoet, P., and Morris, H. P. (1971). Cancer Res. 31, 468–476.
54. Byvoet, P., Shepherd, G. R., Hardin, J. M., and Noland, B. J. (1972). Arch. Biochem. Biophys. 148, 558–567.
55. Candido, E. P. M., and Dixon, G. H. (1971). J. Biol. Chem. 246, 3182–3188.
56. Candido, E. P. M., and Dixon, G. H. (1972). J. Biol. Chem. 247, 3868–3878.
57. Candido, E. P. M., and Dixon, G. H. (1972). Proc. Nat. Acad. Sci. U.S. 69, 2015–2019.
58. Chalkley, G. R., and Maurer, H. R. (1965). Proc. Nat. Acad. Sci. U.S. 54, 498–505.
59. Chambon, P., Gissinger, F., Kedinger, C., Mandel, J. L., and Meilhac, M. (1973). In "The Cell Nucleus" (H. Busch, ed.). Academic Press, New York (in press).
60. Chaudhuri, S., Stein, G., and Baserga, R. (1972). Proc. Soc. Exp. Biol. Med. 139, 1363–1366.
61. Chytil, F., and Spelsberg, T. C. (1971). Nature New Biol. 233, 215–218.
62. Clark, R. J., and Felsenfeld, G. (1971). Nature New Biol. 229, 101–106.
63. Comings, D. E. (1972). Advan. Human Genet. 3, 237–431.
64. Crippa, M. (1970) Nature (London) 227, 1138.
65. Cuatrecasas, P. (1971). J. Agr. Food Chem. 19, 600–604.
66. Cuatrecasas, P. (1972). Advan. Enzymol. 36, 29–89.
67. Davis, R. H., Copenhaver, J. H., and Carver, M. J. (1972). J. Neurochem. 19, 473–477.
68. DeLange, R. J., Fambrough, D. M., Smith, E. L., and Bonner, J. (1969). J. Biol. Chem. 244, 319–334.
69. DeLange, R. J., Fambrough, D. M., Smith E. L., and Bonner, J. (1969). J. Biol. Chem. 244, 5669–5679.
70. DeLange, R. J., Hooper, J. A., and Smith, E. L. (1972). Proc. Nat. Acad. Sci. U.S. 69, 882–884.
71. Dick, C., and Johns, E. W. (1969). Biochim. Biophys. Acta 175, 414–418.
72. Diczfalusy, E. (1972). "Gene Transcription in Reproductive Tissue." Bogtrykkeriet Forum, Copenhagen.
72a. Dijkstra, J., and Weide, S. S. (1972). Exp. Cell Res. 71, 337–381.
73. Dingman, C. W., and Sporn, M. B. (1964). J. Biol. Chem. 229, 3483–3492.
74. Dounce, A. L. (1971). Amer. Sci. 59, 74–83.
75. Dounce, A. L., Chandra, S. K., Ickowicz, R., Volkman, O., Palemiti, M., and Turk, R. (1972). In "Gene Transcription in Reproductive Tissue" (E. Diczfalusy, ed.). pp. 84–111. Bogtrykkeriet Forum, Copenhagen.
76. Dounce, A. L., Umana, R. (1962). Biochemistry 1, 811–819.

77. DuPraw, E. J., (1968). "DNA and Chromosomes." Holt, New York.
78. Edelman, I. S., and Fanestil, D. D. (1970). In "Biochemical Actions of Hormones" (G. Litwack, ed.), pp. 324–331. Academic Press, New York.
79. Elgin, S. C. R., and Bonner, J. (1970). Biochemistry 9, 4440–4446.
80. Elgin, S. C. R., and Bonner, J. (1972). Biochemistry 11, 772–781.
81. Elgin, S. C. R., Froehner, S. C., Smart, J. S., and Bonner, J. (1971). Advan. Cell Mol. Biol. 1, 1–57.
82. Epifanova, O. L. (1971). In "The Cell Cycle and Cancer" (R. Baserga, ed.), pp. 143–190. Dekker, New York.
83. Evans, J. H., Holbrook, D. J., and Irvin, J. L. (1962). Exp. Cell Res. 28, 126–132.
83a. Farina, F. A., Adelman, R. C., HoLo, C., Morris, H. P., and Weinhouse, S. (1968). Cancer Res. 28, 1897–1900.
84. Flamm, W. G., and Birnstiel, M. L. (1964). Biochim. Biophys. Acta 87, 101–110.
85. Frearson, D. M., and Kirby, K. S. (1964). Biochem. J. 94, 578–583.
86. Frenster, J. H. (1965). Nature (London) 206, 680.
87. Frenster, J. H., Allfrey, V. G., and Mirsky, A. E. (1963). Proc. Nat. Acad. Sci. U.S. 50, 1026.
88. Gabel, N. W. (1972). Perspect. Biol. Med. 15, 640–643.
89. Gallwitz, D., and Mueller, G. C. (1969). J. Biol. Chem. 244, 5947–5952.
90. Gallwitz, D., and Mueller, G. C. (1969). Science 163, 1351–1353.
91. Gallwitz, D., and Mueller, G. C. (1970). FEBS Lett. 6, 83–85.
91a. Gallwitz, D., and Sekeris, C. E. (1969). Hoppe-Seyler's Z. Physiol. Chem. 350, 150–154.
92. Georgiev, G. P. (1969). Ann Rev. Genet. 3, 155–180.
93. Georgiev, G. P., Anenieva, L. A., and Kozlov, Y. U. (1966). J. Mol. Biol. 22, 365–371.
94. Gershey, E. L., Haslett, G. W., Vidali, G., and Allfrey, V. G. (1969). J. Biol. Chem. 244, 4871–4877.
95. Gershey, E. L., Vidali, G., and Allfrey, V. G. (1968). J. Biol. Chem. 243, 5018–5022.
96. Gilbert, W., and Müller-Hill, B. (1966). Proc. Nat. Acad. Sci. U.S. 56, 1891–1898.
97. Gilmour, R. S., and Paul, J. (1969). J. Mol. Biol. 40, 137–139.
98. Gilmour, R. S., and Paul, J. (1970). FEBS Lett. 9, 242.
99. Gissinger, F., and Chambon, P. (1972). Eur. J. Biochem. 28, 277–282.
100. Goldstein, L. (ed.) (1967). "The Control of Nuclear Activity." Prentice-Hall, Englewood Cliffs, New Jersey.
101. Goldstein, L., and Prescott, D. M. (1967). J. Cell Biol. 33, 637–644.
102. Goldstein, L., and Prescott, D. M. (1968). J. Cell Biol. 36, 53–61.
103. Gronow, M., and Griffiths, G. (1971). FEBS Lett. 15, 340–344.
104. Gross, P. R. (1968). Ann. Rev. Biochem. 37, 631–660.
105. Gurley, L. R., and Hardin, J. M. (1968). Arch. Biochem. Biophys. 128, 285–292.
105a. Gurley, L. R., Enger, M. D., and Walters, R. A. (1973). Biochemistry 12, 237–245.
105b. Gutierrez-Cernosek, R. M., and Hnilica, L. S. (1971). Biochim. Biophys. Acta 247, 348–354.
106. Hadler, S. C., Smart, J. E., and Bonner, J. (1971). Biochim. Biophys. Acta 236, 253–258.
107. Hamilton, T. H., and Teng, C.-S. (1969). Genetics Suppl. 61, 382–389.
108. Hancock, R. (1969). J. Mol. Biol. 40, 457–466.
109. Hardin, J. M., Noland, B. J., and Shepherd, G. R. (1971). Exp. Cell Res. 68, 459–462.
110. Hardin, J. W., and Cherry, J. H. (1972). Biochem. Biophys. Res. Commun. 48, 299–306.
111. Hardin, J. W., O'Brien, T. J., and Cherry, J. H. (1970). Biochim. Biophys. Acta 224, 667–670.
112. Hayashi, T., and Iwai, H. (·1970). J. Biochem. 68, 415–417.
113. Hearst, J. E., and Botchan, M. (1970). Ann. Rev. Biochem. 39, 151–182.
114. Hempel, K., Lange, H. W., and Birkhofer, L. (1968). Naturwissenschaften 55, 37.
115. Hempel, K., Lange, H. W., and Birkhofer, L. (1968). H.S.Z. Physiol. Chem. 349, 603.
116. Hnilica, L. S. (1964). Experientia 20, 13–14.
117. Hnilica, L. S. (1967). Progr. Nucl. Acid Res. Mol. Biol. 7, 25–106.

118. Hnilica, L. S. (1972). "The Structure and Biological Functions of Histones." Chem. Rubber Co. Press, Clevland, Ohio.
119. Hohmann, P., and Cole, R. D. (1971). *J. Mol. Biol.* **58**, 533–540.
120. Holbrook, D. J., Evans, J. H., and Irvin, J. L. (1962). *Exp. Cell Res.* **28**, 120–125.
121. Holbrook, D. J., Irvin, J. L., Irvin, E. M., and Rotherham, J. (1960). *Cancer Res.* **20**, 1329–1337.
122. Huang, R. C. C., and Bonner, J. (1962). *Proc. Nat. Acad. Sci. U.S.* **48**, 1216–1222.
123. Huang, R. C. C., and Huang, P. C. (1969). *J. Mol. Biol.* **39**, 365–378.
124. Itzhaki, R. (1970). *Biochem. Biophys. Res. Commun.* **41**, 25–32.
125. Iwai, K., Hayashi, H., and Ishikawa, K. (1972). *J. Biochem. (Tokyo)* **72**, 357–367.
126. Jensen, E. V., and DeSombre, E. R. (1972). *Ann. Rev. Biochem.* **41**, 203–230.
127. Jensen, E. V., Numata, M., Brecher, P. I., and DeSombre, E. R. (1971). *In* "The Biochemistry of Steroid Hormone Action" (R. M. S. Smellie, ed.), pp. 133–159. Academic Press, New York.
128. Jensen, E. V., Suzuki, Y., Haroashima, T., Stumpf, W., Jungblut, P., and DeSombre, E. R. (1968). *Proc. Nat. Acad. Sci. U.S.* **59**, 632–638.
129. Jobe, A., Riggs, A. D., and Bourgeois, S. (1972). *J. Mol. Biol.* **64**, 181.
130. Johns, E. W. (1971). *In* "Histones and Nucleohistones" (D. M. P. Phillips), pp. 1–83. Plenum Press, New York.
130a. Johns, E. W., and Forrester, S. (1969). *Eur. J. Biochem.* **8**, 547–551.
130b. Johns, E. W., and Hoare, T. A. (1970). *Nature (London)* **226**, 650–651.
131. Jones, O. W., and Berg, P. (1966). *J. Mol. Biol.* **22**, 199–209.
132. Jungmann, R. A., and Schweppe, J. S. (1972). *J. Biol. Chem.* **247**, 5535–5542.
133. Jungmann, R. A., and Schweppe, J. S. (1972). *Cancer Res.* **32**, 952–959.
134. Kawashima, K., Izawa, M., and Sato, S. (1971). *Biochim. Biophys. Acta* **232**, 192–206.
135. Kaye, A. M., and Sheratzky, D. (1969). *Biochim. Biophys. Acta* **190**, 527–538.
136. Kedinger, C., and Chambon, P. (1972). *Eur. J. Biochem.* **28**, 283–290.
137. Kedinger, C., Gissinger, F., Gniazdowski, M., Mandel, J.-L. and Chambon, P. (1972). *Eur. J. Biochem.* **28**, 269–276.
138. Keller, P. C. (1972). "The Role of Chromosomes in Cancer Biology." Springer-Verlag, New York.
139. Ketterer, B. (1971). *Biochem. J.* **126**, 3P-4P.
140. Kleiman, L., and Huang, R. C. C. (1971). *J. Mol. Biol.* **55**, 503–521.
141. Klein, A., and Bonhoeffer, F. (1972). *Ann. Rev. Biochem.* **41**, 301–332.
142. Kleinsmith, L. J., Allfrey, V. G., and Mirsky, A. E. (1966). *Proc. Nat. Acad. Sci. U.S.* **55**, 1182–1189.
142a. Kleinsmith, L. J., Heidema, J., and Carroll, A. (1970). *Nature (London)* **226**, 1025–1026.
143. Klyszekjo-Stefanowicz, L., and Polanowska, Z. (1971). *Post. Biochem.* **17**, 601–629.
144. Knecht, M. E., and Busch, H. (1971). *Life Sci.* **10**, 1297–1309.
145. Kossel, A. (1884). *Z. Physiol. Chem.* **8**, 511.
146. Kostraba, N. C., and Wang, T. Y. (1971). *Cancer Res.* **31**, 1663–1668.
147. Kostraba, N. C., and Wang, T. Y. (1972). *Cancer Res.* **32**, 2348–2352.
147a. Kuroki, T., and Heidelberger, C. (1972). *Biochemistry* **11**, 2116–2124.
148. Langan, T. A. (1966). *In* "Regulation of Nuclei Acid and Protein Biosynthesis" (V. V. Konigskerger and L. Bosch, eds.), pp. 233. Elsevier, Amsterdam.
149. Langan, T. A. (1968). *Science* **162**, 579–580.
150. Langan, T. A. (1969). *J. Biol. Chem.* **244**, 5763–5765.
151. Langan, T. A. (1969). *Proc. Nat. Acad. Sci. U.S.* **64**, 1276–1283.
152. Langan, T. A., Rall, S. C., and Cole, R. D. (1971). *J. Biol. Chem.* **246**, 1942–1944.
152a. LeStourgeon, W. M., and Rusch, H. P. (1971). *Science* **174**, 1233–1236.
153. Levy, S., Simpson, R. T., and Sober, H. A. (1972). *Biochemistry* **11**, 1547–1554.
154. Levy, R., Levy, S., Rosenberg, S. A., and Simpson, R. T. (1973). *Biochemistry* **12**, 224.
155. Li, H.-J., and Bonner, J. (1971). *J. Biochem.* **10**, 1461–1470.

156. Libby, P. R. (1970). *Biochim. Biophys. Acta* **213**, 234–236.
157. Liew, C. C., Haslett, G. W., and Allfrey, V. G. (1970). *Nature (London)* **226**, 414–417.
158. Littau, V. C., Allfrey, V. G., Frenster, J. H., and Mirsky, A. E. (1964). *Proc. Nat. Acad. Sci. U.S.* **52**, 93.
158a. Loeb, J. (1968). *C. R. Acad. Sci. Paris* **262**, 2183–2186.
158b. Losick, R. (1972). *Ann. Rev. Biochem.* **41**, 409–446.
159. Lotlikar, P. D., and Paik, W. K. (1971). *Biochem. J.* **124**, 443–445.
160. Louie, A. J., and Dixon, G. H. (1972). *Proc. Nat. Acad. Sci. U.S.* **69**, 1975–1979.
161. Lukanidin, E. M., Georgiev, G. P., and Williamson, R. (1971). *FEBS Lett.* **19**, 152–156.
162. Lukanidin, E. M., Zalmanzon, E. S., Komaromi, L., Samarina, O.P., and Georgiev, G. P. (1972). *Nature New Biol.* **238**, 193–197.
163. MacGillivray, A. J., Cameron, R. J., Krauze, D., Rickwood, D., and Paul, J. (1972). *Biochim. Biophys. Acta* **277**, 384–402.
164. MacGillivray, A. J., Paul, J., and Threlfall, G. (1972). *Advan. Cancer Res.* **15**, 93–162.
165. Malamud, D. (1971). *In* "The Cell Cycle and Cancer" (R. Baserga, ed.), pp. 129–142. Marcel Dekher, New York.
166. Mandal, R. C. (1968). *Sci. Cult.* **34**, 78–84.
167. Marushige, K., and Bonner, J. (1966). *J. Mol. Biol.* **15**, 160–174.
168. Marushige, K., and Dixon, G. H. (1969). *Develop. Biol.* **19**, 397–414.
169. Marushige, K., Ling, V., and Dixon, G. H. (1969). *J. Biol. Chem.* **244**, 5953–5958.
170. Marver, D., Goodman, D., and Edelman, I. S. (1972). *Kidney Int.* **1**, 210–223.
170a. Maskos, K. (1971). *Acta Biochim. Polon.* **18**, 57–65.
170b. McClure, M. E., and Hnilica, L. S. (1970). *Int. Cancer Congr. 10th, Houston, 1970* Abs. #441.
171. Meilhac, M., Tysper, Z., and Chambon, P. (1972). *Eur. J. Biochem.* **28**, 291–300.
172. Menon, I. A. (1972). *Brain Res.* **42**, 529–533.
173. Miescher, F. (1897). "Die Histochemischen und Physiologischen Arbeiten" Vogel Vlg., Leipzig.
174. Mirsky, A. E., and Silverman, B. (1972). *Proc. Nat. Acad. Sci. U.S.* **69**, 2115–2119.
175. Morey, K. S., and Litwack, G. (1969). *Biochemistry* **8**, 4813–4821.
176. Murray, K. (1964). *Biochemistry* **3**, 10–15.
177. Murray, K., and Milstein, C. (1967). *Biochem. J.* **105**, 491–495.
178. Neelin, J. M., Callahan, P. X., Lamb, D. C., and Murray, K. (1964). *Can. J. Biochem.* **42**, 1743–1752.
179. Nemer, M., and Lindsay, D. (1969). *Biochem. Biophys. Res. Commun.* **35**, 156–160.
180. Nohara, H., Takahashi, T., and Ogata, K. (1966). *Biochim. Biophys. Acta* **127**, 282–284.
180a. Nohara, H., Takahashi, T., and Ogata, K. (1968). *Biochim. Biophys. Acta* **154**, 529–539.
181. Nunez, E., Engelmann, F., Benassayag, C., Savu, L., Crepy, O., and Jayle, M.-F. (1971). *C. R. Acad. Sci. Paris* **272**, 2396–2399.
182. Ogawa, Y., Quagliarotti, G., Jordan, J., Taylor, C. W., Starbuck, W. C., and Busch, H. (1969). *J. Biol. Chem.* **244**, 4387–4392.
182a. Olins, D. E. (1969). *J. Mol. Biol.* **43**, 439–460.
183. Olson, M. O. J., Sugano, N., Yeoman, L. C., Johnson, B. R., Jordan, J., Taylor, C. W., Starbuck, W. C., and Busch, H. (1972). *Physiol. Chem. Phys.* **4**, 10–16.
184. O'Malley, B. W., and Means, A. (1974). *In* "The Cell Nucleus" (H. Busch, ed.), Vol. III. Academic Press, New York (in press).
185. O'Malley, B. W., Rosenfeld, G., Comstock, J. P., and Means, A. R. (1972). *In* "Gene Transcription in Reproductive Tissue" (E. Diczfalusy, ed.), pp. 281–395. Karolinska Inst., Stockholm.
185a. O'Malley, B. W., Sherman, R. M., Toft, D. O., Spelsberg, W. T., and Steggles, A. W. (1971). *Advan. Biosci.* **7**, 213–231.
186. O'Malley, B. W., Spelsberg, T. C., Schrader, W. T., Chytil, F., and Steggles, A. W. (1972). *Nature (London)* **235**, 141–144.
187. O'Malley, B. W., McGuire, W. L., Hohler, P. O., and Koreman, S. G. (1969). *Rec. Progr. Hormone Res.* **25**, 105.

188. O'Malley, B. W., Taft, D. O., and Sherman, M. R. (1971). *J. Biol. Chem.* **246**, 1117–1122.
189. Ord, M. G., and Stocken, L. A. (1966). *Biochem. J.* **98**, 5P.
189a. Ord, M. G., and Stocken, L. A. (1968). *Biochem. J.* **107**, 403–410.
190. Orrick, L., Olson, M. O. J., and Busch, H. (1973). *Proc. Nat. Acad. Sci. U.S.* **70**, 1316–1320.
191. Paik, W. K., and Kim, S. (1970). *Biochim. Biophys. Res. Commun.* **40**, 224–229.
192. Paik, W. K., and Kim, S. (1970). *J. Biol. Chem.* **245**, 88–92.
193. Paik, W. K., and Kim, S. (1970). *J. Biol. Chem.* **245**, 6010–6015.
194. Paine, P. L., and Feldherr, C. M. (1972). *Exp. Cell Res.* **74**, 84–98.
195. Palau, J., Pardon, J. F., and Richards, B. M. (1967). *Biochim. Biophys. Acta* **138**, 633–636.
196. Panyim, S., Bilek, D., and Chalkley, R. (1971). *J. Biol. Chem.* **246**, 4206–4215.
197. Panyim, S., and Chalkley, R. (1969). *Arch. Biochem. Biophys.* **130**, 337–346.
198. Panyim, S., and Chalkley, R. (1969). *Biochemistry* **8**, 3972–3979.
199. Panyim, S., and Chalkley, R. (1969). *Biochem. Biophys. Res. Commun.* **37**, 1042–1049.
200. Pardon, J. F., and Wilkins, M. H. F. (1972). *J. Mol. Biol.* **68**, 115–124.
200a. Patel, G. L. (1972). *Life Sci.* **11**, 1135–1142.
201. Patel, G., and Wang, T.-Y. (1965). *Biochim. Biophys. Acta* **95**, 314–320.
202. Patel, G., Howk, R., and Wang, T.-Y. (1967). *Nature (London)* **215**, 1488–1489.
203. Paul, J., and Gilmour, R. S. (1966). *J. Mol. Biol.* **16**, 242–244.
203a. Paul, J., and Gilmour, R. S. (1968). *J. Mol. Biol.* **34**, 305–316.
204. Paul, J., and Gilmour, R. S. (1966). *Nature (London)* **210**, 992.
205. Phillips, D. M. P. (1963). *Biochem. J.* **87**, 258–263.
206. Phillips, D. M. P. (1968). *Biochem. J.* **107**, 135–138.
207. Phillips, D. M. P. (1968). *Experientia* **24**, 668–669.
208. Phytila, M. J., and Sherman, F. G. (1968). *Biochem. Biophys. Res. Commun.* **31**, 340–344.
208a. Pietsch, P. (1969). *Cytobios* **1**, 375.
209. Pitot, H. C. (1968). *Cancer Res.* **28**, 1880–1888.
210. Platz, R. D., Kishi, M., and Kleinsmith, L. J. (1970). *FEBS Lett.* **12**, 38–40.
211. Pogo, B. G. T. (1966). *Proc. Nat. Acad. Sci. U.S.* **55**, 805–812.
212. Pogo, B. G. T. (1968). *Proc. Nat. Acad. Sci. U.S.* **59**, 1337–1344.
213. Pogo, B. G. T., Pogo, A. O., and Allfrey, V. G. (1969). *Genetics Suppl.* **61**, 373–379.
214. Potter, M. (1968). *Cancer Res.* **28**, 1891–1896.
215. Potter, V. R. (1968). *Cancer Res.* **28**, 1901–1907.
216. Prescott, D. (1966). *J. Cell. Biol.* **31**, 1–9.
217. Prestayko, A. W., and Busch, H. (1973). *In* "Methods in Cancer Research" Vol. IX, pp. 154–194. Academic Press, New York.
218. Prestayko, A. W., Lewis, B. C., and Busch, H. (1972). *Biochim. Biophys. Acta* **269**, 90–103.
219. Rall, S. C., and Cole, R. D. (1971). *J. Biol. Chem.* **246**, 7175–7190.
220. Reid, B. R., and Cole, R. D. (1964). *Proc. Nat. Acad. Sci. U.S.* **51**, 1044–1050.
221. Reid, B. R., Stellwagen, R. H., and Cole, R. D. (1968). *Biochim. Biophys. Acta* **155**, 593–602.
222. Riggs, A. D., Bourgeois, S., Newby, R. F., and Cohn, M. (1968). *J. Mol. Biol.* **34**, 365–368.
223. Ro, T. S., and Busch, H. (1964). *Cancer Res.* **24**, 1630–1633.
224. Robbins, E., and Borun, T. W. (1967). *Proc. Nat. Acad. Sci. U.S.* **57**, 409–416.
225. Roeder, R. G., and Rutter, W. J. (1969). *Nature (London)* **224**, 234–237.
226. Rovera, G., and Baserga, R. (1971). *J. Cell Physiol.* **77**, 201–212.
227. Ruddon, R. W., and Rainey, C. H. (1971). *FEBS Lett.* **14**, 170–174.
228. Sadgopal, A., and Bonner, J. (1969). *Biochim. Biophys. Acta* **186**, 349–357.
229. Salas, T., and Green, H. (1971). *Nature (London)* **229**, 165–169.
230. Scherzinger, E., Herrlich, P., and Schweiger, M. (1972). *Mol. Gen. Genet.* **118**, 67–77.

231. Schjeide, O. A. (1970). *In* "Cellular Differentiation (O. A. Schjeide and J. de Vellis, ed.), pp. 169–200. Van Nostrand Reinhold, Princeton, New Jersey.
231a. Sedwick, W. D., Wang, T. S.-F., and Korn, D. (1972). *J. Biol. Chem.* **247**, 5026–5033.
232. Seifart, K. H., Benecke, B. J., and Juhasz, P. P. (1972). *Arch. Biochem. Biophys.* **151**, 519–532.
233. Sekeris, C. E., Sekeris, K. E., and Gallwitz, D. (1967). *H.S.Z. Physiol. Chem.* **348**, 1660.
234. Sharma, A. K., and Sharma, A. (1972). "Chromosomal Techniques." Univ. Park Press, Baltimore, Maryland.
235. Shaw, L. M. J., and Huang, R. C. C. (1970). *Biochemistry* **9**, 4530–4542.
236. Shelton, K. R., and Neelin, J. M. (1971). *Biochemistry* **10**, 2342–2348.
237. Shelton, K. R., and Allfrey, V. G. (1970). *Nature (London)* **228**, 132–134.
238. Shepherd, G. R., Noland, B. J., and Hardin, J. M. (1971). *Arch. Biochem. Biophys.* **142**, 299–302.
239. Shepherd, G. R., Hardin, J. M., and Noland, B. J. (1971). *Arch. Biochem. Biophys.* **143**, 1–5.
240. Sherman, M. R., Corval, P. L., and O'Malley, B. W. (1970). *J. Biol. Chem.* **245**, 6085–6096.
241. Sherod, D., Johnson, G., and Chalkley, R. (1970). *Biochemistry* **9**, 4611–4615.
242. Sherton, C. C., and Wool, I. G. (1972). *J. Biol. Chem.* **247**, 4460–4467.
243. Shih, T. Y., and Bonner, J. (1970). *J. Mol. Biol.* **48**, 469–487.
244. Shih, T. Y., and Bonner, J. (1970). *J. Mol. Biol.* **50**, 333–344.
245. Shih, T. Y., and Fasman, G. D. (1971). *Biochemistry* **10**, 1675–1683.
246. Shih, T. Y., and Fasman, G. D. (1972). *Biochemistry* **11**, 398–404.
247. Shyamala, G., and Gorski, J. (1969). *J. Biol. Chem.* **244**, 1097–1103.
248. Siebert, G. (1967). *In* "Methods in Cancer Research" (H. Busch, ed.), Vol. III, pp. 47–59. Academic Press, New York.
248a. Siebert, G., Ord, M. G., and Stocken L. A. (1971). *Biochem. J.* **122**, 721–725.
249. Siebert, G., Villalobos, J., Jr., Ro, T. S., Steele, W. J., Lindenmayer, G., Adams, H., and Busch, H. (1966). *J. Biol. Chem.* **241**, 71–78.
250. Simpson, R. T. (1972). *Biochemistry* **11**, 2003–2008.
251. Singer, S., and Litwack, G. (1971). *Cancer Res.* **31**, 1364–1368.
252. Smellie, R. M. S. (1971). "The Biochemistry of Steroid Hormone Action." Academic Press, New York.
252a. Sonnenberg, B. P., and Zubay, G. (1965). *Proc. Nat. Acad. Sci. U.S.* **54**, 415–420.
253. Sorof, S., Yong, E. M., Coffey, C. B., and Morris, H. P. (1966). *Cancer Res.* **26**, 81–88.
254. Sorof, S., Young, E. M., McCue, M. M., and Fetterman, P. L. (1963). *Cancer Res.* **23**, 864–882.
255. Spelsberg, T. C., and Hnilica, L. S. (1971). *Biochim. Biophys. Acta* **228**, 202–211.
256. Spelsberg, T. C., and Hnilica, L. S. (1971). *Biochim. Biophys. Acta* **228**, 212–222.
257. Spelsberg, T. C., Steggles, A. W., and O'Malley, B. W. (1971). *J. Biol. Chem.* **246**, 4188–4197.
258. Spelsberg, T. C., Wilhelm, J. A., and Hnilica, L. S. (1971). *In* "Sub-Cellular Biochemistry" (B. D. Roodyn, ed.), pp. 1–107. Plenum Press, New York.
259. Stedman, E., and Stedman, E. (1950). *Nature (London)* **166**, 780–781.
260. Steele, W. J., and Busch, H. (1963). *Cancer Res.* **23**, 1153–1163.
261. Steele, W. J., and Busch, H. (1964). *Exp. Cell Res.* **33**, 68–72.
262. Steggles, A. W., Spelsberg, T. C., and O'Malley, B. W. (1971). *Biochem. Biophys. Res. Commun.* **43**, 20–27.
263. Stein, G. (1972). *In* "The Pathology of Transcription and Translation" (E. Farber, ed.), pp. 21–35. Marcel Dekker, New York.
264. Stein, G., and Baserga, R. (1970). *J. Biol. Chem.* **245**, 6097–6105.
265. Stein, G., and Baserga, R. (1971). *Biochem. Biophys. Res. Commun.* **44**, 218–228.
266. Stein, G. S., and Baserga, R. (1972). *Advan. Cancer Res.* **15**, 287–330.
267. Stein, G. S., and Borun, T. W. (1972). *J. Cell Biol.* **52**, 292–307.

268. Stein, H., and Hausen, P. (1970). *Cold Spring Harbor Symp.* Quant. Biol. **XXXV**, 709–717.
269. Stellwagen, R. H., and Cole, R. D. (1969). *Ann Rev. Biochem.* **38**, 951–990.
270. Stellwagen, R. H., and Cole R. D. (1969). *J. Biol. Chem.* **244**, 4878–4887.
270a. Stevely, W. S., and Stocken, L. A. (1968). *Biochem. J.* **110**, 187–191.
271. Sugano, N., Olson, M. O. J., Yeoman, L. C., Johnson, B. R., Taylor, C. W., Starbuck, W. C., and Busch, H. (1972). *J. Biol. Chem.* **247**, 3589–3591.
272. Sung, M. T., and Dixon, G. H. (1970). *Proc. Nat. Acad. Sci. U.S.* **67**, 1616–1623.
272a. Sung, M. T., Dixon, G. H., and Smithies, O. (1971). *J. Biol. Chem.* **246**, 1358–1364.
273. Teng, C.-S., and Hamilton, T. H. (1970). *Biochem. Boiphys. Res. Commun.* **40**, 1231–1238.
274. Teng. C. S., Teng, C. T., and Allfrey, V. G. (1971). *J. Biol. Chem.* **246**, 3597–3609.
275. Tidwell, T., Allfrey, V. G., and Mirsky, A. E. (1968). *J. Biol. Chem.* **243**, 707–715.
276. Tobey, R. A., Peterson, D. F., and Anderson, E. C. (1971). *In* "The Cell Cycle and Cancer (R. Baserga, ed.), pp. 309–353. Dekker, New York.
277. Ursprung, H., Smith, K. D., Sofer, W. H., and Sullivan, P. T. (1968). *Science* **160**, 1075–1081.
278. Vendrely, R., Knobloch-Mazen, A., and Vendrely, C. (1960). *Biochem. Pharm.* **4**, 19–28.
279. Venis, M. A. (1972). *Biochem. J.* **127**, 29P.
280. Vidali, G., Boffa, L. C., and Allfrey, V. G., (1972). *J. Biol. Chem.* **247**, 7365–7373.
280a. Vidali, G., Gershey, E. L., and Allfrey, V. G. (1968). *J. Biol. Chem.* **243**, 6361–6366.
281. Von Hahn, H. P. (1971). *Beitr. Pathol. Bd.* **144**, 327–343.
282. Von Hippel, P. H., and McGhee, J. D. (1972). *Ann. Rev. Biochem.* **41**, 231–300.
283. Vorbrodt, A. (1974). *In* "The Cell Nucleus" (H. Busch, ed.). Academic Press, New York.
284. Wagner, T., and Spelsberg, T. C. (1971). *Biochemistry* **10**, 2599–2605.
285. Wakabayashi, K., and Hnilica, L. S. (1972). *J. Cell Biol.* **55**, 271a.
286. Wang, T. Y. (1966). *J. Biol. Chem.* **241**, 2913–2917.
287. Wang, T. Y. (1968). *Arch. Biochem. Biophys.* **127**, 235–240.
288. Wang, T. Y. (1972). *Exp. Cell Res.* **69**, 217–219.
289. Weaver, R. F., Blatti, S. P., and Rutter, W. J. (1971). *Proc. Nat. Acad. Sci. U.S.* **68**, 2294.
289a. Wilchek, M. (1972). *Biochem. J.* **127**, 7–9.
290. Wilhelm, J. A., Ansevin, A. T., Johnson, A. W., and Hnilica, L. S. (1972). *Biochim. Biophys. Acta* **272**, 220–230.
291. Wilhelm, J. A., Groves, C. M., and Hnilica, L. S. (1972). *Experientia* **28**, 514–516.
292. Wilhelm, J. A., and McCarty, K. S. (1970). *Cancer Res.* **30**, 418–425.
293. Williams, D. L., and Gorski, J. (1972). *In* "Gene Transcription in Reproductive Tissue." (E. Diczfalusy, ed.), pp. 420–438. Bogtrykkeriet Forum, Copenhagen.
294. Wittliff, J. L., Hilf, R., Brooks, W. F., Jr., Savlov, E. D., Hall, T. C., and Orlando, R. A. (1971). *Cancer Res.* **32**, 1983–1992.
294a. Wong, K.-Y., Patel, J., and Krause, M. O. (1972). *Exp. Cell Res.* **69**, 456–460.
295. Yeoman, L. C., Olson, M. O. J., Sugano, N., Jordan, J., Taylor, C. W., Starbuck, W. C., and Busch, H. (1972). *J. Biol. Chem.* **247**, 6018–6023.
296. Yeoman, L. C., Taylor, C. W., and Busch, H. (1973). *Biochem. Biophys. Res. Commun.* **51**, 956–966.
296a. Yeoman, L. C., Taylor, C. W., Jordan, J. J., and Busch, H. (1973). *Biochem. Biophys. Res. Commun.* **53**, 1067–1076.
297. Yoshida, M., and Shimura, K. (1972). *Biochim. Biophys. Acta* **263**, 690–695.
298. Zbarsky, I. B., and Georgiev, G. P. (1959). *Biochim. Biophys. Acta* **32**, 301–302.
299. Zhelabovskaya, S. M., and Berdyshev, G. D. (1972). *Exp. Geront.* **7**, 313–320.
300. Zubay, G., and Doty, P., (1959). *J. Mol. Biol.* **1**, 1–20.
301. Zubay, G., Morse, D. E., Schrenk, W. J., and Miller, J. H. M. (1972). *Proc. Nat. Acad. Sci. U.S.* **69**, 1100–1103.

CHAPTER IX

Protein Synthesis

A. CLARK GRIFFIN

I. Introduction

The fundamental reaction of protein synthesis, the synthesis of a peptide bond between two amino acids, is not difficult to achieve in the laboratory. However, the functional groups of the amino acids must be preserved and the addition of each amino acid requires several steps. Through ingenuity and perseverance several of the peptide hormones including oxytocin, vasopressin, α-melanocyte-stimulating hormone, and adrenocorticotrophin have been chemically synthesized. The two chains of insulin have also been synthesized and recently automated solid-phase techniques were developed in which the repetitive steps are programmed. It has been possible to chemically synthesize complicated polypeptides and even proteins such as pancreatic ribonuclease (124 residues). Many days were required for this ingenious synthesis and the formation of each peptide bond is still measured in hours. Most living cells have

355

the potential for the biosynthesis of an almost unlimited number of proteins of varying degree of complexity, at a rate less than one second per peptide bond and with an accuracy of less than one misplaced amino acid in 5000–10,000.

Protein synthesis in living cells encompasses a range of events in which the information encoded in the genes is translated into ordered arrangements of amino acid in the many specific polypeptides and proteins required for the cellular and body composition and function. As this information was expanded, aspects of protein synthesis became important in genetics, evolution, embryogenesis, differentiation, mitosis, regulation, cellular physiology, and pathology including neoplasia. A perusal of almost any of the journals of biology or biochemistry reveals that many articles are concerned with some aspect of protein synthesis.

The direct relationship, if any, that the above translational events may have on either the origin of cancer cells or their subsequent behavior has not been clearly established. If cancer results from somatic mutations, oncogenes, protoviruses, or other causes that are gene or chromosome related, it is quite possible that the mechanistic stages of translations proceed in a normal manner. Even if there are observable differences at one or more of the stages of protein synthesis, they may be secondary to the mutational changes. On the other hand, it is possible that alterations in translational events may have a more direct or primary role in carcinogenesis and the abnormal behavior of the cancer cells. Most of this chapter will be concerned with the polysomal system of protein synthesis which does appear to be functional in all living cells. Comparative and evolutionary aspects of this system will be presented including studies employing cancer cells. Protein synthesis in the cell nucleus and cytoplasm will be considered as well as some other mechanisms of peptide bond formation. Attention is directed to some of the recent comprehensive reviews covering protein synthesis (3, 9, 39, 58, 62).

Space limitations make it impossible to give credit to the many investigators who have contributed to our present knowledge of the translational mechanism. However, most of the major developments have been achieved during the past decade. It may be of interest to point out that one of the first cell-free amino acid incorporating systems was isolated from Ehrlich mouse ascites tumor (65). While there was considerable speculation during the 1950's as to the existence and nature of a genetic code for protein synthesis, the establishment of the triplet code was not made until 1961 (16, 77). The complete nucleotide sequence of yeast alanyl-tRNA was reported in 1965 (47) (see Chapter VI).

II. Systems for Protein Biosynthesis

A. Polysomal System

Approximately 80% or even more of the total cellular capacity for protein synthesis takes place on messenger RNA-polysomal complexes. It is relatively easy to demonstrate the incorporation of radio-labeled amino acids into an acid-insoluble fraction by employment of disrupted cellular preparations such as the combination of the high-speed ultracentrifuge supernatant fractions and the pH 5.0 insoluble proteins of the cytoplasm. On the other hand, it has been essential to utilize a variety of techniques in order to resolve the multiple components of the cell involved in protein synthesis. The *in vitro* reconstitution of these components has made it possible to establish many of the reactions and events involved in protein synthesis in the intact cell. Much of our present knowledge and understanding of protein synthesis has been obtained from studies involving the components isolated from microbial cells. Extension of this investigative approach to mammalian systems has provided considerable indication that the same overall mechanism is operative. Some comparative aspects will be considered later in this chapter. The *in vitro* findings which have been invaluable in studying the components and individual reactions do have limitations. The reactions have been removed from the organizational and regulatory influences of the intact cell or the organism. Any difference that may exist between the normal and cancerous cells may be at this higher level and would not be apparent in the usual *in vitro* approaches.

Protein biosynthesis involving the polysomal system may be conveniently subdivided into three categories: polypeptide chain initiation, chain elongation, and chain termination.

1. CHAIN INITIATION

The components or factors include initiating aminoacyl-tRNA; initiating factors, F_1, F_2, and F_3; ribosomes; mRNA; and GTP and Mg^{2+}. Peptide chain initiation requires a specific tRNA that will combine with methionine: $tRNA_F^{M \circ}$ in bacteria, mitochondria, and chloroplasts and $tRNA_1^{Met}$ in eukaryotes. The initiator tRNA is characterized by a different arrangement of the complementary bases than is observed in the other tRNA's that are involved in peptide chain elongation. In the former, the first complementary base pair is position 6 (from the 3' terminal), while base pairing starts at position 5 for the latter (19, 92). Formation of $Met-tRNA_F^{Met}$ and other aminoacyl-tRNA probably occurs by a two-stage mechanism (79):

$$\text{Aminoacyl synthetase}(E) + \text{methionine} + ATP \rightarrow E\text{-Met-AMP} + PP$$
$$E\text{-Met-AMP} + tRNA_F^{Met} \rightarrow \text{Met-}tRNA_F^{Met} + E + AMP$$

Loftfield (65a) has reviewed the mechanisms of the aminoacylation of transfer RNA. He believes that the generally accepted mechanism of tRNA esterification (as presented in this chapter) is not acceptable for many amino acids. Loftfield concludes: "For the physiological situation, where almost all enzyme is associated with tRNA and where the concentration of spermine may be greater than Mg^{2+}, we propose a concerted reaction in which tRNA, amino acid enzyme, and ATP react to form aminoacyl tRNA, AMP, PPi, and free enzyme with no discrete intermediates."

In bacteria and chloroplasts, the methionine is formylated after aminoacylation (69).

$$\text{Met-tRNA}_{\text{F}}^{\text{Met}} \xrightarrow[\text{Met-tRNA formylase}]{N^{10}\text{-formyltetrahydrofolic acid}} \text{fMet-tRNA}_{\text{F}}^{\text{Met}}$$

The formylase has been obtained in a high degree of purity from *E. coli*. The molecular weight of this enzyme is approximately 25,000 and its sedimentation constant is 2.02, which is about the same size as part of its substrate. In eukaryotes, the initiating tRNA (met-tRNA^{Met}) does not have to undergo formylation for chain initiation (92).

The codons for tRNA$_{\text{F}}^{\text{Met}}$ or tRNA$_{\text{I}}^{\text{Met}}$ are AUG and GUG and the *N*-formyl Met-tRNA selects the first codon within the mRNA to be translated. It has been established that subsequent translation is from the 5' to the 3' end of the mRNA, and it would appear that the initiator codon should occupy the 5' terminus. Analysis of the base sequence of the RNA of bacteriophage R17 indicated that the initiator codons for coat proteins, RNA synthetase, and maturation protein started from nucleotides at considerable distances from the 5' end of the R17 RNA (98). Initiation can also take place with a high efficiency upon a single-stranded DNA molecule (10).

Washing of *E. coli* ribosomes with 0.5 to 2.0 *M* NH$_4$Cl releases several protein factors from the 30 S subunit that are required for the initiation events. These factors designated F$_1$, F$_2$, and F$_3$ have been highly purified employing polyacrylamide gels and the molecular weights determined are F$_1$ (crystalline), 9400 daltons; F$_2$, 80,000 daltons; and F$_3$ a heat stabile, single polypeptide chain, 21,000 daltons. Comparable factors appear to be involved in mammalian systems; however, this has not been investigated as thoroughly as for the microbial systems. Three factors, M$_1$, M$_2$, and M$_3$, have been observed in the reticulocyte system (83). Mg^{2+} in the microbial cell-free system should be 4–8 m*M*/liter for fMet-tRNA-dependent initiation. Higher concentrations of Mg^{2+} may lead to a nonspecific initiation.

The two remaining requirements for initiation of protein synthesis are ribosomes and GTP. Ribosomes may be classified as follows:

Prokaryote-bacterial 70 S, 2.8 × 10⁶ daltons
Eukaryotes-cytoplasmic 80 S, 4 × 10⁶ daltons
Mitochondrial (miniribosomes) 55 S

A further characterization of ribosomes follows:

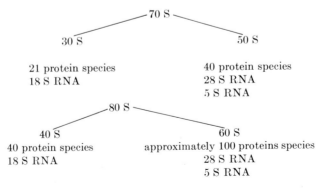

There are at least two binding sites on ribosomes usually designated as the aminoacyl-tRNA acceptor site (A) and the peptidyl donor site (P). Actually, these sites may be distinguished by the addition of puromycin, a structural analog of the terminal aminoacyl adenosine of an aminoacyl-tRNA. Puromycin reacts with the peptidyl-tRNA attached to the ribosome to form peptidyl puromycin and tRNA. No further amino acid can be linked to the peptidyl puromycin and chain termination occurs. *In vitro* amino acid-incorporating systems with added poly U direct the biosynthesis of polyphenylalanine which initially is bound to the ribosome. It was observed that two forms of polyphenylalanyl-tRNA ribosomes occurred in these systems. One of these would react directly with puromycin and the other required the supernatant factors (described below) and GTP. Only when the peptidyl-tRNA is attached to the donor site (P) can the peptidyl residue react with puromycin. When it is attached to the aminoacyl-tRNA acceptor site, transfer factors and GTP are required for the shift to the peptidyl donor site.

The scheme proposed by Lengyel and Söll (58) provides the basis for the following diagram used to illustrate chain initiation.

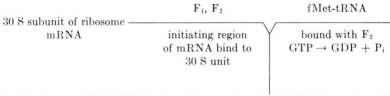

Recently, a similar initiation sequence was demonstrated in rabbit reticulocyte preparation (12). Met-tRNA$_1^{Met}$ is specific for the 40 S subunit. A two-stage mechanism has been proposed for the initiation and translation of polycistronic messengers (78).

2. CHAIN ELONGATION

Additional requirements are Mg^{2+}, K^+, or NH_4^+; binding factor (T); translocase (G); peptidyl transferase (inherent in larger ribosomal subunit); and GTP.

The elongation factors G and T were isolated from the high speed supernatant fraction of *E. coli* (see 62). Both factors have been crystallized. Factor G (84,000 daltons) is inactivated by reagents which react with sulfhydryl groups. T factors from *E. coli* and *P. fluorescens* have been separated into chemically stable or unstable forms designated Ts and Tu. *In vitro* incorporating systems have a relatively high requirement for monovalent cation in addition to a Mg^{2+} requirement. GTP is required for the binding of aminoacyl-tRNA and for translocation of peptidyl-tRNA from acceptor to the peptidyl donor site.

Various designations for the transferases isolated by different investigators have appeared in the literature. Felicetti and Lipmann (24) separated the factors from rat liver and proposed a common nomenclature for identification—T_1 to be associated with the GTP-linked binding of aminoacyl-tRNA to the ribosomes

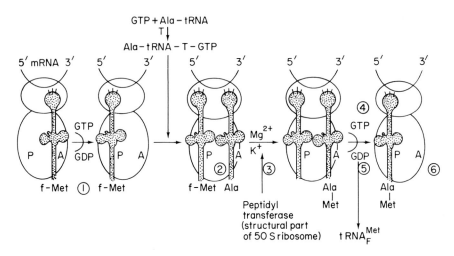

Fig. 9.1. Initiation and elongation of peptidyl chain. Blocking sites are 1, puromycin—preliminary chain termination; 2, tetracycline—inhibits binding of aminoacyl-tRNA to site A on ribosomes; 3, sparsomycin—peptidyl transferase; 4, fusidic acid—translocation; 5, diphtheria toxin—specifically inhibits rat liver T-2; and 6, chloroamphenicol—inhibits polypeptide release in microbial systems.

and T_2 with the translocation function. A new soluble protein factor, distinct from T_1, catalyzes the codon-specific binding of some aminoacyl-tRNA's to mammalian 40 S subunits (31).

Elongation of the peptidyl chain is shown in Fig. 9.1. The next aminoacyl-tRNA (Ala-tRNA) is bound to the acceptor site (A) after forming a complex with factor T and GTP. fMet is released from the fMet-tRNA on the donor site and simultaneously transferred to the α-amino group of the Ala-tRNA forming a peptide bond. Peptidyl transferase, a structural part of the 50 S ribosome, is responsible for this key reaction. The newly formed Met-Ala-tRNA still on site A is translocated to site P. This step requires factor G and GTP. $tRNA_F^{Met}$ must be released or ejected before translocation can occur. A specific factor promotes the ejection of deacylated initiator tRNA from ribosomes (90) and this differs from release of the noninitiating tRNA (66). During translocation, the ribosomes move through the mRNA nucleotides from the 5' to 3' direction and site A is clear for the next designated aminoacyl-tRNA. Some of the steps that are blocked or inhibited by antibiotics or other compounds are also indicated in Fig. 9.1.

3. CHAIN TERMINATION AND RELEASE

The requirements are UAA, ochre codon; UAG, amber codon; UGA, opal codon; and release factors, R_1 and R_2.

The "nonsense" codons observed in bacteriophage mutants were shown later to terminate protein synthesis. Several investigators established that the three codons, UAA, UAG, and UGA, were involved in this function. Release factors R_1 and R_2 present in the cytoplasm, are nondialyzable, inactivated by trypsin, not affected by RNase, and their molecular weights are about 44,000 and 47,000 daltons, respectively. R_1 appears to be specific for UAA and UAG and R_2 for UAA and UGA. When the terminator trinucleotides and the release factors are incubated with the N-formyl-Met-tRNA-AUG-ribosome complex there is release of free N-formylmethionine from the ribosomal intermediate (13). The R_1 and R_2 interact with the terminator codons resulting in the release of polypeptidyl-tRNA and dissociation of mRNA and ribosome. There is also evidence that another factor is required for the dissociation of 70 S ribosomes into 30 S and 50 S subunits. This factor may be identical to one of the initiating factors, F_3.

These mechanisms have been established largely from investigations involving microbial systems. There are many aspects of protein synthesis that require further elucidation, i.e., peptide bond formation, initiation, and release, intramolecular binding sites on tRNA's, ribosomes, ribosomal structure, etc. Considerably less is known concerning mammalian systems than the microbial systems. However, the elaborate studies of Schweet and his co-workers have revealed that the polysomal systems in reticulocytes closely resemble that of microbial systems. In fact, the studies involving liver cells, brain tissues, tumor cells, and other mammalian tissues and organs seem to provide strong indication that the above described mechanism of protein synthesis has evolved as a generally universal one. Evolutionary aspects of peptide biosynthesis have been evaluated (63). Comparative aspects of protein synthesis with emphasis on the cancer cell will be considered in further detail in Section III,B.

B. Mitochondrial Systems

Mitochondria contain a protein-synthesizing system distinct from that of the cytoplasm. This has been observed in studies involving *Neurospora* (5) and rat liver (6, 43). Aminoacyl synthetases and tRNA's are present in mitochondria. Reverse phase chromatography shows the presence of distinct and separable species of mitochondrial and cytoplasmic tRNA's for 15 amino acids in *Neurospora* (21). While the mechanism of this protein-synthesizing system has not been elucidated it appears to be more bacterialike in nature. Mitochondrial preparations from *Neurospora* contain a tRNA$_F^{Met}$ as well as another tRNA^{Met}. The former can be formylated by an enzyme present in mitochondrial extracts. Mitochondrial protein synthesis requires a formylated methionine for initiation which is analogous to the microbial systems (22) (Section II,A,1). However, addition of polyuridylic or polyadenylic acids had no stimulating effect on the incorporation of labeled amino acids into protein by isolated rat liver mitochondria (43).

There still remains considerable doubt as to the exact nature of proteins synthesized in the mitochondria. Several investigators have reported that this system produces several of the structural proteins and more specifically certain of the insoluble proteins of the inner membrane. Beattie *et al.* (6) concluded, however, that rat liver mitochondria *in vitro* do not incorporate amino acids into such major proteins of the structural protein fraction as cytochromes b and c_1, cytochrome oxidase, or ATPase.

C. Nuclear Systems

A review of the biosynthetic reactions in the cell nucleus (2) indicates that the mechanism of amino acid incorporation into the proteins of the nucleus is similar in many respects to the cytoplasmic system. Many of the proteins synthesized in the nucleus may be included in the regulation of gene activity. Nuclear ribosomes have been isolated and studied. These particles have sedimentation coefficients of 78 S. The nuclear system also utilizes activating enzymes and specific tRNA's. Nuclear ribosomal preparations have a Mg^{2+} and GTP requirement for amino acid incorporation. This system is also responsive to synthetic polynucleotides and is inhibited by the addition of puromycin or ribonuclease. While the isolated nuclear ribosomal system is stimulated by the addition of DNA, there are indications that protein synthesis in the nucleus depends upon mRNA. Recently, Liew *et al.* (61) have made the important observation that N-acetylseryl-tRNA is involved in the initiation of synthesis of f2a histones which have in common the acetylated amino-terminal peptide, N-acetyl-serylglcylarginine. It is generally considered that histones are synthesized in the cytoplasm (see Chapter VIII).

Nucleoli isolated from various sources have been shown to incorporate amino acids into proteins. Recently, Lamkin and Hurlbert (56) reported that incorporation of amino acids into proteins of nucleoli from Novikoff ascites tumor. The authors concluded that nucleoli contain the amino acid-activating enzymes, tRNA's, and other components for total protein synthesis. Liau *et al.* (60) have found several tRNA methylases in the Novikoff tumor nucleoli.

D. Aminoacyl-tRNA Protein Transferases

With tumor and liver *in vitro* amino acid-incorporating systems an apparent incorporation of several amino acids was observed in nonribosomal fractions of cytoplasm. Significant amounts of labeled arginine and lesser quantities of glutamic acid, phenylalanine, lysine, and valine were present in a hot TCA-insoluble form following incubation of the pH 5.0 insoluble fraction of Novikoff ascites tumor (38). With *E. coli* S100 soluble fractions, it was observed that leucine and phenylalanine were also incorporated in the absence of ribosomes (49). Further study provided indications that tRNA may be involved in these phenomena. During the last 2–3 years the mechanism for this apparent incorporation was found with the discovery of a new group of enzymes, the amino-acyl-tRNA protein transferases (95).

Arginyl-tRNA protein transferase was first obtained from the soluble fraction of sheep thyroid cytoplasm. Its activity was measured by the transfer of [^{14}C]Arg-tRNA into the hot TCA-insoluble fraction in the absence of Mg^{2+}. As the enzyme was purified it became apparent that an acceptor protein was needed. Serum albumin filled this requirement; however, not all the proteins possessed this acceptor activity. Further investigation of the requirements for this reaction established the need for monovalent cation (K^+ was not effective) and for SH. GTP and the usual transfer factors were not required and puromycin had no effect upon the reaction. The reaction mechanism involves the transfer of arginine into a peptide bond with the N-terminal aspartic or glutamic acid residues of the acceptor protein. A similar enzyme was found in the cytoplasm of rabbit liver cells and in E. coli. Another aminoacyl-tRNA protein transferase was obtained from E. coli that catalyzes the transfer of either leucine or phenylalanine to acceptor protein. This transferase appears to be a single enzyme. An amino terminal arginine is required in the acceptor protein transferase (57, 93).

Arginyl-tRNA protein transferase has been obtained in a highly purified form from rabbit liver. This enzyme catalyzes the transfer of one mole of arginine (Arg-tRNA) to the amino terminal aspartic acid of a mole of albumin and two arginines per mole of bovine thyroglobulin. Studies with other acceptor proteins, including several immunoglobulins, have indicated that there are specific acceptors (94). The role played by this class of enzymes in physiological activities or in the function of the cancer cell must await further investigations. The early observations that the Novikoff ascites tumor has an apparent active tRNA protein transferase warrant additional study.

E. Peptide Synthesis Not Involving Nucleic Acids

Two fractions required for the in vitro synthesis of gramicidin S, a cyclic decapeptide, were isolated from B. brevis (51, 63). The heavier fraction obtained from Sephadex G-200 chromatography (approximate MW 200,000 daltons) contained the enzymic function for the activation of four L-amino acids (L-Pro, L-Val, L-Orn, L-Leu) as revealed by amino acid dependent ATP-PP$_i^{32}$ exchanges. A lighter fraction II with an approximate molecular weight of 100,000 daltons contained an enzyme for activation of D- or L-phenylalanine.

The four amino acids are activated by a polyenzyme system that is charged with its four substrates, first as aminoacyl adenylates and then in a subsequent form. The bound derivatives will not enter into peptidation reactions unless the activating enzyme (II) is present which is carrying the bound phenylalanine. The apparent initiating event involves an association of the amino acid-charged enzymes and leads to polymerization and cyclization of the prebound amino acids. The organization of the enzyme complex directs the amino acid sequence.

A similar system is responsible for the synthesis of tyrocidins obtained from the above organism. Whether comparable systems are involved in the biosynthesis of small polypeptides in mammalian cells has not been ascertained. The specificity of amino acid charging is of a lower order than that achieved by the nucleic acid-coded system. Several amino acid substitutions have been observed in both gramacidin and tyrocidine.

III. Mammalian Amino Acid-Incorporating Systems

A. Normal Tissues and Organs

The properties and function of the polysomal system of protein synthesis in normal cellular systems, while not identical, are remarkably similar to those already described in Section II, A for microbial systems. Reticulocytes obtained from phenylhydrazine-treated rabbits have proved to be an invaluable source of ribosomes and the other factors involved in protein synthesis. The general procedures employed for isolation of the components of this system have been reviewed (39). Two factors, TF-I and TF-II (corresponding to bacterial T and G), have been purified to homogeneity. TF-I has a MW of 186,000 and TF-II, a MW of 70,000.

Cell-free amino acid-incorporating systems from liver have been studied in considerable detail (24, 28, 39, 52, 85). The liver ribosomal systems, while considerably less active than the microbial or the reticulocyte systems in amino acid incorporation, have provided further indication of the similarity of polypeptide biosynthesis to the already described microbial system. Amino acid incorporating-systems have been isolated from many other mammalian tissues and organs including skeletal muscle, (26), brain, (36, 68), pancreas, (18), chick oviduct, (72, 81), testis, (71), and heart (73).

Several human tissues (tonsil, placenta, adrenals, spleen) have been utilized for *in vitro* studies of protein synthesis. The general mechanisms of the polysomal synthesis of proteins on these tissues is similar to that already described for microbial and also other mammalian systems. However, the systems derived from human tissues have not been studied as intensively as the *E. coli* and the reticulocyte systems (7, see 39 for general procedures employed).

B. Cancer Cells

A protein-synthesizing system was isolated from L-1210 mouse ascites leukemia (80). An efficient amino acid-incorporating system is also obtainable from Novikoff ascites tumor (39). By employing highly purified ribosomes from this tumor it was possible to demonstrate that two factors, T_1 and T_2, are also involved in protein synthesis (8). A ribosomal-polysomal system for amino acid incorporation was prepared from Krebs II ascites carcinoma (23) and a cell-free system was obtained from rat lymphosarcoma (53). The cell-free system from Krebs II ascites tumor could translate several purified mRNA's of both mammalian and viral origin (70).

The immunoglobulin-producing plasma cell tumors (myelomas) of mice represent an invaluable source of cells for the study of protein synthesis (82). These tumors are programmed for the synthesis of specific immunoglobulins and could provide the basis for investigation into the regulation of specific aspects of protein synthesis (Chapter XIV). An interesting clinical corollary has been reported (80a). Several myeloma patients, successfully treated by chemotherapeutic methods, later developed monocytic leukemia and simultaneously began to excrete large quantities of the enzyme lysozyme. This finding raises the question of possible relations between myeloma and monocytic leukemia and also regulatory mechanisms that direct the synthesis of relatively large quantities of specific proteins in cells.

C. Comparative Aspects and Specificity

The general description of the amino acid-incorporating systems placed emphasis upon the similarity of the polysomal systems from the range of tissues and cells that have been investigated. From the *in vitro* studies involving components isolated from mammalian, microbial, and plant sources it would appear that this basic mechanism may be operative in all living cells. The findings and interpretations have been obtained from *in vitro* studies in which the components have been isolated from the many organizational and regulatory mechanisms inherent in the intact cell or organism; the artifactual nature of the isolated *in vitro* systems has been pointed out (44).

There are many indications that the quantities, as well as the type of proteins that are synthesized may be regulated at one or more of the translational stages. A model has been proposed with evidence for posttranscriptional control of protein synthesis (101). Hormones, such as testosterone and insulin, chalones, glycoproteins such as fibroblast growth factors (46, 64), or erythropoietin (54), play a major role in protein synthetic activities. The transfer RNA's may also be involved in the regulation of protein synthesis (Section IV, A, 1).

Many of the components involved in the *in vitro* synthesis of polypeptides are interchangeable from one species to another (39, 59). Ribosomes and the transfer factors, T-1 and T-2, of normal rat liver, ascites tumor cells, and reticulocytes are completely interchangeable. Studies on *in vitro* components from liver, Novikoff tumor and *E. coli* showed that the microbial T factor could be substituted for the comparable mammalian factor T-1 (55). However, the microbial G factor did not replace the mammalian T-2. Conversely, neither mammalian T-1 or T-2 was functional in the *E. coli*-incorporating system.

In cell-free systems, the factors required for hemoglobin chain initiation were found to be present in reticulocytes but absent in Landschutz ascites cells (15). The reticulocyte ribosomes could be inactivated by ascites ribosomes and it was suggested that in specialized cells as reticulocytes and muscle cells (myosin synthesis) there is no destruction of the mRNA, whereas in less specialized cells such as the ascites cells the ribosome destroys the mRNA after translation. However, liver ribosomes do possess a high ribonuclease activity specific for the breakdown of a nonribosomal high molecular weight RNA.

There are major differences in the ribosomal structure from microbial and mammalian sources (Section II,A,1). Differences in the largest molecular species of ribosomal RNA (28 S) between the human and mouse were demonstrated employing polyacrylamide gel electrophoresis. An extension of these observations also revealed that the 28 S RNA's from human and mouse could be distinguished between those of the Syrian hamster and the African green monkey (20). A comprehensive review of ribosomal specificity of protein synthesis (14) shows there are no definitive data on differences of major components of protein synthesis in any correlative manner with respect to neoplasia. Definitive answers must await a characterization of the many functional sites upon the ribosomes as well as more precise structural information on the component proteins and the RNA moieties. Busch and associates have initiated this monumental task of the complete sequential analysis of the 28 S RNA subunit of the mammalian ribosome (see Chapter V).

IV. Specific Aspects of Protein Synthesis as Related to the Cancer Cell

A. Transfer Ribonucleic Acids

1. ROLE OF tRNA IN PROTEIN SYNTHESIS

This aspect of the polysomal system of protein biosynthesis is included in view of the many reports (103) that altered tRNA patterns, as measured by various chromatographic procedures, have been observed during sporulation, embryogenesis, differentiation, viral and chemical carcinogenesis, viral infections, etc. In addition, the aminoacyl-tRNA patterns of several tumors differ from the normal tissue or organ pattern (see also Chapter VI).

The complete nucleotide sequences of approximately 50 tRNA's have been established (39, 103). The structure of one of the rat liver seryl-tRNA's is illustrated in Fig. 9.2. With the sequential nucleotide analysis of the increasing numbers of tRNA's some interesting structural characteristics are beginning to emerge. The nucleotide content ranges from 77 to 87. All tRNA's have the common sequence CCA at the 3′ or amino acid acceptor terminal. In addition, all tRNA's whose structures are known have four common nucleotides, GTΨC (shown in Fig. 9.2) which may be one of the ribosome recognition or binding sites. Initiator transfer RNA$_F^{Met}$ from eukaryotic cells may differ in structure from the tRNA$_F^{Met}$ of prokaryotic cells as reported in this chapter. Originally it was believed that all tRNA's have the common nucleotide sequence, –G–T–Ψ–C– in the so-called TΨC loop or region. Simsek and RajBhandary (91a) have now reported that yeast initiator transfer RNA$_F^{Met}$ does not contain this sequence and it is replaced by –G–A–U–C–.

P. Piper and B. Clark (81a) found that tRNA$_F^{Met}$ from myeloma cells also contain this same sequence, –G–A–U–C–.

It should also be pointed out that R. J. Roberts (88a) observed that the structures of tRNA$_{I_A}^{Gly}$ and tRNA$_{I_B}^{Gly}$ of S. epidermidis in this same region is –G–U–G–C–. These tRNA's are not involved in protein synthesis but participate in

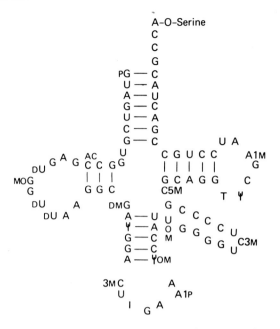

Fig. 9.2. Structure of rat liver seryl-tRNA (97).

peptidoglycan synthesis. Infection of *E. coli* with defective transducing bacteriophage leads to the synthesis of three suppressor tRNA's that differ in the base adjacent to the anticodon (32). fMet-tRNA has an A in the 5th position from the 3' terminal which does not hydrogen bond with the 5' terminal C. The nucleotides of other tRNA's involved in the placement of tRNA in the polypeptide chain are complementary in this respect.

In addition to the four major nucleosides, the tRNA's contain approximately 15% minor nucleosides (42). At least 20 of these minor or modified nucleosides have been isolated from tRNA. Most are methylated derivatives. Cytokinins that promote cell division have been found as integral components of tRNA's. $N^6(\Delta^2\text{-isopentenyl})$adenosine occurs in all species as a component of the tRNA (41) and can inhibit the growth of certain lines of cancer cells and also human blood lymphocytes (86). Many methods are available for the fractionation and sequential analysis of the tRNA's (103). By employing various chromatographic or countercurrent distribution procedures many investigators have accumulated considerable evidence suggesting that there is a multiplicity of tRNA's for many amino acids. As pointed out by von Ehrenstein (103), separate tRNA's are required when 2 codons specifying one amino acid begin with different bases (codons for leucine, serine, arginine). However, a single tRNA can recognize three codons if these have the first two bases in common and U, C, or A as the third base. The redundant species of tRNA may have regulator or suppressor functions.

From chromatographic data as well as sequential nucleotide analysis, there is evidence for species specificity in tRNA's for a given amino acid. There are major differences, for example, in the nucleotide sequence of tRNA^{Tyr} of yeast and *E. coli* and between tRNA^{Ser} of yeast and rat liver. However, comparative studies of the chromatographic profiles of a specific aminoacyl-tRNA of various tissues and organs from several mammalian sources reveal a striking similarity. Alterations in certain of these profiles which occur during cancer induction or differences which appear in the cancer cell will be discussed later in this section. While there is some degree of multiplicity in the tRNA's, a single amino-acyl synthetase appears to recognize all of the tRNA's specific for a given amino acid. Aminoacyl synthetase preparations from one mammalian source will usually recognize and charge tRNA's from other mammalian sources and even from nonmammalian species. A highly purified arginyl synthetase charged the 4–5 isoaccepting species of tRNA^{Arg} present in rat, hamster, and mouse liver, and in Novikoff ascites tumor. This enzyme preparation also catalyzed the formation of Arg-tRNA with *E. coli* and yeast tRNA (48). However, tRNA from one species is not always charged by the corresponding enzyme from another species. The aminoacylation reaction is a unique and highly significant event in that this represents the translation stage between the nucleotides and the amino acids. A high degree of accuracy is required at this stage to maintain the high fidelity of protein synthesis (see Section IV,B).

2. tRNA PATTERNS IN NORMAL AND CANCER CELLS

Many investigators have reported differences in the chromatographic profiles of specific aminoacyl-tRNA's of tumors and normal tissues or organs. A partial listing of these and some related findings are presented in Table 9.1 (9, 104). There are some apparent discrepancies in the findings from different laboratories which may be attributed in some part to the different procedures employed, strain differences, etc. However, the continued reports of differences in profiles of certain aminoacyl-tRNA's (aspartyl-, tyrosyl-, phenylalanyl- and seryl-) would indicate they may have some role in cancer induction or in neoplasia in general.

The aspartyl-tRNA pattern (Fig. 9.3) is representative of the differences that may be observed between normal and cancerous cells. In this study tRNA was isolated from an SV40-induced tumor and also from the livers of normal hamsters (11). The tumor tRNA was charged with [^{14}C]aspartic acid and amino-acylation of the liver tRNA was carried out with [^{3}H]aspartic acid. The two preparations were cochromatographed by an accelerated reverse phase chroma-tography system (50). Fractions from the column were analyzed for radioactivity and the elution profiles were plotted. The late eluting Asp-tRNA peak, evident in the tumor tRNA, has been observed in other virus-induced tumors. These preliminary findings posed several questions: (a) are virus-induced tumors char-acterized by this third Asp-tRNA peak; (b) what mechanism(s) is involved in the appearance of this peak; (c) how does the late eluting peak differ struc-turally from the other two major Asp-tRNA peaks; and (d) does this unusual profile offer any possibility for ascertaining viral involvement in human tumors. Hybridization studies (91) showed that none of the altered Asp-tRNA's were encoded in the SV40 genome. The pattern of Asp-tRNA may be due to selective cellular gene expression (29). Studies are in progress in our laboratory to obtain

TABLE 9.1
ALTERATIONS IN TRANSFER RNA PROFILES ASSOCIATED WITH NEOPLASIA

Tissues or cells	Differences observed	Reference
SV40-induced tumor	New Tyr-tRNA	45
Mouse tissues and tumors	Several tRNA's	100
Rat liver and Novikoff hepatomas	His-tRNA, Tyr-tRNA	4
Plasma cell tumor	tRNA patterns	106
Plasma cell tumor	tRNA patterns	67
Rat liver and hepatoma	Phe-tRNA	34
Plasma cell tumors	Leu-tRNA	75
Rat liver and Morris hepatomas	Ser-tRNA, Phe-tRNA, His-tRNA	102
Ehrlich ascites tumor-HN-2 resistant	Phe-tRNA	87
Normal and leukemic lymphoblasts	Tyr-tRNA, Glu-tRNA	30
Livers of azo dye fed rats	Lys-tRNA, Leu-tRNA, Phe-tRNA, Tyr-tRNA	33
Rat liver and Morris hepatomas	Phe-tRNA	35
Rat liver and Novikoff hepatomas	Leu-tRNA	88
Liver and Morris hepatomas	Tyr-tRNA	
	His-tRNA, Asn-tRNA	96
Human myeloma cells	Asp-tRNA, Tyr-tRNA	27
SV40 transformed cells	Asp-tRNA, Asn-tRNA	
	His-tRNA	91
Polyoma and SV40 transformed cells	Asp-tRNA	29
SV40 tumors	Asp-tRNA	11

sufficient quantities of each of the three major peak components for initial structural and functional studies. From preliminary observations, the second and third peaks have the same codon response (GAU) indicating that their chromatographic behavior results from other structural modifications. With larger quantities of the purified Asp-tRNA peaks it will be possible to determine if the third peak is functional in an *in vitro* amino acid-incorporating system. It will also be possible to compare oligonucleotide profiles from DEAE-cellulose columns following the ribonuclease T₁ digestion of each of the Asp-tRNA's, and thin layer chromatography (84) could also be utilized for comparison of the base compositions of these chromatographically separable Asp-tRNA's. From these studies it should be possible to determine whether the third Asp-tRNA is the result of an altered nucleotide sequence or some modification of one or more of the bases.

It is premature to speculate as to whether altered tRNA profiles of specific tRNA's have any direct involvement in neoplasia. With the many reports suggesting that the tRNA's may be involved in differentiation, growth control, and other cellular regulatory activities (99), further studies along these lines are indeed warranted. The tRNA's, the smallest of the biologically active nucleic acids, can be isolated and subjected to extensive structural characterizations. This approach offers an opportunity to study the mechanisms involved in the transformation of normal cells to cancer cells. Many carcinogens are first metabolized into more reactive forms (see Chapter X). These ultimate carcinogens

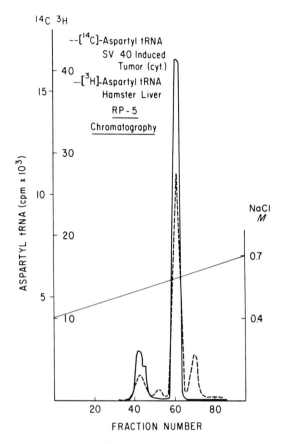

Fig. 9.3. Reverse phase chromatography (RP-5) patterns of aspartyl-tRNA's from hamster liver and SV40-induced tumors.

react with tissue components including the tRNA's. Administration of 3'-methyl-4-dimethylaminoazobenzene alters the chromatographic profile of several of the aminoacyl-tRNA's of rat liver (34). A purified tRNA^Phe isolated from the livers of rats fed diets containing this hepatocarcinogen was characterized by the presence of several nucleoside-azo metabolite interaction components as well as an alteration in the nucleoside composition (A. H. Daoud and A. C. Griffin, unpublished data).

A change in the primary nucleotide sequence of a specific tRNA could reflect the effects of the carcinogen or its metabolites upon the DNA. Alternatively, it is possible that the carcinogens react directly with the tRNA and modify their structure and function (1, 25). Recently, it was reported (74) that tetrahydrohydroxynaphthyl cysteine (THN-cysteine), formed by the interaction of cysteine and polycyclic hydrocarbon, undergoes esterification with yeast valyl- and isoleucyl-tRNA. It also appears that the aminoacyl synthetases for valine and isoleucine are the activating enzymes involved. Furthermore, the THN-cysteine-tRNA^Ile and THN-cysteine-tRNA^Val are incorporated by an *in vitro* yeast ribosomal system into a hot TCA-precipitable form. It is not difficult to visualize the havoc that could occur in terms of cellular function or regulation when a compound such as THN-cysteine is substituted for valine and isoleucine in enzymes and other proteins.

B. Fidelity—Accuracy of Protein Synthesis

Most codons are translated with relatively little error, i.e. 0.1–0.01% error or less (76). However, the error with some codons may be considerably higher. Some of the factors that may affect codon recognition include: temperature, Mg^{2+}, pH, antibiotics, polyamines, and other substances. Increasing the Mg^{2+} concentration, lowering the temperature, or addition of streptomycin, spermine, or spermidine did not appreciably enhance the ability of synthetic polynucleotides to code for leucine or isoleucine in mammalian *in vitro* systems such as rat liver or reticulocyte (105). The fidelity of the translational mechanism of mammalian cells is higher than is observed in bacterial (*in vitro*) systems (104, 105).

Relative concentrations of the various species of tRNA's may affect the accuracy of codon translation (40). Streptomycin induces miscoding in sensitive strains of *E. coli* and other microorganisms (17, 37). This antibiotic binds to the 30 S portion of the ribosomes and interferes with the codon-aminoacyl-tRNA complex. Streptomycin can cause the misreading of U as C and C as U or A in the first or second positions of the mRNA codon. The aminoglysidic antibiotics related to streptomycin (kanamycin, paramycin, neomycin) may also affect the codon translation. The phenotypic reversal of an amber alkaline phosphatase has been shown to be the consequence of 5-fluorouracil mispairing as cytosine during translation (89).

Aminoacyladenylate formation and the biosynthesis of aminoacyl-tRNA may be isolated and studied as separate reactions. Recognition and interaction between an aminoacyl synthetase for one amino acid and another occurs infrequently. However, highly purified isoleucyl-tRNA synthetase has been shown to form an aminoacyladenylate with valine as well as isoleucine. However, no valine was transferred to tRNA^{Ile}. Actually the tRNA^{Ile} enhanced the breakdown of the enzyme valyladenylate to valine. Thus, it would appear that the amino acid specificity of this step is even greater than the first reaction and reduces the chance of esterification of a wrong amino acid to the tRNA (79, 103, 107). While this general area of translational fidelity is relatively unexplored, there is no conclusive evidence at present that would link neoplasia and any generalized errors of protein synthesis.

V. Summary

As indicated in the introductory section most of our knowledge of the biosynthesis of proteins has evolved during the last decade. While many of the specific aspects of synthesis still remain to be established, the general mechanistic pattern of the mRNA-polysomal system appears to be functional in all living cells. At the present time there is no conclusive indication that protein synthesis in cancer cells differ in any fundamental respect from the mechanism presented earlier in this chapter. Most of the studies of proteins synthesis have been conducted employing *in vitro* techniques utilizing the purified components isolated from microbial or mammalian cells. Thus, the data obtained were under conditions wherein the organizational and other regulatory mechanisms of the cell or the body had been disrupted or removed. It is reasonable to assume that it is at these regulatory levels that cancer cells may differ from normal cells. While the necessity for study of the individual events in protein synthesis, utilizing the isolated components under controlled conditions is most obvious, the artifactual nature of these *in vitro* systems should be realized. Hoagland noted: "Indeed, we are now becoming aware that the simplified systems we study in the test tube are but sad reflections of intracellular capabilities. The triumph of mechanistic universality may in fact result from too assiduous efforts to discard those elements of the machinery which contribute to diversity" (44).

While there are no concrete indications at present linking patterns or alterations of protein synthesis with neoplasia, it is of interest to speculate what may emerge during the next decade. Many investigators are studying the structure and function of the multiple protein and RNA species that comprise the 40 S and 60 S subunits of mammalian ribosomes. A better understanding of the regulatory mechanisms will be attained. Subtle changes in one or more of these structures, in the transfer RNA's, or the enzymes or factors that are involved in the initiation, elongation, or release stages of protein synthesis, may result in an altered response to the usual cellular control mechanisms. Other promising approaches include the further investigations of the interaction of the carcinogens or their activated metabolites with the components of the protein-synthesizing systems. Such interactions may have drastic consequences in terms of the fidelity and regulation of translational events. A study of the production of and the amino acid sequences of immunoglobulins in the cancer patient may provide new insight into the fundamental aspects of cellular differentiation and neoplasia (108).

Acknowledgments

The author is an American Cancer Society Professor of Biochemistry. Studies included in this chapter were supported by grants from the American Cancer Society and The Robert A. Welch Foundation.

References

1. Agarwal, M. K., and Weinstein, I. B. (1970). *Biochemistry* 9, 503–508.
2. Allfrey, V. G. (1970). *In* "Aspects of Protein Synthesis" (C. B. Anfinsen, Jr., ed.), Part A, pp. 247–365. Academic Press, New York.

3. Anfinsen, C. B., Jr. (1970). "Aspects of Protein Synthesis," Part A. Academic Press, New York.
4. Baliga, B. S., Borek, E., Weinstein, I. B., and Srinivasan, P. R. (1969). *Proc. Nat. Acad. Sci. U.S.* **62**, 899–905.
5. Barnett, W. E., and Brown, D. H. (1967). *Proc. Nat. Acad. Sci. U.S.* **57**, 452–458.
6. Beattie, D. S., Patton, G. M., and Stuchell, R. N. (1970). *J. Biol. Chem.* **245**, 2177–2184.
7. Bermek, E., and Matthaei, H. (1970). *FEBS Lett.* **10**, 121–124.
8. Black, D. D., and Griffin, A. C. (1970). *Cancer Res.* **30**, 1281–1286.
9. Borek, E., and Kerr, S. J. (1972). *Advan. Cancer Res.* **15**, 163–190.
10. Bretscher, M. S. (1968). *Nature (London)* **220**, 1088–1091.
11. Briscoe, W. T., Taylor, W., Griffin, A. C., Duff, R., and Rapp, F. (1972). *Cancer Res.* **32**, 1753–1755.
12. Cashion, L. M., Kolb, A. J., and Stanley, Jr., W. M. (1972). *Biochim. Biophys. Acta* **262**, 525–534.
13. Caskey, C. T., Tompkins, R., Scolnick, E., Caryk, T., and Nirenberg, M. (1968). *Science* **162**, 135–138.
14. Ciferri, O., and Parisi, B. (1970). *Prog. Nucleic Acid Res. Mol. Biol.* **10**, 121–144.
15. Cohen, B. B. (1971). *Biochim. Biophys. Acta* **247**, 133–140.
16. Crick, F. H. C., Barnett, L., Brenner, S., and Watts-Tobin, R. J. (1961). *Nature (London)* **192**, 1227–1232.
17. Davies, J. (1966). *Cold Spring Harbor Symp. Quant. Biol.* **31**, 665–670.
18. Dickman, S. R., and Bruenger, E. (1969). *Biochemistry* **8**, 3295–3303.
19. Dube, S. K., Rudland, P. S., Clark, B. F. C., and Marcker, K. A. (1969). *Cold Spring Harbor Symp. Quant. Biol.* **34**, 161–166.
20. Eliceiri, G. L., and Green, H. (1970). *Biochim. Biophys. Acta* **199**, 543–544.
21. Epler, J. L. (1969). *Biochemistry* **8**, 2285–2290.
22. Epler, J. L., Shugart, L. R., and Barnett, W. E. (1970). *Biochemistry* **9**, 3573–3579.
23. Fais, D., Shakulov, R. C., and Klyachko, E. V. (1971). *Biochim. Biophys. Acta* **246**, 530–541.
24. Felicetti, L., and Lipmann, F. (1968). *Arch. Biochem. Biophys.* **125**, 548–557.
25. Fink, L. M., Nishimura, S., and Weinstein, I. B. (1970). *Biochemistry* **9**, 496–502.
26. Florini, J. R., and Breuer, C. B. (1966). *Biochemistry* **5**, 1870–1876.
27. Fujioka, S., and Gallo, R. C. (1971). *Blood* **38**, 246–252.
28. Galasinski, W., and Moldave, K. (1969). *J. Biol. Chem.* **244**, 6527–6532.
29. Gallagher, R. E., Ting, R. C., and Gallo, R. C. (1972). *Biochim. Biophys. Acta* **272**, 568–582.
30. Gallo, R. C., and Pestka, S. (1970). *J. Mol. Biol.* **52**, 195–219.
31. Gasior, E., and Moldave, K. (1972). *J. Mol. Biol.* **66**, 391–402.
32. Gefter, M. L., and Russell, R. L. (1969). *J. Mol. Biol.* **39**, 145–157.
33. Goldman, M., and Griffin, A. C. (1970). *Cancer Res.* **30**, 1677–1680.
34. Goldman, M., Johnston, W. M., and Griffin, A. C. (1969). *Cancer Res.* **29**, 1051–1055.
35. Gonano, F., Chiarugi, V. P., Pirro, G., and Marini, M. (1971). *Biochemistry* **10**, 900–908.
36. Goodwin, F., Shafritz, D., and Weissbach, H. (1969). *Arch. Biochem. Biophys.* **130**, 183–190.
37. Gorini, L., Jacoby, G. A., and Breckenridge, L. (1966). *Cold Spring Harbor Symp. Quant. Biol.* **31**, 657–664.
38. Griffin, A. C. (1967). *Advan. Cancer Res.* **10**, 83–116.
39. Griffin, A. C., and Black, D. D. (1971). *In* "Methods in Cancer Research" (H. Busch, ed.) Vol. VI, pp. 189–251. Academic Press, New York.
40. Grunberg-Manago, M., and Dondon, J. (1965). *Biochem. Biophys. Res. Commun.* **18**, 517–522.
41. Hall, R. H. (1970). *Progr. Nucleic Acid Res.* **10**, 57–86.
42. Hall, R. H. (1971). "The Modified Nucleosides in Nucleic Acids." Columbia Univ. Press, New York.
43. Hänninen, O., and Alanen-Irjala, K. (1968). *Acta Chem. Scand.* **22**, 3072–3080.

44. Hoagland, M. B. (1969). *Symp. on Polypeptides* Sponsored by Miles Lab., New York.
45. Holland, J. J., Taylor, M. W., and Buck, C. A. (1967). *Proc. Nat. Acad. Sci. U.S.* **58**, 2437–2444.
46. Holley, R. W., and Kiernan, J. A. (1968). *Proc. Nat. Acad. Sci. U.S.* **60**, 300–304. .
47. Holley, R. W., Apgar, J., Everett, G. A., Madison, J. T., Marquisee, M., Merrill, S. H., Penswick, J. R., and Zamir, A. (1965). *Science* **147**, 1462–1465.
48. Ikegami, H., and Griffin, A. C. (1969). *Biochim. Biophys. Acta* **178**, 166–174.
49. Kaji, A., Kaji, H., and Novelli, G. D. (1965). *J. Biol. Chem.* **240**, 1185–1191.
50. Kelmers, A. D., and Heatherly, D. E. (1971). *Anal. Biochem.* **44**, 486–495.
51. Kleinkauf, H., Gevers, W., and Lipmann, F. (1969). *Proc. Nat. Acad. Sci. U.S.* **62**, 226–233.
52. Klink, F., Kramer, G., Nour, A. M., and Petersen, K. G. (1967). *Biochim. Biophys. Acta* **134**, 360–372.
53. Koka, M., and Nakamoto, T. (1972) *Biochim. Biophys. Acta* **262**, 381–392.
54. Krantz, S. B., and Jacobsen, L. O. (1970). "Erythropoietin and the Regulation of Erythropoiesis." Univ. Chicago Press, Chicago, Illinois.
55. Krisko, I., Gordon, J., and Lipmann, F. (1969). *J. Biol. Chem.* **244**, 6117–6123.
56. Lamkin, A. F., and Hurlbert, R. B. (1972). *Biochim. Biophys. Acta* **272**, 321–326.
57. Leibowitz, M. J., and Soffer, R. L. (1970). *J. Biol. Chem.* **245**, 2066–2073.
58. Lengyel, P., and Söll, D. (1969). *Bacteriol. Rev.* **33**, 264–301.
59. Li, C-C, and Yu, C-T (1971). *Biochemistry* **10**, 3009–3013.
60. Liau, M. C., O'Rourke, C. M., and Hurlbert, R. B. (1972). *Biochemistry* **11**, 629–636.
61. Liew, C. C., Haslett, G. W., and Allfrey, V. G. (1970). *Nature* (*London*) **226**, 414–417.
62. Lipmann, F. (1969). *Science* **164**, 1024–1031.
63. Lipmann, F. (1971). *Science* **173**, 875–884.
64. Lipton, A., Klinger, I., Paul, D., and Holley, R. W. (1971). *Proc. Nat. Acad. Sci. U.S.* **68**, 2799–2801.
65. Littlefield, J. W., and Keller, E. B. (1957). *J. Biol. Chem.* **224**, 13–30.
65a. Loftfield, R. B. (1972). *Progr. Nucl. Acid Res. Mol. Biol.* **12**, 87–127.
66. Lucas-Lenard, J., and Haenni, A. (1969). *Proc. Nat. Acad. Sci. U.S.* **63**, 93–97.
67. Mach, B., Koblet, H., and Gros, D. (1968). *Proc. Nat. Acad. Sci. U.S.* **59**, 445–452.
68. Mahler, H. R., and Brown, B. J. (1968). *Arch. Biochem. Biophys.* **125**, 387–400.
69. Marcker, K., and Sanger, F. (1964). *J. Mol. Biol.* **8**, 835–840.
70. Mathews, M. B. (1972). *Biochim. Biophys. Acta* **272**, 108–118.
71. Means, A. R., and Hall, P. F. (1969). *Biochemistry* **8**, 4293–4298.
72. Means, A. R., Abrass, I. B., and O'Malley, B. W. (1971). *Biochemistry* **10**, 1561–1569.
73. Morgan, H. E., Jefferson, L. S., Wolpert, E. B., and Rannels, D. E. (1971). *J. Biol. Chem.* **246**, 2163–2170.
74. Morrison, J. C., Whybrew, D. W., Trass, T. C., Sohby, C. M., Morrison, W. C., and Bucovaz, E. T. (1971). *Proc. Amer. Ass. Cancer Res.* **12**, 47.
75. Mushinski, J. F., and Potter, M. (1969). *Biochemistry* **8**, 1684–1691.
76. Nirenberg, M. (1970). *In* "Aspects of Protein Biosynthesis" (C. B. Anfinsen, Jr., ed.), Part A, pp. 215–246. Academic Press, New York.
77. Nirenberg, M. W., and Matthaei, J. H. (1961). *Proc. Nat. Acad. Sci. U.S.* **47**, 1588–1602.
78. Noll, M., and Noll, H. (1972). *Nature New Biol.* **238**, 225–228.
79. Norris, A. T., and Berg, P. (1964). *Proc. Nat. Acad. Sci. U.S.* **52**, 330–337.
80. Ochoa, M., Jr., and Weinstein, I. B. (1964). *J. Biol. Chem.* **239**, 3834–3842.
80a. Osserman, E. F. (1971). 3rd Meeting Amer. Cancer Soc. Res. Professors, Virgin Islands, Dec. 1971.
81. Palmiter, R. D., Christensen, A. K., and Schimke, R. T. (1970). *J. Biol. Chem.* **245**, 833–845.
81a. Piper, P. W., and Clark, B. F. C. (1973). *FEBS Lett.* **30**, 265–267.
82. Potter, M. (1972). *Physiolog. Rev.* **52**, 631–719.
83. Prichard, P. M., Gilbert, J. M., Shafritz, D. A., and Anderson, W. F. (1970). *Nature* (*London*) **226**, 511–514.

84. Randerath, K., Rosenthal, L. J., and Zamecnik, P. C. (1971). *Proc. Nat. Acad. Sci. U.S.* **68**, 3233–3237.
85. Rao, P., and Moldave, K. (1969). *J. Mol. Biol.* **46**, 447–457.
86. Rathbone, M. P., and Hall, R. H. (1972). *Cancer Res.* **32**, 1647–1650.
87. Richie, R. C., English, M. G., and Griffin, A. C. (1970). *Proc. Soc. Exp. Biol. Med.* **134**, 1156–1161.
88. Ritter, P. O., and Busch, H. (1971). *Physiol. Chem. Phys.* **3**, 411–425.
88a. Roberts, R. J. (1972). *Nature New Biol.* **237**, 44–45.
89. Rosen, B., Rothman, F., and Weigert, M. G. (1969). *J. Mol. Biol.* **44**, 363–375.
90. Rudland, P. S., and Klemperer, H. G. (1971). *J. Mol. Biol.* **61**, 377–385.
91. Sekiya, T., and Oda, K. (1972). *Virology* **47**, 168–180.
91a. Simsek, M., and RajBhandary, U. L. (1972). *Biochem. Biophys. Res. Commun.* **49**, 508–515.
92. Smith, A. E., and Marcker, K. A. (1970). *Nature (London)* **226**, 607–610.
93. Soffer, R. L. (1970). *J. Biol. Chem.* **245**, 731–737.
94. Soffer, R. L. (1971). *J. Biol. Chem.* **246**, 1481–1484.
95. Soffer, R. L., Horinishi, H., and Leibowitz, M. J. (1969). *Cold Spring Harbor Symp. Quant. Biol.* **34**, 529–533.
96. Srinivasan, D., Srinivasan, P. R., Grunberger, D., Weinstein, I. B., and Morris, H. P. (1971). *Biochemistry* **10**, 1966–1973.
97. Staehelin, M., Rogg, H., Baguley, B. C., Ginsberg, T., and Wehrli, W. (1968). *Nature (London)* **219**, 1363–1365.
98. Steitz, J. A. (1969). *Cold Spring Harbor Symp. Quant. Biol.* **34**, 621–633.
99. Sueoka, N., and Kano-Sueoka, T. (1970). *Prog. Nucleic Acid Res. Mol. Biol.* **10**, 23–55.
100. Taylor, M. W., Granger, G. A., Buck, C. A., and Holland, J. J. (1967). *Proc. Nat. Acad. Sci. U.S.* **57**, 1712–1719.
101. Tomkins, G. M., Levinson, B. B., Baxter, J. D., and Dethlefsen, L., (1972). *Nature New Biol.* **239**, 9–14.
102. Volkers, S. A. S., and Taylor, M. W. (1971). *Biochemistry* **10**, 488–497.
103. von Ehrenstein, G. (1970). *In* "Aspects of Protein Biosynthesis" (C. B. Anfinsen, Jr., ed.), Part A, pp. 139–214. Academic Press, N. Y.
104. Weinstein, I. B., and Fink, L. M. (1969). *In* "Methods in Cancer Research" (H. Busch, ed.), Vol. VI, pp. 311–343, Academic Press, New York.
105. Weinstein, I. B., Ochoa, M. Jr., and Friedman, S. M. (1966). *Biochemistry* **5**, 3332–3339.
106. Yang, W. K., and Novelli, G. D. (1968). *Proc. Nat. Acad. Sci. U.S.* **59**, 208–215.
107. Yarus, M. (1972). *Proc. Nat. Acad. Sci. U.S.* **69**, 1915–1919.
108. Zamecnik, P. C. (1969). *Cold Spring Harbor Symp. Quant. Biol.* **34**, 1–16.

CHAPTER X

Biochemical Mechanisms of Chemical Carcinogenesis

ELIZABETH C. MILLER AND JAMES A. MILLER

I. Gross Aspects of Chemicals as Carcinogens

Chemical carcinogens are nonviral and nonradioactive substances which, under appropriate circumstances, cause malignant tumors to develop in multicellular organisms in significantly greater incidences than would occur spontaneously. These substances may also induce the formation of benign tumors. The ability of some benign tumors to progress to malignancy (32) makes it unlikely that, with adequate tests, chemicals will be found which induce only benign or only malignant tumors.

The chemical carcinogens now known comprise a large and structurally diverse group of synthetic and naturally occurring organic and inorganic compounds with various species and tissue selectivities (19, 42, 43, 133). The majority of these chemical carcinogens are small organic molecules with molecular weights of less than 500. These chemicals include such diverse structures as simple alkylating agents, aromatic amines and amides, aliphatic nitrosamines and nitrosamides, polycyclic aromatic hydrocarbons, halogenated aliphatic and alicyclic hydrocarbons, complex pyrrolizidine alkaloids, and aflatoxins B_1 and G_1. Some of these structures are shown in Figs. 10.1–10.3. The chemical carcinogens also include a small group of compounds of certain metals (beryllium, cadmium, chromium, cobalt, lead, and nickel) and certain complex silicates (asbestos) (19). The carcinogenic potentials of many classes of organic compounds and of most of the metals and their derivatives are not known.

Historically and to the present time chemical carcinogenesis has been studied primarily *in vivo* in mammals. However, malignant tumors have been induced by chemicals in a wide variety of animal species. Furthermore, studies of the past decade have clearly established that chemicals can induce high incidences of malignant transformations in cell cultures in a reproducible manner (11, 24, 45, 64). While most of the studies on carcinogenesis *in vitro* have resulted in the production of sarcomas in cultures consisting only or primarily of fibroblasts, transformation of epithelial cells has also been reported to occur as a consequence of treatment with chemicals (21, 143). These simplified cellular systems *in vitro* permit quantitative experiments not possible in the whole animal, but the malignancy of the transformed cells from these systems must still be monitored in whole animals.

II. Chemical Carcinogenesis in Man

The induction of tumors by chemicals was first discovered two centuries ago in man through the observations of Hill (107) on nasal cancer in snuff users and the findings of Pott (100) on the relatively high incidence of scrotal cancer in chimney sweeps. Today a variety of chemicals and mixtures of chemicals are known to be carcinogenic in man (Table 10.1) (19, 89). These conclusions have usually been obtained from epidemiological studies of small groups exposed to large amounts of the chemical(s) for many years. The most widespread known carcinogenic exposure is due to the inhalation of cigarette smoke (147). Most of the other known exposures occurred in industrial situations, but one chemical [N,N-bis(2-chloroethyl)-2-naphthylamine, chlornaphazin] was administered as a drug (33).

Many other chemicals and mixtures of chemicals are suspected of being human carcinogens. A recent example is diethylstilbestrol which has been implicated in the etiology of vaginal carcinomas in young women whose mothers were administered large doses of the hormone because of threatened abortion (46). The suspicion that some of the aflatoxins are carcinogenic in man is based on the high potencies of aflatoxins B_1 and G_1 as liver carcinogens for a wide variety of animal species and on the high incidence of carcinoma of the liver in man in parts of the world where contamination of food with these fungal metabolites is known to occur. Preliminary studies on liver carcinoma incidences and aflatoxin contamination of food in Thailand and parts of Africa have suggested that there could be a relationship between these two situations (49, 117), but further epidemiological studies are necessary before firm conclusions

TABLE 10.1

CHEMICALS RECOGNIZED AS CARCINOGENS IN MAN AS WELL AS
IN EXPERIMENTAL ANIMALS

Carcinogen	Target
2-Naphthylamine	Urinary bladder
Benzidine	Urinary bladder
4-Aminobiphenyl	Urinary bladder
4-Nitrobiphenyl	Urinary bladder
N,N-Bis(2-chloroethyl)-2-naphthylamine	Urinary bladder
Bis(2-chloroethyl)sulfide	Lungs
Nickel compounds	Lungs, nasal sinuses
Chromium compounds	Lungs
Asbestos	Lungs, pleura
Soots, tars, oils	Skin, lungs
Cigarette smoke	Lungs, other sites
Betel nut	Buccal mucosa

can be drawn. For example, a closely related and strongly hepatocarcinogenic mold metabolite, sterigmatocystin, may be even more widely distributed in the environment than the aflatoxins (105). In a similar manner, the occurrence of small amounts of secondary nitrosamines in some foods and the potent carcinogenicities of many of these compounds in several tissues in many species has focussed attention on these compounds as possible human carcinogens (68, 75, 145). These compounds may also be formed in the stomach from nitrites and

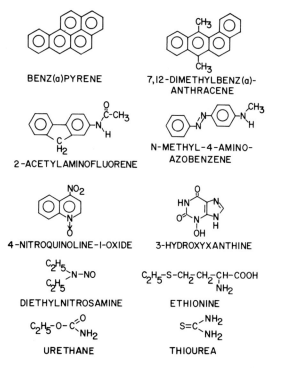

Fig. 10.1. Some synthetic chemical carcinogens.

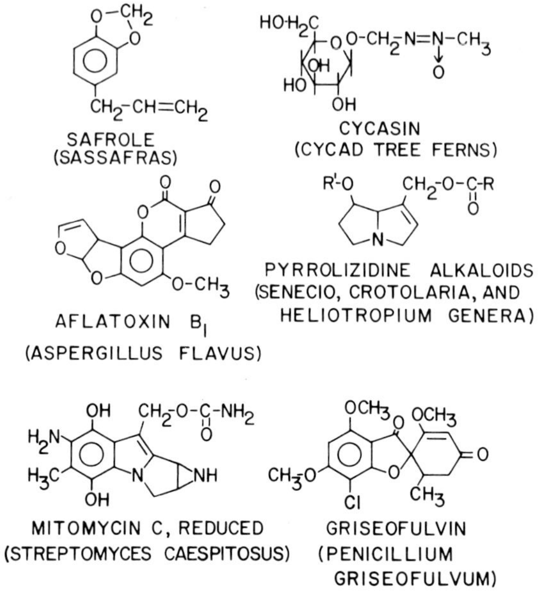

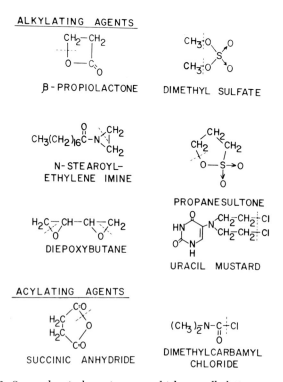

Fig. 10.2. Some naturally occurring carcinogens (91, 93).

ALKYLATING AGENTS

β-PROPIOLACTONE   DIMETHYL SULFATE

N-STEAROYL-
ETHYLENE IMINE

PROPANESULTONE

DIEPOXYBUTANE

URACIL MUSTARD

ACYLATING AGENTS

SUCCINIC ANHYDRIDE   DIMETHYLCARBAMYL
                                       CHLORIDE

Fig. 10.3. Some chemical carcinogens which are alkylating or acylating agents.

secondary amines. Sodium nitrite is employed as a preservative to inhibit the growth of *Cl. botulinum* spores and as a color fixative in cured meats and fish (145). An interesting and controversial situation is the implication of some inorganic trivalent arsenic compounds in the induction of tumors of the skin and possibly other organs after prolonged and high medical, industrial, or environmental exposures (1). These compounds of arsenic, however, have so far proven inactive as carcinogens in experimental animals.

Other general environmental aspects suggest an even greater importance of carcinogenic chemicals in the etiology of human cancer. Modern epidemiological studies show that large differences exist in the incidence of many important cancers in man between and within various countries (47, 60, 113, 147) and that migrants tend to assume the cancer incidences characteristic of their new habitats (41). A striking example concerns primary tumors of the stomach and colon. The incidence of stomach cancer·in the United States has declined for the past forty years and is now one-third of that in 1930, whereas the incidence of colon cancer in the United States at present is among the highest in the world. In Japan the opposite situation occurs, viz., the incidence of stomach cancer is the highest in the world and the incidence of colon cancer is low. The experience of Japanese migrants to the United States clearly indicates that environmental factors are of major importance, since these migrants, especially the second generation, exhibit large reductions in the incidence of stomach cancer and large increases in the incidence of colon cancer. These data and the great variations in the incidences of many important tumors around the world are the basis for the conclusion that a high percentage, perhaps as much as 80–90%, of human cancer has strong environmental elements in its etiology (47). The importance of genetic factors has been discounted because of the fact that the changes in incidence have occurred within one to a few generations.

Similarly, variations in the exposures to carcinogenic radiations, other than ultraviolet light in the induction of skin cancer in man (135), are not considered to be sufficient to explain the geographical differences noted. Thus chemicals, and possibly viruses, are the principal agents under suspicion, and certain chemicals in the environment—in food, water, air, drugs, etc.—may well be decisive elements in the etiology of many important tumors that occur in man. These chemicals include not only man-made chemical agents but also naturally occurring compounds (Fig. 10.2). An increasing number of chemical carcinogens are being found in green plants and fungi (90, 92). The prevention of many cancers in man has become an increasingly attractive and, perhaps, attainable goal.

These considerations of chemicals as carcinogens in experimental animals and in man emphasize the importance of further research on chemical carcinogenesis. Great improvements are needed in the sensitivity of methods for the detection of chemical carcinogens in the environment and for the extrapolation of the data to man. Similarly, considerable progress is needed in our understanding of processes of chemical carcinogenesis at the molecular level to permit further approaches toward reducing *in vivo* the carcinogenic impact of chemical agents which cannot be avoided in daily life (95).

III. The Nature of Chemical Carcinogenesis

Tumors, regardless of the causative agent, are made up of clones and subclones of altered somatic cells plus normal vascular and stromal tissue. Tumor cells clearly contain heritable defects in growth control since they can be transplanted, even with single cells, and grow as tumors from normal host to normal host. Chemical carcinogens are required for only a fraction of the long latent period which elapses after the first application of these agents and before tumors appear. Thus chemical carcinogens are not needed for the continued growth of the tumors they induce. However, the prolonged administration of a carcinogen and the use of larger doses lead to higher incidences of tumor-bearing animals and larger total numbers of tumors until toxic effects of the chemical carcinogens intervene. Thus, as for other pharmacological and toxic substances, dose-response relationships exist for a variety of chemical carcinogens (26).

Some of the cellular alterations needed for the eventual formation of tumors may be caused by doses of chemical carcinogens too low for completion of the carcinogenic process within the life span of the animal (10, 14, 137). These alterations may remain latent in tissues for a long time. This is evident in the gross stages of *initiation* and *promotion* in skin carcinogenesis and in similar but less defined stages in chemical carcinogenesis in the liver and some other tissues. For example, sufficient dosages of certain polycyclic aromatic hydrocarbons can cause the complete carcinogenic process in mouse skin with the appearance of papillomas and then carcinomas within a few months. Yet a single sufficiently low dose of these compounds, which will not cause the appearance of gross tumors in the lifetime of the mouse, may still initiate early stages in the process of skin carcinogenesis. The process can be completed by subsequent applications of essentially noncarcinogenic promoters such as croton oil or its phorbol ester components (44). The initiation stage in skin carcinogenesis appears to be completed rapidly and to be essentially irreversible, since periods of almost a year between initiation and promotion did not alter the rate of appearance of the tumors or their incidence (14, 137). Promotion, however, appears to require considerable time and to be reversible. Many other parameters such as dose, frequency and route of administration, species, sex, age, hormonal status, presence of viral information, intrinsic species susceptibility, etc. control the incidence and rate of appearance of tumors induced by chemical carcinogens. Some of these factors control the activation and deactivation of chemical carcinogens as discussed below.

IV. Metabolism and Reactivity of Chemical Carcinogens

A. General Considerations

Like other chemicals, chemical carcinogens are subject to metabolism by the animals to which they are administered. In most cases the major share of the metabolism is probably toward deactivation, and most of the administered carcinogen is eventually excreted as noncarcinogenic derivatives. However, with most chemical carcinogens other than the carcinogenic alkylating and acylating agents (see Fig. 10.3), metabolism to proximate carcinogens (metabolites closer to the final active form than the administered compound) and ultimate carcinogens (the final active forms) is apparently necessary for their activity. In many cases this metabolism toward proximate and ultimate carcinogenic derivatives may be only a small fraction of the total metabolism. The realization that this metabolic activation is an essential feature of carcinogenesis by many chemicals and information on the nature of some of these metabolic activations have constituted important recent advances in the knowledge of chemical carcinogenesis (89).

The available data can be generalized to suggest that the ultimate carcinogenic forms of most, if not all, chemical carcinogens are strong electron-deficient or electrophilic reactants (89, 94). This generalization is an important unifying concept of the fundamental nature of chemicals which react with cellular constituents to induce neoplastic transformations. It has also been important in focusing attention on particular portions of chemical structures for making more knowledgeable predictions on the possible carcinogenic activities of chemicals.

The electrophilic nature of the ultimate chemical carcinogens was inferred in part from our knowledge of the carcinogenic activity of certain alkylating agents since these compounds are electrophilic reactants per se (111). In the case of the simple carcinogenic alkylating agents such as dimethyl sulfate, it is difficult to conceive of any other reactive species which could be derived from them. In other cases the electrophilic natures of the ultimate reactive (and presumably carcinogenic) species have been derived in part from the structures of the protein- and nucleic acid-bound derivatives formed from them *in vivo,* especially in the target tissues (89). Thus, alkylation, arylation, arylamidation, or arylamination of N-7, C-8 and the oxygen atom on C-6 of guanine, N-1 and N-3 of adenine, and N-3 of cytosine in the nucleic acids and of the sulfur atoms of methionine and cysteine residues in proteins indicate that the attacking species for these nucleophilic centers must have been electrophilic (88).

In a few cases, especially with carcinogenesis in the liver of the rat by 2-acetylaminofluorene, the identity of the major ultimate carcinogenic form has been established through special metabolic information (see below). These strong electrophilic reactants which appear to be ultimate carcinogenic forms differ in important respects from the normal cellular electrophiles which interact with normal cellular nucleophiles in multitudinous covalent bond-breaking and bond-making events during cellular metabolism. In the latter case the electrophiles and nucleophiles are formed and joined under tight and highly ordered control at enzyme surfaces. In contrast, the strongly reactive electrophilic forms of chemical carcinogens are capable of attacking nucleophiles in the cell with relatively little discrimination and usually without the aid of enzymes. Some of these attacks apparently initiate the malignant transformation, while other attacks of the ultimate carcinogens and a variety of enzymic reactions lead to the destruction or inactivation of a part of the dose of carcinogen.

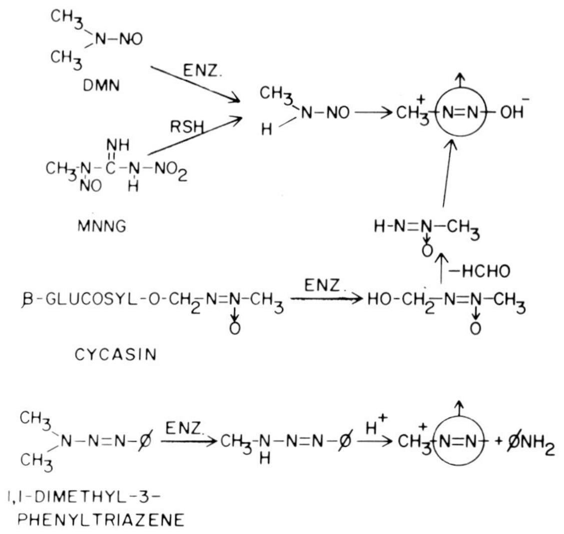

Fig. 10.4. The mechanisms of activation for carcinogenesis and electrophilic reactivity of some potential alkylating agents.

B. Potential Alkylating Agents

The particular combinations of metabolic capacities of the tissues of an animal play a major role in determining its susceptibility to a chemical and in determining the sites of tumor formation within the animal (Fig. 10.4). Thus, the alkylnitrosamides require only reaction with a nucleophile such as a sulfhydryl group to be converted to alkylating species. As a class the nitrosamides have been distinguished by the wide variety of tissues in which they induce tumors and by the susceptibility of most of the species in which they have been assayed (28, 76). The dialkylnitrosamines have also been impressive carcinogens because of the wide range of structures which are carcinogenic and because of the broad species susceptibility. However, the dialkylnitrosamines are clearly less versatile as carcinogens than the nitrosamides, and the more restricted range of tissues susceptible to their carcinogenic activity appears to be related to the necessity that the dialkylnitrosamines be enzymically dealkylated to monoalkylnitrosamines (27, 74, 76). The monoalkylnitrosamines decompose essentially spontaneously to yield alkylating species. The mixed function oxygenases of the endoplasmic reticulum are, at least primarily, responsible for the dealkylations, and the high susceptibility of liver to the carcinogenic activity of the dialkylnitrosamines appears to be related to the high mixed function oxygenase activity in liver.

Similarly, the carcinogenic activities of the dialkylaryltriazenes and of the dialkylazo, azoxy, and hydrazo compounds appear to depend on their enzymic dealkylation to intermediates which decompose spontaneously to alkylating agents (102). A different type of enzymic activation which leads to the formation of a methylating agent is the hydrolysis of orally administered cycasin by bacterial β-glucosidase in the intestinal lumen of rats (79, 121). The aglycone (methylazoxymethanol) thus formed is a methylating agent at pH 7, but it is apparently stable enough to be absorbed and transported to various tissues, especially the liver and kidney, where it induces tumors. Because of this requirement for hydrolysis of the glucosidic linkage and the virtual absence of β-glucosidase in rat tissues after weaning, cycasin is not carcinogenic when administered orally to germfree rats or parenterally to normal or germfree rats after the 25th day of age. The small intestine of preweaning rats does contain β-glucosidase, and rats given a single injection of cycasin prior to 20 days of age developed high incidences of tumors, especially in the kidney (79). Still another pathway for the enzymic formation of a simple alkylating agent and ultimate carcinogen may be the conversion of the hepatic carcinogen ethionine to S-adenosylethionine. The latter compound can transfer its S-ethyl group to cellular constituents by the enzyme machinery used for methylation in normal metabolism (98, 128).

Alkylating intermediates are also apparently formed as the ultimate carcinogenic metabolites of a variety of other structures which, in the forms administered, appear to have limited chemical similarity. Thus, it seems likely that the hepatic carcinogen carbon tetrachloride is oxidized by the mixed function oxygenases to an alkylating species which attacks cellular proteins and nucleic acids (36, 81, 108). The pyrrolizidine alkaloids, which are allylic esters with weak alkylating activity, are oxidized by the mixed function oxygenases to pyrrole derivatives, which are much more reactive and toxic allylic esters (20, 80, 82) under physiological conditions. These pyrrolic esters seem very likely to be ultimate carcinogenic metabolites. Similarly, recent evidence has shown that the hepatocarcinogen safrole is metabolized by rats and mice to 1'-hydroxysafrole (13). The greater carcinogenic activity of this allylic and benzylic alcohol as compared to that of the parent compound indicates that it is a proximate carcinogenic metabolite (12). An ester of 1'-hydroxysafrole has been suggested as the ultimate carcinogenic metabolite on the basis of the reactivity and carcinogenicity of the synthetic acetic acid ester of 1'-hydroxysafrole and by analogy with the central role of the sulfuric acid ester of N-hydroxy-2-acetylaminofluorene in hepatic carcinogenesis by 2-acetylaminofluorene in the rat liver.

C. Aromatic Amines, Amides, and Nitro Derivatives

Among the best understood of the chemical carcinogens in terms of its metabolic activation is 2-acetylaminofluorene (Figs. 10.5 and 10.6). This carcinogen, which induces tumors especially in the liver, sebaceous ear duct gland, mammary gland, and epithelium of the small intestine, in the rat is N-hydroxylated *in vivo*, apparently primarily in the liver, to N-hydroxy-2-acetylaminofluorene (93, 94). This N-hydroxy metabolite is a much more potent carcinogen than the parent compound at the sites at which 2-acetylaminofluorene is carcinogenic. In addition, it induces tumors at sites of application where 2-acetylaminofluorene has little or no activity; these include especially the subcutaneous tissue and

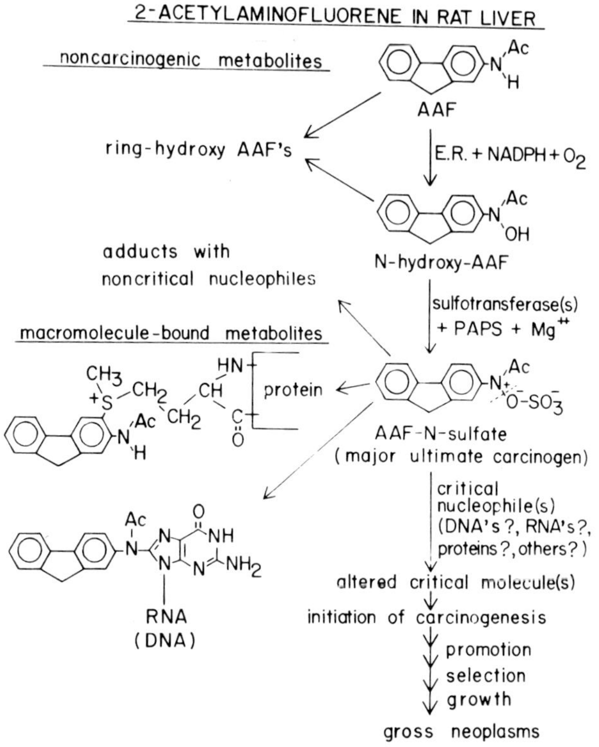

Fig. 10.5. The major routes for the activation and deactivation of 2-acetylaminofluorene in the male rat liver. Abbreviations: AAF, 2-acetylaminofluorene; Ac, acetyl; E. R., endoplasmic reticulum; PAPS, 3′phosphoadenosine-5′-phosphosulfate.

the forestomach of the intact rat and rat fibroblasts in culture (114, 93, 94).

Further study revealed that N-hydroxy-2-acetylaminofluorene can be esterified to yield the sulfuric acid ester by a rat liver sulfotransferase system which utilizes 3′-phosphoadenosine-5′-phosphosulfate (22, 59). Correlations between the carcinogenicities of 2-acetylaminofluorene and N-hydroxy-2-acetylamino-fluorene and the sulfotransferase activity of the livers of rodents indicated that the high susceptibility of the livers of male random-bred rats of the Charles River stock and of male and female Fischer rats to the carcinogenicity of these fluorene derivatives was related to their hepatic sulfotransferase activity for N-hydroxy-2-acetylaminofluorene (22, 40). By making the amount of sulfate ion limiting *in vivo* through administration of p-hydroxyacetanilide the reactivity and toxicity of N-hydroxy-2-acetylaminofluorene for rat liver were correlated with its ability to synthesize the sulfuric acid ester (23). Similar chronic experiments revealed that the hepatocarcinogenicity of N-hydroxy-2-acetylamino-fluorene was greatly inhibited by the administration of acetanilide (which is oxidized to p-hydroxyacetanilide *in vivo*) and that this inhibition was partially prevented by the simultaneous administration of excess sulfate ion (140).

While the sulfuric acid ester of N-hydroxy-2-acetylaminofluorene appears to

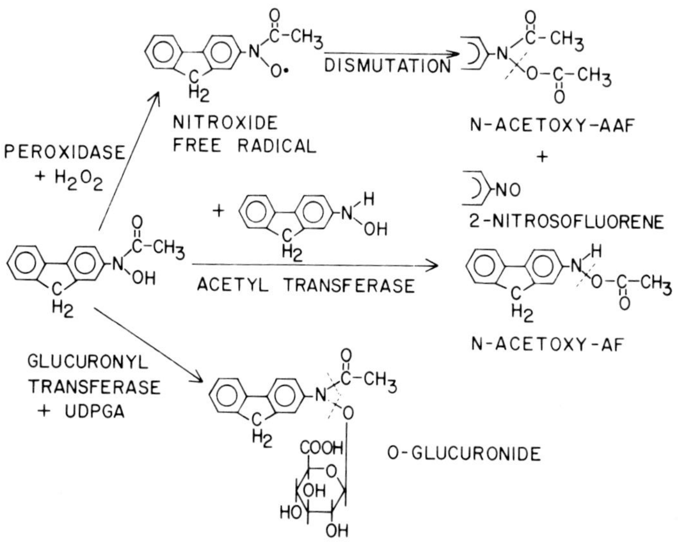

Fig. 10.6. Enzymic mechanisms, in addition to those shown in Fig. 10.5, for the metabolism of N-hydroxy-2-acetylaminofluorene to electrophilic reactants. The roles of these derivatives in the carcinogenicity of N-hydroxy-2-acetylaminofluorene have not been determined. Abbreviations: AF, 2-aminofluorene; AAF, 2-acetylaminofluorene; UDPGA, uridine diphosphate glucuronic acid.

be the major ultimate carcinogenic metabolite of N-hydroxy-2-acetylamino-fluorene in rat liver, it appears likely that other ultimate carcinogenic derivatives of N-hydroxy-2-acetylaminofluorene play some role (probably minor) in hepatic carcinogenesis. Other ultimate carcinogenic metabolites must play major roles in carcinogenesis at other sites. Attempts to demonstrate sulfotransferase activity for N-hydroxy-2-acetylaminofluorene in subcutaneous tissue, sebaceous ear duct gland, or the mammary tissue of the rat have not been successful, even though these are important targets for carcinogenesis by this agent (22, 52). A number of metabolic mechanisms have been discovered in addition to the formation of the sulfuric acid ester for the formation of reactive derivatives of N-hydroxy-2-acetylaminofluorene and N-hydroxy-2-aminofluorene (Fig. 10.6). Each of these reactive electrophilic metabolites, if it reaches and reacts with a critical target, might induce tumors.

One of these other candidates is the glucuronide of N-hydroxy-2-acetylamino-fluorene, which is a normal urinary metabolite of the carcinogen. This glucuronide, although quite stable, has some electrophilic reactivity toward nucleic acids and guanine and methionine derivatives (55, 83) at pH 7, and its reactivity increases markedly at slightly alkaline pH. The synthetic derivative N-hydroxy-2-aminofluorene-O-glucuronide is much more reactive than the N-acetyl glucuronide (53). While there is no evidence for the formation of the nonacetylated glucuronide in vivo, it is a likely metabolite and a candidate ultimate metabolite.

Similarly, mechanisms have been proposed for the possible formation of the phosphoric and acetic acid esters of N-hydroxy-2-acetylaminofluorene through esterifications with adenosine triphosphate, carbamyl phosphate or S-acetyl co-enzyme A (22, 59, 71, 72). The necessary enzymic machinery for the formation of these esters metabolically has not been demonstrated. The acetic acid ester of N-hydroxy-2-acetylaminofluorene can be formed through one-electron oxidation, nonenzymically or via a peroxidase, of N-hydroxy-2-acetylaminofluorene to a free radical; dismutation of two of these radicals yields one molecule of N-acetoxy-2-acetylaminofluorene and one molecule of 2-nitrosofluorene (7, 8). The enzymic O-acetylation of N-hydroxy-2-aminofluorene by transacetylation from N-hydroxy-2-acetylaminofluorene has been demonstrated with the soluble fraction from liver and certain other rodent tissues (5, 6). The roles of these metabolic activation mechanisms in the induction of carcinogenesis by N-hydroxy-2-acetylaminofluorene are not known.

Synthetic esters of N-hydroxy-2-acetylaminofluorene react with guanine derivatives to yield N-(guan-8-yl)-2-acetylaminofluorene derivatives, and the acetic acid ester of N-hydroxy-2-aminofluorene yields the corresponding 2-aminofluorene derivative (6, 63). The glucuronide of N-hydroxy-2-acetylaminofluorene, although reacting to a much smaller extent, yields a mixture of these two products and the proportion of the deacetylated derivative increases as the pH of the reaction mixture is increased (83). In similar fashions these esters and glucuronides react with methionyl residues to yield sulfonium derivatives which decompose to give 1- and 3-methylmercapto-2-aminofluorene or their N-acetyl derivatives (6, 73, 83). Thus, these esters and glucuronides are both arylamidating or arylaminating and arylating reagents. Each of the above-mentioned guanine and methionine derivatives has also been identified as a degradation product of the hepatic nucleic acids or proteins from rats administered 2-acetylaminofluorene or N-hydroxy-2-acetylaminofluorene (4, 22, 54, 61). These findings thus support the conclusion that esters of the N-hydroxy derivatives or metabolites with similar reactivities are ultimate reactive and carcinogenic derivatives of the fluorene carcinogens.

A variety of other carcinogenic aromatic amines and amides are known. As far as we know, they appear to follow a similar metabolic activation to that shown for 2-acetylaminofluorene. Thus, the N-hydroxylation in vivo of 4-acetylaminostilbene, 2-acetylaminophenanthrene, and 4-acetylaminobiphenyl in rats and of 4-aminobiphenyl, 1-aminonaphthalene, and 2-aminonaphthalene in dogs have been demonstrated through detection of the N-hydroxy metabolites in the urine (93, 106). Each of these N-hydroxy derivatives has proved to be more carcinogenic than the parent amine or amide in one or more assays (93). N-Hydroxy-4-acetylaminobiphenyl and N-hydroxy-4-acetylaminostilbene are both substrates for the rat hepatic sulfotransferase system (22). By analogy with the data on the fluorene derivatives N-(guan-8-yl)-4-aminobiphenyl, N-(guan-8-yl)-4-acetylaminobiphenyl, and 3-methylmercapto-4-acetylaminobiphenyl have been detected in the liver nucleic acids and protein of rats administered N-hydroxy-4-acetylaminobiphenyl (22, 62). Both the biphenyl and stilbene compounds are, however, more carcinogenic at extrahepatic sites than in the liver.

Indirect evidence points to an ester of N-hydroxy-N-methyl-4-aminoazobenzene as an ultimate carcinogenic metabolite of N-methyl-4-aminoazobenzene, even though neither N-hydroxy-N-methyl-4-aminoazobenzene nor an ester of the hydroxylamine has been characterized as either an *in vivo* or an *in vitro* metabolite (99). The evidence for the formation of an ester *in vivo* rests on the identity of the methionyl, tyrosinyl, and guanyl derivatives formed on reaction nonenzymically at neutrality of the synthetic ester N-benzoyloxy-N-methyl-4-aminoazobenzene with methionine, tyrosine, or guanine derivatives and products isolated from the liver protein and nucleic acids from rats administered N-methyl-4-aminoazobenzene-³H (69, 70, 89).

In a manner similar to some of the above hydroxamic acids, 3-hydroxyxanthine, which induces sarcomas on subcutaneous injection and some liver carcinomas on administration of higher doses, is esterified by a liver system which requires 3′-phosphoadenosine-5′-phosphosulfate. Esters of 3-hydroxyxanthine react readily with nucleophilic sites to yield 8-substituted xanthine derivatives (125, 126).

The carcinogencity of a variety of nitroaromatic compounds is probably attributable to their reduction *in vivo* to aromatic hydroxylamines, which are then further metabolized to ultimate carcinogenic derivatives. This situation is exemplified by the finding that the carcinogen 4-nitroquinoline-1-oxide is reduced by rat liver and subcutaneous tissue to N-hydroxy-4-aminoquinoline-1-oxide and to 4-aminoquinoline-1-oxide (78, 127). While the latter compound was inactive as a carcinogen, N-hydroxy-4-aminoquinoline-1-oxide is more carcinogenic than the parent nitro compound (118). Furthermore, evidence has been presented for the enzymic esterification by an ascites hepatoma system of N-hydroxy-4-aminoquinoline-1-oxide by an ATP-requiring system (130). Both this presumed phosphoric acid ester and the synthetic diacetate of N-hydroxy-4-aminoquinoline-1-oxide are electrophilic reactants and yield *in vitro* products with nucleic acids which appear to be very similar to those obtained from mice and rats administered 4-nitroquinoline-1-oxide or N-hydroxy-4-aminoquinoline-1-oxide (29, 51, 131).

D. Polycyclic Aromatic Hydrocarbons

The carcinogenic polycyclic aromatic hydrocarbons include a relatively large class of compounds which, for the most part, contain four or more fused ring systems and are essentially planar. Their carcinogenic activities cover a wide range, and a number of approaches have been made toward systematizing their carcinogenicity through calculations of electronic structure, particularly at the K regions (the phenanthrene double bonds) (2, 19, 104). Some members of this class have very high potencies [e.g., 7,12-dimethylbenz(a)anthracene], and this fact together with their carcinogenic activities at sites of administration (subcutaneous tissue and skin) led earlier to suggestions that these compounds are carcinogenic in the forms administered. However, the *in vitro* binding of the polycyclic aromatic hydrocarbons to macromolecules is weak and does not correlate with their carcinogenicities (66).

Early studies revealed that the carcinogenic polycyclic hydrocarbons undergo extensive metabolism *in vivo* to phenols and dihydrodiols which are conjugated and excreted (46). Where they have been tested these derivatives have proved to be noncarcinogenic, and this route of metabolism was considered for many years to be one of detoxification. However, the metabolism of aromatic rings by the mixed function oxygenases has been dissected in considerable detail in the past few years, and the primary mode of attack has been shown to be epoxidation (37, 57, 115). The epoxides can rearrange (apparently primarily nonenzymically) to yield phenols, react with water through the mediation of epoxide hydrase to yield dihydrodiols, react enzymically with the sulfhydryl group of glutathione, or react nonenzymically with a variety of nucleophilic centers. The multiplicity of phenols and dihydrodiols which have been found as metabolites of certain of the hydrocarbon carcinogens, as well as of other aromatic compounds, indicates that the epoxidative attack can occur at many or most of the possible sites on the aromatic rings (15, 119, 120).

In early studies the K-region epoxides of several hydrocarbons were assayed by topical application to mouse skin or by subcutaneous injection and were found to be much less carcinogenic than the parent compounds (17, 86, 138). However, recent reexamination of this problem has revealed that the K-region epoxides of benz(a)anthracene, dibenz(a,h)anthracene, 3-methylcholanthrene, and benz(a)pyrene are much more active than the parent hydrocarbons or the corresponding phenols or dihydrodiols in the malignant transformation of fibroblast cultures *in vitro* (38, 48, 77). These data, together with the direct demonstration that these hydrocarbons can be converted to epoxides by liver preparations (37, 115) suggest that epoxides are important ultimate carcinogenic derivatives of the polycyclic hydrocarbons. The relative roles of the various possible epoxides remain to be explored; the one non-K-region epoxide which has been tested for ability to induce malignant transformation *in vitro* was not active (48, 77). The possible key role of the K-region epoxides would be consistent with the emphasis which has been placed on this portion of the molecule by correlations of electronic structure with carcinogenic activity and with the *in vivo* data on the carcinogenicities of fluorinated benz(a)anthracene derivatives (84, 91, 104). The latter data point to the importance of an unsubstituted 3-position for carcinogenic activity.

The marked enhancement of the carcinogenicity of benz(a)anthracene by substitution of a methyl group in position 7 or, especially, of methyl groups in both positions 7 and 12 has raised the question of the role of these methyl groups in the activity of the methylated derivatives. These methyl groups are oxidized by the mixed function oxygenases (16, 56). 7-Hydroxymethyl-12-methylbenz(a)anthracene and 7-methyl-12-hydroxymethylbenz(a)-anthracene are both carcinogenic for rats and mice, but they are less active than the parent hydrocarbon (17, 31). The interest in benzylic esters as ultimate carcinogenic metabolites of certain other carcinogens has focused additional attention on these methyl groups and has led to the synthesis of halomethyl derivatives and esters of the hydroxymethyl compounds. Both types of compounds have electrophilic reactivity and are carcinogenic, but their carcinogenicities appear to be less than those of the parent compounds (17, 25, 31, 48, 77). These data suggest that the methyl groups may not be directly involved in the carcinogenic action of the hydrocarbons and may exert steric or other effects which enhance the ability of the hydrocarbon or a derivative to react at some other site of the molecule. The possibility that the methylated hydrocarbons have some special activation mechanism has also been suggested by the recent observation that, unlike the epoxides of the other carcinogenic hydrocarbons which have been assayed for induction of malignant transformation *in vitro,* the K-region epoxide of 7-methylbenz(a)anthracene has no more activity than the parent hydrocarbon (48, 77).

The possible routes of activation of these hydrocarbons also include the formation of electrophilic radical cations by one-electron oxidation; these free radicals react readily *in vitro* with cellular macromolecules (35, 66, 142). Metabolites such as 6-hydroxybenz(a)pyrene can also serve as sources of free radicals (97).

V. Critical Targets of Chemical Carcinogens

The growth of tumors into gross clones of similar cells appears to require at least a quasi-permanent alteration in the phenotype of the cells of the tumor as compared to the normal cells of origin. It has therefore appeared to be axiomatic that the ultimate carcinogenic derivatives of chemical carcinogens must interact in some manner with one or more of the informational molecules of the cell—DNA's, RNA's, or proteins.

The electrophilic nature of at least most ultimate carcinogens places emphasis on the nucleophilic centers in cellular constituents as targets of the chemical carcinogens. Such nucleophilic centers are available in both the nucleic acids and proteins (Fig. 10.7), and both nucleic acid- and protein-bound derivatives of chemical carcinogens are formed in target tissues on administration of chemi-

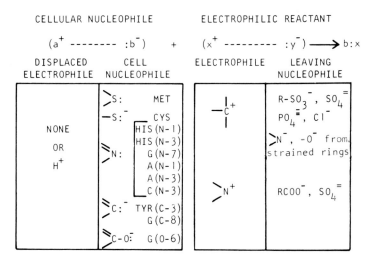

Fig. 10.7. Cellular nucleophiles known to be attacked *in vivo* by electrophilic metabolites of chemical carcinogens.

cal carcinogens (18, 85). As one approach to determining which targets are critical in carcinogenesis, the amounts of covalent binding of various chemical carcinogens (aminoazo dyes, 2-acetylaminofluorene, alkylating agents, polycyclic aromatic hydrocarbons) have been studied in target tissues as a function of the likelihood of tumor development under various conditions. In specific instances the data on the binding of a carcinogen to one or another of these macromolecules has appeared to correlate better with the carcinogenic potential than the binding to other macromolecules. However, the data have not been definitive, and it is not possible to conclude from any of these correlations that a reaction with a specific macromolecule is of key importance.

Probably one of the greatest difficulties in these studies has been the lack of really sophisticated analyses. In most cases the amount of bound carcinogen residue has been determined for all or a major class of a particular macromolecule in a large population of cells, most of which were probably not destined to be progenitors of tumors. Analysis of DNA from whole cells may include both nuclear and mitochondrial DNA, and even the nuclear DNA is markedly heterogeneous. Both RNA's and proteins are composed of many different species with different properties, functions, and half-lives. Further, each of these macromolecules is subject to attack at a number of sites, either with respect to different kinds of residues or the same type of residue at different locations in the macromolecule. Some ultimate carcinogens can react with a given nucleic acid base or amino acid residue to yield more than one chemical structure (for instance, N-7 and O-6 alkylation of guanine residues). Further, if a carcinogen is metabolized to more than one ultimate carcinogenic and reactive form, two or more types of carcinogen residues may be linked to the nucleic acids and proteins. Thus, as noted above, administration of N-hydroxy-2-acetylaminofluorene leads to the formation of bound 2-aminofluorene and bound 2-acetylaminofluorene residues in both the nucleic acids and proteins of the rat liver (see Chapter IV).

While the emphasis has been placed on covalent bindings, it is clear that tight non-covalent interactions might alter the function of a macromolecule for a sufficient time to redirect the status of the cell and its descendants (for instance, by causing a frameshift mutation through intercalation between the bases in the DNA helix of a cell in S phase). Likewise, a chemical interaction which resulted in an altered macromolecule without retention of a portion of the carcinogen molecule, although difficult to detect, could have as far-reaching effects on the behavior of the cell and its descendants as an alteration for which retention of a portion of the carcinogen served as a marker.

The protein- and RNA-bound derivatives of chemical carcinogens have generally had half-lives of no more than a few days, and usually little of these bound forms has been detectable after one or two weeks. The DNA-bound derivatives are more stable; after an initial rapid loss of one-half or more of the DNA-bound derivatives, the residual DNA-bound fraction appears to be relatively stable and to persist in some cases for several months (30, 129, 139). Because of the possible causal importance of mutations to carcinogenesis, considerable significance has been attached to this "persistent binding" to DNA (Chapter IV).

Altered cells can remain apparently dormant for a considerable time before proliferation to a gross clone (14, 137), and this fact could be explicable in terms of the ultimate error-prone division of a cell containing damaged DNA. On the other hand, the persistent binding of carcinogens to DNA as compared to their more labile binding to RNA's and proteins may not reflect a role of DNA in carcinogenesis; it may only be related to the major differences in the half-lives of these molecules.

VI. Molecular Mechanisms of Chemical Carcinogenesis

The lack of definitive data on the identity of the critical target in even one instance of chemical carcinogenesis and the difficulty of obtaining decisive data on this point have led to much speculation on the essential nature of carcinogenesis. These speculations have, in general, been based on the dual importance of the information coded in the genome and the controlled expression of the genomic information in determining the phenotypes of populations of cells. From studies on nuclear transplantation it is apparent that the nuclei of at least some differentiated frog cells contain all of the information which is needed for the development of a fertilized egg to a swimming tadpole (39). On the other hand, the fact that the cells of each tissue produce many more generations of the same kinds of cells *in vivo* and, in some cases, in culture emphasizes that these various differentiated expressions of a genotype become essentially fixed under specific sets of circumstances (see Chapters I and VIII).

The genetic mechanisms involved may lead to an altered base sequence in the DNA of the progeny cells. In most cases the change would be expected to occur in the nuclear DNA, but the observation that certain mutations in fungi, such as the petite mutants of yeast (112), result from mutations of the mitochondrial DNA suggests that critical mutations leading to neoplasia could

TABLE 10.2
Possible Mechanisms of Chemical Carcinogenesis

I. Genetic mechanisms which result in heritable modifications of the DNA genome via:
    1. Direct modification of the DNA
    2. Modification of RNA which is subsequently transcribed into DNA that becomes integrated into host DNA
    3. Alterations of molecules other than DNA which decrease, at least temporarily, the fidelity of copying of DNA
II. Epigenetic mechanisms, which, through nongenomic changes, give rise to:
    1. Quasi-permanent changes in the transcription of DNA (including integrated virus genomes and oncogenes)
    2. The preferential proliferation and progression toward malignancy of previously existing preneoplastic or neoplastic cells

occur in this organelle. The carcinogen N-methylnitrosourea was found to alkyl-ate rat liver mitochondrial DNA more extensively than the nuclear DNA (146). As indicated in Table 10.2 there are several mechanisms through which such alterations in the base sequence in DNA might occur. The most widely recog-nized is the classic situation in which the chemical causes an alteration in the DNA which is expressed in the next generation by an inexact copy of the original nucleotide sequence. These mutational alterations may be of various types—point mutations, frameshift mutations, small or large deletions of sections of the DNA, or losses, additions, or rearrangements of chromosomes. The type of mutation which occurs depends in part on the chemical properties of the mutagen, and the nature of the lesion induced will also affect the probability that it will be repaired (34). The repair of mutations can be essentially error-free under some circumstances and error-prone under others; in the latter situation the repair itself can be a source of mutational events (144). Finally the capacity for some types of repair depends on the genetic properties of the host, as empha-sized by the very limited repair of ultraviolet light-induced and some chemically induced lesions by cells from xeroderma pigmentosum patients (116, 124, see also Chapter IV).

Reactions with specific proteins or RNA's could also, at least theoretically, lead to heritable changes in the DNA genome. The existence of RNA-directed DNA polymerase activity in the RNA tumor viruses and in certain apparently uninfected cells provides a means by which the misinformation in a chemically altered RNA could be transcribed to yield an abnormal DNA (132). Likewise, the chemical alteration of a protein, especially a DNA polymerase, could de-crease the fidelity of copying of DNA and thus introduce critical and heritable changes in the DNA. A precedent for this model is the high mutation frequency of certain strains of bacteriophage T4 because of their mutant error-prone DNA polymerase (122).

The somatic mutation concept of the origin of cancer has been disputed for many years. It is an attractive concept since carcinogenesis and mutagenesis are grossly similar in that each leads to heritable changes in phenotype. The time scales on which these processes operate appear to be widely different in most cases. The attractiveness of the somatic mutation concept has been enhanced in recent years by observations on the chemical similarities between carcinogens and mutagens (87). Thus, as noted above, the active forms of most, if not all, chemical carcinogens are electrophilic; similarly, the ultimate forms of most, but not all, chemical mutagens are electrophilic. The exceptions in the latter group appear to be the frameshift-inducing mutagens and the muta-genic base analogs. Further, as information accrues on the active forms of chemi-cal carcinogens and as host-mediated assays for mutagenicity are developed (65), much better correlations between the mutagenic and carcinogenic activities of chemicals can be expected.

These findings on the similar chemical natures of ultimate chemical carcino-gens and mutagens have also emphasized that correlations between the muta-genicity and carcinogenicity of a series of chemicals cannot be taken as evidence for the mutagenic nature of carcinogenesis. Thus, a correlation may be merely a reflection of the nucleophilicity of the targets for both carcinogenesis and mutagenesis (87). The exact relationships between carcinogenesis and mutagenesis by chemicals will remain unsolved until these processes can be studied at the molecular level in the same cells and a cause-effect relationship proved or denied (see Chapter I).

The reactions of ultimate chemical carcinogens with proteins and RNA's in cells require that epigenetic mechanisms of chemical carcinogenesis also be considered (Table 10.2). The first of these epigenetic mechanisms is the altered expression of a part of the genomic information as a consequence of changes in other molecules which affect the readout of the DNA. The mechanism is based on models of cell differentiation in which nongenomic changes lead to quasi-permanent alterations in the transcription of the genome, presumably through effects on repressors or derepressors. This epigenetic model is consistent with the expressions of fetal antigens and fetal-type enzymes in a number of chemically induced neoplasms (101, 123). Such changes in gene expression might affect not only presumably normal portions of the genome, but they might also cause the transcription of a part or all of integrated virus genomes or oncogenes (134). Indirect epigenetic effects might be alterations in the hormonal balance, immunological capacity, or other competence of the host so that previously existing preneoplastic or neoplastic cells, which had been relatively quiescent, were given a proliferative advantage.

VII. On the Roles of Viruses or Integrated Viral Genomes in Chemical Carcinogenesis

The demonstrations in the late 1950's of the presence of transmissible murine leukemia virus in the leukemias induced in certain strains of mice by X-irradiation suggested that the role of irradiation was to permit the emergence of active leukemia virus (58). The subsequent demonstrations of gs antigens for the murine leukemia and sarcoma viruses in the leukemias and sarcomas induced by 3-methylcholanthrene suggested that the role of the hydrocarbon in these instances might be to permit the expression and/or replication of the integrated viral information (50, 141). This possibility has received further support from the recent reports that, in fibroblast cultures which had been infected with murine leukemia viruses, malignant transformation by polycyclic hydrocarbons, diethylnitrosamine, or smog extracts occurred with markedly increased efficiency and with much lower doses of the chemicals (103, 109, 110, see also Chapter XI).

A somewhat similar situation has been suggested for the induction of mammary carcinomas in mice by chemicals (9). In this case it appears that a repressor produced by a regulator gene controls the rate of release of genetically transferred mammary tumor virus information and that this repression can be abrogated by treatment of low mammary tumor strains with the carcinogen urethan.

Although the possible importance of carcinogenic chemicals in facilitating the release and/or expression of the murine leukemia and mammary tumor viruses has been recognized only quite recently, the fact that certain strains of mice carry and transmit these specific tumor-inducing viruses has been known for several decades. It is not possible at this time to relate these situations in a meaningful way to other types of tumors which are induced by chemicals and for which no viral agent has been detected.

VIII. Tumor-Specific Transplantation Antigens in Chemically Induced Tumors

Tumors induced by chemical carcinogens usually, but not always, possess unique transplantation antigens, which differ from tumor to tumor even for multiple tumors induced by the same chemical in the same host or from the same clone of cells in culture (3, 96). The transplantation antigens of chemically induced tumors differ from the strong transplantation antigens of virally induced tumors in that the latter are specific for the virus and thus cross-react with the antigens of other tumors induced by the same or closely related viruses. Whether the apparent difference in the individuality of the antigens of chemically and virally induced tumors is real is not clear; with special technics individual tumor-specific antigens have recently been detected in some virus-induced tumors (136). The specific antigens may be only a reflection of the variety of the indiscriminate attacks of ultimate chemical carcinogens on the many vulnerable points in the informational macromolecules of the cell and may or may not have an important role in the genesis or development of the tumor, except in the determination of its growth rate.

IX. Summary

The nearly one-half century which has elapsed since the discovery of the carcinogenic activity of the first pure chemical carcinogen (dibenz(a,h)-anthracene) has seen an accelerating rate of increase in our knowledge of the induction of neoplasia by chemicals. The major advances of the past two or three decades include a much broader knowledge of the types of chemicals which can induce cancer in man and experimental animals, evidence that many human cancers are determined by environmental factors (including chemicals), the determination that most chemical carcinogens require metabolic conversion to strong electrophiles before they can induce neoplasia, and the ability to induce malignancy with chemicals in cell cultures.

At the same time, we are still far from a real understanding of the molecular mechanisms involved in the induction of malignancy by chemicals, viruses, or radiations. In no instance of carcinogenesis have the molecular mechanisms responsible for its induction or the nature of the critical molecular target(s) been elucidated. Likewise, the essential molecular phenotype has not been defined for any malignant cell. Importantly, for all of these issues there is no certainty that there is only one answer. Thus, there is no basis at present on which to propose that all tumors induced by a given chemical in a given tissue arise by the same molecular mechanism or have the same critical phenotype. In fact, if the tumor-specific transplantation antigens do play a role in neoplasia, their specificity may suggest that there is not a unitary mechanism.

When the molecular mechanisms of carcinogenesis are known in detail, there should be stronger bases on which to work toward the interruption or slowing down of some of the processes of chemical carcinogenesis. In the meantime the information which has already accrued forms a solid base for work toward the prevention or reduction of the incidences of some cancers of man. The realization that chemicals can induce cancers in man (Table 10.1) and the indication that as many as 80% of human cancers may be determined by environmental factors strongly support the idea that chemicals have an important role in the etiology of many human cancers. For instance, knowledge of the potent carcinogenicity of the mold metabolites aflatoxin B_1, aflatoxin G_1, and sterigmatocystin for a variety of species and the surveys which show that these metabolites are contaminants of the food of man and livestock in many areas of the world has caused concern about this aspect of the human diet (49, 105, 117). Likewise, in spite of our lack of knowledge of the structures of the causative chemicals and of the molecular mechanisms of carcinogenesis, the data on the major etiological role of cigarette smoke in the development of bronchial carcinoma in man give adequate information on which the incidence of bronchial carcinomas could be reduced in a dramatic fashion (147). Thus, while studies are directed toward a better understanding of chemical carcinogenesis at the molecular level, the knowledge available should be increasingly applied for the benefit of mankind.

Current knowledge should also be applied to the development of better and quicker screens for the detection of possible environmental carcinogens. The finding that chemical carcinogens and chemical mutagens in their ultimate forms have similar electrophilic reactivity has suggested that the detection of mutagenic activity can be developed as a preliminary screen for possible carcinogenic activity. If such assays are coupled with host-mediated systems, in which human tissues metabolize the putative mutagen and carcinogen to ultimate reactive forms, these mutagenicity assays might have sufficient predictive value to warrant their use on a wide scale. Similarly, the ability to induce malignant transformations by chemicals in cell cultures, particularly when such systems can be developed with human cells, should provide another very useful assay for the detection of human carcinogens.

With continued incisive fundamental research at the biological and molecular levels and with imaginative applications of this knowledge to the human problem, real progress should continue to be made toward the prevention and, possibly, the interruption of carcinogenic processes in man. However, the final attainment of our goal will also require strong and constant public support to disseminate knowledge of the human hazards, to educate the populace on the importance of prevention, and to enforce measures for human protection.

Acknowledgments

The research of the authors and their collaborators in chemical carcinogenesis has been supported by funds from CA 07175 and CRTY 5002 of the National Institutes of Health, USPHS.

References

1. Anon. (1972). *Food Cosmet. Toxicol.* **10,** 100–102.
2. Arcos, J. C., and Argus, M. F. (1968). *Advan. Cancer Res.* **11,** 305–471.
3. Baldwin, R. W. (1970). *Eur. J. Clin. Biol. Res.* **15,** 593–598.
4. Barry, E. J., Malejka-Giganti, D., and Gutmann, H. R. (1969–70). *Chem.-Biol. Interactions* **1,** 139–155.
5. Bartsch, H., Dworkin, C., Miller, E. C., and Miller, J. A. (1973). *Biochim. Biophys. Acta* **304,** 42–55.
6. Bartsch, H., Dworkin, M., Miller, J. A., and Miller, E. C. (1972). *Biochim. Biophys. Acta* **286,** 272–290.
7. Bartsch, H., and Hecker, E. (1971). *Biochim. Biophys. Acta* **237,** 567–578.
8. Bartsch, H., Traut, M., and Hecker, E. (1971). *Biochim. Biophys. Acta* **237,** 556–566.
9. Bentvelzen, P., Daams, J. H., Hageman, P., and Calafat, J. (1970). *Proc. Nat. Acad. Sci. U.S.* **67,** 377–384.
10. Berenblum, I., and Shubik, P. (1947). *Brit. J. Cancer* **1,** 383–391.
11. Berwald, Y., and Sachs, L. (1965). *J. Nat. Cancer Inst.* **35,** 641–661.
12. Borchert, P., Miller, J. A., Miller, E. C., and Shires, T. K. (1973). *Cancer Res.* **33,** 590–600.
13. Borchert, P., Wislocki, P. G., Miller, J. A., and Miller, E. C. (1973). *Cancer Res.* **33,** 575–589.
14. Boutwell, R. K. (1964). *In* "Progress in Experimental Tumor Research" (F. Homburger, ed.), Vol. 4, pp. 207–250. Karger, Basel.
15. Boyland, E. (1964). *Brit. Med. Bull.* **20,** 121–126.
16. Boyland, E., and Sims, P. (1965). *Biochem. J.* **95,** 780–787.
17. Boyland, E., and Sims, P. (1967). *Int. J. Cancer* **2,** 500–504.
18. Brookes, P. (1966). *Cancer Res.* **26,** 1994–2003.
19. Clayson, D. B. (1962). "Chemical Carcinogenesis." Little, Brown, Boston, Massachusetts.
20. Culvenor, C. C. J., Downing, D. T., Edgar, J. A., and Jago, M. V. (1969). *Ann. N.Y. Acad. Sci.* **163,** 837–847.
21. Dao, T. L., and Sinha, D. (1972). *J. Nat. Cancer Inst.* **49,** 591–593.
22. DeBaun, J. R., Miller, E. C., and Miller, J. A. (1970). *Cancer Res.* **30,** 577–595.
23. DeBaun, J. R., Smith, J. Y. R., Miller, E. C., and Miller, J. A. (1970). *Science* **167,** 184–186.
24. DiPaolo, J. A., Donovan, P., and Nelson, R. (1969). *J. Nat. Cancer Inst.* **42,** 867–876.
25. Dipple, A., and Slade, T. A. (1970). *Eur. J. Cancer* **6,** 417–423.
26. Druckrey, H. (1967). *In* "Potential Carcinogenic Hazards from Drugs" (R. Truhaut, ed.), pp. 60–77, Springer-Verlag, Berlin.
27. Druckrey, H., Preussmann, R., and Ivankovic, S. (1969). *Ann. New York Acad. Sci.* **163,** 676–695.
28. Druckrey, H., Preussmann, R., Ivankovic, S., Schmahl, D., Afkham, J., Blum, G., Mennel, H. D., Müller, M., Petropoulos, P., and Schneider, H. (1967). *Z. Krebsforsch.* **69,** 103–201.
29. Enomoto, M., Sato, K., Miller, E. C., and Miller, J. A. (1968). *Life Sci.* **7,** (part II), 1025–1032.

30. Epstein, S. M., Benedetti, E. L., Shinozuka, H., Bartus, B., and Farber, E. (1969/70) *Chem.-Biol. Interactions* 1, 113–124.
31. Flesher, J. W., and Sydnor, K. L. (1971). *Cancer Res.* 31, 1951–1954.
32. Foulds, L. (1969). "Neoplastic Development," Vol. 1, pp. 41–89. Academic Press, New York.
33. Fraumeni, J. F., and Miller, R. W. (1972). *J. Nat. Cancer Inst.* 48, 1267–1270.
34. Freese, E. (1971). *In* "Chemical Mutagens—Principles and Methods for Their Detection" (A. Hollaender, ed.), Vol. 1, pp. 1–56. Plenum Press, New York.
35. Fried, J., and Schumm, D. E. (1967). *J. Amer. Chem. Soc.* 89, 5508–5509.
36. Garner, R. C., and McLean, A. E. M. (1969). *Biochem. Pharmacol.* 18, 645–650.
37. Grover, P. L., Hewer, A., and Sims, P. (1971). *FEBS Lett.* 18, 76–80.
38. Grover, P. L., Sims, P., Huberman, E., Marquardt, H., Kuroki, T., and Heidelberger, C. (1971). *Proc. Nat. Acad. Sci. U.S.* 68, 1098–1101.
39. Gurdon, J. B. (1963). *Quart. Rev. Biol.* 38, 54–78.
40. Gutmann, H. R., Malejka-Giganti, D., Barry, E. J., and Rydell, R. E. (1972). *Cancer Res.* 32, 1554–1561.
41. Haenszel, W., and Kurihara, M. (1968). *J. Nat. Cancer Inst.* 40, 43–68.
42. Hartwell, J. L. (1951). Survey of Compounds Which Have Been Tested for Carcinogenic Activity. U.S. Public Health Serv. Publ. No. 149, 2nd ed., Washington, D.C.
43. Hartwell, J. L., and Shubik, P. (1957, 1959). Survey of Compounds Which Have Been Tested for Carcinogenic Activity, Suppl. 1 and 2. U.S. Public Health Service Publ. No. 149, Washington, D.C.
44. Hecker, E. (1968). *Cancer Res.* 28, 2338–2348.
45. Heidelberger, C. (1970). *Eur. J. Cancer* 6, 161–172.
46. Herbst, A. L., Ulfelder, H., and Pozkanzer, D. C. (1971). *New England J. Med.* 284, 878–881.
47. Higginson, J. (1969). *Can. Cancer Conf.* 8, 40–75.
48. Huberman, E., Kuroki, T., Marquardt, H., Selkirk, J. K., Heidelberger, C., Grover, P. L., and Sims, P. (1972). *Cancer Res.* 32, 1391–1396.
49. Hutt, M. S. R. (1969). *In* "Liver Cancer," IARC Sci. Publ. No. 1, pp. 21–29. Int. Agency for Res. on Cancer, Lyon.
50. Igel, H. J., Huebner, R. J., Turner, H. C., Kotin, P., and Falk, H. L. (1969). *Science* 166, 1624–1626.
51. Ikegami, S., Nemoto, N., Sáto, S., and Sugimura, T. (1969/70). *Chem.-Biol. Interactions* 1, 321–330.
52. Irving, C. C., Janss, D. H., and Russell, L. T. (1971). *Cancer Res.* 31, 387–391.
53. Irving, C. C., and Russell, L. T. (1970). *Biochemistry* 9, 2471–2476.
54. Irving, C. C., and Veazey, R. A. (1969). *Cancer Res.* 29, 1799–1804.
55. Irving, C. C., Veazey, R. A., and Hill, J. T. (1969). *Biochim. Biophys. Acta* 179, 189–198.
56. Jellinck, P. H., and Smith, G. (1969). *Biochem. Pharmacol.* 18, 679–682.
57. Jerina, D. M., Daly, J. W., Witkop, B., Zaltzman-Nirenberg, P., and Udenfriend, S. (1970). *Biochemistry* 9, 147–156.
58. Kaplan, H. S. (1967). *Cancer Res.* 27, 1325–1340.
59. King, C. M., and Phillips, B. (1968). *Science* 159, 1351–1353.
60. Kmet, J., and Mahboudi, E. (1972). *Science* 175, 846–853.
61. Kriek, E. (1969–70). *Chem.-Biol. Interactions* 1, 3–17.
62. Kriek, E. (1971). *Chem.-Biol. Interactions* 3, 19–28.
63. Kriek, E., Miller, J. A., Juhl, U., and Miller, E. C. (1967). *Biochemistry* 6, 177–182.
64. Kuroki, T., and Sato, H. (1968). *J. Natl. Cancer Inst.* 41, 53–71.
65. Legator, M. S., and Malling, H. V. (1971). *In* "Chemical Mutagens—Principles and Methods for Their Detection," (A. Hollaender, ed.), Vol. 2, pp. 569–589. Plenum Press, New York.
66. Lesko, S. A., Jr., Smith, A., Ts'o, P. O. P., and Umans, R. S. (1968). *Biochemistry* 7, 434–447.

67. Lesko, S. A., Jr., Ts'o, P. O. P., and Umans, R. S. (1969). *Biochemistry* **8**, 2291–2298.
68. Lijinsky, W., and Epstein, S. S. (1970). *Nature (London)* **225**, 21–23.
69. Lin, J.-K., Miller, J. A., and Miller, E. C. (1968). *Biochemistry* **7**, 1889–1895.
70. Lin, J.-K., Miller, J. A., and Miller, E. C. (1969). *Biochemistry* **8**, 1573–1582.
71. Lotlikar, P. D., and Luha, L. (1971). *Biochem. J.* **124**, 69–74.
72. Lotlikar, P. D., and Luha, L. (1971). *Mol. Pharmacol.* **7**, 381–388.
73. Lotlikar, P. D., Scribner, J. D., Miller, J. A., and Miller, E. C. (1966). *Life Sci.* **5**, 1263–1269.
74. Magee, P. N. (1969). *Ann. N.Y. Acad. Sci.* **163**, 717–729.
75. Magee, P. N. (1971). *Food Cosmet. Toxicol.* **9**, 207–218.
76. Magee, P. N., and Barnes, J. M. (1967). *Advan. Cancer Res.* **10**, 163–256.
77. Marquardt, H., Kuroki, T., Huberman, E., Selkirk, J. K., Heidelberger, C., Grover, P. L., and Sims, P. (1972). *Cancer Res.* **32**, 716–720.
78. Matsushima, T., Kobuna, I., Fukuoka, F., and Sugimura, T. (1968). *Gann* **59**, 247–250.
79. Matsumoto, H., Nagata, Y., Nishimura, E. T., Bristol, R., and Haber, M. (1972). *J. Nat. Cancer Inst.* **49**, 423–434.
80. Mattocks, A. R. (1968). *Nature (London)* **217**, 723–728.
81. McLean, A. E. M., and McLean, E. K. (1966). *Biochem. J.* **100**, 564–571.
82. McLean, E. K. (1970). *Pharmacol. Rev.* **22**, 429–483.
83. Miller, E. C., Lotlikar, P. D., Miller, J. A., Butler, B. W., Irving, C. C., and Hill, J. T. (1968). *Mol. Pharmacol.* **4**, 147–154.
84. Miller, E. C., and Miller, J. A. (1960). *Cancer Res.* **20**, 133–137.
85. Miller, E. C., and Miller, J. A. (1966). *Pharmacol. Rev.* **18**, 805–838.
86. Miller, E. C., and Miller, J. A. (1967). *Proc. Soc. Exp. Biol. Med.* **124**, 915–917.
87. Miller, E. C., and Miller, J. A. (1971). *In* "Chemical Mutagens—Principles and Methods for Their Detection" (A. Hollaender, ed.), Vol. 1, pp. 83–119. Plenum Press, New York.
88. Miller, E. C., and Miller, J. A. (1972). *In* "Environment and Cancer." The University of Texas M. D. Anderson Hospital and Tumor Inst. at Houston, *Annu. Symp. Fundamental Cancer Res., 24th,* pp. 5–39. Williams & Wilkins, Baltimore, Maryland.
89. Miller, J. A. (1970). *Cancer Res.* **30**, 559–576.
90. Miller, J. A. (in press). *In* "Toxicants Occurring Naturally in Foods" (F. M. Strong, ed.), 2nd ed. Nat. Acad. of Sci.—Nat. Res. Council, Washington, D.C.
91. Miller, J. A., and Miller, E. C. (1963). *Cancer Res.* **23**, 229–239.
92. Miller, J. A., and Miller, E. C. (1965). *Cancer Res.* **25**, 1292–1304.
93. Miller, J. A., and Miller, E. C. (1969). *In* "Progress in Experimental Tumor Research" (F. Homburger, ed.), Vol. 11, pp. 273–301. Karger, Basel.
94. Miller, J. A., and Miller, E. C. (1969). *In* "The Jerusalem Symposia on Quantum Chemistry and Biochemistry" (E. D. Bergmann and B. Pullman, eds.), Vol. 1, Physiochemical Mechanisms of Carcinogenesis, pp. 237–261. Israel Acad. of Sci. and Humanities, Jerusalem.
95. Miller, J. A., and Miller, E. C. (1971). *J. Nat. Cancer Inst.* **47**, V–XIV.
96. Mondal, S., Iype, P. T., Griesbach, L. M., and Heidelberger, C. (1970). *Cancer Res.* **30**, 1593–1597.
97. Nagata, C., Tagashira, Y., Inomata, M., and Kodama, M. (1971). *Gann* **62**, 419–421.
98. Pegg, A. E. (1972). *Biochem. J.* **128**, 59–68.
99. Poirier, L. A., Miller, J. A., Miller, E. C., and Sato, K. (1967). *Cancer Res.* **27**, 1600–1613.
100. Pott, P. (1775). "Chirurgical Observations Relative to Cancer of the Scrotum." London. Reprinted in *Nat. Cancer Inst. Monograph* **10**, 7–13.
101. Potter, V. R., Walker, P. R., and Goodman, J. I. (1972). *Gann Monograph No. 13,* 123–136.
102. Preussmann, R., Druckrey, H., Ivankovic, S., and von Hodenberg, A. (1969). *Ann. N.Y. Acad. Sci.* **163**, 697–714.
103. Price, P. J., Freeman, A. E., Lane, W. T., and Huebner, R. J. (1971). *Nature New Biol.* **230**, 144–146.

104. Pullman, A., and Pullman, B. (1955). *Advan. Cancer Res.* **3**, 117–169.
105. Purchase, I. F. H., and van der Watt, J. J. (1970). *Food Cosmet. Toxicol.* **8**, 289–295.
106. Radomski, J. L., and Brill, E. (1970). *Science* **167**, 992–993.
107. Redmond, E. R., Jr. (1970). *New England J. Med.* **282**, 18–23.
108. Reynolds, E. S. (1967). *J. Pharmacol. Exp. Therap.* **155**, 117–126.
109. Rhim, J. S., Cho, H. Y., Rabstein, L., Gordon, R. J., Bryan, R. J., Gardner, M. B., and Huebner, R. J. (1972). *Nature (London)* **239**, 103–107.
110. Rhim, J. S., Vass, W., Cho, H. Y., and Huebner, R. J. (1971). *Int. J. Cancer* **7**, 65–74.
111. Ross, W. J. C. (1962). "Biological Alkylating Agents." Butterworth, London and Washington, D.C.
112. Schwaier, R., Nashed, N., and Zimmermann, F. K. (1968). *Mol. Gen. Genet.* **102**, 290–300.
113. Segi, M., Kurihara, M., and Matsuyama, T. (1969). "Cancer Mortality for Selected Sites in 24 Countries, No. 5 (1964–1965)." Sanko Printing, Sendai, Japan.
114. Sekely, L. I., Malejka-Giganti, D., Gutmann, H. R., and Rydell, R. E. (1973). *J. Nat. Cancer Inst.* **50**, 1337–1345.
115. Selkirk, J. K., Huberman, E., and Heidelberger, C. (1971). *Biochem. Biophys. Res. Commun.* **43**, 1010–1016.
116. Setlow, R. B., and Reagan, J. D. (1972). *Biochem. Biophys. Res. Commun.* **46**, 1019–1024.
117. Shank, R. C., Bhamarapravati, N., Gordon, J. E., and Wogan, G. N. (1972). *Food Cosmet. Toxicol.* **10**, 171–179.
118. Shirasu, Y. (1965). *Proc. Soc. Exp. Biol. Med.* **118**, 812–814.
119. Sims, P. (1967). *Biochem. Pharmacol.* **16**, 613–618.
120. Sims, P. (1970). *Biochem. Pharmacol.* **19**, 795–818.
121. Spatz, M. (1969). *Ann. N.Y. Acad. Sci.* **163**, 848–859.
122. Speyer, J. F., Karam, J. D., and Lenny, A. B. (1966). *Cold Spring Harbor Symp. Quant. Biol.* **31**, 693–697.
123. Stanislawski-Berencwajg, M., Uriel, J., and Grabar, P. (1967). *Cancer Res.* **27**, 1990–1997.
124. Stich, H. F., San, R. H. C., Miller, J. A., and Miller, E. C. (1972). *Nature New Biol.* **238**, 9–10.
125. Stöhrer, G., and Brown, G. B. (1970). *Science* **167**, 1622–1624.
126. Stöhrer, G., Corbin, E., and Brown, G. B. (1972). *Cancer Res.* **32**, 637–642.
127. Sugimura, T., Okabe, K., and Nagao, M. (1966). *Cancer Res.* **26**, 1717–1721.
128. Swann, P. F., Pegg, A. E., Hawks, A., Farber, E., and Magee, P. N. (1971). *Biochem. J.* **123**, 175–181.
129. Szafarz, D., and Weisburger, J. H. (1969). *Cancer Res.* **29**, 962–968.
130. Tada, M., and Tada, M. (1972). *Biochem. Biophys. Res. Comm.* **46**, 1025–1032.
131. Tada, M., Tada, M., and Takahashi, T. (1970). *In* "Genetic Concepts and Neoplasia" (M. D. Anderson Hospital and Tumor Institute), pp. 214–227, Williams and Wilkens Co., Baltimore.
132. Temin, H. M. (1971). *J. Nat. Cancer Inst.* **46**, III–VII.
133. Thompson, J. I., and Co. (1972). "Survey of Compounds Which Have Been Tested for Carcinogenic Activity," 1968–69 volume, Public Health Service Publication No. 149. Washington, D.C.
134. Todaro, G. J., and Huebner, R. J. (1972). *Proc. Nat. Acad. Sci., U.S.*, **69**, 1009–1015.
135. Urbach, F. (1969). *In* "The Biologic Effects of Ultraviolet Radiation (with Emphasis on the Skin)" (J. Urbach, ed.), pp. 635–650, Pergamon Press, Oxford and New York.
136. Vaage, J., Kalinovsky, T., and Olson, R. (1969). *Cancer Res.* **29**, 1452–1456.
137. Van Duuren, B. L. (1969). *In* "Progress in Experimental Tumor Research" (F. Homburger, ed.), Vol. 11, pp. 31–68. Karger, Basel.
138. Van Duuren, B. L., Langseth, L., Goldschmidt, B. M., and Orris, L., (1967). *J. Nat. Cancer Inst.* **39**, 1217–1228.
139. Warwick, G. P., and Roberts, J. J. (1967). *Nature (London)* **213**, 1206–1207.

140. Weisburger, J. H., Yamamoto, R. S., Williams, G. M., Grantham, P. H., Matsushima, T., and Weisburger, E. K. (1972). *Cancer Res.* **32**, 491–500.
141. Whitmire, C. E., Salerno, R. A., Rabstein, L. S., Huebner, R. J., and Turner, H. C. (1971). *J. Nat. Cancer Inst.* **47**, 1255–1265.
142. Wilk, M., and Girke, W. (1969). *In* "The Jerusalem Symposia on Quantum Chemistry and Biochemistry" (E. D. Bergmann and B. Pullman, eds.), Vol. 1, Physiochemical Mechanisms of Carcinogenesis, pp. 91–105. Israel Acad. of Sci. and Humanities, Jerusalem.
143. Williams, G. M., Elliott, J. M., and Weisburger, J. H. (1973). *Cancer Res.* **33**, 606–612.
144. Witkin, E. M., and Ferquharson, E. L. (1969). *In* "Mutation as Cellular Process" (G. E. W. Wolstenholme and M. O'Connor, eds.), pp. 36–49. Churchill, London.
145. Wolff, I. A., and Wasserman, A. E. (1972). *Science* **177**, 15–19.
146. Wunderlich, V., Schütt, M., Böttger, M., and Graffi, A. (1970). *Biochem. J.* **118**, 99–109.
147. Wynder, E. L., and Mabuchi, K. (1972). *Preventive Med.* **1**, 300–334.

CHAPTER XI

Oncogenic Viruses

MATILDA BENYESH-MELNICK AND JANET S. BUTEL

I. Introduction

Ample evidence obtained by research on transformation of cells *in vitro* indicates that cancer originates in a single cell. Once altered, the cell possesses new and heritable properties which may be expressed as morphological, metabolic, and antigenic alterations, ultimately coupled with the development of oncogenicity. In the animal, the outcome of these phenomena may be one of two kinds: either the altered cells may invade the surrounding tissue and metastasize to distant organs and result in host death or the host may retain its homeostasis through humoral or cellular immune control mechanisms.

Whatever the outcome *in vivo*, one of the central problems in cancer entails the identification of the molecular mechanisms by which a cell is rendered malignant.

The past several decades have witnessed concomitantly the ups and downs of various "exclusive" or "unifying" theories of carcinogenesis as well as the overwhelming realization of the molecular and genetic complexity of the vertebrate cell. The advances made in recent years in defining the genetic composition of oncogenic viruses and in elucidating the interactions between viral and cell genes are providing significant insights into the problem of carcinogenesis at the cellular level.

Although the viral origin of avian leukemia was discovered early in this century (162), the field of viral oncology has only recently received wide attention. Intensified research has led to the discovery of the viral etiology of many common tumors in lower animals. Recent contributions have been possible largely because of technological advances in tissue culture methods, the use of newborn animals of defined genetic constitution for assays, and the application of modern biophysical, biochemical, and immunological methodology.

The oncogenic viruses can be classified into two main groups with differing physical, chemical, and biological properties: those which contain RNA as their genetic material (RNA viruses or oncornaviruses) and those which contain DNA as their genetic material (DNA viruses). The mechanism by which oncogenic viruses render cells malignant and how they differ in this respect from ordinary cytocidal viruses are questions which have not yet been fully answered. Infection of a cell by a cytocidal virus results exclusively in cell death, whereas infection by a tumor virus leads to a synchronous virus-cell coexistence which results in profound changes in the properties of the infected cells. The application of quantitative methods to the study of virus-cell interactions in tissue culture and for the detection of viral-induced macromolecules integrated into the genome of cells they have rendered malignant has brought some understanding of the mode of action of oncogenic viruses.

Those interested in the detailed historical background and development of the area of viral oncology should consult the recently revised monograph "Oncogenic Viruses" (234). In addition, several reviews dealing with both groups of viruses have been published in recent years (120, 150, 175, 227, 474). This chapter deals with selected aspects of *in vivo* and *in vitro* carcinogenesis by representative members of the RNA and DNA groups of viruses in an attempt to evaluate present day work on viral carcinogenesis and its implication to the possible role of viruses in carcinogenesis in man.

II. Oncogenic RNA Viruses (Oncornaviruses)

A. General Consideration and Classification

The oncogenic RNA viruses have been termed leukoviruses (175), thylaxoviridiaee (saclike viruses) (119), and more recently (424) oncornaviruses. The terms "C-type" and "B-type" oncornaviruses, originally based only on morphological distinction alone (see Section II,B) and more recently based also on certain antigenic and enzymic differences (see Sections II,D and II,E), are also in use. As the field has developed, several comprehensive reviews have appeared on the oncornaviruses (234, 588, 625) as well as excellent reviews on the avian (628) and murine (69, 74, 491) oncornaviruses.

The oncornaviruses listed in Table 11.1 are similar in structure, chemical composition, and mode of replication. They are widespread in nature and are known to cause natural tumors in the host of origin. With the exception of the murine mammary tumor virus and some more recently recognized viruses (see below), the oncornaviruses fall into species-specific groups of agents inducing either leukemias or sarcomas. For these, the term leukemia-sarcoma complex will be used. The usual mode of transmission of those which induce leukemias is vertical (congenital) rather than horizontal (postnatal). Those viruses which have been well studied can be divided into 6 groups on the basis of antigenic makeup, host range, and type of malignancy.

1. AVIAN LEUKEMIA-SARCOMA COMPLEX

Since the first demonstration of the infectious nature of avian leukemia (162) and of avian (Rous) sarcoma (507), numerous antigenically related strains of avian leukemia virus (ALV) and Rous sarcoma virus (RSV) have been recognized (234, 628). Many of the ALV and RSV isolates have been found in the past to consist of mixtures of strains (628). The use of viruses derived by means of passage at limiting dilution in tissue culture (628) has facilitated a more contemporary classification. Four major antigenic subgroups (A–D) have been recognized, each including different ALV and RSV strains as well as different nontransforming Rous-associated viruses, termed RAV, which can form pseudotypes with certain defective RSV genomes (see Section II,G). This classification, based on antigenic cross reactions in neutralization and immunofluorescence tests with antisera prepared in chickens, is in agreement with a classification based on virus host range and virus interference in cells of genetically defined avian species (Table 11.2). A dominant cell gene governs the susceptibility of such cells (C/O, C/A, C/B, C/AB, C/BC) to avian oncornaviruses (450). In susceptible cells, viruses within the one antigenic subgroup interfere with each other but do not interfere with viruses of the other antigenic subgroups (see 631). A fifth subgroup E (451, 646) is comprised of Rous-associated viruses, RAV-0 and RAV-60, and nontransforming avian agents that are released from avian cells following induction with irradiation or carcinogens (see Section II,H).

2. MURINE LEUKEMIA-SARCOMA COMPLEX

Since the first isolation of a murine leukemia virus (MuLV) by Gross in 1951, many other MuLV strains have come to light (234, 491). Four of these have been most prominently used for classification purposes; they bear the name

TABLE 11.1

SOME PROPERTIES OF RNA-CONTAINING TUMOR VIRUSES (ONCORNAVIRUSES)

Virus	Abbreviations used	Host of origin	Natural tumors (host of origin)[b]	Experimental host range		Virion morphology (C- or B-type particles)[c]
				in Vivo tumor[b]	in Vitro cell transformation	
Avian complex						
Leukemia	ALV[a]	Chicken	Yes	Chicken, turkey	Chicken[d]	C
Sarcoma (Rous)	RSV	Chicken	Yes	Avian, rodent, monkey	Avian, rodent, bovine, monkey, man	C
Murine complex						
Leukemia	MuLV	Mouse	Yes	Mouse, rat, hamster		C
Sarcoma	MSV	Mouse	No	Mouse, rat, hamster	Mouse, rat, hamster	C
Murine mammary tumor (Bittner)	MTV	Mouse	Yes	Mouse		B
Feline complex						
Leukemia	FeLV	Cat	Yes	Cat		C
Sarcoma	FeSV	Cat	Yes	Cat, dog, rabbit, monkey	Cat, dog, monkey, man	C
Other						
Viper		Viper	Yes			C
Hamster, leukemia?	HaLV	Hamster				C
Rat, leukemia?	RaLV	Rat				C
Guinea pig, leukemia		Guinea pig	Yes			C
Bovine, lymphoma		Cow	Yes			
Primate						
Sarcoma (Woolly monkey, gibbon)		Monkey, ape	Yes	Monkey	Monkey	C
Mammary carcinoma (Mason-Pfizer)		Monkey				B

[a] The term RAV has been used for ALV strains associated with the defective Bryan strain of RSV.

[b] Usually there is a persistence of infectious virus in the tumor.

[c] Size ranges from 70 to 100 nm; virus matures at cell membrane by a process of budding.

[d] Attained with avian myeloblastosis virus only.

TABLE 11.2

CLASSIFICATION OF AVIAN ONCORNAVIRUSES BY HOST RANGE

Antigenic subgroup	Representative viruses[a]		Ability of viruses within antigenic subgroups to grow in:						
	Leukemia strains	Rous sarcoma strains	Genetically defined chick embryo cells						Japanese quail cells
			C/O	C/A	C/B	C/AB	C/BC	C/E	
A	RAV-1 AMV-1 RIF-1	SR-RSV-A MH-RSV PR-RSV-A	+[b]	0	+	0	+	+	+
B	RAV-2 AMV-2 RIF-2	SR-RSV-B HA-RSV	+	+	0	0	0	+	0
C	RAV-7 RAV-49	PR-RSV-C[c] B77[c]	+	+	+	+	0	+	±
D	RAV-50	SR-RSV-D[c] CZ-RSV-D[c]	+	+	±	±	±	+	0
E	RAV-0 RAV-60 ILV	None	+	+	0	0	0	0	+

[a] *Abbreviations:* RSV = Rous sarcoma virus; RAV = Rous-associated virus; AMV = avian myeloblastosis virus; RIF resistance-inducing factor) = field strains of avian leukemia viruses that interfere with the focus-forming capacity of RSV; ILV = induced leukemia viruses (see Section II,H); SR = Schmidt Ruppin strain; MH = Mill Hill strain; PR = Prague strain; HA = Harris strain; B77 = Bratislava 77 strain of RSV; and CZ = Carr-Zilber strain.

[b] + = cells fully susceptible; ± = intermediate cell susceptibility; 0 = cells resistant.

[c] Strains of RSV capable of inducing tumors in rodents and of transforming rodent cells.

of the investigator first reporting the strain and shall be designated here as follows: G-MuLV (232); F-MuLV (185); M-MuLV (402); and R-MuLV (483). On the basis of type-specific antigens, found both on the virion surface and on the surface of infected cells, the existing MuLV strains have been divided into 2 main antigenic groups, one carrying the protein coat antigens of the Friend-Moloney-Rauscher (FMR) viruses and the other the antigens of the Gross (G) virus (196, 430, for review see also, 447). This classification has been supported by virus neutralization, complement fixation, immunofluorescence, and cytotoxic tests (see reviews 286, 431, 447, 491). A new grouping of these agents into N-tropic, B-tropic, and NB-tropic viruses has recently been suggested based on virus host range in genetically defined mouse embryo cells; the first group contains agents capable of replicating mainly in cells derived from NIH/Swiss (N) mice, the second group of viruses replicates mainly in cells derived from BALB/c (B) mice, and the third group, composed of laboratory strains only, replicates equally well in both types of cells. Unlike the avian oncornavirus system, this grouping is not in accord with the above antigenic classification since viruses of the G group can be either N- or B-tropic and viruses of both FMR and G groups have been found to be NB-tropic (254).

Furthermore, unlike the avian oncornavirus system, a dominant cell gene governs resistance to MuLV rather than susceptibility (456, 457).

Five different strains of murine sarcoma virus (MSV) have been recognized to date: H-MSV (255); FJB-MSV (177); M-MSV (403); Ki-MSV (330); and GZ-MSV (194). All five strains exist as mixtures of MSV and MuLV and bear the antigenicity of the associated MuLV.

3. MURINE MAMMARY TUMOR VIRUS (MTV)

This virus is also known as the Bittner milk agent (61a). Several different strains of MTV have been identified, all transmitted through the milk and all responsible for mammary carcinomas in certain strains of mice (69, 234). Different strains of MTV share protein coat antigens and fall into one major antigenic group, distinct from the other murine oncornaviruses (see reviews 69, 70, 423).

4. FELINE LEUKEMIA-SARCOMA COMPLEX

This represents a newly evolving group of antigenically related feline leukemia viruses (FeLV), which can cause leukemias in the cat (299, 493), and feline sarcoma viruses (FeSV), which cause sarcomas in the cat (191, 560), as well as in other species including dogs (191) and marmoset monkeys (124). The protein coat antigens of the different FeLV and FeSV isolates are not well defined as yet, but these agents are antigenically distinct from the other oncornaviruses.

5. HAMSTER LEUKEMIA-SARCOMA COMPLEX

This is also a newly recognized group of antigenically related agents. The hamster leukemia viruses (HaLV) appear to be indigenous to the hamster (224, 568). They have been best characterized in tissue culture as nontransforming agents present in stocks of hamster-specific sarcoma viruses (318, 320). The hamster-specific sarcoma viruses (HaSV) have been derived from hamster sarcomas induced by different strains of MSV and are oncogenic in hamsters but not in mice (36, 318, 341, 454). They are considered to consist of the MSV genome in the envelope of the helper HaLV, which is responsible for the altered host range and protein coat antigenicity (317, 341). It remains to be seen whether more than one serotype of HaLV exists. However, sufficient evidence does indicate that both HaLV and the HaSV (pseudotypes of the original MSV) are antigenically distinct from the other murine C-type viruses (317, 319, 435, 436).

6. PRIMATE ONCORNAVIRUSES

Recently, three viruses have been isolated from cell lines derived from spontaneous tumors of subhuman primates. The Mason-Pfizer virus, identified as a B-type virus, was derived from a rhesus monkey mammary tumor (104, 301),

and is serologically distinct from other simian viruses and the known oncornaviruses (425, 549, 550). The other two are C-type viruses and have been isolated
from a woolly monkey fibrosarcoma (599, 651) and from a gibbon ape lymphosarcoma (314), respectively. Serological studies indicate that the latter two
agents are closely related to each other, but are unrelated to other simian viruses
and are distinct from the known oncornaviruses (444, 549, 550).

7. Other Oncornaviruses

Particles with the morphology of C-type oncornaviruses have been detected
by electron microscopy in malignancies of snakes (654), rats (103), guinea
pigs (see 234, 297), and in phytohemagglutinin-stimulated lymphocytes of cattle
with lymphosarcoma (398, 573). The snake agent (viper sarcoma virus) isolated
from a spleen cell line of a myxofibroma-bearing Russell's viper (654) has the
biophysical properties of other oncornaviruses, but appears to be antigenically
distinct from them (208). The rat virus, termed rat leukemia virus (RaLV),
bears a similarity to the HaLV described above in that it has been detected
in tissue culture as a nonfocus-forming agent that serves as a helper virus for
a rat-tropic (but not mouse-tropic) strain of MSV and is antigenically distinct
from the murine oncornaviruses (2, 209, 600).

C-type particles have also been detected in various malignancies of man (see
234), and B-type particles that appear to have some properties in common
with the murine mammary tumor virus (see Section IV,A) have been recently
associated with human breast cancer (407).

More recently, two C-type viruses have been reported, allegedly from human
malignancies. The first, ESP-1 virus, isolated from a cell line derived from a
child with lymphoma, was originally thought to be of human origin (464).
It was subsequently reported that ESP-1 virus is apparently a contaminant of
murine origin as it has a species-specific gs* antigen (211) and reverse transcriptase (550) virtually indistinguishable from those of the murine leukemia viruses.
The second, RD-114 virus, isolated from an embryonal human rhabdomyosarcoma after passage through fetal cats (388), appears at present to be unrelated
to the known feline or other oncornaviruses; it has been shown to possess a
species-specific gs-1 antigen (see Section II,E) that is unrelated to that of cat,
mouse, rat, or hamster oncornaviruses (390, 437) and its reverse transcriptase
(see Section II,D) is also unrelated to that of the above 4 oncornaviruses (550)
or to that of the 3 primate oncornaviruses (549). Thus on the basis of available
data, it is impossible at present to determine the species of origin of the RD-114
virus, and further study is needed to identify this agent.

B. Virion Structure

Ultrastructural studies have revealed many similarities between the various
oncornaviruses (53, 79, 119, 130, 371, 424, 529, 530). The mature virions are

* gs = group specific.

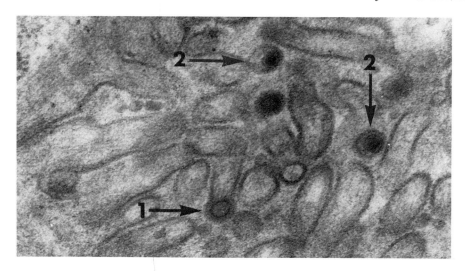

Fig. 11.1. Electron micrograph of murine mammary tumor virus (MTV) particles (75,000×). A budding particle (1) and typical mature B-type particles (2) are seen in the alveolar lumen of a mammary gland from an infected mouse. Courtesy of D. Medina and M. Klima, Department of Cell Biology, Baylor College of Medicine, Houston, Texas.

nearly spherical structures (100–120 nm in size) comprised of an RNA and protein-containing electron-dense nucleoid (presumably the nucleocapsid) that is enclosed in a glycoprotein and lipid-containing envelope (see reviews: 137, 496). The envelope is derived from the cellular membrane during the process of budding which is the characteristic mode of release from infected cells for all oncornaviruses (53, 119, 130). Unlike the nucleoids of mature virions, those of budding or freshly released particles are electroluscent and are separated by two concentric rings from the envelope (53, 119, 130). A difference exists between the B-type particles of the murine mammary tumor virus (Fig. 11.1) and the C-type particles of the remaining oncornaviruses (Fig. 11.2) in that the nucleoids are eccentric in the former and central in the latter. In addition, unlike in the C-type particles, the envelope of negatively stained B-type particles has been shown to have surface projections (530).

Disruption of the lipid-containing envelope by mild treatment with nonionic detergents or ether results in the liberation of the nucleoids which have a higher buoyant density (1.22–1.27 gm/cm^3) than the buoyant density (1.16–1.18 gm/cm^3) of the intact virion (25, 126, 530). The structure of the nucleoids (whether within the intact virion or after isolation) is not fully understood at present. There is increasing evidence which suggests a helical nucleocapsid structure (26, 126, 307, 370, 529, 530). Different models have been proposed to explain the transition of the highly ordered double ringed form of the nucleoid in the budding (or freshly released) virion into the amorphous or filamentous-appearing nucleoid of the extracellular mature virion. It is thought that during virus maturation supercoiled helical ribonucleoprotein strands form a hollow sphere and, due to structural (or thermal) instability after maturation, uncoil

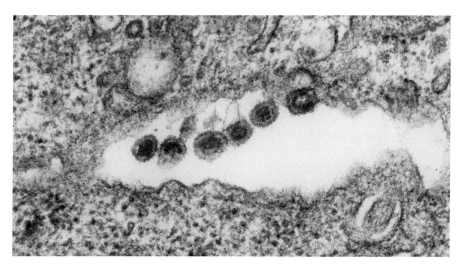

Fig. 11.2. Electron micrograph of C-type virus particles in the intracellular space of rat fibroblasts infected with murine leukemia virus (75,000×). Courtesy of R. McCombs, Department of Virology, Baylor College of Medicine.

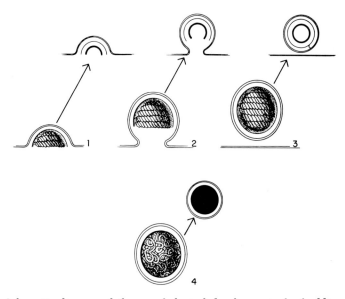

Fig. 11.3. Schematic diagram of the morphological development of a budding C-type virus particle to a mature extracellular form. The nucleocapsid helix starts forming a shell immediately below the site of viral budding (stage 1), which in thin section will appear as a crescent-like structure. Ultimately, a hollow sphere is formed (stage 3) which in section appears as 2 concentric closed rings. At this stage, the virus is budded-off from the cell membrane and the hollow, spherical nucleoid undergoes a rapid structural transition to yield a condensed nucleoid (stage 4). (Courtesy of N. H. Sarkar, R. C. Nowinski, and D. H. Moore: *J. Virol.* **8**, 564, 1971.)

and fill the interior of the nucleoid (Fig. 11.3). However, the complete substantiation of helical nucleocapsid structure awaits further study.

Chemical analysis of purified virions has revealed a remarkable similarity in composition between different oncornaviruses (see reviews 137, 496). Analysis of MuLV, ALV, RSV, and MTV indicates that lipids (30–40%) and proteins (60–70%) comprise over 90% of the dry mass of the virus, the remainder of the particle consisting of RNA (1–2.5%) and small amounts of carbohydrates which exist primarily as glycoproteins (78, 137, 303, 371, 467, 496). More recent studies (see below) indicate that some of the oncornaviruses contain a small amount of DNA within the highly purified virions in addition to the RNA.

C. Viral Nucleic Acids

In its native form, the nucleic acid isolated from purified oncornavirions consists of a major single-stranded RNA component with a sedimentation constant of 60–70 S (corresponding to a molecular weight of $1–2 \times 10^7$ daltons) and variable amounts of slower sedimenting (4–10 S) single-stranded RNA molecules, as well as small amounts of 18 S and 28 S ribosomal RNA (26, 112, 137, 227, 496, 588, 625).

The 4–10 S molecules were originally thought to be fragments of the high molecular weight RNA produced by degradation (24). Further studies with avian myeloblastosis virus revealed that the 4 S RNA is methylated (168) and can be acylated with various amino acids (80, 169, 612) and thus is indistinguishable from host-cell transfer RNA (tRNA). However, it appears that the amino acid-accepting activity of the 4 S viral RNA is different from that of host cell tRNA (161, 612, 613), and differences in base composition have been found between host cell tRNA and the 4 S RNA of avian myeloblastosis virus (473) and of RSV (57). A strain-specific, single-stranded 7 S RNA that is not methylated and is thus different from tRNA has been detected in purified virions of RSV (56). The role that these native low molecular weight (4–10 S) RNA species may play in virus replication is not clear.

The fast sedimenting 60–70 S RNA of the oncornaviruses appears to be an aggregated structure that can be dissociated by heat or dimethylsulfoxide into several (3–4) major subunits with a sedimentation constant each of 30–40 S, corresponding to a molecular weight of $3–4 \times 10^6$ daltons (24, 58, 71, 136, 137, 139, 168, 405, 496) and smaller subunits, the most prominent of which is a 4 S RNA that has the properties of tRNA (60, 170, 391, see also Chapter VI).

The finding of hydrogen-bonded 30–40 S subunits in the 60–70 S RNA of oncornaviruses is taken as an indication that their genome is segmented like that of influenza virus and reovirus. Recent evidence showing a recombination frequency between avian oncornaviruses (312, 633) as high as that reported for influenza virus (281) and for reovirus (176) lends further support to this assumption. It remains to be determined whether the 30–40 S subunits differ in physicochemical properties and what is the manner by which they assemble into the 60–70 S RNA of the complete virion. However, more recent studies indicate the existence of two functionally different subunits that can be separated by polyacrylamide gel electrophoresis. This stems from work with spontaneous (632), radiation-induced (219, 223, 611) or mutagen-induced temperature-sensitive (22, 62, 310, 382) mutants of RSV that can replicate but cannot transform cells. Heat-dissociated 60–70 S RNA of transforming RSV yields both subunits ("a" and "b"); the larger one (subunit "a") appears to contain the genetic information for transformation as it is absent in similarly treated RNA of non-transforming RSV (140, 384). The segmented nature of the genome of oncornaviruses may be one of the reasons that most attempts to demonstrate infectivity for the viral RNA have not been successful (588).

Recent investigations have shown that highly purified murine (60, 61, 501) and avian (358, 359, 494) oncornavirions contain a small amount (about 2.5% of the total viral nucleic acid) of a low molecular weight (7 S) DNA that can be resolved into two components with different densities in CsCl (60, 61, 358). The significance of these small viral DNA molecules has not been established but preliminary evidence suggests that they may be of cellular origin (359).

D. Viral Enzymes

The finding that purified preparations of murine and avian oncornaviruses contain an RNA-dependent DNA polymerase (reverse transcriptase) capable of transcribing viral RNA *in vitro* into DNA (28, 592) was soon confirmed for all the known oncornaviruses (549, 550, 565). Subsequent work on the mechanism of the *in vitro* transcription of viral RNA into DNA (588, 591) indicates the following:

(1) Purified oncornavirions contain several nucleic acid-related enzymes, the two most thoroughly studied being an RNA-dependent DNA polymerase (28, 592) and a DNA-dependent DNA polymerase (566). The modes of action of others, such as DNA endonuclease, DNA ligase (400) and RNase H or hybridase (401), have only begun to be studied. These enzymic activities appear to be associated with the virion cores (77, 107, 205, 577) and they may all be involved in oncornavirus replication should the *in vitro* model of RNA to DNA transcription hold true for the *in vivo* system.

(2) The "endogenous" *in vitro* reaction (which employs nonionic detergent-treated virions as the source for both enzymic activity and viral RNA template) yields DNA products which are small (6–8 S) molecules and represent a mixture of sequentially synthesized RNA-DNA hybrids, single-stranded DNA, and double-stranded DNA (189, 375); both the reaction and the product are specified by the viral RNA as pretreatment of disrupted virions with RNase (but not with DNase) abolishes the reaction (28, 592), and the product is composed of sequences complementary to the viral RNA (138, 144, 189, 501, 565). Whether the entire viral genome is transcribed into complementary DNA molecules (144) or this is true only for selected sequences of the viral RNA (621) is uncertain at present.

(3) In the "exogenous" reaction, purified virion-derived enzyme(s) which has been freed from the endogenous viral RNA template utilizes a variety of natural nucleic acids as templates, the most potent being the 60–70 S viral RNA (142, 143, 352). A wide variety of synthetic polynucleotides are also utilized (142, 143, 294, 352, 566, 567). Unlike other DNA polymerases, the virion poly-merase(s) has a preference for ribohomopolymers over deoxyhomopolymers as templates (29). The preferential utilization of oligomer-homopolymer complex $dT_{10} \cdot poly \, rA$ over oligomer-homopolymer complex $dT_{10} \cdot poly \, dA$ has been used to specifically distinguish the viral enzyme from other cell DNA poly-merases (221).

(4) Like other DNA polymerases the viral enzyme(s) is unable to synthesize DNA *de novo* but requires both a template and a primer (hydrogen-bonded to the template) in order to carry out polymerization of nucleotides comple-mentary to single-stranded regions of the template (29). Both in the exogenous and in the endogenous reactions the enzyme(s) catalyzes chain elongation through repairlike reactions in which nucleotides are added to the 3'-OH end of the primer (294, 352, 559). The primer has been found to be covalently linked to the newly synthesized DNA in the *in vitro* reaction (99, 352, 559, 624). Experiments with 60–70 S RNA used as a template indicate that the primer is a small (~4 S) RNA molecule (99, 352, 624). This ~4 S RNA can be isolated from the heat-dissociated 60–70 S viral RNA and, when added (under annealing conditions) to purified 30–40 S RNA subunits, renders them capable of template activity (99). The latter authors suggest that the ~4 S RNA primer molecule differs from the transfer RNA-like 4 S viral subunit (170) as its dissociation temperature from the 60–70 S viral RNA is higher. The 4 S cellular RNA is free of priming activity under their experimental conditions. Further work is needed to clarify the function of these small (~4 S) subunits of the 60–70 S RNA both in the *in vitro* reaction as well as during virus replication.

Although it was originally thought that reverse transcriptase activity was unique for oncornaviruses, several other RNA viruses, which are free from demonstrable oncogenicity but cause latent infections in their host of origin, possess the enzyme. This is true for two antigenically related viruses inducing "slow" infections of sheep, visna virus, and progressive pleuropneumonia virus (PPV) and for syncytium-forming ("foamy") viruses of primate, bovine, and feline origin (443, 445, 547, 574, 575). In addition to the presence of reverse transcriptase, these agents share other biological and biophysical properties with oncornaviruses. Visna virus and PPV have been shown to transform mouse cells *in vitro* (583), and their RNA genome was found to be a 60–70 S molecule with the same physicochemical properties as that of oncornavirions (575); the syncytium-forming viruses have not been shown to transform cells, but are resis-tant to inactivation by ultraviolet light and their replication is also inhibited by actinomycin D and thymidine analogs (443, 445). Unless these above agents are shown to be oncogenic, it would appear that both the presence of reverse transcriptase within virions and their possible replication through a DNA inter-mediate are phenomena with broader implications for pathogenesis.

The development of procedures for partial purification of the DNA polymerase from solubilized virions has not only led to the characterization of their physicochemical properties (142, 306, 365, 503) and antigenic properties (6, 446, 550), but also to their physical separation from other cellular DNA polymerases (365, 503). Currently, the partially purified enzyme appears to be a protein with a molecular weight of about 110,000 that is separable from the major group-specific (gs) antigen (molecular weight of about 30,000, see Section II,E). Enzyme inhibition experiments with purified IgG from sera of tumor-bearing animals or from rabbit antisera prepared against partially purified enzymes indicate that, like the gs antigen (see Section II,E), the polymerases of mammalian C-type oncornavirions carry species-specific and interspecies antigenic determinants (6, 446, 550). Antisera to the MuLV and to the FeLV enzymes strongly inhibit the homologous polymerase activity, have partial reciprocal inhibition, and partly inhibit the activity of rat and hamster C-type viruses; thus there is both species-specific and interspecies reactivity. In contrast, antisera to the polymerase of the avian oncornaviruses have only species-specific reactivity and the avian enzyme is not inhibited by antisera to the MuLV or FeLV polymerase (446, 550). The enzymes of the viper virus, MTV, visna virus, foamy virus, and 3 primate viruses (Mason-Pfizer, Woolly monkey, gibbon) and the RD-114 virus of human extraction appear to be unrelated to any of the above as they are not inhibited by antisera to the polymerases of either murine, feline, or avian viruses (446, 550). Cross-inhibition tests with antisera to the enzymes of the 3 primate viruses and of the RD-114 virus indicate that the enzymes of the Woolly monkey and the gibbon virus are closely related, whereas those of the Mason-Pfizer virus and the RD-114 virus are distinct (549). Further cross-inhibition experiments are needed to clarify the exact antigenic relatedness, but the availability of antisera to partially purified enzymes appears to offer a fruitful means of grouping the polymerase-bearing viruses. Furthermore, such antisera allow the distinction between virion and cellular polymerases as it has been shown that antiserum to the MuLV polymerase will inhibit the viral polymerase activity but not the cell polymerase activity of infected cells (503).

Various other enzymes, such as hexokinase, protein kinase, RNA methylase, etc., have been associated with purified oncornavirions (188, 400, 576). However, these may turn out to be cell enzymes incorporated within the viral envelope during the process of maturation as was shown earlier to be the case for the enzyme adenosinetriphosphatase (ATPase) of avian myeloblastosis virus (628).

E. Viral Proteins

1. BIOPHYSICAL AND BIOCHEMICAL PROPERTIES

In addition to similarities in virion structure and nucleic acid composition, all oncornaviruses share a great deal of similarity in protein composition (see reviews 137, 424, 496, 625 for references to earlier work). Polyacrylamide gel electrophoresis (PAGE) of purified and disrupted virions revealed the presence of 5 major polypeptides in MTV (423, 426), 6 polypeptides in the mammalian C-type viruses (408, 427, 435, 542–544), and 7 polypeptides in the avian oncorna-viruses (40, 75–77, 141, 183, 293). There is a remarkable similarity in PAGE profiles of the different oncornaviruses with polypeptides ranging in molecular weight from about 12,000 to 100,000 daltons; these results correspond well with those obtained by gel filtration of disrupted virions in the presence of 6 M guanidine hydrochloride (183, 427).

Two of the major polypeptides of the avian and mammalian C-type viruses (molecular weight 100,000 and 37,000 daltons, respectively) have been shown to be glycoproteins with type-specific antigenicity (see below) and to reside in the viral envelope (76, 141, 183, 293, 408, 427). One of the 5 polypeptides of MTV (molecular weight 23,000 daltons) has also been localized in the viral envelope and found to possess type-specific activity (423, 426). The remaining polypeptides, comprising 60–80% of the total viral protein, are internal compo-nents of the virions (137, 231) and have been shown to represent the group-spe-cific (gs) antigen(s) of oncornaviruses (see below). Unlike those associated with the viral envelope, the internal proteins are resistant to ether, and the usual mode of their liberation from intact virions is Tween-ether treatment (231). The complete identification of the internal polypeptides of the various oncornaviruses awaits further study, but it appears that, in the avian and mam-malian C-type oncornaviruses, the major polypeptide with gs antigenicity is a basic protein with a molecular weight of about 30,000 (75, 183, 231, 427, 435, 542) while that of MTV (B-type) has a higher molecular weight of about 50,000 (423, 426). Current efforts on the determination of the amino acid se-quence of the polypeptides of the avian (11, 13) and mammalian (206) oncorna-viruses may shed further light as to more refined differences between those of the various groups of viruses.

2. ANTIGENIC PROPERTIES

As indicated above, two types of antigens have been described for oncorna-viruses—type-specific (or subgroup-specific) antigens associated with the viral envelope and group-specific (gs) antigens that are internal components of the virion. In addition, tumor-specific transplantation antigens (TSTA) are elicited by oncornaviruses.

a. TYPE-SPECIFIC ANTIGENS. The antigens associated with the viral envelope are characteristic for individual strains, or groups of strains, within oncornavi-ruses of each species (Table 11.3). They are detectable by neutralization, com-plement fixation, immunodiffusion, and immunofluorescence tests with sera of animals bearing virus-producing tumors or with antisera against intact virions (196, 253, 286, 317, 430, 431, 447, 491, 534, 628, 631). No cross-reactions have been observed between the type-specific (envelope) antigens of the avian on-cornaviruses and those of the mammalian oncornaviruses or between oncornavi-ruses of different mammalian species (424, 625, 628). Furthermore, there is

TABLE 11.3

ANTIGENS OF ONCORNAVIRUSES

Antigens	Location	Chemical properties of major antigens	Specificity	Detection	
				Most common methods	Reagents
Type-(subgroup-)specific	Virion envelope; virus-infected cells	Glycoproteins (MW 23,000–100,000 daltons); ether-sensitive	Cross-reaction between strains within a subgroup[a]; lack of cross-reaction outside a subgroup within a species or between species	Neutralization; complement fixation[b]; immunofluorescence; immunodiffusion	Sera of animals bearing virus-producing tumors; antisera against intact virions
Group-specific	Virion core; virus-infected cells; virus-free tumor (transformed) cells; certain normal cells	Basic polypeptides (MW 25,000–50,000 daltons); ether-resistant	gs-1, species-specific; gs-3, interspecies-specific; shared by mammalian C-type viruses	Complement fixation; immunofluorescence; immunodiffusion; radioimmunoassay	Sera of animals bearing virus-free tumors; antisera to disrupted virions; monospecific antisera to purified polypeptides

[a] Five subgroups for the avian C-type viruses; 2 subgroups for the murine C-type viruses.

[b] COFAL (complement fixation avian leukosis) test for ALV; COMUL (complement fixation murine leukemia) test for MuLV; COCAL (complement fixation cat leukosis) test for FeLV.

[c] See Table 11.4 for further details on specificity of gs-1 and gs-3 cross-reactivities.

no cross-reaction between the murine mammary tumor virus (B-type) and leukemia-sarcoma complex of viruses (C-type) of this species (69, 70, 423). (See Section II,A for classification of oncornaviruses on the basis of type-specific envelope antigens.)

b. GROUP-SPECIFIC (gs) ANTIGENS. These antigens have been found in oncornaviruses of each host species. They are detectable by complement fixation, immunodiffusion, and immunofluorescence tests using either sera of animals of heterologous species that bear virus-induced (but usually virus-free) tumors or antisera prepared against Tween-ether disrupted virions (see Table 11.3). Monospecific antisera to individual polypeptides, separated and purified in their native form by either Sephadex G-200 chromatography (426, 427) or by isoelectrofocusing (434, 436), have afforded a more precise antigenic analysis of the gs antigens of oncornavirions.

Several internal polypeptides have gs antigenic reactivity, the major gs antigen being a basic polypeptide with molecular weight varying from 25,000 to 50,000 daltons. The major gs antigen, termed gs-1 antigen (231), is shared by and is species-specific for the C-type viruses within a host species (avian, feline, hamster, murine, primate, rat, viper); the same is true for different strains of the B-type murine MTV (see Tables 11.3 and 11.4). No cross-reactions have been observed between the gs-1 antigen of the avian oncornaviruses and that of the mammalian oncornaviruses (197, 542). Furthermore, there is no cross-reaction between the gs-1 antigen of the C-type and the B-type viruses within the murine (423, 426) or primate (444) species (Table 11.4).

TABLE 11.4

CROSS-REACTIONS BETWEEN GROUP-SPECIFIC ANTIGENS OF ONCORNAVIRUSES[a]

Viruses[b]	Species-specific antigens (gs-1)										Interspecies-specific antigens (gs-3)									
	C-type viruses							B-type viruses			C-type viruses							B-type viruses		
	A	M	F	R	H	P	V	M	P		A	M	F	R	H	P	V	M	P	
C-type																				
Avian	+	−	−	−	−	−	−	−	−		−	−	−	−	−	−	−	−	−	
Murine	−	+	−	−	−	−	−	−	−		−	+	+	+	+	+	−	−	−	
Feline	−	−	+	−	−	−	−	−	−		−	+	+	+	+	+	−	−	−	
Rat	−	−	−	+	−	−	−	−	−		−	+	+	+	+	+	−	−	−	
Hamster	−	−	−	−	+	−	−	−	−		−	+	+	+	+	+	−	−	−	
Primate	−	−	−	−	−	+	−	−	−		−	+	+	+	+	+	−	−	−	
Viper	−	−	−	−	−	−	+	−	−		−	−	−	−	−	−	−	−	−	
B-type																				
Murine	−	−	−	−	−	−	−	+	−		−	−	−	−	−	−	−	−	−	
Primate	−	−	−	−	−	−	−	−	+		−	−	−	−	−	−	−	−	−	

[a] A = avian, M = murine, F = feline; R = rat, H = hamster, P = primate, and V = viper.
[b] See Table 11.1 for further details on viruses in each group.

Recent studies have revealed that the gs antigens of the mammalian C-type viruses carry, in addition to the species-specific determinant (gs-1 antigen), an interspecies antigenic determinant and also, the gs-3 antigen (197) or "gs-interspec" (542). The gs-3 antigen (Table 11.4) is shared by all the mammalian C-type viruses; the avian oncornaviruses and the B-type mammalian oncornaviruses are free of such interspecies antigenic reactivity (423, 444, 542). Complement fixation and immunodiffusion studies (542) have suggested that the gs-1 and gs-3 antigens of the FeLV are in two different polypeptides with molecular weights of 15,000 and 30,000 daltons, respectively. However, immunodiffusion tests (210, 434, 436) or radioimmunoassay (444) have shown that both the gs-1 species-specific reactivity and the gs-3 interspecies reactivity reside in the same major internal polypeptide with molecular weight of 30,000 daltons.

i. Avian oncornaviruses. The gs antigen shared by all the viruses of this group can be detected with sera of rodents bearing RSV-induced but virus-free tumors (289) or with antisera prepared against purified gs antigen from disrupted virions (40). The most common tests for detection of gs antigen are a COFAL (complement fixation avian leukosis) test (532), an immunodiffusion test (41, 52), and an immunofluorescence test (316, 449). The gs antigen detected in disrupted virion preparations is identical to that found in virus-infected cells (41) (Table 11.3). The same type of antigen is present in virus-induced but virus-free tumor cells (289). The methodology developed to detect gs antigens in the virion as well as in infected cells has led to the discovery of the same antigen as a heritable property of cells derived from certain normal virus-free avian species (see Sections II,G and II,H for references and discussion on the implications of these findings).

ii. Murine oncornaviruses. The gs-1, species-specific antigen, shared by all the murine leukemia and sarcoma viruses can be detected with sera of rats bearing transplantable virus-induced lymphomas (196), or MSV-induced (virus-free) sarcomas (286), as well as with antisera against purified antigen from disrupted virions (231). The most common tests for gs antigen detection are the COMUL [complement fixation murine leukemia test (252, 253, 286)] and the immunodiffusion test (196). As with the avian oncornaviruses (see Table 11.3), the gs antigen of the virion is identical to that found in virus-infected cells and in most of the MSV-induced but virus-free rat sarcomas (252, 253, 286). As in the avian system, gs antigen is also detected in certain normal murine cells (see Section II,H for further details).

iii. Murine mammary tumor virus (MTV). All MTV strains share a common soluble gs antigen (MTV-S1) that can be detected with antisera to disrupted virions and is distinct from the gs antigen of the other murine oncornaviruses (423, 426). MTV lacks the interspecies gs antigen described above for the C-type mammalian oncornaviruses (423, 424).

iv. Feline oncornaviruses. A species-specific gs antigen, detectable by a COCAL (complement fixation cat leukosis) test (534), immunodiffusion (197,

542), or immunofluorescence (619) with antisera to disrupted virions, is shared by members of this group. The viruses also contain the interspecies gs antigen (see Table 11.4) that cross-reacts with the other C-type mammalian oncornaviruses (197, 210, 444, 542).

v. Hamster oncornaviruses. The leukemia viruses in this group (HaLV) have species-specific gs-1 antigenicity that is different from that of the murine or other mammalian C-type viruses (317, 319, 435, 444). The major gs-1 antigen of the HaSV pseudotypes is identical to that of the HaLV and does not cross-react with that of the murine or other C-type oncornaviruses (319, 435). All the HaLV isolates and the HaSV pseudotypes have the interspecies gs-3 antigen shared (see Table 11.4) by the mammalian C-type viruses (197, 444).

vi. Primate oncornaviruses. As indicated earlier (see Section II,A), the Woolly monkey and gibbon C-type viruses appear to be antigenically distinct from the B-type Mason-Pfizer virus as well as from other mammalian oncornaviruses. The two C-type viruses share a gs antigen (444), while the gs antigen of the B-type Mason-Pfizer virus is distinct (425, 444).

vii. Other oncornaviruses. The precise antigenic makeup of the less well studied oncornaviruses is yet to be established. However, a species-specific (gs-1) antigen has been detected for the viper (208) and rat (209) oncornaviruses described in Section II,A.

c. TUMOR-SPECIFIC TRANSPLANTATION ANTIGENS (TSTA). TSTA are nonvirion antigens detectable in virus-induced tumors or transformed cells. Assessment of TSTA in the oncornavirus systems studied has been difficult, especially in the case of leukemia-inducing viruses, since carcinogenesis *in vivo* or *in vitro* is accompanied by the continuous production of virions and virion antigens. The major aspects of TSTA induction as well as humoral and cell immune mechanisms are basically the same for carcinogenesis by oncornaviruses and by the DNA tumor viruses. Assessment of TSTA in the latter system has been facilitated by the fact that both virus-induced tumors or transformed cells are virion-free. Section III,E,3 reviews TSTA in the DNA tumor virus system and several excellent reviews describe TSTA of oncornaviruses (70, 237, 258, 263, 264, 335, 336, 429, 447, 553).

F. Tumor Induction with Oncornaviruses

1. AVIAN LEUKEMIA-SARCOMA COMPLEX

a. AVIAN LEUKEMIA VIRUSES (ALV). Leukemic diseases are common in chickens, and the leukemia-inducing viruses are widespread in normal and in diseased chicken populations. The main types of viral leukemias encountered are lymphoid, myeloid, and erythroid. They derive their names from the characteristic primitive cells (lymphoblast, myeloblast, erythroblast) found in large quantities in the blood of the diseased animal, and from this terminology the names of the viruses have evolved: avian lymphomatosis virus, myeloblastosis virus, and erythroblastosis virus (234, 628).

Infectious virus and physical particles of the virus may be found in high concentration in tumor cells, peripheral blood, and other organs of the affected animals, a phenomenon not encountered with the DNA tumor viruses. Myeloblasts or erythroblasts taken from diseased birds and grown in tissue culture continue to release virus, which can induce the malignancy on inoculation into chickens (234, 628).

Malignancy can be induced in newborn or adult animals by inoculation with cell-free virus derived from diseased animals, or from leukemic cells grown in culture. Serial transplantation can also be made with leukemic cells; the resulting malignancy is eventually composed of cells of the recipient host, which suggests that it is virus-induced (234, 628).

Almost all flocks of chickens have been found to be infected with various strains of ALV, especially avian lymphomatosis virus. The virus is transmitted horizontally through the saliva and feces, producing an infection in the adult animal characterized by transitory viremia and enduring antibodies. Relatively few adult birds develop clinical disease. Vertical transmission from the viremic hen (not from the viremic rooster) results in congenitally infected viremic chickens, tolerant to the virus, free of antibodies, and permanent shedders of the virus. The incidence of leukemia in congenitally infected animals is much higher than in animals infected by contact (518, 519; also see review 628).

b. Rous Sarcoma Viruses (RSV). Rous sarcoma virus has undergone countless passages experimentally since it was first isolated in 1911, and it probably now differs from the naturally occurring virus. Several strains of RSV exist which differ in their oncogenicity, antigenic structure, and host range (628, 631).

RSV causes sarcoma in birds of all ages and in chick embryos; unlike lymphomatosis virus, however, it is not naturally transmitted. RSV also induces tumors in ducks, turkeys, pigeons, and other birds (628). Certain virus strains (Schmidt-Ruppin and other strains described in Table 11.2) also induce tumors when inoculated into newborn rats, Syrian and Chinese hamsters, rabbits, mice, guinea pigs, and even monkeys. The presence of infectious virus and of physical particles of the virus is a common finding in avian but not in mammalian tumors (see reviews 578, 628, 655).

2. Murine Leukemia-Sarcoma Complex

a. Murine Leukemia Viruses (MLV). To date, numerous leukemogenic murine viruses have been isolated. The types of leukemia vary. For example, in mice of certain lines, the Graffi virus causes mainly myeloid forms of leukemia, whereas in others lymphatic leukemia occurs in a high percentage of cases. In certain experiments, Gross virus causes almost all known types of leukemic disease: lymphatic, stem cell, myeloid and monocytic leukemia, erythroblastosis, chloroleukemia, lymphosarcoma, and reticulum cell sarcoma. Most leukemia viruses have proved to be pathogenic in rats and, with the Moloney virus, in hamsters (for reviews see 234, 491).

Newborn animals are most susceptible to the effect of leukemogenic viruses, but the disease can also be produced in young and adult animals. Genetic factors play an important role in the susceptibility of mice to the virus, the nature of the disease caused, and the transmission of the virus. Thymectomy reduces the attack rate of lymphatic leukemia but not that of the myeloid forms; it has no effect on the multiplication of the viruses in other organs. In infected animals, large amounts of infectious virus and of virus particles occur in the blood and in tumor tissue. Some MuLV strains can be transmitted through the milk, the ovum, and the sperm (see reviews 234, 491).

The murine leukemia viruses are also widespread in nature (253). In certain "high-leukemia" strains (AKR), the Gross virus is the cause of the natural disease and is vertically transmitted from mother to offspring in an infectious form (for review see 234); the congenitally infected animals are tolerant to the virus (196). Certain "low-leukemia" strains of mice, such as C57BL, harbor vertically transmitted MuLV genetic information; irradiation or X-ray treatment results in the production of lymphoid leukemia, yielding infectious MuLV which is capable of inducing leukemia in other hosts and has been named radiation-induced leukemia virus (RadLV) (234, 308).

b. MURINE SARCOMA VIRUS (MSV). Different strains of MSV have been recognized that bear the antigenicity of the MuLV with which they are associated. Unlike MuLV, the MSV virions cause rhabdomyosarcomas in newborn mice, rats, and hamsters (177, 194, 255, 330, 403).

3. MURINE MAMMARY TUMOR VIRUS (MTV)

Tumorigenesis by different strains of MTV is a result of a complex interplay between the virus and the genetic constitution of the host and hormonal factors (for review see 69, 234). The virus is found naturally in certain "high-mammary cancer" strains of inbred mice in which mammary adenocarcinomas develop early in life, with large amounts of infectious virus and B-type particles in the tumor, milk, blood, and other tissues. In such animals the virus is transmitted vertically through the milk, the ovum, and the sperm (69, 234). Inoculation of MTV into newborn mice by various routes (oral, subcutaneous, intraperitoneal) results in the production of mammary adenocarcinomas or subclinical infection; both the cancerous and subclinically infected animal can then transmit the virus to the offspring through the milk. More recent work with different highly inbred strains of mice indicates that the distribution of MTV is ubiquitous. Electron microscopic, immunological, and biological investigations have revealed the presence of MTV in various "low-mammary cancer" strains of mice. In some strains, the virus could be detected in an overt form and, in others, after irradiation or treatment with carcinogens; Mendelian analysis indicates that vertical transmission of viral information and resistance to superinfection by MTV is controlled by the same or similar genes (49, 50). See also Section II,H.

4. FELINE LEUKEMIA-SARCOMA COMPLEX

Several isolates of feline leukemia virus (FeLV) and feline sarcoma virus (FeSV) have been derived from cats with leukemia and fibrosarcoma, respectively. When inoculated into newborn kittens, FeLV induces transmissible leukemia and FeSV induces transmissible fibrosarcoma. The virus is found in the tumor cells, bone marrow cells, and blood of the infected animals (191, 299, 493, 560). FeSV causes sarcomas also in dogs, rabbits, and monkeys (124, 191).

5. OTHER ONCORNAVIRUSES

The hamster leukemia virus (HaLV) (224, 568), has not been shown to induce leukemia in its host of origin (318, 320). The hamster-specific sarcoma viruses (HaSV) which have been isolated from MSV-induced hamster sarcomas, have the antigenicity of the indigenous HaLV and induce sarcomas in hamsters but not in mice (36, 318, 341, 454). The same pattern appears to exist with indigenous rat leukemia virus (RaLV), that has not been shown as yet to induce leukemia in the rat, but has rendered a strain of MSV oncogenic for the rat but not for the mouse by virtue of supplying the MSV genome with its own envelope (2, 600). The primate oncornaviruses have been best studied in tissue culture, except for the Woolly monkey fibrosarcoma virus which has been shown to induce sarcomas in marmosets (599, 651).

G. Virus Replication and Cell Transformation

1. GENERAL CONSIDERATIONS

a. VIRUS REPLICATION. A characteristic property of the RNA tumor viruses is that they are not cytocidal for the cells in which they replicate. Like other viruses, oncornaviruses pass through an eclipse phase. The infected cell then produces new infectious virus, continues to multiply, and may or may not undergo malignant transformation depending upon the virus or the cell used. Infectious virus and virus particles are readily detected in most of the tumor cells or cells transformed in vitro. As shown by electron microscopic studies (see Section II,B), the virions mature at the cellular membrane and are released from it by a process of budding. Virus particles and viral coat antigens are usually detected in the cytoplasm or on the surface of infected cells (625, 628), however it has been suggested that synthesis of the group-specific antigen may be initiated in the cell nucleus (449, 625). More recent studies also suggest a nuclear site for viral RNA replication; hybridization experiments revealed the presence of virus-specific RNA molecules in the nuclei of oncornavirus-infected cells (58, 190, 230, 353). In addition, it has been recently found that the 60–70 S RNA of oncornaviruses contains adenylic acid-rich (A-rich) sequences that are covalently linked to the 30–40 S subunits (212, 228, 348, 504). Similar to the poly A regions of mRNA of eukaryotic cells, the A-rich sequences of oncornaviral RNA may be involved in the transport of the RNA from the nucleus to the cytoplasm (348), further supporting the notion that oncornavirus replication may begin in the nucleus.

Early studies revealed that metabolic inhibitors of DNA synthesis (including 5-fluorodeoxyuridine, 5-bromodeoxyuridine, 5-iododeoxyuridine, cytosine arabinoside, thymidine, and aminopterin) prevented the replication of oncornaviruses and cell transformation if applied within 8–12 hours after infection but not thereafter. Low doses of actinomycin D (an inhibitor of DNA transcription) were inhibitory throughout the replicative cycle (for review see 227, 588, 625). Neither virus replication nor cell transformation was affected by inhibitors of protein synthesis, such as puromycin or cycloheximide (above reviews and 21). These findings indicated that transient DNA synthesis and DNA transcription are required for replication and transformation and led to the assumption that oncornaviruses may replicate through a DNA intermediate. According to the "provirus" theory (587), the entering viral RNA is transcribed to DNA early after infection. The RNA-DNA hybrid is then further transcribed to a double-stranded DNA which, during cell division, integrates into the host-cell DNA. The newly integrated viral-specific DNA (provirus) serves both as a permanent template for the transcription of progeny viral RNA molecules and as a heritable gene for transformation (588). All of the newly synthesized DNA molecules may become integrated into the cell chromosomes. An alternative model suggests that part of the virus-specific DNA integrates into cell DNA as a provirus and part remains extrachromosomal and is transcribed into viral RNA independently (21).

The observation that viral RNA hybridized with DNA of cells transformed by RSV to a greater extent than with DNA of normal cells was taken as indirect evidence for the existence of provirus in the transformed cells (see 588 for review). However, more recent findings render the interpretation of hybridization studies with cell DNA much more complex. The DNA of normal avian and murine cells contains nucleotide sequences homologous to the corresponding oncornavirus. Using avian oncornaviral RNA in RNA-DNA hybridization studies, it has been shown that a variety of avian cells contain DNA complementary to the viral RNA even though the amount of such DNA was higher in virus-infected cells (30, 502). On the other hand, DNA–DNA hybridization experiments with labeled double-stranded DNA made *in vitro* by the DNA polymerase of the virion have failed to show quantitative differences in virus-specific nucleotide sequences between normal or infected cells. RSV-specific nucleotide sequences have been detected in equal numbers in the DNA of RSV-infected cells and of various normal chick cells (including those free of gs antigen) but not in DNA of other species (623). Similarly, equal amounts of MuLV-specific DNA sequences have been found in normal and in virus-transformed mouse and rat cells (198), and no difference in MTV-specific nucleotide sequences could be found in cells of mice with high or low incidence of mammary tumor (622). Even though these latter experiments have contributed to the understanding of the heritable nature of oncornaviral genes, the interpretation of both RNA–DNA and DNA–DNA hybridization studies should still be considered with caution, especially in view of recent findings that oncornaviral RNA contains A-rich sequences similar to those of cell mRNA (212, 228, 348, 504).

A more direct evidence for the assumption that oncornaviruses replicate through a DNA intermediate has come from experiments on the apparent incorporation of the thymidine analogue 5-bromodeoxyuridine (5-BUdR) into the genome of RSV; growth of RSV in stationary cultures (under conditions of minimal cell DNA synthesis) in the presence of 5-BUdR followed by exposure to visible light has resulted in intracellular inactivation of focus formation (27, 72), and growth of RSV in cells exposed to 5-BUdR during the early stages of replication has resulted in the derivation of conditionally lethal, temperature-sensitive mutants, incapable of transforming cells at elevated temperatures (23).

The discovery of the enzyme reverse transcriptase, present in purified virions and capable of transcribing viral RNA to DNA in an *in vitro* reaction system, has strengthened the assumption that oncornaviruses replicate through a DNA intermediate. The question as to the exact biological role of the viral DNA polymerase is yet to be answered. The finding that noninfectious variants of RSV (243) and of MSV (385, 452) are deficient in the enzyme suggests such an activity, but others (497) have reported conflicting results.

The most convincing evidence to date stems from the isolation of infectious DNA from chicken (404) or mammalian (274, 275, 277) fibroblasts transformed by RSV but virus-free; transfer of the isolated DNA into chick embryo fibroblasts resulted in cell transformation and the production of infectious RSV biologically and antigenically identical to the original RSV strain used to transform the cells from which the DNA was derived. Especially convincing is the recovery of a temperature-sensitive mutant of RSV from chicken cells exposed to DNA extracted from hamster cells that had been transformed by the same mutant (275). Confirmation of these experiments is important to substantiate the existence of an infectious provirus.

The availability of a virus-specific DNA product, synthesized *in vitro* by the viral polymerase, has opened new avenues to examine the mode of replication of oncornaviral RNA in infected and transformed cells. After it was found that single-stranded DNA synthesized by the RNA-directed polymerase of RSV is entirely complementary to the 70 S RNA (189, 190), the same group of workers (353) used this DNA as an annealing probe; with it heterogeneous species of viral-specific RNA were detected in the nuclei and cytoplasm of RSV-producing cells. In similar experiments, virus-specific RNA species were detected in avian and rat cells infected with RSV (108), in the nucleus and cytoplasm of virus-producing mouse and rat cells transformed by MSV (230), in hamster cells transformed by MSV but free of infectious virus (617), and in the nuclear and polysomal fractions of mouse mammary tumor cells (19). The precise RNA species detected by these procedures remain to be elucidated. However, the nucleotide sequences of the RNA species detected are identical to those of the viral RNA (plus strands), and RNA species complementary to viral RNA (minus strands) have not been detected. The polysomal (messenger) RNA detected in these experiments is transcribed from virus-specific DNA.

Other studies have suggested that at least part of the viral RNA may replicate through an RNA intermediate. The cytoplasm of cells infected with avian myeloblastosis virus has been reported to contain a virus-specific RNA-dependent RNA polymerase (639). MSV-producing transformed rat cells (78A1) were found to contain two nuclear RNA species, a single-stranded 31–36 S RNA and a partially double-stranded 18–22 S RNA, complementary to viral RNA (58, 59); double-stranded RNA has been detected by others in the nuclei of the same MSV-transformed (78A1) rat cells but not in the nuclei of uninfected cells (620). The single-stranded complementary RNA molecules in the 78A1 cells may represent the minus strand of the replicating virus and the virus-specific partially double-stranded nuclear RNA may represent a replicative intermediate. However, much evidence indicates that oncornaviral RNA is transcribed from a DNA template. Should the studies suggesting an RNA intermediate be confirmed by others, a possibility exists that a dual pathway of replication of oncornaviral RNA may exist. Taking into consideration the subunit structure of oncornaviral RNA and the fact that the major intracellular virus-specific RNA species, whether detected by RNA–RNA hybridization (58, 59) or by DNA–RNA hybridization (230, 617), are close in size to the major 30–40 S viral RNA subunit, it is conceivable that the 60–70 S viral RNA does not replicate as a unit; independent pathways of replication may exist for different 30–40 S subunits, one part replicating through a DNA intermediate and one part through an RNA intermediate with the newly synthesized molecules being assembled into the 69–70 S viral RNA prior to virus maturation. Studies on the mode of RNA replication of nontransforming oncornaviral mutants that have been shown to lack a major RNA subunit (140, 384) may shed further light on this problem.

b. CELL TRANSFORMATION. With few exceptions (cited below), transformation of cells in culture is attained only with the sarcoma-inducing oncornaviruses. Transformation is expressed as heritable changes in cell phenotype, the most prominent being: loss of contact inhibition, altered morphology, increase in growth rate, acquisition of new antigens, and tumorigenicity. These and other changes in cells transformed by oncornaviruses—such as growth under soft agar, increased glycolysis, increases in acid mucopolysaccharide and hyaluronic acid production, and decrease in serum requirement for growth and for glycolysis, etc. (372, 588, 625, 628)—appear to be basically similar to those induced in cells transformed by DNA viruses and to be related to functional changes in cell membranes during the process of transformation. Increase in the rate of uptake of various sugars by cells infected with transforming oncornavirions is being taken as a pathognomonic early marker for transformation (22, 256, 257). Transformation by oncornaviruses occurs with high efficiency, especially in the presence of polyanions such as diethylaminoethyldextran (589, 625), and conditions where 90% of chick embryo cells are transformed by RSV within 24 hours have been described (240).

The exact mechanism by which oncornaviruses transform susceptible cells is not clear as yet, and the number of viral genes required for virus replication and for transformation is not known. However, recent studies with nontransforming mutants of RSV suggest that the replicating and cell transforming capacities may reside in different subunits of the viral genome (140, 384). Work with temperature-sensitive mutants of RSV that fail to transform cells but can replicate at the nonpermissive temperature (22, 62, 310, 382) is beginning to elucidate the viral functions required for the initiation of cell transformation and for maintenance of the transformed state. Although different mutants and different criteria for assessing the phenotype of the transformed cells have been used, it was found that cells transformed with a particular mutant at the permissive temperature lose their transformed phenotype within a few hours after shift to the nonpermissive temperature and cells that have lost their transformed phenotype at the nonpermissive temperature regain it after shift to the permissive temperature. These results suggest that the continuous presence of a functional viral gene product is necessary for maintenance of the transformed state. Furthermore, since with these mutants viral replication is unperturbed at the nonpermissive temperature, the gene product necessary for cell transformation is evidently not required for virus replication. For two of these mutants (62, 310) the viral gene product required for maintenance of the transformed state in a temperature-sensitive ("transforming") protein: reappearance of the transformed phenotype after shift of mutant-infected cells from the nonpermissive to the permissive temperature was prevented by inhibitors of protein synthesis but not by inhibitors of DNA synthesis or of DNA-dependent RNA synthesis. Furthermore, it appears from complementation studies with several different temperature-sensitive mutants of RSV that at least two different virus-induced proteins are involved in cell transformation (313).

Mutants of RSV that are temperature-sensitive for both virus replication and for cell transformation have been described with similar results (186). However, these mutants fail to replicate at the nonpermissive temperature and do not offer the possibility for separation of viral functions required for replication and for transformation. Undoubtedly, further work with mutants capable of replication but not of transformation at the nonpermissive temperature will elucidate the biochemical events associated with cell transformation. RSV functions involved in change of cell morphology could be separated from those involved in increased sugar uptake and hyaluronic acid synthesis (22). Similar studies are in progress with temperature-sensitive mutants of murine sarcoma virus (551).

The temperature shift experiments described above of cells infected with temperature-sensitive transforming oncornaviruses have opened new avenues for study of the problem of reversion of transformed cells. Earlier studies with the Schmidt-Ruppin strain of RSV demonstrated that reversion of transformed cells was accompanied by loss of viral genes (372, 373). Similar results were recently reported for reversion of cells that had been transformed by murine sarcoma virus (181, 420). Work with the temperature-sensitive mutants described above indicates the importance of altered expression of viral genes. It is premature at present to generalize as to the implication of the phenomenon of reversion of transformed cells *in vitro* in relation to potential reversion of the malignant state *in vivo*. With one RSV temperature-sensitive mutant, "*in vivo*" experiments were described in which the mutant failed to induce pocks in the chorioallantoic membrane of embryonated eggs at the nonpermissive temperature, and pocks (tumors) produced in the membrane at the permissive temperature disappeared after shift to the nonpermissive temperature (62). An increasing amount of evidence has been also mounted in recent years on reversion of cells transformed by DNA tumor viruses (see Section III,D and 372, 373). Undoubtedly, continuing work with conditional lethal mutants of both oncornaviruses and DNA tumor viruses will provide further insights into the aspects of possible reversion of malignant cells *in vivo*.

2. AVIAN LEUKEMIA-SARCOMA COMPLEX

a. LEUKEMIA VIRUSES (ALV). Most of the leukemia viruses multiply in cultures of chick embryo fibroblasts without causing any cytopathic change or cell transformation. Virus replication in such cells can be detected by means of an immunofluorescence focus assay with type-specific chicken antisera or by failure of the cells to transform when exposed to Rous sarcoma virus, a phenomenon termed interference (for review, see 628). The interfering property of the leukosis viruses is utilized to measure their activity in tissue culture in an RIF (resistance-inducing factor) test (517). Cells chronically infected with ALV can be propagated in serial passage, yielding large quantities of virus capable of inducing neoplasia *in vivo* or of inducing interference with Rous sarcoma virus *in vitro* (see above review). A plaque assay for infectivity has been recently described (311) for some strains of ALV making use of cells maintained at 41°C and preinfected with either a temperature-sensitive mutant that replicates but does not transform at this temperature or with the Rous-associated virus RAV-1.

Morphological transformation of susceptible mesenchymal target cells into myeloblastlike cells has been achieved only with the avian myeloblastosis virus. The transformed cells multiply exponentially and produce new virus which in turn is capable of producing neoplasia *in vivo* or of transformation *in vitro*. This *in vitro* transforming ability of avian myeloblastosis virus is a means of quantitatively assaying the virus (31, 628).

b. ROUS SARCOMA VIRUSES (RSV). Unlike the leukemia viruses, with which they share many physical and antigenic properties, the Rous sarcoma viruses are unique among tumor viruses in the speed and high frequency with which they induce malignant transformation of the infected cell (240, 588, 628). Infection of chick embryo cells with RSV results in foci of transformed cells, the morphology of which varies for the virus strain used. Virus activity is measured as the number of focus-forming units (FFU) per unit volume (588, 593, 628). *In vitro*, transformed chick or duck cells usually continue to release virus; both transformed cells and virus released from them can induce tumors *in vivo* (588, 628).

The Schmidt-Ruppin (SR-RSV), Carr-Zilber (CZ-RSV), Prague (PR-RSV), and the B77 strains of RSV (see Table 11.2), which have been shown to induce tumors in mammals (including macaque and marmoset monkeys), can induce transformation in chick embryo cells as well as in mouse, rat, hamster, and human fibroblast cells (see reviews 578, 628, 655). The transformed chick embryo cells continue to produce infectious virus. Infectious virus cannot be demonstrated in cell-free extracts from transformed cells of mouse, rat, or hamster origin by conventional methods. However, these cells usually contain the gs antigen characteristic for the avian oncornaviruses and, in some instances, virus particles as well. Infectious RSV can be rescued from viable nonpermissive transformed cells either by their implantation into chickens or by their cocultivation *in vitro* with susceptible chick embryo cells, usually in the presence of ultraviolet-inactivated Sendai virus which facilitates the formation of heterokaryons (578, 625). The mechanism of rescue by cocultivation with susceptible cells is not completely understood at present. Virus production occurs in the heterokaryons and there is a good correlation between the number of heterokaryons formed (this being enhanced over 100-fold in the presence of inactivated Sendai virus) and the extent of virus rescue (578). The incidence of virus-producing heterokaryons depends on the gs antigen content of the transformed mammalian cells but not on the presence of gs antigen in the avian cells, as both gs⁻ and gs⁺ can be successfully used in rescue experiments (578, 579, 626). Nondividing avian cells, including chick embryo erythrocytes, have been shown to be incapable of rescue, although capable of heterokaryon formation (579). However, a recent study reported virus rescue when rat cells transformed by the B77 strain of RSV (and free of gs antigen) were fused in the presence of Sendai virus with either irradiated (nondividing) chick embryo fibroblasts or with chicken erythrocytes (106). Further work is needed to identify the factors in avian cells responsible for the release and production of infectious virus from RSV-transformed mammalian cells.

Some important features of RSV-cell interaction have come to light from work with the "defective" Bryan high-titer strain of RSV (B-RSV): (1) Cell transformation is a function of the RSV genome and (2) antigenicity, host range, and sensitivity to specific interference by ALV strains are governed by the protein coat in which the RSV genome is encapsidated. Stocks of B-RSV contain a 10-fold excess of a nontransforming ALV—hence the term Rous-associated virus or RAV for the ALV in such preparations. When plated at limiting dilution in the presence of RAV antiserum, cells transformed individually by the B-RSV genome were obtained. Upon continuous passage they maintained their transformed phenotype and malignant characteristics but failed to produce infectious RSV or protein coat antigen, so were designated nonproducer (NP) cells. Superinfection of continuously propagated NP cells with a nontransforming RAV resulted through phenotypic mixing in the production of infectious RSV which possessed the antigenicity of the RAV helper virus but was capable of transforming new cells *in vitro* and of inducing sarcoma *in vivo*. These observations suggested that the B-RSV genome was defective (244). Different antigenically distinct RAV strains, such as RAV-1, RAV-2, RAV-3, RAV-50, etc., have been used and the resulting infectious pseudotypes RSV (RAV-1), RSV (RAV-2), RSV (RAV-3), RSV (RAV-50), etc. have been shown to possess the antigenicity, host range, and interference properties of the corresponding helper RAV virus

(242, 244; see also reviews 241, 634). This experimental alteration of the viral envelope of B-RSV was further evidence that the RSV genome in the pseudotypes remains unaltered even though the host range is strictly dependent upon the viral protein coat. The enclosure of the genome of the Schmidt-Ruppin strain of RSV (SR-RSV) in the viral protein coat of RAV-1 [SR-RSV (RAV-1)] rendered it incapable of inducing tumors in mammals. Conversely, enclosure of the genome of the B-RSV in the protein coat of RAV-50 [B-RSV (RAV-50)] conferred on it the property of tumor induction in mammals. However, such alteration in the viral envelope did not cause a heritable stable change of the virus genome. Infection of chick embryo cells with SR-RSV (RAV-1) in the presence of RAV-1 antiserum led to the occurrence of transformed cells that yielded infectious SR-RSV capable of inducing tumors in mammals or in transforming mammalian cells *in vitro*. Unlike SR-RSV, the B-RSV genome present in the transformed mammalian cells could not be rescued by the mere cocultivation of mammalian cells and chick embryo cells, but it could be elicited by superinfection of the cocultivated cell mixture with RAV virus, yielding infectious B-RSV (RAV) virus (242).

Further studies with NP cells derived after solitary infection with B-RSV revealed that such cells not only contained rescuable RSV but also the group-specific antigen of avian oncornaviruses (316). Over 90% of the different NP cell lines studied were found by electron microscopy to carry virus particles (131). These particles were shown to contain the same high molecular weight RNA characteristic of oncornaviruses (495) and were termed RSV(o) as they were thought to be nondefective and capable of replicating in certain avian cells in the absence of helper virus (629, 643). However, subsequent study indicated that the capacity of RSV(o) to replicate depends upon the host cell used and, in most cases, upon the presence in susceptible cells of helper viruses that have not been recognized in the past. These results stem from the finding that almost all C/A cells and some C/O cells derived from leukemia virus-free chickens contain a group-specific (gs) antigen that is indistinguishable from the gs antigen of the virions and that is genetically transmitted in a simple Mendelian manner as a dominant cell characteristic (132, 448).

Group-specific antigen-positive cells (gs⁺) were also found to contain a factor termed chick cell-associated helper factor (chf) that is inherited in the same manner as the gs antigen (and is presumably coded for by the same gene) and aids the replication of RSV(o) in solitary infection. Thus, chf⁺ gs⁺ chick cells were found to support the replication of RSV(o), whereas chf⁻ gs⁻ cells did not (246, 644, 645). Transformation of gs⁺ C/A cells by RSV(o) led to the recognition of helper virus RAV-O, an unusually unstable nontransforming leukosis virus, that provides the protein coat for the RSV genome and leads to the apparent production of infectious RSV (RAV-O) pseudotype (635). In addition, chf⁺ gs⁺ C/O cells contain the incomplete genome of another helper virus, RAV-60, which cannot code for its own protein coat unless the cells are infected with RSV(o) (or one of the known avian leukemia viruses). Once rescued, however, it provides the protein coat for the RSV genome, and this results in the formation of infectious RSV (RAV-60) pseudotype (245). More recent studies indicate that RAV-60 is also present in chf+ gs⁻ cells (248). It remains to be determined whether RAV-O and RAV-60 are identical or represent two different viruses. Work with C/O cells has also revealed that, in addition to infectious RSV (RAV-60), also termed RSV (f), two other variants·of RSV(o) exist: (1) RSV(−), obtained after transformation of chf⁻ gs⁻ C/O cells by B-RSV; this first variant is noninfectious for any of the avian cells tested but is capable of transforming avian cells under conditions of cell fusion in the presence of ultraviolet-inactivated Sendai virus. (2) RSVα(f), isolated from chf+ gs+ C/O cells transformed by B-RSV [RSVα(f) fails to rescue RAV-60 from these cells]; this second variant is noninfectious for any avian cells examined thus far, even in the presence of Sendai virus. Both RSV(−) and RSVα(f) can make infectious pseudotypes in the presence of a suitable helper RAV (247, 248). It remains to be seen whether RSV(−) and RSVα(f) are truly nondefective in their transforming capacity or whether they require the assistance of another unrecognized helper virus. The report that the noninfectious α form of RSV lacks reverse transcriptase (243), suggested that the enzyme is necessary for productive infection. However, further study is necessary as others (497) have reported conflicting results.

3. MURINE LEUKEMIA-SARCOMA COMPLEX

a. MURINE LEUKEMIA VIRUSES (MuLV). The tissue culture aspects of MuLV–cell interaction are similar to those described above for ALV and earlier studies have been reviewed in detail (74). Virus replication in susceptible cells is not accompanied by overt morphological changes and the infected cells continue to release infectious MuLV for indefinite periods of time. However, the virus released from such chronically infected cells is about 10,000-fold less infectious than virus circulating in the blood of the leukemic animal (74). Virus replication in susceptible cells has been detected by several indirect tests: the complement-fixation (COMUL) test (252, 253), immunofluorescence (653), a viral interference test detecting the prevention of focus formation with MSV by MuLV (533), an enhancement assay, measuring the potentiation of focus formation by certain strains of MSV by MuLV (179), and more recently by a test measuring the development of RNA-dependent DNA polymerase activity in infected cells (321). A recently developed quantitative plaque assay for murine leukemia viruses is widely used. This test is based on the fortuitous observation that rat cells (XC cells) transformed by the Prague strain of Rous sarcoma virus (but are virus-free) can fuse with MuLV-infected mouse cells to form giant cells which are detected as visible plaques (342, 512). In addition, a rapid quantitative tissue culture assay for MuLV has been described that makes use of a transformed, sarcoma virus-positive, leukemia virus-negative (S+L⁻) line of BALB/3T3 mouse cells that contains the MSV genome but is free of detectable infectious virus (see below); upon addition of exogenous MuLV, typical MSV foci appear proportional to the concentration of MLV used for superinfection (39).

b. MURINE SARCOMA VIRUSES (MSV). Infection of mouse, rat, hamster, or human embryo cells with MSV results in foci of transformed cells and virus activity can be measured in focus-forming units (FFU) per unit volume (251). A certain degree of similarity exists between the various strains of MSV and the defective Bryan strain of RSV (B-RSV). Similar to B-RSV, MSV preparations have been found to contain a 10- to 100-fold excess of nontransforming murine leukemia virus (MuLV) and phenotypic mixing between MSV and MuLV results in the formation of infectious MSV (MuLV) pseudotypes (286, 290). As with the B-RSV system, the host range and antigenicity of the MSV pseudotypes is governed by the helper MuLV used. Unlike the B-RSV system, under usual conditions of infection in mouse embryo cells, MSV was shown to require the helper MuLV not only for the formation of infectious progeny but also for initiation of cell transformation; focus formation followed a "two-hit" dose response curve, which converted to a "one-hit" curve upon addition of exogenous MuLV (251, 442). However, subsequent reports indicate that MSV can induce transformation of mouse cells singly but requires the helper MuLV for replication of infectious particles (3, 37).

In rat cells MSV does not require helper MuLV for transformation as it follows a one-hit dose response (442). This confirmed an earlier observation that a nondefective MSV termed MSV(o) exists which replicates in rat cells in the absence of helper MuLV; a rat tumor induced by the Moloney strain of MSV (M-MSV) was propagated in tissue culture and cell clones were found to release MSV(o) which was antigenically distinct from the Moloney leukemia virus (present in the original M-MSV) and was infectious for rat embryo cells but not for mouse embryo cells (600). However, subsequent work revealed the presence of a rat leukemia virus (RaLV) in stocks of MSV(o) that appears to serve as helper for the replication of MSV in rat cells with the apparent production of an MSV (RaLV) pseudotype (2). This is a situation similar to the hamster-specific sarcoma viruses (Section II,A) which appear to be pseudotypes of the MSV genome used to induce the original hamster tumor with the acquired antigenicity of the helper hamster leukemia virus (317, 318, 341, 435).

Several different defective MSV–cell interaction systems have been described dealing with the presence of the MSV genome in the absence of release of infectious sarcoma virus; in all cases, the MSV genome is rescuable by super-infection with a helper MuLV. Several distinct phenotypes of cells transformed by MSV and propagated in culture in the absence of detectable MuLV are described below.

i. Nonproducer (NP) cells of hamster or mouse origin. The former derive from MSV-induced hamster fibrosarcomas (290) and the latter appear after infection in tissue culture (3, 508). Both hamster and mouse NP cells are free of detectable virions or MuLV gs antigen. Infectious MSV can be rescued from the hamster NP cells by cocultivation with permissive mouse cells in the presence of helper MuLV (286, 290) and from the mouse NP cells by mere superinfection with MuLV (3, 508). Various strains of MuLV have been used in rescue experiments and the resulting pseudotypes have the host range and antigenicity of the helper MuLV; of particular interest in this respect are experiments with the Kirsten leukemia virus which, unlike other MuLV strains, forms pseudotypes capable of infecting and transforming human cells (5). The feline leukemia virus (FeLV) has also been used for rescue of MSV from NP cells with a resulting MSV (FeLV) pseudotype capable of transforming feline cells and other cells susceptible to FeLV but not mouse cells (536). These experiments complement earlier studies in which the MSV could be encapsidated in a FeLV envelope by means of physical aggregation of virions in the ultracentrifuge; substitution of the FeLV envelope with that of MuLV results in MSV (MuLV) pseudotype infectious for mouse cells (180). More recent studies indicate that the primate Woolly monkey and gibbon oncornaviruses may also rescue MSV from NP cells (550). This phenotypic mixing between oncornaviruses of unrelated species deserves further study for it may open avenues to elucidate possible defective viral genomes in human tumor cells.

ii. MSV-transformed mouse cells. These cells are termed "sarcoma positive, leukemia-negative" (S^+L^-), which, unlike the NP cells, have the MuLV gs antigen and release noninfectious virions that apparently possess a faulty RNA (37, 38, 182). As with the NP cells, the MSV genome can be rescued from S^+L^- cells by superinfection with various strains of MuLV and this has led to a convenient quantitative assay for the detection of MuLV (39).

iii. Hamster cells. Hamster cells transformed by the newly recognized (194) Gazdar strain of MSV (GZ-MSV) that contain the MSV genome, the MuLV gs antigen, release noninfectious particles which have the 60–70 S RNA characteristic of oncornavirions but appear to lack reverse transcriptase; these cells have been termed "sarcoma-positive, helper-negative" (S^+H^-) as they appear to be free of detectable helper leukemia virus of either murine or hamster origin, and the MSV genome can be rescued by either cosedimentation of the noninfectious virions released by the cells with MuLV or by superinfection of the cells with MuLV (193, 195, 452).

iv. MSV-transformed normal rat kidney cells: MSV-1 (NRK). These cells have characteristics similar to the S^+H^- cells described above in that the cells contain the MuLV gs antigen, release 60–70 S RNA-containing virions that lack reverse transcriptase and are noninfectious for mouse cells. The particles can transform normal rat kidney cells, but the transformed cells do not produce MSV that can infect either rat or mouse cells. Superinfection with MuLV results in the production of pseudotypes infectious for both mouse and rat cells (385, 562). An MSV-transformed clone of normal rat kidney cells has been found from which the MSV genome cannot be rescued (385, 562).

The studies described above confirm the notion that under certain experimental conditions MSV can transform cells singly, resulting in cell populations with varying degrees of MSV genome expression; a helper leukemia virus is needed for the replication of infectious MSV. Virions free of reverse transcriptase appear to be defective for replication and this function can be restored by a helper leukemia virus.

4. OTHER ONCORNAVIRUSES

The tissue culture aspects of the feline oncornaviruses are similar to those of the avian and murine agents. The feline leukemia viruses (FeLV) replicate in feline, canine, monkey, and human cells without the causation of morphologic changes. The infected cells release infectious virus leukemogenic for the newborn kitten (239, 301, 535, 537). The feline sarcoma viruses (FeSV) have been found to transform cultures of feline, canine, monkey, and human origin (392, 531, 535). Similar to the avian and murine systems, cells infected with FeLV are resistant to transformation by FeSV or the MSV (FeLV) pseudotypes discussed above. This interference test is being used as a quantitative *in vitro* assay for the detection of FeLV strains (531) in addition to the commonly used complement fixation, COCAL, test (534). Propagation of the murine mammary tumor virus in culture has been generally unsuccessful (69).*

H. Inheritance and Activation of Oncornavirus Genes

Work with genetically defined strains of mice and chickens has provided ample evidence that some of the naturally occurring malignancies are caused by oncornaviruses, including the C-type murine and avian leukemia viruses and the B-type murine mammary tumor virus. Infectious virus can be isolated from various tissues prior to occurrence of malignancy and from the tumor itself when it appears. Evidence exists that in such animals ("high-cancer" or "high-leukemia" strains) the virus is transmitted vertically, predominantly from the infected mother to the offspring. In addition, vertical transmission of latent C-type or B-type oncornaviruses has been invoked to explain transmissible murine leukemias and mammary carcinomas, respectively, that were induced by irradiation, chemicals, or hormones (49, 234, 308, 491, 628).

A great majority of the inbred animals studied to date are of the low-cancer type in that they are virtually free of oncornavirus-associated malignancies. However, experimental evidence has accumulated during the past several years which suggests the inheritance of genetic information for oncornaviruses in animals of both murine and avian species, even when overt viral expression (such as infectious virions or virus particles) is not recognized. This development stems from work in two main areas: (1) the ability to identify the gs antigen of oncornaviruses in cells transformed by these agents which appear to be virus-free (see above sections dealing with RSV and MSV) and (2) the delineation of host genes in inbred strains of mice and chickens which govern their susceptibility or resistance to oncornaviruses.

---

* Information on the tissue culture aspects of the remaining viruses in the oncornavirus group which have been isolated recently (see Section II,A) is too premature to be discussed here.

Earlier studies with mice showed that some spontaneous tumors which occur in old age as well as some of the tumors induced by irradiation or chemical carcinogens contain C-type particles and, occasionally, fully infectious virus capable of inducing leukemia in other animals. However, most of the above tumors are free of detectable C-type particles. Further work revealed that such tumors free of virus particles contain the gs antigen of murine oncornaviruses (291).

The gs antigen of the murine C-type oncornaviruses is present in embryonic tissues of virtually all strains of mice as well as in rapidly replicating postnatal tissues and in normal tissues of old mice (8, 291). Similarly, the gs antigen of avian oncornaviruses is present in a high proportion of embryos from genetically defined and leukemia virus-free chickens (132, 448). The finding that chickens, mice, hamsters, and cats are capable of developing antibodies to the coat protein antigen but not to the species-specific gs antigen of the homologous oncornavirus following either infection or immunization has been taken as evidence of tolerance in these animals to the homologous gs antigen and as further support for its heritable nature (292). This assertion has been questioned by others who, using more sensitive detection procedures, have detected antibodies to homologous gs antigen both in chickens (133, 505) and in mice (381, 432). Further work is needed to delineate the type of tolerance being detected, but these differences do not detract from the fact that gs antigen information is heritable in nature.

Genetic studies with inbred strains of chickens and mice indicate that gs antigen expression is controlled by a single dominant autosomal host cell gene that is inherited in a simple Mendelian manner (448, 586). As indicated in Section II,G, gs antigen-positive (gs^+) chick embryo cells have been found to also contain a chick-cell-associated helper factor (chf) that is regarded as the precursor of RAV-60 or RAV-0. This factor is also heritable and appears to be genetically linked to the same gene controlling gs antigen expression (645). More recent studies (248) indicate that the presence of the heritable helper factor is more ubiquitous as it has also been detected in chick embryo cells which lack the gs antigen ($chf^+ gs^-$ cells). These latter data correlate well with hybridization studies (see Section II,G) which indicate that gs^+ and gs^- normal chick embryo cells contain equal amounts of DNA complementary to the RNA of the avian oncornaviruses (502, 623). Similar results have been reported in the murine system for MuLV-specific DNA sequences in normal mouse cells (198) and MTV-specific nucleotide sequences in cells of mice with low incidence of mammary tumor (622).

The most direct evidence for the presence of heritable viral genes in normal avian or murine cells has come from activation experiments in tissue culture. Exposure of normal chick cells derived from leukemia virus-free embryos (including those of red jungle fowl captured wild and considered to be the predecessors of domestic animals) to ionizing radiation, chemical carcinogens, or various mutagens resulted in the production of a C-type RNA virus with all the tissue culture characteristics of an avian leukemia virus; this activation was achieved with chick embryo cells that were $chf^+ gs^+$ or $chf^- gs^-$ (646). Similarly, exposure of virus-free mouse embryo cells to 5-iododeoxyuridine (IUdR) or to 5-bromodeoxyuridine (BUdR) resulted in the production of a C-type RNA virus with the tissue culture characteristics of a murine leukemia virus; the same results were observed whether the virus-free embryo cells were derived from the AKR high-leukemia mouse strain (367, 513) or from the low-leukemia BALB/c mouse strain (7, 569). Similar findings have been reported for the XC rat cells (see Section II,G); they are free of rat or murine gs antigen and, upon BUdR treatment, yielded C-type virus with the antigenic properties of the rat oncornavirus (343). The mechanism by which the halogenated pyrimidines induce C-type viruses from normal cells remains unclear at present, but it appears that incorporation of the drugs into DNA is required since inhibition of DNA synthesis during exposure to the drugs prevents activation (515). These activation experiments led to the conclusion that normal murine and avian cells have the complete genetic potential for specifying a C-type RNA virus. The final interpretation of these findings rests with the biological characterization of these vertically inherited and inducible viruses, such as tests for their oncogenic potential *in vivo* and the role they may play in spontaneous carcinogenesis. None of the rescued virions have yet been shown to transform cells *in vitro*.

These recent developments tend to reinforce the oncogene hypothesis (287, 606) which states that the entire genome of oncornaviruses (the virogene) is an intrinsic part of the heritable genetic material of vertebrate cells. According to the hypothesis, the oncogene is the segment of the virogene that codes for the production of "transforming protein(s)" responsible for tumorigenesis; the remaining segments code for the production of gs antigens, envelope antigens, and enzymes involved in virus replication. The degree of expression of different components of the viral genome is controlled by host cell regulatory genes and by environmental factors such as physical and chemical carcinogens. The hypothesis thus invokes the integration of the oncornaviral genome into cell DNA (provirus) and the existence of repressors, coded for by regulatory genes in normal cells, that control the expression of the endogenous virus information. There is no experimental evidence as yet supporting the existence of either a repressor or a transforming protein, and as indicated above, induced C-type viruses have not yet been shown to be oncogenic either *in vivo* or *in vitro*. There appears to be little difference between the oncogene hypothesis and the provirus hypothesis (587) inasmuch as they both invoke integration of viral genetic material into cell DNA even though the former deals with the concept of endogenous viral information and the latter with exogenous. Temin's recent protovirus hypothesis (589, 590), which attempts to explain the common features of carcinogenesis and cell differentiation, states that regions of cell DNA serve as templates for the synthesis of RNA which, through the reverse transcriptase, serve as templates for new DNA synthesis; the new DNA then becomes integrated into the DNA of the original or adjacent cells of the organism resulting in gene amplification and modification of the original information. Since the theory assumes that this modification takes place only in somatic cells but not in germ cells, it infers that an occasional somatic cell on a random basis could contain all the information for a C-type virus.

The high degree with which induction of C-type viruses from somatic cells occurs would tend to argue against the protovirus theory in terms of explaining the heritable nature of oncornavirus information. However, if heritable oncorna-virus information is as ubiquitous as it appears to be, then the mechanism by which an exogenous oncornavirus renders a cell malignant remains unsolved. More recent genetic studies being conducted with the high leukemia AKR strain of mice may lead to an answer to this question since AKR mice possess two independently segregating chromosomal loci (AKV-1 and AKV-2), either of which leads to the spontaneous appearance of infectious MuLV early in life or to the synthesis of infectious MuLV after induction with IUdR; these results suggest AKV-1 and AKV-2 are chromosomally integrated viral genetic determi-nants (509, 510). Further genetic mapping has identified the chromosomal loca-tion of the virus-inducing locus AKV-1 on the same linkage group, 12 map units apart, from the gene for the isozymes of glucose phosphate isomerase (Gpi-1) whose phenotype is independent of virus expression; both AKV-1 and Gpi-1 expressions were amenable to measure *in vivo* as well as in tissue culture (514). The finding of close linkage between AKV-1, a viral gene, and Gpi-1, a gene independent of the viral genome, offers possibilities for further genetic studies which may lead to the identification of a locus for the integration of a superinfecting MuLV genome.

III. Oncogenic DNA Viruses

A. General Consideration and Classification

The known DNA-containing tumor viruses are a more diverse group of agents than the RNA tumor viruses described in the preceding sections, all of which are remarkably similar in structure and chemical composition. DNA viruses with proven oncogenic capabilities range from the small, comparatively simple papovaviruses to members of the much larger, much more complex poxvirus group (see Table 11.5). The papovaviruses (SV40 and polyoma) and the adeno-viruses induce tumors in species different from the host of origin. In contrast, the papilloma viruses, poxviruses, and some of the herpesviruses do initiate tumor formation in the natural host. Another noteworthy property of the DNA tumor viruses is that, in general, infectious virus is not continuously produced and released by the tumor cells in contradistinction to the virus–cell interaction result-ing from transformation mediated by most of the oncornaviruses. Cells trans-formed by DNA viruses do express several virus-specific markers however, and these will be described in following sections of this review. The productive and transforming cycles of a DNA tumor virus are compared schematically in Fig. 11.4.

The diversity among the DNA viruses makes it impossible to describe in detail here the chemical and physical properties of the DNA-containing virions themselves and contrast the basic parameters of their cycles of replication with

TABLE 11.5

SOME PROPERTIES OF DNA-CONTAINING TUMOR VIRUSES

Virus	Host of origin	Natural Tumors (host of origin)	Experimental host range		Size (nm)	Structure	Site of virus maturation	Persistence of infectious virus in tumor
			in Vivo tumors	in Vitro cell transformation				
PAPOVAVIRUSES								
Papilloma					40–55	Icosahedral symmetry	Nucleus	Yes
Human	Man	Yes	Man					
Rabbit	Rabbit	Yes	Rabbit					
Bovine	Cow	Yes	Cow	Bovine				
Canine	Dog	Yes	Dog					
Polyoma	Mouse	No	Mouse, hamster, other rodents	Mouse, hamster, rat				No
SV40	Monkey	No	Hamster	Hamster, mouse, monkey, man				
ADENOVIRUSES					70–80	Icosahedral symmetry	Nucleus	No
Human types 3, 7, 11, 12, 14, 16, 18, 21, 31	Man	No	Hamster, rat, mouse	Hamster, rat, man				
Simian (some)	Monkey	No	Hamster, rat, mouse	Hamster, rat, man				
Bovine type 3	Cow	No	Hamster, rat, mouse	Hamster, rat, man				
Avian (CELO)	Chicken	No	Hamster, rat, mouse	Hamster, rat, man				
HERPESVIRUSES					100	Icosahedral symmetry	Nucleus	No
Human Type 2	Man		Hamster	Hamster				
EB viruses	Man			Man				
Monkey (Melendez)	Monkey	No	Monkey					
Avian (Marek)	Chicken	Yes	Chicken					
Frog (Lucké)	Frog	Yes	Frog					
Rabbit (Hinze)	Rabbit	No	Rabbit					
POXVIRUSES					230 × 300	Complex symmetry	Cytoplasm	Yes
Molluscum contagiosum	Man	Yes	Man					
Yaba	Monkey	Yes	Monkey					
Fibroma-myxoma	Rabbit, squirrel, deer	Yes	Rabbit, squirrel, deer					

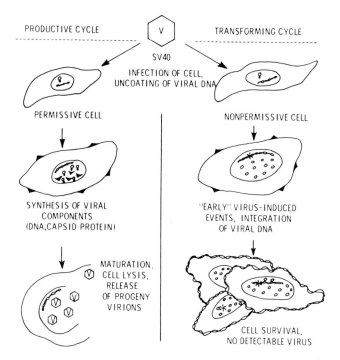

Fig. 11.4. Schematic comparison of two types of interaction between a DNA tumor virus and a host cell (productive and transforming cycles).

what is known of the process of cell transformation by the same agents. There-fore, attempts will be made to unify the data obtained from different virus systems to form general basic concepts where it is feasible to do so. The inter-ested reader is urged to consult recent reviews for further information pertaining to specific virus groups (64, 98, 123, 227, 339, 474–476, 545, 561), as well as appropriate chapters in books (120, 175, 360, 376).

1. PAPOVAVIRUSES

The designation for this group is composed of the first two letters of the names of some of its member viruses: *pa*pilloma viruses of man, rabbit, cow, and dog; *po*lyoma virus of mice; and *va*cuolating virus (simian virus 40 or SV40) of monkeys (395). The papilloma viruses form a natural subgroup in that they are approximately 10 nm larger in diameter (114) and contain a larger molecule of DNA than the other members of the group (e.g., SV40, polyoma). Typical SV40 virions are shown in Fig. 11.5.

Human papilloma virus was the first tumor virus to be isolated and transmitted in a cell-free filtrate (105). Papilloma viruses were recovered from cows, dogs, and rabbits in rapid succession (115, 125, 552, respectively). Unfortunately, no tissue culture systems are available for the propagation of the papilloma vi-

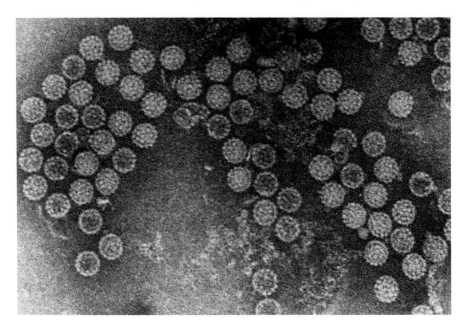

Fig. 11.5. Electron micrograph of purified papovavirus SV40 (176,000×). Courtesy of R. McCombs, Department of Virology, Baylor College of Medicine.

ruses *in vitro* (94), so studies with these potentially important agents are greatly hampered.

In contrast, members of the other papovavirus subgroup can be readily propagated in tissue culture and represent the most well-studied DNA tumor viruses today. Polyoma virus was first recovered from mice (233) and later isolated in pure form (570). Plaque-purified polyoma virus was able to induce a variety of types of tumors in various organs after inoculation of newborn mice, rats, and hamsters (158, 159, 570).

SV40 was isolated (580) from cultures of rhesus and cynomolgus monkey kidney cells which exhibited no obvious cytopathic effects. However, the presence of SV40 can be easily recognized in African green monkey kidney cells, the commonly used host cell system, due to the extensive cytoplasmic vacuolization which occurs. SV40 became of medical interest when it was inadvertantly administered to millions of people as a contaminant of poliovirus vaccines. Viable SV40 was recovered from both live and inactivated poliovirus vaccines (217, 580). Fortunately, no known adverse effects to the recipients have been attributed to this accidental exposure to SV40. The oncogenic potential of SV40 is manifest upon introduction of the virus into newborn hamsters.

2. ADENOVIRUSES

The adenovirus group is comprised of a large number of agents which are distributed widely in nature and have been recovered from many species. At least 31 distinct antigenic types have been isolated from man, 16 from monkeys,

8 from chickens, 7 from cattle, 4 from swine, and 2 each from dogs and mice (422). Adenoviruses, as a rule, are quite species-specific and will replicate only in cells derived from the same species as the host of origin. On occasion, an abortive (incomplete) cycle of adenovirus replication occurs following infection of cells derived from a heterologous species.

The first adenovirus isolates were obtained from humans in the early 1950's (276, 511). Although many adenovirus infections in man are inapparent, certain antigenic types have been found to be frequently associated with various syndromes such as acute respiratory disease, pharyngoconjunctival fever, acute febrile conjunctivitis, keratoconjunctivitis, and viral pneumonia (15).

The adenoviruses have received much attention from viral oncologists because they were the first isolates of human origin proved to be oncogenic for newborn hamsters (614). The human adenoviruses have been grouped on the basis of their oncogenic potential in newborn hamsters (227). Group A contains the "highly oncogenic" viruses (types 12, 18 and 31) which induce tumors in a high proportion of animals within 2 months after inoculation. "Weakly oncogenic" group B members (types 3, 7, 11, 14, 16, 21) ultimately induce tumors in only a small proportion of animals and these after 4–18 months. Group C agents (e.g., types 1, 2, 5, 6) are nononcogenic in newborn hamsters, but are able to morphologically transform rat embryo cells *in vitro*. Several simian, bovine, and avian adenoviruses have also been shown to be tumorigenic in newborn hamsters.

3. HERPESVIRUSES

The herpesviruses are the most recent group of DNA-containing viruses to gain prominence due to suspected oncogenic ability. The prototype virus for the group is human herpes simplex virus type 1 (HSV-1), which is the causative agent of fever blisters as well as acute stomatitis and eczema herpeticum in children, keratoconjunctivitis, and meningoencephalitis. A characteristic feature of the pathogenicity of herpes simplex virus is that it induces a latent infection which may be activated by various stimuli, such as infections, fever, wind, sunlight, or stress. Many individuals, therefore, are subject to recurrent herpes throughout their lifetimes (15, 485). There are no indications that HSV-1 possesses oncogenic properties. However, it appears that the virus can transform hamster cells in tissue culture (149).

A serologically related virus, designated herpes simplex virus type 2 (HSV-2), commonly induces genital infections and is transmitted venereally (413, 485, 487). There is serological evidence which suggests that HSV-2 may play a role in the development of cervical carcinoma (17, 412, 486). Recently, it has been found that UV-irradiated HSV-2 can induce malignant transformation of hamster cells *in vitro* (148).

EB virus was first observed microscopically in lymphoblasts established in culture from Burkitt tumor tissue (167). The herpes-type particles proved to be biologically inert and serologically distinct from known members of the herpes family (164, 165). EB virus is intimately associated with Burkitt's lymphoma, but an absolute etiological relationship has not yet been established. However, there is strong evidence that EB virus is the etiological agent of infectious mononucleosis (271). On the basis of serological data, EB virus has been associated with postnasal (nasopharyngeal) carcinoma (273), but also with several other nonmalignant immunoproliferative disorders of man (see Section IV,D for further discussion and pertinent references).

Two oncogenic herpesviruses have recently been isolated from monkeys, herpesvirus saimiri (HVS) and herpesvirus ateles (HVA) (394). HVS was isolated from spontaneously degenerating primary squirrel monkey kidney cultures (393); the virus is apparently latent in the *Saimiri* species. HVA was recovered from a primary kidney cell culture derived from a spider monkey (394). These two viral isolates are serologically distinct from each other and all other known herpesviruses. HVS induces the development of malignant lymphomas in marmosets, owl and spider monkeys, and of reticuloproliferative diseases in Cebus and African green monkeys. HVA was found to be oncogenic in marmoset monkeys. In contrast to EB virus, both HVS and HVA undergo productive cycles of replication in a variety of cell types in tissue culture.

A herpesvirus causes Marek's disease, a lymphoproliferative disease of chickens (415). Marek's disease virus (MDV) is carried by most chicken flocks, but generally only a few birds develop the disease (55). Several different strains of MDV have been isolated which display slight differences in antigenicity, virulence, and tissue tropism (some strains are basically viscerotropic while others are neurotropic). The virus undergoes an abortive cycle of replication *in vivo* in most tissues of the chicken with the exception of feather follicle epithelium in which the infection results in the production of complete infectious progeny virus. An antigenically related herpesvirus (HVT) which has been recovered from turkeys (315, 650) is apathogenic in chickens and has been used successfully as a vaccine to reduce the incidence of Marek's disease in infected flocks (465).

The first herpesvirus to be implicated as the etiological agent of a tumor (368), was that observed by electron microscopy in nuclear inclusion-bearing cells of a renal adenocarcinoma of frogs, *Rana pipiens* (226). Semipurified herpesvirus particles, extracted from Lucké tumors, have been shown to be oncogenic in *R. pipiens* embryos (399). Unfortunately, conclusive proof that the Lucké herpesvirus (LHV) is actually the etiologic agent of the renal tumor is lacking for two reasons: (a) all attempts to isolate and propagate LHV in tissue culture have failed and (b) several other viruses have been recovered from the tumor cells. These include a polyhedral cytoplasmic deoxyribovirus (PCDV), at least one other herpesvirus distinct from LHV and designated frog virus 4 (FV4), and a small virus tentatively classified as a papovavirus. All these latter isolates failed to induce tumors in developing frog embryos (226).

A herpesvirus (*Herpesvirus sylvilagus*), indigenous in wild cottontail rabbits, has been recently recognized by Hinze (278) as a new and antigenically distinct member of the herpesvirus group. When inoculated into weanling cottontail rabbits (but not in domestic rabbits), the virus induces generalized hyperplasia of lymphoid elements and in some instances malignant lymphomas as well (279).

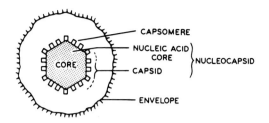

Fig. 11.6. Schematic diagram illustrating the components of a complex virus particle (the virion). (From "Review of Medical Microbiology" with permission of Lange Medical Publications, Los Altos, Calif.).

4. POXVIRUSES

This group contains the largest known DNA-containing viruses; they carry a large complement of genetic information and possess a complex virion structure (304). Molluscum contagiosum of man, Yaba virus of monkeys, and Shope fibroma virus of rabbits are agents which cause tumorlike growths *in vivo* and are classified in the poxvirus group (15, 120). With the latter two agents, spontaneous regression of the tumor frequently occurs.

B. Virion Structure

The DNA tumor viruses under consideration all exhibit cubic symmetry, the basic structure being that of an icosahedron with the number of structural capsomeres being distinct for each major virus group. Only the herpesviruses possess a lipid-containing envelope. A complete virus particle with its components designated is shown schematically in Fig. 11.6. Details of icosahedral symmetry are presented in Table 11.6.

The number of capsomeres in the papovavirus capsid has been the subject of some controversy, but the strongest evidence indicates that the agents fall into the T = 7 series of icosahedra and that 72 is the correct capsomere figure. The member viruses can be placed into two general size classes: the papilloma-

TABLE 11.6

DETAILS OF ICOSAHEDRAL SYMMETRY RELEVANT TO DNA-CONTAINING TUMOR VIRUSES

Virus group	n^a	T^b	No. of capsomeres	Envelope
Papova[c]	3	7	72	0
Herpes	5	16	162	+
Adeno	6	25	252	0

[a] $N = 10(n - 1)^2 + 2$ in which N = total number of capsomeres and n = number of capsomeres on one side of each of 20 equilateral triangle faces of the icosahedron.

[b] $M = 10T + 2$ in which M = number of morphologic units (capsomeres) and T = triangulation number, the number of small triangles formed on a single face of the icosahedron when each adjacent morphologic unit is connected by a line.

[c] Capsomeres are in a skew arrangement.

viruses have an average diameter of about 50–55 nm, approximately 10 nm larger than the other agents, such as polyoma and SV40. The papillomaviruses have an approximate sedimentation coefficient of 300 S in sucrose, while for the smaller particles the value is 240 S. Tubular, filamentous forms have been observed by the electron microscope in some virus preparations (585). The papovaviruses do not contain any essential lipid.

The adenoviruses are also naked icosahedrons; the capsid is composed of 252 capsomeres and is 65–80 nm in diameter. The structure of the adenoviruses is more complex in that the vertex (penton) capsomeres carry projections called fibers which end in a terminal knob. The length of the fiber varies from one adenovirus serotype to the next and is probably involved in the attachment of the virus particle to a susceptible cell. There is also an internal protein associated with the viral DNA in the virion (213, 422).

The herpesvirus group is also characterized by icosahedral capsids, comprised of 162 capsomeres, but differs from the two groups described above in that the complete virion includes a lipid-containing envelope. The naked nucleocapsid (DNA plus capsid) is approximately 100 nm in diameter while the enveloped particles range in size from 150 to 180 nm. There is currently conflicting inconclusive data pertaining to the question of whether the envelope is essential for viral infectivity (499).

C. Chemical Composition

1. Nucleic-Acids

Although the tumor viruses under discussion all contain DNA as their genetic material, the molecular size and structural configuration of the DNA varies markedly with the different virus groups. The reader may consult reviews (112, 227, 440, 93) for further details regarding the nucleic acids of these tumor viruses.

The papovaviruses contain approximately 12% DNA; the molecular weight of the polyoma and SV40 genomes averages about 3 million daltons each. SV40 DNA reportedly contains 41% guanine + cytosine (G + C), while the base composition of polyoma DNA has been calculated to be 48% G + C (112). The DNA extracted from polyoma or SV40 separates upon zonal sedimentation into two components (I and II) with sedimentation coefficients of 20 S and 16 S, respectively (113, 153, 627, 641). Component I exists in a twisted supercoiled circular configuration while component II is a relaxed circular form of the same molecule. The conversion of form I to II occurs whenever a single-strand break is introduced into the supercoiled structure (627). Both form I and form II structures are recovered when DNA is extracted from purified virions. The supercoiled component I configuration represents 60–90% of the total DNA (32, 153, 641). Whether form II DNA exists as such in the mature virions or is produced during the extraction procedures due to a single-strand break in component I molecules is unknown.

Both forms I and II are infectious, as are single-stranded rings prepared by alkaline denaturation of form II DNA (153, 616). It has been calculated that 10^5 to 10^6 form I SV40 DNA molecules are required for one plaque-forming unit in the DEAE-dextran plaque assay (4, 440, 616). The infectivity of the supercoiled form is retained after heating at 100°C for 5 minutes in 0.15 M NaCl followed by rapid cooling, but if the DNA has been nicked several times by DNase, boiling does inactivate its infectivity (153, 640). These results are all compatible with the model for papovavirus DNA being that of two intertwined circles, only one ring of which must be intact in order for the molecule to be infectious.

In spite of their many biophysical similarities, there does not appear to be any homology between the DNA from polyoma virus and that from SV40 virus or Shope rabbit papilloma virus (112). Cyclic structures similar to those described above have been described for the DNA's isolated from the papilloma virus members of the papovavirus group, including human papilloma virus (111), Shope rabbit papilloma virus (110, 340), and bovine papilloma virus (84). Papilloma virus DNA's average approximately 5 million daltons in molecular weight and this larger size is reflected in sedimentation coefficients of about 28 S and 21 S for forms I and II, respectively. The papilloma virus DNA's range from 41 to 47% G + C. No homology between the different agents has been detected using nucleic acid hybridization (112). The DNA from Shope papilloma virus is infectious *in vivo* in domestic rabbits (298).

To date, no virus which morphologically resembles a papovavirus has failed to yield a circular DNA genome. The description of circular DNA and a survey of its distribution in eukaryotic as well as prokaryotic systems has been recently reviewed (268).

The term "pseudovirion" is used to designate papovavirus particles which contain host cell DNA rather than the viral genome (397). Pseudovirions were first detected in preparations of polyoma virus grown in mouse kidney cells (397, 648, 649). What was originally designated as form III DNA extracted from purified polyoma virus with a sedimentation coefficient of ~14 S was shown to consist of linear fragments of mouse cellular DNA. SV40 pseudovirions have also been described (356, 615). The linear, 14 S DNA was able to hybridize with cellular DNA, but not with viral DNA and, as would be expected, was not infectious under the conditions used to detect infectious SV40 DNA. To date, no pseudovirions have been detected in any virus preparations other than those of papovaviruses.

The host cell exerts a profound influence on the production of pseudovirions. Pseudovirions form following infection by SV40 of primary GMK cells but not after infection of two other stable monkey cell lines, BSC-1 and CV-1 (356). A mouse hamster hybrid cell line produces primarily pseudovirions after infection with polyoma virus (34). The reason(s) responsible for this variable production of pseudovirions in different host cells remains obscure.

Pseudovirions are of interest because of their inherent potential for gene transfer. They could conceivably act as transducing particles in mammalian cells and, as such, would resemble "generalized transducing" bacteriophage in that no specific region of the cellular genome appears to be preferentially incorporated into the papova viral capsids (222, 649). Host cell DNA carried by pseudovirions can be delivered into the nucleus of a recipient host cell, but it is not known whether it is functional (222, 466). There are too few genetic markers currently available for mammalian cells which could be utilized to detect expression by the transduced DNA. When such experiments become technically feasible, pseudovirions may be of use in the treatment of human genetic defects by means of gene transfer. It will be necessary, of course, to devise conditions under which specific sequences of DNA are incorporated into pseudovirions rather than the random, heterogeneous incorporation of host cell DNA typically observed.

The human adenoviruses contain linear duplex molecules of DNA, ranging in size from 20 to 25 million daltons (229). This amount of DNA represents 12–13% of the intact virion. There is an interesting correlation between the $G + C$ content of the DNA and the degree of oncogenicity of the human adenoviruses in newborn hamsters (227). The "highly oncogenic" group A members contain DNA with a 48–49% $G + C$ content, the "weakly oncogenic" group B is typified by a $G + C$ value of 50–52%, and "nononcogenic" group C agents contain 55–61% $G + C$. All the members within each group are closely related, sharing 70–100% of their base sequences as determined by viral DNA-DNA hybridization reactions. In contrast, members from different groups share only 10–26% of their base sequences. These common base sequences probably code for characteristics all adenoviruses have in common, such as some virion proteins.

For many years, no infectivity was demonstrated for isolated adenovirus DNA, but the successful isolation of DNA from adenovirus type 1 which retained infectivity for human embryonic kidney cells in tissue culture has recently been reported (417). The infectivity appeared to be a property of DNA in that it was inactivated by DNase, but there was 1–2% residual protein in the DNA preparations. Whether or not this protein played any role in the infectivity of the DNA remains to be elucidated.

The correlation between low $G + C$ content of the DNA and high oncogenic potential of the virus does not extend to the simian adenoviruses. Highly oncogenic isolate SA7 contains 58–60% $G + C$, as compared to a composition of 56% $G + C$ in the DNA from nononcogenic adenovirus SV15. Simian adenoviruses SA7 and SV15 show only 9–23% homology with any of the human adenoviruses (227). SA7 DNA appears to be a linear duplex structure with a molecular weight of approximately 22 million daltons (90); no circular molecules have been detected. Phenol-extracted DNA from SA7 is infectious in monkey cells which have been pretreated with DEAE-dextran, in addition to being oncogenic in suckling hamsters (90, 91).

Herpesviruses contain a linear, double-stranded genome larger than that of the adenoviruses, the reported molecular weights for the DNA's from several members of the group averaging about 100×10^6 daltons (45, 225, 327, 351). No evidence for circular forms of the herpesvirus genome has been presented. The group varies widely in the $G + C$ content of the DNA's, ranging from as low as about 46% for Lucké tumor virus and Marek's disease virus to as high as 74% for pseudorabies virus (500). Using DNA-DNA hybridization, it has been shown that there exists 50 to 70% homology between the DNA's of HSV-1 and HSV-2 and only 8–10% complementarity between pseudorabies DNA and either HSV-1 or HSV-2 DNA (328, 369). No infectivity has yet been demonstrated for purified herpesvirus DNA.

2. VIRION-ASSOCIATED ENZYMES

An endonuclease activity has been detected in purified particles of polyoma virus (118) and SV40 (309, 326). The virion-associated activity produces single-strand nicks which convert form I viral DNA to form II. The localization of the enzymic activity in the virion and the source of genetic information coding for the enzyme (cell or viral) have not yet been established.

Another endonuclease, one which cleaves both strands of viral DNA, has been found associated with adenovirus particles (89). Based on enzyme assays using purified capsid subunits, as well as inhibition of activity by specific antisera, it was established that the enzyme activity resides in the protein of the penton base. Endonuclease activity has also been detected in cells infected with adenovirus (88).

3. VIRAL PROTEINS

SV40 contains 6 distinct structural polypeptides with molecular weights of approximately 43,000 (VP1, representing 70% of virion protein), 32,000 (VP2, 9%), 23,000 (VP3, 10%), 14,000 (VP4, 6%), 12,500 (VP5, 4%), and 11,000 (VP6, 3%) (171). VP1 and VP2 probably form the viral capsid, and VP4, 5, and 6 are complexed with the viral DNA. All or part of VP3 is bound to the viral DNA and is part of a deoxyribonucleoprotein complex (285, 345). Similar results have been obtained using SV40-infected cells (178, 637). At least 6 polypeptides have been detected in purified preparations of polyoma virus, the major capsid protein having a molecular weight of 48,000 daltons (498). There is good evidence that the basic, internal proteins derived from polyoma virus and SV40, are actually host cell histones (170a, 184).

The adenoviruses are complex structures composed of at least 9 different viral-specific polypeptides (Fig. 11.7). These proteins are the structural components for the hexon (MW 120,000) which comprise about 50% of the total virion protein, penton base (MW 70,000) which possesses endonuclease activity (see preceding section), and fiber (MW 62,000) antigens. The hexons represent the group-specific antigen of adenoviruses, while pentons are responsible for type-specific activity. In addition, there are three arginine-rich core polypeptides (MW 44,000, 24,000, and 24,000) and two minor polypeptides (MW 13,000 each) which are associated with the hexons. The sum of the molecular weights of the virion peptides represents about 29% of the coding capacity of the viral genome (374).

Purified herpesvirus virions have recently been reported to contain at least 24 structural proteins, 12 of which are glycosylated (563). The proteins range

Appearance	Name	Number Per Virion	Molecular Weight	Antigen	Specificity	Protein Components
Virion	DNA		23,000,000			
	Protein		150,000,000			
○	Hexon	240	210,000 400,000 320,000 360,000	A	Group	II
	Hexons	20	3,600,000			II, VIII, IX
	Penton	12	280,000 1,100,000			III, IV
	Penton Base	12	210,000	B	Subgroup	III
	Fiber	12	70,000	C	Type	IV
Core	DNA	1	23,000,000	P		
	Protein		29,000,000			V, VI, VII
	Protein		13,000			VIII, IX
	Protein		7,500			X

(Header groupings: "Morphological Subunits" spans Appearance, Name, Number Per Virion, Molecular Weight; "Antigenic Subunits" spans Antigen, Specificity; "Protein Components")

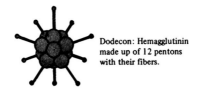

Dodecon: Hemagglutinin made up of 12 pentons with their fibers.

Fig. 11.7. Comparative data on adenovirus type 2 morphological and antigenic subunits and protein components. (From "Review of Medical Microbiology," with permission of Lange Medical Publications, Los Altos, Calif., Modified from Maizel *et al., Virology* 36, 126–136, 1968).

in molecular weight from 25,000 to 275,000 daltons, the sum of the molecular weight being 2.58×10^6 daltons. These structural proteins are organized into a core, a multilayered capsid (inner, middle, and outer capsid layers), and a complex envelope (inner and outer layers) (500). The viral-specific proteins described above have not yet been assigned to any of the morphological components of the virion. Even though DNA homology studies have revealed a certain degree of genetic dissimilarity between HSV-1 and HSV-2 (83, 328), no differences have been as yet detected in the structural proteins of the two viruses either by polyacrylamide gel electrophoresis (541) or by amino acid composition analysis of purified nucleocapsids (134).

D. Viral Tumorigenesis

1. Papovaviruses

The papilloma viruses are the only members of the papovavirus group known to cause natural tumors in their hosts of origin. These same agents have not been grown in tissue culture, so studies with them have been limited to *in vivo* systems. Currently, the only source of papilloma virus particles are extracts prepared from excised papilloma tissues. The successful experimental transmission of warts from man to man by filtered human papilloma tissue extracts has been accomplished by a number of investigators (516). Attempts to induce papillomas in any heterologous species by human papilloma virus have been uniformly unsuccessful (94, 516).

Shope rabbit papilloma virus causes benign tumors in cottontail rabbits which, rarely, progress to malignant carcinomas. Skin papillomas can be induced experimentally in domestic rabbits; these tend to regress spontaneously, but occasionally develop into squamous cell carcinomas. Virus can be recovered in large quantities from cottontail rabbit papillomas, but only very rarely from cottontail rabbit carcinomas or from either type of tumor in the domestic rabbits (474). Purified rabbit papilloma virus DNA is also oncogenic in rabbits (298).

Polyoma virus infection is widespread among laboratory and wild mice, but does not cause detectable tumor formation under natural conditions. However, when virus is inoculated into newborn animals (mice or hamsters), tumors develop rapidly (157, 474). Polyoma is of interest historically as it was the first virus demonstrated to induce tumors in hamsters. The agent was named "polyoma" because a variety of tumors develop in the inoculated animals, both at the site of injection and at distant sites. Parotid carcinomas, adenocarcinomas, spindle cell sarcomas, hemangiomas, and epidermoid carcinomas were found in experimentally infected mice (570). Rats, rabbits, and ferrets have also been reported to be susceptible to the oncogenic effects of polyoma virus (474). Isolated viral nucleic acid is also capable of inducing tumor formation in newborn hamsters (129). In contrast to papillomas, polyoma tumors are virus-free.

SV40 is not known to cause any disease in its natural host, the rhesus monkey. However, it is capable of inducing tumor formation in newborn hamsters (16, 160, 216). The latent period for tumor development ranges from three months to more than a year, depending upon a number of variables such as the concentration of virus inoculum and the age of the recipient hamsters. SV40-induced tumors have been identified as undifferentiated sarcomas and fibrosarcomas (156), although ependymomas have been observed following intracerebral inoculation of virus (329). SV40 DNA is also oncogenic in hamsters (73), but attempts to induce tumors by SV40 in mice, rats, guinea pigs, rabbits, and monkeys have been unsuccessful (156). SV40-induced tumors are similar to those elicited by polyoma virus in that they do not contain infectious virus.

2. ADENOVIRUSES

Adenovirus type 12 was the first human isolate shown to be oncogenic in an experimental animal when newborn hamsters injected intrapulmonarily developed tumors (614). Several other serotypes have subsequently been shown to be oncogenic in neonatal hamsters (157). As pointed out in Section III,A, the human adenoviruses fall into three categories on the basis of their oncogenicity in the hamster system: the "highly oncogenic," "weakly oncogenic," and "nononcogenic" groups (227). Adenovirus-induced tumors are typically friable, necrotic, undifferentiated epithelioid neoplasms. Cells from adenovirus tumors have been notoriously difficult to establish in tissue culture. Simian, avian, canine, and bovine adenovirus isolates have also induced tumor formation in newborn hamsters (157).

Adenovirus-induced tumors do not contain detectable levels of infectious virus. However, as is also the case with polyoma and SV40 tumors, the cells possess certain virus-specific markers which reveal that the transforming viral genome is present in a noninfectious form. The evidence in support of a persistent association between the virus and transformed cell will be discussed in more detail in Section III,E,2.

3. Herpesviruses

Herpesvirus saimiri (HVS) induces in various primates highly malignant disease characterized as lymphomas, reticulum cell infiltrates, and leukemia. Especially surprising is the rapidity with which the disease progresses in cotton-top marmosets, for all the inoculated animals expire within 48 days. The lymphoid cells of the diseased primates do not contain infectious virus, but it is possible to rescue HVS by cocultivation of the neoplastic cells with susceptible cells (394). Herpesvirus ateles (HVA), a new isolate obtained from black spider monkeys, has induced malignant lymphoma in cotton-top marmosets similar to that observed following HVS inoculation (394).

Marek's disease virus (MDHV) causes a highly contagious, malignant lymphomatosis in chickens which was confused for many years with visceral lymphomatosis induced by avian oncornaviruses. During the last decade, a severe form of the disease appeared, designated the "acute form" of Marek's disease, which is having a devastating effect on the poultry industry. Levels of mortality with the acute form have reached as high as 80% of the flock, in contrast to the classic form in which clinical disease occurs only sporadically and is responsible for low levels of mortality. The classic form is characterized by variable degrees of paralysis, whereas with the acute form lymphoid tumors are a common symptom, occurring in gonads, lungs, heart, liver, spleen, kidney, muscle, and skin (55).

Marek's disease is a highly contagious infection and is probably spread by infected saliva, feces, and feathers. Contaminated litter and droppings have remained infectious for surprisingly long periods of time (16 weeks). The severity of the disease is influenced by both the strain of MDHV (some are highly pathogenic) and the genetic constitution of the host. The epizootiology of the disease is complicated by the fact that exposure to mild or apathogenic strains of the virus may have an ameliorative effect on subsequent infection with a virulent strain (55).

E. Properties of Cells Transformed by DNA Viruses

1. Parameters of Transformation

Viral transformation has been defined as an induced inheritable change in the properties of a cell, accompanied by the loss of regulatory controls of cell growth. The criteria for transformation of cells generally include the following (163): (1) Loss of contact inhibition, (2) altered morphology, (3) increased growth rate, (4) increased capacity to persist in serial subcultures, (5) chromosomal abnormalities, (6) increased resistance to reinfection by the transforming virus, (7) emergence of new antigens, and (8) capacity to form neoplasms. The details of various transformation systems were recently summarized (64, 98, 151, 459, 524, 525, 545). Features of transformation by the papovavirus, SV40, will be emphasized in this section of the chapter, as it represents one of the most well-characterized DNA-containing oncogenic agents.

SV40 is maximally oncogenic *in vivo* in newborn hamsters, but the narrow host range of the virus has been widely extended by *in vitro* transformation experiments. In addition to transformation of hamster cells in culture, SV40 can transform cells of human, mouse, rabbit, rat, bovine, guinea pig, and monkey origin. In the hamster species, the most thoroughly studied transformation system for SV40, cells from a variety of organs and tissues have been shown to be susceptible to virus-induced transformation. SV40 exhibits little, if any, particular tissue tropism *in vitro*, since cells derived from 9 different types of differentiated hamster tissue have been successfully transformed (98).

Cells which have been transformed by SV40 fall into three categories: (1) permissive, (2) semipermissive, and (3) nonpermissive. Permissive cells are those which are highly susceptible to SV40 and in which the virus undergoes a typical replicative cycle, such as monkey kidney cells (283, 386). Human cells represent the semipermissive system in which small amounts of infectious virus are produced by the infected cells. However, even when free viral nucleic acid is used to infect the human cells, the yields of virus do not attain the levels produced by monkey cells (333, 581). All other species of cells fall into the nonpermissive category and are not susceptible to SV40 and do not produce detectable amounts of progeny virus. Even after exposure to SV40 DNA, no infectious progeny virus can be detected in cultures of hamster and mouse cells (581).

Nonpermissive cells can be transformed much more readily by SV40 than those derived from permissive species. The mouse 3T3 cell line is sensitive to transformation by SV40 and constitutes the most widely employed quantitative transformation system for the virus (63, 603). In the 3T3 system, one transforming unit of virus corresponds to about 10^3 infectious units and about 10^5 physical particles. When high concentrations of virus are used, at least 10% of the 3T3 population will transform. In contrast, transformation of semipermissive human diploid cells is much less efficient—an equivalent input of virus will transform only about 0.03% of the human cells.

Irradiation experiments indicate that the entire papovavirus genome is not required for transformation. Virus-specific functions probably fall into the following order based on increasing UV-resistance: plaque-forming ability, induction of V antigen, induction of T antigen, and transformation (1, 35, 47, 349). Since only a portion of the genome is needed to mediate transformation, defective particles present in virus populations may be responsible for some of the observed transformation events (95, 98).

Transformation of a given cell by one member of the papovavirus group does not preclude its further transformation by a second member of the same virus group. Colonial morphology showed that SV40 could further transform 3T3 mouse cells initially transformed by polyoma virus (602). Several isolated clones of the doubly transformed 3T3 cells were shown to contain specific T antigens of both viruses (608). SV40-induced hamster tumor cells became doubly transformed after superinfection with polyoma virus (582). TSTA and T antigens (see Section III,E,3) were induced by both viruses in the doubly transformed cells.

Cells can be doubly transformed by SV40 and a human adenovirus, as well. Cells transformed either *in vivo* or *in vitro* by the PARA (defective SV40)-adenovirus hybrid populations sometimes contain both SV40 and adenovirus T antigens and generally induce antibody against both SV40 and adenovirus T antigens in tumor-bearing hamsters (66, 97, 145, 480, 482, 492). The morphology of the tumors and transformed cells are sometimes characteristic of either adenovirus or SV40-transformed cells or, on occasion, histologically intermediate (67, 295, 481). The most convincing evidence, however, that both SV40 and adenovirus information can be present in the cultures of PARA-transformed cells is that both adenovirus 7 and SV40 specific RNA's were detected in such cultures after cloning (355). The PARA system is unique because the defective SV40 and the defective adenovirus 7 DNA's appear to be linked (42, 43, 322, 355). Therefore, integration of the SV40 portion of the PARA genome would also carry into the chromosome the adenovirus 7 region. However, cells transformed by a transcapsidant PARA-adenovirus 12 population sometimes contained both adenovirus 7- and adenovirus 12-specific RNA in addition to the SV40-specific RNA (355). This observation indicates that both the PARA and adenovirus 12 genomes can be integrated into the same host cell.

One important facet of multiple transformation by viruses has not yet been studied. That area concerns the number of *different* genetically defined viral genomes which can be present in the same transformed cell. Such information would indicate how many different integration sites there are for a given virus in a single cell.

Transformation of hamster and/or rat cells has been reported for various human and simian adenoviruses (459, 545). Hamster embryo fibroblasts have also been transformed *in vitro* by UV-irradiated herpes simplex virus type 2 (148).

2. State of the Viral Genome

SV40-transformed cells produce infectious virus only very rarely, if at all, so attempts were made to determine the state of the viral genome in such cells. Assays of nucleic acid isolated from SV40-transformed cells failed to reveal the presence of any free, infectious viral DNA (81, 332, 521).

SV40-transformed hamster cells were first shown to contain DNA with homology to SV40 mRNA prepared *in vitro* (488). With RNA prepared from highly purified component I virus DNA as template, it was estimated that the number of viral DNA equivalents per transformed cell ranged from 7 to 58 (647). Recent estimates are that there are only 1–9 SV40 DNA equivalents per transformed cell (199, 357), but whether some of the "equivalents" might be defective (incomplete) viral genomes is uncertain.

The next step was to determine the state of the multiple copies of viral nucleic acid within the transformed cells. Using the DNA-RNA hybridization technique and an SV40-transformed line of mouse 3T3 cells, the following points were found about the physical state of the viral DNA (526, 647): (a) It is in the nucleus; no hybridizable DNA was detected in cytoplasmic extracts. (b) It is associated with the cellular chromosomes. Chromosomes were isolated from metaphase cells and the DNA isolated from the chromosomes was shown to hybridize to the same extent as DNA from interphase cells. (c) It is not in the form of circular molecules. Following centrifugation to equilibrium in cesium chloride in the presence of ethidium bromide, the hybridizable material was found in the cellular DNA band in the gradient. (d) It is not present in the form of free molecules the size of a single SV40 genome. The Hirt salt precipitation method (282), which separates large and small molecules of DNA, showed that the hybridizable regions were found in the precipitate of cellular DNA. (e) The viral and cellular DNA's are not separated by alkaline denaturation and centrifugation in a sucrose gradient.

Therefore, the main conclusion to be drawn from these studies is that the SV40 DNA is apparently covalently bound to the chromosomal DNA of the transformed cell. The site (or sites) of insertion of the multiple copies of the genome is still unknown. Identical findings were obtained for polyoma DNA in similar experiments carried out in parallel with polyoma-transformed 3T3 cells (647).

The use of interferon has also suggested the integration of the viral genome into that of the host cell. The induction of T antigen by SV40 in 3T3 cells is sensitive to inhibition by interferon, but serial passage of SV40-transformed 3T3 cells in the presence of interferon had no effect on the synthesis of T antigen (438). Previous investigations had established that fixation of the transformed state in the infected cell required only one cell generation (604) and that treatment of the cells at the time of infection with interferon would prevent transformation (601). The use of synchronized cell cultures revealed that if the cells were not synthesizing DNA, transformation remained interferon-sensitive, but if the cells were rapidly synthesizing cellular DNA (S phase), transformation readily became interferon-resistant (605). Since there is evidence that interferon blocks translation of viral mRNA (305, 377), these observations can be explained by the assumption that the viral DNA becomes integrated into the cellular chromosomes during the S phase of cell growth. Once integrated, the viral mRNA is masked by attached regions of cell mRNA so that interferon no longer recognizes it as being viral in origin.

Numerous studies have attempted to determine the degree to which transcription of viral genes occurs in transformed cells. A small fraction of pulse-labeled RNA from polyoma or SV40-transformed cells was able to hybridize with the DNA of the corresponding virus (48). With the SV40 system, the mRNA formed during lytic infection prior to viral DNA synthesis ("early" RNA) was different from the mRNA present after the onset of viral DNA replication ("late" RNA). Approximately one-third of the SV40 genome was represented in the early RNA whereas at least 75% of the genome was represented in the late RNA (14, 428, 540). Competition experiments between virus-specific RNA from transformed cells and late RNA from infected cells suggested that only about one-third of the genome was transcribed in the transformed cells. Interestingly, approximately 80% of the SV40 genome appeared to be transcribed in one transformed green monkey kidney cell line. In all cases, it appeared that the lack of expression of certain viral genes in transformed cells was at the level of transcription.

A more recent study of the regulation of SV40 gene activity in transformed cells utilized a series of SV40-transformed mouse cell lines (383). The extent of transcription in the individual lines varied, ranging from 30 to 100% of that seen during lytic infection. This study emphasized that the extent of transcription of the SV40 genome is variable from one transformed cell line to the next, even within a single species of host cell. In an SV40-transformed green monkey kidney cell line, production of late viral mRNA sequences was not prevented when DNA synthesis was inhibited (539). This was in contrast to a productive infection by SV40 in which inhibitors of DNA synthesis prevented the appearance of late mRNA. The mechanism(s) responsible for the apparent differences in transcriptional control is not known at this time.

High molecular weight heterogenous RNA that contains viral-specific RNA has been detected in the nucleus of transformed mouse cells (363). Polysomal mRNA of lower molecular weight also contained viral-specific RNA; thus the large nuclear molecules may be precursors of the cytoplasmic mRNA (see Chapter V). Interestingly, the largest molecules containing SV40 sequences were longer than one SV40 genome. These molecules were subsequently shown to carry both viral and cellular base sequences (636). Polycistronic "viral-cell" hybrid RNA molecules have also been detected in adenovirus 2-transformed rat embryo cells and adenovirus 7-induced hamster tumor cells (618). The presence of cellular mRNA regions adjacent to viral-specific sequences is supportive evidence of the concept of integration of the viral genome into that of the host cell.

Recent results from studies on the transcription of SV40 DNA during productive infection complicate interpretations of regulatory mechanisms at the transcriptional level. It appears that there is a strand switch during *in vivo* transcription. Early RNA, synthesized prior to viral DNA synthesis, is transcribed from one DNA strand. After DNA replication has started, "late" message is transcribed from the other strand (324, 364, 527). *E. coli* DNA polymerase copies only the "early," or minus, strand and that in its entirety. Transformed cells contain primarily early sequences copied from the minus strand. However, in mouse cells abortively infected with SV40, the extent and pattern of transcription was almost identical to that seen in permissive cells late in infection (325). Controls at the transcriptional and posttranscriptional level during productive and abortive infections by SV40 and their relevance to transcription of viral information in transformed cells are currently unresolved, but are the subject of intense investigation.

No discussion of transcription in virus-transformed cells is complete without reference to the patterns delineated in adenovirus-transformed cells (227). Comparison of transcription of virus-specific genes in cells transformed by representatives of the three different groups of human adenoviruses showed that viral genes were transcribed in preference to cellular genes. Although only about 0.01% of the total DNA of the transformed cell was adenovirus 12 DNA, at least 2% of the messenger RNA's associated with the polyribosomes contained viral sequences. Interestingly, the mRNA's in cells transformed by *any* adenovirus serotype had G + C contents of 47–51%, even though the G + C content of some of the viral DNA's were as much as 8% higher than that value. Therefore, either the regions of the viral genomes with an average G + C content of 47–51% are integrated or those regions are transcribed selectively in the transformed cells.

In addition, the virus-specific mRNA from cells transformed by group A, B, and C adenoviruses did not share base sequences even though the respective viral DNA's showed 10–25% homology. Viral mRNA from group A-transformed cells would hybridize only with DNA from a member group A virus, and not with group B or C viral DNA's. Likewise, mRNA's from group B and C transformed cells were specific for those subgroups. It does not appear that any detectable viral genes common to the A, B, and C subgroups are transcribed in human adenovirus-transformed cells (227).

3. Antigens Associated with Transformed Cells

Cells transformed by DNA tumor viruses possess several virus-induced antigens distinct from virion structural proteins (Table 11.7). The presence of these antigens indicates that at least some of the viral-specific messenger RNA species detected in transformed cells are functional and are translated into recognizable proteins.

TABLE 11.7

ANTIGENS AND SURFACE CHANGES OBSERVED AFTER TRANSFORMATION BY SV40[a]

Antigen	Location in cell	Virus-specific	Species-specific	Transformed cells	Productive infection	Cryptic in normal cells
Tumor (T)	Nucleus	+	0	+	+	0
Transplantation (TSTA)	Surface	+	0	+	+	0
Surface (S)	Surface	+	0	+	?	0
Normal cell	Surface	0	0	+	?	+
Embryonic	Surface	0	?	+	?	0
Agglutination sites	Surface	0	0	+	+	+

[a] + = present, 0 = absent, ? = not known.

The tumor (T) antigen was first localized in the nucleus of transformed cells using the immunofluorescence technique and sera from SV40 tumor-bearing hamsters (460, 477). The existence of the T antigen had previously been recognized using the complement fixation test (288). T antigen was then shown to be synthesized during the SV40 replicative cycle, thereby directly relating the antigen found in transformed cells to the transforming virus (478, 522). T antigen is synthesized early in the replicative cycle prior to viral DNA synthesis (479). Although the same T antigen is present in all species of cells infected or transformed by SV40, its biological function is obscure. T antigen with the properties described above for the SV40 system is also induced by polyoma virus and by adenovirus (see reviews 123, 237, 545).

A presumably new SV40-specific antigen, designated the U antigen (362), accumulates in the perinuclear region of cells infected with a strain of adenovirus type 2 carrying a defective SV40 genome ($Ad2^+ND_1$). However, U-positive antisera (from monkeys immunized with cells infected with $Ad2^+ND_1$) react with an intranuclear antigen which has the typical distribution of T antigen in both SV40-transformed and SV40-infected cells (361). Antibodies to both T and U antigens are present in sera from SV40 tumor-bearing hamsters. The only feature which distinguishes U antigen from T antigen is that the former is more heat-stable. Before it can be established that U antigen is a unique gene product of SV40, further study is required.

The existence of tumor-specific-transplantation antigen (TSTA) on papovavirus-transformed cells was demonstrated first with polyoma virus (236, 554) and subsequently with the SV40 system (122, 238, 323, 344). There are special reviews on TSTA of papovaviruses and of adenoviruses (123, 237, 258, 263, 545, 553). For brevity, the findings with the SV40 system will be emphasized. TSTA is specific for the transforming virus, being distinct from the TSTA induced by any heterologous, unrelated virus. The presence of TSTA is detected by the transplantation rejection test which involves immunizing animals, e.g. hamsters, with live virus, followed by the subsequent challenge of immune and nonimmune animals with varying numbers of transplantable tumor cells. The results can be expressed as the number of cells required to produce tumors in 50% of the animals (TPD_{50}). A tenfold difference in the TPD_{50} of the immune animals when compared to that of the control group is indicative of the presence of TSTA in the tumor cells.

In addition to the transplantation rejection test, SV40 TSTA on transformed cells can be detected by immunogenicity tests. Transformed cells, as well as virus, can immunize hamsters against tumor cell challenge and can prevent oncogenesis if inoculated prior to tumor appearance in animals which had received virus as newborns (214, 350).

TSTA is localized at the surface of transformed cells as evidenced by the facts that (a) lymphocytes must be in contact with tumor cells to kill them, and (b) isolated cell membranes can immunize against tumor cell challenge (109, 594, 598). Finally, SV40 TSTA has been detected during the viral replicative cycle in monkey cells (215). It appeared to be an early antigen in that its synthesis was not prevented by inhibitors of DNA synthesis.

A number of *in vitro* tests have been devised in efforts to detect SV40 TSTA. The antigen(s) detected by these *in vitro* tests will be designated collectively as surface or "S" antigen(s). SV40 S antigen was first demonstrated on the surface of viable SV40-transformed cells using the indirect immunofluorescence test and sera from hamsters which had rejected transplants of SV40-transformed cells (595). S antigen was specific for SV40; the antibody did not react with either normal cells or those transformed by heterologous viruses. S antigen has since been demonstrated using the mixed hemadsorption technique (259, 396), colony inhibition assays (597), and cytotoxicity tests (558, 652). It has been distinguished from TSTA since some transplantable hamster cell lines exist which carry S activity but lack detectable amounts of TSTA (596, 652).

Some derepressed embryonic antigens are present on the surface of SV40-transformed cells, as well. Sera from normal pregnant hamsters reacted with the S antigen of SV40-transformed cells (146). Other recent studies (260) have suggested that one S antigen reaction is due to a normal cell antigen which is specifically unmasked during transformation. After brief treatment with trypsin, spontaneously oncogenic or polyoma virus-transformed cells were found to react with SV40 S antibody. Also shown to be cryptic in normal cells were the "tumor-specific" surface sites demonstrated by agglutination tests using agglutinin isolated from wheat germ lipase (85). The agglutinin binding sites could be unmasked in normal cells by treatment with trypsin. They were not specific for any given tumor virus (for a detailed discussion of the relationship of the S antigen(s) to each other and TSTA, see 98).

4. Rescue of the Transforming Viral Genome

Cells transformed either *in vivo* or *in vitro* by SV40 are generally virus-free. However, it is possible to occasionally recover small amounts of infectious virus from some transformed cell lines (Table 11.8). Occasional tumors and cell lines spontaneously release small amounts of infectious virus (16, 65, 202, 520, 521). Minute amounts of virus found in extracts of such tumors amounted at most to $10^{3.3}$ tissue culture infectious dose 50 ($TCID_{50}$)/gm of tumor tissue. Induction

TABLE 11.8
SPECTRUM OF ABILITY TO RESCUE VIRUS FROM SV40-TRANSFORMED CELLS

Category of virogenic state of transformed cells	Detection of infectious SV40				
	Spontaneous release	Induction by chemicals	Cell contact	Cell fusion	DNA transfer
1	+	+	+	+	+
2	0	+	+	+	+
3	0	0	+	+	+
4	0	0	0	+	+
5	0	0	0	0	+
6	0	0	0	0	0

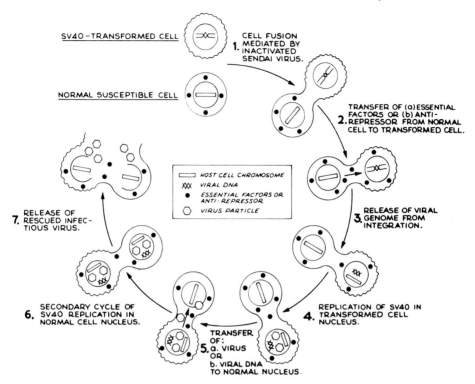

Fig. 11.8. Process of rescue of infectious SV40 from transformed cells following fusion with susceptible cells. (From "Review of Medical Microbiology," with permission of Lange Medical Publications, Los Altos, Calif.).

attempts using procedures known to induce lysogenic bacteria to produce infectious bacteriophages, such as exposure to mitomycin C, proflavine, hydrogen peroxide, and X-irradiation, were only minimally effective when applied to SV40 tumor cells (200, 506, 521). Combinations of inducing agents were not more effective at induction of infectious SV40 than were the individual agents alone. In addition, there was no dose-response relationship between the concentration of inducer employed and the yield of virus (506). Yields of SV40 following induction of mitomycin C were in the range of 10–1000 PFU/10^6 cells. Thus, only the very rare tumor cell had been induced to release infectious virus in those experiments.

Recovery of infectious SV40 was more efficient if the tumor cells were placed in direct contact with susceptible indicator cells, such as primary African green monkey cells (201). The sensitivity of the indicator cell system was increased by the use of inactivated Sendai virus to form heterokaryons (250) of tumor and indicator cells (201, 346, 638) (Fig. 11.8). The fusion technique increased the yield of virus about 1000-fold over simple cocultivation, but the vast majority of the heterokaryons were nonproductive (346, 638). Although one of the most sensitive means of virus rescue currently available, it only rarely succeeds in inducing a tumor cell to produce virus. The frequency of successful virus recoveries and the amount of virus rescued in the fusion experiments has been observed (a) to vary widely between clonal lines of transformed cells derived from the same parental cell line (638), (b) to vary at different passage levels of the same clone (638), (c) not to correlate with the number of viral DNA equivalents estimated to be present in each transformed cell (647), and (d) not to be dependent upon the multiplicity of infection at the time transformation occurred (331).

It is possible to rescue infectious SV40 by the inoculation of chromosomal DNA from an SV40-transformed cell line into permissive simian cells in the presence of diethylaminoethyl (DEAE)-dextran (81). The actual DNA extraction procedure employed varied but relatively large amounts of the transformed cell DNA were required (>10 μg/culture of 10^6 cells) to effect rescue of SV40 by passage in monkey cells. Virus was recovered from three different species of SV40-transformed cells by the "DNA transfer" method; the efficiency of virus recovery varied from about 50 to 80% of the trials using various cell lines as the source of the donor DNA. It appeared that the DNA transfer method was recovering the integrated viral genome because (1) the infectious DNA from transformed cells was found in the "Hirt pellet" (282) of precipitated cellular DNA rather than the supernate where free SV40 DNA appears, and (2) the infectivity was inactivated by boiling which does not destroy free SV40 circular DNA. The DNA transfer method succeeded in rescuing virus from a number of cell lines which were nonyielders in fusion experiments. The mechanism of rescue of the integrated viral genome, as well as the applicability of the method to other transformed cell systems, remains to be determined.

"Partial" induction of one SV40-transformed cell line has been achieved by heat shock. Exposure to 45°C for 30 minutes induced the synthesis of SV40 viral antigen, but not infectious virus, in transformed BSC-1 cells (378). The mechanism of this heat induction phenomenon is not clear, but a plausible explanation is that only a portion of the transforming viral genome has been derepressed and possibly only one of the viral coat protein polypeptides synthesized (379). It is not yet known whether the heat induction procedure results in the detachment of an integrated viral genome prior to capsid antigen synthesis.

In general, virus which has been recovered from tumor cells has resembled the parental transforming virus (135, 584, 610). However, distinctive genetic markers were not available for those studies. In one interesting exception (607), rescued virus was more efficient at transformation than the parental type. It was then postulated that the enhanced efficiency of transformation of the rescued virus could be due either to a selection of more efficient transforming viruses from the original stock or to some host-induced modification of the virus.

An important question crucial to an understanding of the process of viral carcinogenesis is the mechanism by which transformed cells prevent the completion of the virus replicative cycle. Four hypotheses can be proposed: (a) A virus-specific "repressor" is synthesized and the presence of this material blocks the replicative cycle. (b) The transformed cells lack some essential factor required by the virus for replication. (c) Defective viral genomes which are inherently unable to replicate because of a lack of certain genetic information are

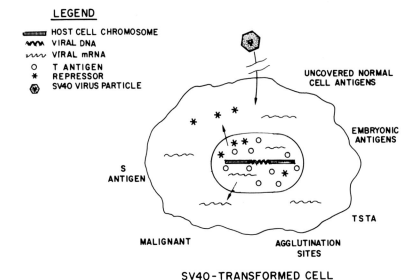

Fig. 11.9. Schematic representation of an SV40-transformed cell. (From Butel *et al.*, *Advan. Cancer Res.* **15**, 1, 1972).

the transforming agents. (d) An excision system required to release the viral genome from integration is absent. Based on the information available regarding transformed permissive cells, it is difficult to distinguish between the alternate hypotheses.

A specific "repressor," protein in nature, was found in cells of different species transformed by SV40, as well as in cells productively or abortively infected by SV40 (100, 101). However, other investigators have failed to obtain results compatible with the existence of a cytoplasmic virus-specific repressor (33, 96, 300, 334, 581).

The majority of transformed monkey and human cell lines were susceptible to superinfection by SV40 DNA even though some were resistant to challenge with complete SV40. Therefore, it appears that transformed cells can possess all the necessary SV40 replication factors. Some SV40-transformed monkey kidney cell lines, as well as many SV40-transformed human cell lines, yield infectious virus under appropriate rescue conditions (16, 81, 333, 346). Therefore, one cannot conclude that permissive cells can be transformed only by defective particles. The mechanisms by which the transformed state and the integration of the viral genome are maintained have not yet been defined with certainty and are presently the subject of intense investigation.

To summarize the studies described above, an SV40-transformed cell is presented diagrammatically in Fig. 11.9.

5. Reversion of Transformed Cells

The transformation of a normal cell into a cancer cell has generally been held to be an irreversible change. However, examples from experimental systems ranging from plants to frogs, newts, mice, hamsters, and humans, show that the reversal of the neoplastic state can and does occur (82). For this chapter, only those tumors induced by viruses will be considered with respect to the property of reversion.

Treatment of transformed cells with FUdR at different cell densities resulted in the selection of certain cell variants which exhibited a flattened morphology, attained lower saturation densities, and, with the two variants tested, reduced tumor-producing capacity *in vivo* (458). This particular study included 3T3 mouse cells transformed by either SV40 or polyoma and a hamster tumor cell line originating from a polyoma virus-induced tumor. The variant clones retained the virus-specific T antigens and, with at least one derivative cell line, still yielded infectious SV40 following fusion with monkey kidney cells. Similar contact-inhibited variants were isolated from SV40-transformed 3T3 cells by treatment with the plant lectin, concanavalin A (116). These revertants synthesized SV40 T antigen and yielded virus after fusion with monkey cells. It would be informative to determine the transforming capabilities of the rescued viruses. Such experiments would indicate whether the observed reversion was due to a mutation of one or more essential genes of the transforming virus or whether reversion was due, instead, to an alteration in the expression of the essential virus genes in the transformed cells.

Hamster embryo fibroblasts transformed by polyoma virus have reportedly undergone a reversion of properties characteristic of transformation (296, 468–472). These variants showed a decreased cloning efficiency in soft agar, a decreased saturation density, and a loss of the ability to multiply at 41°C. The variants also acquired the ability to form colonies on glutaraldehyde-fixed normal cells, manifested contact inhibition toward one another, and inhibited the parental transformed cells. The variant cells had an altered cell surface membrane in that they were no longer agglutinated by the carbohydrate-binding protein concanavalin A. The variants produced *in vitro* were less tumorigenic than the parental transformed cells, while those produced *in vivo* were more tumorigenic. All the variant cells continued to synthesize polyoma T antigen. Eight different variant cell lines were shown to have suffered a partial or complete loss of detectable levels of polyoma-specific transplantation antigen. Further, it was observed that the reversion was initially unstable but that it could be stabilized by inhibiting cell multiplication to prevent a crowded condition.

Some revertant cells support the hypothesis (523) that the presence of the transplantation antigen on the cell surface results in a change in the control mechanism for cell replication. However, there are published observations which do not support that hypothesis. Hare (249) reported that the lp-D strain of polyoma virus does not induce virus-specific transplantation immunity in weanling hamsters, yet it is oncogenic. Furthermore, cells derived from lp-D-induced tumors do not contain polyoma transplantation antigen. The sp-D strain of polyoma virus, also lacking the marker for TSTA, was able to efficiently transform cells *in vitro*. A variety of cell lines were analyzed for maximum population density, inhibition by normal cells, serum requirement, and growth in soft agar, and attempts were made to correlate such properties with heterotransplantability

(154). It was concluded that none of the properties studied was a valid *in vitro* criterion for predicting tumorigenicity. However, it would be interesting to do such a study within a single species, e.g., SV40-transformed hamster cells, the *in vitro* properties of which could then be correlated with transplantability *in vivo* in weanling hamsters.

Some revertant cells (380) appeared to have lost the viral genes present in the parental cells. The revertant cells were less tumorigenic and both polyoma-specific T and transplantation antigens were lost or reduced. The cells could be retransformed by polyoma virus. This latter fact ruled out the possibility that reversion was a consequence of the loss of cell genes required for the expression of the transformed phenotype.

The involvement of cellular genes in the phenotypic expression of the transformed state was directly implicated (490) when mutagenized SV40 was used to transform 3T3 cells, followed by a procedure employing FUdR to select for cells temperature-sensitive (ts) for the transformed phenotype. It was hoped that such a procedure would select cells transformed by viral mutants affected in genes for transformation. Several cell lines were isolated which were ts for several parameters of cell transformation. However, when infectious SV40 was recovered from the ts cells by fusion, it was similar to wild-type virus with respect to growth and transforming abilities. These results suggest, then, that the selected cells were mutated in a host cell gene, rather than a viral gene. A more recent study has revealed that the ts cells can be transformed by M-MSV under nonpermissive conditions (489). These data reveal that the ts cells have not irreversibly lost their ability to express any transformed phenotype at the elevated temperature.

The value of studying cells transformed by a ts virus is illustrated by the elegant studies with the Ts-a mutant of polyoma virus (630); 3T3 cells transformed by Ts-a display a transformed phenotype at 38.5°C. However, when shifted to the permissive temperature of 31°C, a large proportion of the cells start producing virus. Of interest is the observation that 40% of the viral DNA synthesized after such induction is in the form of oligomeric molecules (117). Although the Ts-a function has not been identified, it is apparently required both for activation of virus in the transformed cell and for the initiation of DNA replication.

"Reversion" of certain properties was observed when cells transformed by a ts mutant of polyoma virus were shifted to the nonpermissive temperature. Mouse cells transformed by mutant ts-3 were found to be temperature-dependent with respect to loss of contact inhibition as measured by DNA synthesis. Two other properties of transformed cells (growth in soft agar and serum requirements) were not rendered temperature-dependent (152). Hamster cells transformed by the same mutant displayed the cell surface alteration characterized by enhanced agglutination by concanavalin A only at the permissive temperature; the surface alteration reverted to normal when the cells were grown at the elevated temperature (155). These results suggest that the two properties studied above are under the control of the viral genome.

From the few scattered reports available, one can conclude that reversion of virus-transformed cells probably can and does occur. Some appear to have detected complete reversion, possibly as a consequence of the loss of the transforming viral genes. Some of the other observed cases of reversion would more accurately be denoted partial reversion in that some phenotypic properties were altered but viral-specific antigens were still present. In these latter examples, transplantability of the cells was sometimes lessened and sometimes increased. The available data are too few and too preliminary at this time to prompt any generalizations about either the properties of cells which have reverted, or the mechanisms of the observed reversion.

IV. Viruses and Human Cancer

The progress made in understanding viral carcinogenesis in animals has offered new approaches in the quest for the possible viral etiology of at least some human cancers. Several reviews dealing with the possible role of viruses in human carcinogenesis have been published in recent years (12, 68, 165, 387, 484) and the subject has been discussed in detail by Gross (234). Some of the more recent developments in these areas are discussed below.

A. Studies Based on the Models of Oncornavirus Tumorigenesis in Animals

Early studies on human leukemias and human solid tumors revealed some similarities to animal malignancies induced by oncornaviruses. Particles similar to C-type oncornaviruses were detected by electron microscopy in cells or plasma of patients with leukemia and in solid tumors of man such as Hodgkin's lymphoma, lymphosarcomas, and sarcomas (see review 234). Similar particles have been reported in some cell lines derived from human malignancies by electron microscopy (234, 410) or by labeling the cells with radioactive uridine and measuring the release of particles with a density in sucrose gradients of 1.16–1.18 gm/cm^3 (609). However, the significance of these findings has been disputed and the biological activity of the particles resembling C-type virions and detected in either tumor tissue or in cultured tumor cells is yet to be demonstrated (51, 387, 416, 455, 463, 557).

Following the model of activation experiments in the animal model systems described in Section II,H, similar findings were reported with cell lines derived from human sarcomas (571, 572). Treatment of the cultured cells with IUdR and dimethyl sulfoxide resulted in the detection by electron microscopy of particles resembling C-type oncornavirions. However, information is insufficient to evaluate these findings, especially since, unlike C-type oncornavirions, the particles were found to bud from the endoplasmic reticulum and their biological activity remains unknown.

It was recently reported that cells derived from an embryonal human rhabdomyosarcoma (and free of C-type particles) induced disseminated rhabdomyosarcomas (with a chromosomal pattern indicating human origin) in kittens following prenatal inoculation. A cell line derived from one of these tumors revealed C-type virus that appears to be different from the known feline oncornaviruses (388). The agent, named RD-114 virus (see Sections II,A, D, and E), has been propagated in cultures of diverse origin including feline, human, and rodent cells (390). As discussed earlier (see above 3 sections), serological and enzyme studies indicated that the virus is distinct from the known oncornaviruses. However, on the basis of available data, it is impossible at present to ascertain that RD-114 virus is of human origin, especially since unpublished observations (564) show that the viral RNA appears to have nucleotide sequences complementary to the DNA of feline cells but not to the DNA of human cells.

Particles resembling the murine mammary tumor virus (B-type particles) were recently detected in human mammary cancer and in the milk of Parsi women (a population in India with a very high incidence of mammary cancer) and of American women with a family history of mammary cancer (407). However, later studies by the same group (528) seem to question the validity of the morphological observations. Even though the infectious nature of these particles remains to be determined, evidence suggests that they contain high molecular weight RNA (70 S) and reverse transcriptase enzyme activity characteristic of oncornaviruses (548). This work has been aided by the development of a method for simultaneous detection of the enzyme activity and the high molecular weight RNA of known oncornavirions (546). Preliminary data suggest a relationship between the human particles and the murine mammary tumor virus (MTV). Sera of women with mammary cancer were reported to neutralize the activity of MTV (102), and rabbit antisera to purified MTV were reported to precipitate a soluble antigen in sera of women with mammary cancer (411). Furthermore, the DNA synthesized *in vitro* by the enzyme of MTV (using MTV RNA as a template) was found to hybridize with polysomal RNA obtained from human mammary adenocarcinomas. No such hybridization was observed with RNA derived from other human malignancies or normal tissues, and in addition the DNA product of the reverse transcriptases of the Rauscher strain of murine leukemia virus (R-MuLV) or of avian myeloblastosis virus failed to hybridize with the RNA from the human mammary adenocarcinoma (18). It was further reported that the RNA in extracts from human mammary adenocarcinomas is a 70 S component encapsidated together with RNA-directed DNA polymerase in a particle with the density characteristic of oncornavirions. The DNA synthesized *in vitro* by the human 70 S RNA-enzyme complex hybridized specifically with the RNA of MTV (20).

Using the same procedures, the above group of workers reported the presence of RNA complementary to the RNA of R-MuLV (but not to that of MTV) in other human malignancies unrelated to breast cancer. DNA obtained from R-MuLV by the use of reverse transcription *in vitro* was found to hybridize with RNA obtained from cells of various leukemias (261), lymphomas (262), and sarcomas (347). Further, the RNA in cells from various human leukemias is a 70 S RNA complexed with reverse transcriptase and the DNA synthesized from the complex hybridized specifically with the RNA of R-MuLV but not with the RNA of MTV or of avian myeloblastosis virus (44). These results appear to corroborate the reports (187, 538) on the presence of reverse transcriptase in cells of patients with acute lymphoblastic leukemia. However further work is needed to characterize the enzyme found in leukemic cells as the possibility that it may be a cellular enzyme has not been ruled out (538).

As indicated earlier, the role that the reverse transcriptase of the known animal oncornaviruses may play in viral carcinogenesis is not clear at present. The above findings with human malignancies tend to suggest the presence of virus-related information. Further experiments are needed in which different known strains of oncornaviruses are used as a probe to ascertain the ultimate significance of virus-related RNA and enzymes in human malignancies. However, the methodology now at hand is leading to a further search for enzymic evidence of possible human oncornaviruses in human malignancies.

B. Studies Based on the Models of DNA Virus Tumorigenesis in Animals

In view of the finding that, with few exceptions, solid tumors induced in experimental animals by papovaviruses and adenoviruses are free of infectious virus or of infectious nucleic acid, it is not surprising that innumerable attempts to isolate viruses from a variety of solid human tumors have met with failure (234, 387).

Following the finding of the presence of virus-specific messenger RNA (mRNA) in DNA virus-induced (but virus-free) tumors, a search in human tumor tissues for mRNA hybridizable with the DNA of the known oncogenic virus was attempted. Special attention was given to the adenoviruses since they are oncogenic in experimental animals and are so widespread in man. However, the results to date have failed to give indication that any of the human tumors examined contain adenovirus-specific mRNA (387, 389). Further study with these and other human viruses, especially the herpesviruses known to exist in a latent state in man, may yield more definitive information.

Recently, several new agents morphologically typical of papovavirions have been isolated from patients suffering either from progressive multifocal-leukoencephalopathy (439, 642) or, in a single case, from ureteric obstruction following a renal transplant (192). The new isolates are serologically unrelated to the other papovavirus of human origin, human papilloma virus, but several have exhibited varying degrees of cross-reaction with SV40. The role these new isolates may play in human disease remains to be determined.

C. Immunological Studies

The finding of virus-induced T antigens in tumors (or in transformed cells) and of T antibodies in the tumor-bearing animals has led to similar immunological studies in cancer of man. Attempts made to test the sera of cancer patients for the presence of complement-fixing or immunofluorescence antibodies to the T antigens of SV40 or adenovirus have thus far yielded negative results (207).

Patients with melanomas, osteosarcomas, or liposarcomas develop antibodies that react by immunofluorescence with a cytoplasmic antigen present in imprints of autochthonous and homologous tumors (409, 410). The antibody has been found to react by immunofluorescence and complement fixation (employing human complement) with antigens derived from cells of such tumors propagated in tissue culture (161, 410). Similar reactivity has been found in sera of the patients' family contacts with a much greater frequency than in sera of the population at large (410). The latter finding suggests that the antibody reactions attained may be directed to a viral antigen present in the tumor cell rather than a T-type antigen. Preliminary evidence suggested the presence of leukemia C-type particles in liposarcoma cultures and a capacity of supernatant fluids from such cultures to transform normal human embryo fibroblasts (410). However, the significance of these findings awaits further study.

Carcinomas of the gastrointestinal tract have been found to contain an antigen which is absent from normal adult gut cells but present in embryonal gut cells. This antigen has been named carcinoembryonic antigen (CEA), and it is believed that its appearance in gastrointestinal carcinomas is due to genetic derepression (218, 220). The antigen can be isolated and purified from the tumor or embryonic tissue and can be detected by means of several different tests with antisera prepared in goats or rabbits. Patients with gastrointestinal carcinomas have circulating CEA presumably released from the tumor cells (218). The exact nature of this antigen and the antibody response monitored in the cancer patient remain to be determined, especially in view of contradictory results obtained by others (92, 366). Preliminary findings also suggest that tumor cells from different patients with Hodgkin's disease may contain a common antigen detectable with antisera prepared in heterologous animals (433), but further study is needed to verify these results. It also appears that cells from patients with leukemia possess antigens to which autologous humoral and cell-mediated immune reactions develop (54, 235, 354). However, it remains to be seen whether or not these reactivities are of viral nature.

The knowledge that transplantation type antigens in virus-induced tumors can be detected by an *in vitro* colony inhibition test (for review see 263) has been recently applied to the elucidation of similar antigens in some human tumors. Lymphocytes from children bearing neuroblastomas have been found to inhibit the plating efficiency of their tumor cells grown in culture. Lymphocytes of their mothers but not from unrelated controls had the same inhibitory effect (265, 266). The reaction observed is reminiscent of that mentioned above for the virus-induced animal tumor systems. However, evidence is still lacking that the antigens being measured in the neuroblastoma cells are indeed virus-induced.

Transplantation type antigens have been recently detected in various other human tumors using the colony inhibition tests with the patient's lymphocytes and cells from the autologous tumor. Tumors of certain histological types in different patients share transplantation type antigens (267). However, further well-controlled studies are needed before it can be concluded that such tumors possess common antigens. Evidence is accumulating that, similar to the animal model systems described above, patients with advanced cancer have circulating serum factors that can block the *in vitro* reaction of autologous lymphocytes in the colony inhibition test (267, 555). Further studies in this direction may lead to an understanding of the mechanisms involved in tumor progression or regression *in vivo*.

D. Herpesviruses and Human Malignancies

In recent years a great deal of attention has been focused on herpesviruses of man as potential oncogenic agents. The recently isolated and characterized herpes simplex virus type 2 has been found to be venereally transmitted in man (413, 485, 487). Seroepidemiologic studies revealed a high degree of association between infection with this virus and invasive carcinoma of the cervix. The prevalence of herpes type 2 antibody in women with the disease was found to be much higher than in matched controls (9, 10, 17, 414, 486). In some of these studies, women with cervical dysplasia and carcinoma *in situ* (considered by some to be premalignant lesions leading to invasive carcinoma) had an increased prevalence of herpes type 2 antibody. Careful follow-up of such patients as well as prospective seroepidemiologic surveys of different populations may shed further light on whether the association found is covariable or etiologic. Further support for the oncogenic potential of herpes type 2 virus has been provided in recent reports which indicate that this virus can cause malignant transformation of hamster embryo cells (147, 148).

The EB (Epstein-Barr) virus, a newly recognized and antigenically distinct member of the herpesvirus group, has been found in association with several immunoproliferative disorders of man. The virus was detected initially by electron microscopy (167) and subsequently by immunofluorescence (269) in lymphoid cell lines derived from Burkitt's lymphoma, a tumor with a predilection for the jaw and peculiar for children in Central Africa (86, 87). There are numerous reviews on the viral and immunological aspects of EB virus infection in man (164, 166, 172, 337–339, 556).

A strong association has been observed between the EB virus and two human malignancies: Burkitt's lymphoma (86, 87) and postnasal (nasopharyngeal) carcinoma, found in Chinese male populations in Southeast Asia (284). The finding of high incidence and high titers of EB antibody detectable by several different tests (338) in patients with Burkitt's lymphoma (272) and postnasal carcinoma (273) led to the assumption that the association may be etiologic.

However, subsequent seroepidemiologic surveys showed that infection with EB virus in normal populations is widespread not only in Africa and Asia, but all over the world (419, 453, 462). Furthermore, it was demonstrated that EB virus has an extreme predilection for cells of lymphoid origin. The virus has been detected with great regularity in cell lines derived not only from Burkitt's lymphoma (269) and postnasal carcinoma (127) but also those derived from peripheral blood leukocytes of patients with infectious mononucleosis (128) and various other disease entities (164) as well as from normal individuals (164, 203, 406).

A much stronger case has been made for the etiologic association between EB virus infection and infectious mononucleosis, a benign immunoproliferative disorder, for such patients reveal a seroconversion to EB virus (172, 173, 271, 418). An association has also been observed betwen EB virus and Hodgkin's disease (302), sarcoidosis (280), lupus erythematosus (174), and lepromatous leprosy (441).

The question as to whether EB virus is etiologically related to the above 2 malignancies, Burkitt's lymphoma and postnasal carcinoma, or a passenger virus present in lymphoid cells trapped within the tumor, remains unanswered at present. Indeed, other viruses, such as herpes simplex virus and reovirus, have been frequently isolated from Burkitt's lymphomas (46). On the other hand, one cannot exclude the possibility that EB virus is indeed the prime agent responsible for the induction of malignant cells *in vivo. In vitro* experiments reveal that the virus can convert virus-free normal peripheral blood leukocytes or fetal leukocytes into virus-positive cells capable of continuous growth (204, 270, 461). Some of these virus-positive cells were heterotransplantable when given in high doses to newborn mice (121).

In DNA-DNA hybridization studies, small quantities of EB viral DNA have been detected in virus-free biopsy specimens of Burkitt's lymphoma and postnasal carcinoma (657). These findings are similar to those obtained with cell lines derived from the same tumors (421, 656, 658) but at present they still do not answer the question whether the partial viral genome detected is the cause of the malignancy or results from a secondary infection of the tumor cells by the virus.

The techniques for searching for viruses in human cancer have become more sophisticated than those used in the virus diagnostic laboratory. However, investigators must still contend with the problem of identifying "passenger" viruses present in the cancer but not in a causal relationship. Of even greater concern is the converse, the problem of identifying a virus no longer present in the cancer that it may have caused. Some of the modern approaches that have proved fruitful in the study of viral carcinogenesis in animals have been outlined in this chapter.

Acknowledgment

The authors acknowledge the able assistance of Mrs. Connie Dunn in the preparation of this manuscript.

Dr. Butel is the recipient of Faculty Research Award PRA-95 from the American Cancer Society.

References

1. Aaronson, S. A. (1970). *J. Virol.* **6**, 393–399.
2. Aaronson, S. A. (1971). *Virology* **44**, 29–36.
3. Aaronson, S. A., and Rowe, W. P. (1970). *Virology* **42**, 9–19.
4. Aaronson, S. A., and Todaro, G. J. (1969). *Science* **166**, 390–391.
5. Aaronson, S. A., and Weaver, C. A. (1971). *J. Gen. Virol.* **13**, 245–252.

6. Aaronson, S. A., Parks, W. P., Scolnick, E. M., and Todaro, G. J. (1971). *Proc. Nat. Acad. Sci. U.S.* **68**, 920–924.

7. Aaronson, S. A., Todaro, G. J., and Scolnick, E. M. (1971). *Science* **174**, 157–159.

8. Abelev, G. I., and Elgort, D. A. (1970). *Int. J. Cancer* **6**, 145–152.

9. Adam, E., Levy, A. H., Rawls, W. E., and Melnick, J. L. (1971). *J. Nat. Cancer Inst.* **47**, 941–951.

10. Adam, E., Sharma, S. D., Zeigler, O., Iwamoto, K., Melnick, J. L., Levy, A. H., and Rawls, W. E. (1972). *J. Nat. Cancer Inst.* **48**, 65–72.

11. Allen, D. W. (1969). *Virology* **38**, 32–41.

12. Allen, D. W., and Cole, P. (1972). *New England J. Med.* **286**, 70–82.

13. Allen, D. W., Sarma, P. S., Niall, H. D., and Sauer, R. (1970). *Proc. Nat. Acad. Sci. U.S.* **67**, 837–842.

14. Aloni, Y., Winocour, E., and Sachs, L. (1968). *J. Mol. Biol.* **31**, 415–429.

15. Andrewes, C., and Pereira, H. G. (1967). "Viruses of Vetebrates," 2nd ed. Williams and Wilkins, Baltimore, Maryland.

16. Ashkenazi, A., and Melnick, J. L. (1963). *J. Nat. Cancer Inst.* **30**, 1227–1265.

17. Aurelian, L., Royston, I., and Davis, H. J. (1970). *J. Nat. Cancer Inst.* **45**, 455–464.

18. Axel, R., Schlom, J., and Spiegelman, S. (1972). *Nature (London)* **235**, 32–36.

19. Axel, R., Schlom, J., and Spiegelman, S. (1972). *Proc. Nat. Acad. Sci. U.S.* **69**, 535–538.

20. Axel, R., Gulati, S. C., and Spiegelman, S. (1972). *Proc. Nat. Acad. Sci. U.S.* **69**, 3133–3137.

21. Bader, J. P. (1972). *Virology* **48**, 485–493.

22. Bader, J. P. (1972). *J. Virol.* **10**, 267–276.

23. Bader, J. P., and Brown, N. R. (1971). *Nature New Biol.* **234**, 11–12.

24. Bader, J. P., and Steck, T. L. (1969). *J. Virol.* **4**, 454–459.

25. Bader, J. P., Brown, N. R., and Bader, A. V. (1970). *Virology* **41**, 718–728.

26. Bader, J. P., Steck, T. L., and Kakefuda, T. (1970). *Current Topics Microbiol. Immunol.* **51**, 105–113.

27. Balduzzi, P., and Morgan, H. R. (1970). *J. Virol.* **5**, 470–477.

28. Baltimore, D. (1970). *Nature (London)* **226**, 1209–1211.

29. Baltimore, D., and Smoler, D. (1971). *Proc. Nat. Acad. Sci. U.S.* **68**, 1507–1511.

30. Baluda, M. A. (1972). *Proc. Nat. Acad. Sci. U.S.* **69**, 576–580.

31. Baluda, M. A., and Goetz, I. E. (1961). *Virology* **15**, 185–199.

32. Barbanti-Brodano, G., Swetly, P., and Koprowski, H. (1970). *J. Virol.* **6**, 78–86.

33. Barbanti-Brodano, G., Swetly, P., and Koprowski, H. (1970). *J. Virol.* **6**, 644–651.

34. Basilico, C., and Burstin, S. J. (1971). *J. Virol.* **7**, 802–812.

35. Basilico, C., and Di Mayorca, G. (1965). *Proc. Nat. Acad. Sci. U.S.* **54**, 125–127.

36. Bassin, R. H., Simons, P. J., Chesterman, F. C., and Harvey, J. J. (1968). *Int. J. Cancer* **3**, 265–272.

37. Bassin, R. H., Tuttle, N., and Fischinger, P. J. (1970). *Int. J. Cancer* **6**, 95–107.

38. Bassin, R. H., Phillips, L. A., Kramer, M. J., Haapala, D. K., Peebles, P. T., Nomura, S., and Fischinger, P. J. (1971). *Proc. Nat. Acad. Sci. U.S.* **68**, 1520–1524.

39. Bassin, R. H., Tuttle, N., and Fischinger, P. J. (1971). *Nature (London)* **229**, 564–566.

40. Bauer, H., and Bolognesi, D. P. (1970). *Virology* **42**, 1113–1126.

41. Bauer, H., and Janda, H. (1967). *Virology* **33**, 483–490.

42. Baum, S. G., and Fox, R. I. (1971). *Proc. Nat. Acad. Sci. U.S.* **68**, 1525–1529.

43. Baum, S. G., Reich, P. R., Hybner, C. J., Rowe, W. P., and Weissman, S. M. (1966). *Proc. Nat. Acad. Sci. U.S.* **56**, 1509–1515.

44. Baxt, W., Hehlmann, R., and Spiegelman, S. (1972). *Nature New Biol.* **240**, 72–75.

45. Becker, Y., Dym, H., and Sarov, I. (1968). *Virology* **36**, 184–192.

46. Bell, T. M. (1967). *Prog. Med. Virol.* **9**, 1–34.

47. Benjamin, T. L. (1965). *Proc. Nat. Acad. Sci. U.S.* **54**, 121–124.

48. Benjamin, T. L. (1966). *J. Mol. Biol.* **16**, 359–373.

49. Bentvelzen, P., Daams, J. H., Hageman, P., and Calafat, J. (1970). *Proc. Nat. Acad. Sci. U.S.* **67**, 377–384.
50. Bentvelzen, P., Daams, J. H., Hageman, P., Calafat, J., and Timmermans, A. (1972). *J. Nat. Cancer Inst.* **48**, 1089–1094.
51. Benyesh-Melnick, M., Smith, K. O., and Fernbach, D. J. (1964). *J. Nat. Cancer Inst.* **33**, 571–579.
52. Berman, L. D., and Sarma, P. S. (1965). *Nature (London)* **207**, 263–265.
53. Bernhard, W. (1960). *Cancer Res.* **20**, 712–727.
54. Bias, W. B., Santos, G. W., Burke, P. J., Mullins, G. M., and Humphrey, R. L. (1972). *Science* **178**, 304–306.
55. Biggs, P. M. (1970). *In* "Comparative Leukemia Research 1969" (R. M. Dutcher, ed.), pp. 198–209. Karger, Basel.
56. Bishop, J. M., Levinson, W. E., Sullivan, D., Fanshier, L., Quintrell, N., and Jackson, J. (1970). *Virology* **42**, 927–937.
57. Bishop, J. M., Levinson, W. E., Quintrell, N., Sullivan, D., Fanshier, L., and Jackson, J. (1970). *Virology* **42**, 182–195.
58. Biswal, N., and Benyesh-Melnick, M. (1969). *Proc. Nat. Acad. Sci. U.S.* **64**, 1372–1379.
59. Biswal, N., and Benyesh-Melnick, M. (1970). *Virology* **42**, 1064–1072.
60. Biswal, N., McCain, B., and Benyesh-Melnick, M. (1970). *In* "The Biology of Oncogenic Viruses" (L. G. Silvestri, ed.), pp. 221–231. North-Holland Pub., London.
61. Biswal, N., McCain, B., and Benyesh-Melnick, M. (1971). *Virology* **45**, 697–706.
61a. Bittner, J. J. (1936). *Science* **84**, 162.
62. Biquard, J.-M., and Vigier, P. (1972). *Virology* **47**, 444–455.
63. Black, P. H. (1966). *Virology* **28**, 760–763.
64. Black, P. H. (1968). *Ann. Rev. Microbiol.* **22**, 391–426.
65. Black, P. H., and Rowe, W. P. (1963). *Proc. Nat. Acad. Sci. U.S.* **50**, 606–613.
66. Black, P. H., and White, B. J. (1967). *J. Exp. Med.* **125**, 629–646.
67. Black, P. H., Berman, L. D., and Dixon, C. B. (1969). *J. Virol.* **4**, 694–703.
68. Black, P. H., Burns, W. H., and Hirsch, M. S. (1971). *In* "Viruses Affecting Man and Animals" (M. Sanders and M. Schaeffer, eds.), pp. 191–205. Green, St. Louis, Missouri.
69. Blair, P. B. (1968). *Current Topics Microbiol. Immunol.* **45**, 1–69.
70. Blair, P. B. (1971). *Israel J. Med. Sci.* **7**, 161–186.
71. Blair, C. D., and Duesberg, P. H. (1968). *Nature (London)* **220**, 396–399.
72. Boettiger, D., and Temin, H. M. (1970). *Nature (London)* **228**, 622–624.
73. Boiron, M., Levy, J. P., and Thomas, M. (1965). *Ann. Inst. Pasteur* **108**, 298–305.
74. Boiron, M., Levy, J. P., and Peries, J. (1967). *Progr. Med. Virol.* **9**, 341–391.
75. Bolognesi, D. P., and Bauer, H. (1970). *Virology* **42**, 1097–1112.
76. Bolognesi, D. P., Bauer, H., Gelderblom, H., and Hüper, G. (1972). *Virology* **47**, 551–566.
77. Bolognesi, D. P., Gelderblom, H., Bauer, H., Mölling, K., and Hüper, G. (1972). *Virology* **47**, 567–578.
78. Bonar, R. A., and Beard, J. W. (1959). *J. Nat. Cancer Inst.* **23**, 183–197.
79. Bonar, R. A., Heine, U., and Beard, J. W. (1964). *Nat. Cancer Inst. Monogr.* **17**, 589–614.
80. Bonar, R. A., Sverak, L., Bolognesi, D. P., Langlois, A. J., Beard, D., and Beard, J. W. (1967). *Cancer Res.* **27**, 1138–1157.
81. Boyd, V. A. L., and Butel, J. S. (1972). *J. Virol.* **10**, 399–409.
82. Braun, A. C. (1970). *Amer. Sci.* **58**, 307–320.
83. Bronson, D. L., Graham, B. J., Ludwig, H., Benyesh-Melnick, M., and Biswal, N. (1972). *Biochim. Biophys. Acta* **259**, 24–34.
84. Bujard, H. (1967). *J. Virol.* **1**, 1135–1138.
85. Burger, M. M. (1969). *Proc. Nat. Acad. Sci. U.S.* **62**, 994–1001.
86. Burkitt, D. (1962). *Brit. Med. J.* **2**, 1019–1023.
87. Burkitt, D. P. (1969). *J. Nat. Cancer Inst.* **43**, 19–28.

88. Burlingham, B. T., and Doerfler, W. (1972). *Virology* **48**, 1–13.
89. Burlingham, B. T., Doerfler, W., Pettersson, U., and Philipson, L. (1971). *J. Mol. Biol.* **60**, 45–64.
90. Burnett, J. P., and Harrington, J. A. (1968). *Proc. Nat. Acad. Sci. U.S.* **60**, 1023–1029.
91. Burnett, J. P., and Harrington, J. A. (1968). *Nature (London)* **220**, 1245.
92. Burtin, P., Martin, E., Sabine, M. C., and von Kleist, S. (1972). *J. Nat. Cancer Inst.* **48**, 25–32.
93. Butel, J. S. (1973). *Methods Cancer Res.* **8**, 287–338.
94. Butel, J. S. (1972). *J. Nat. Cancer Inst.* **48**, 285–299.
95. Butel, J. S., and Melnick, J. L. (1972). *Exp. Mol. Pathol.* **17**, 103–119.
96. Butel, J. S., Richardson, L. S., and Melnick, J. L. (1971). *Virology* **46**, 844–855.
97. Butel, J. S., Tevethia, S. S., and Nachtigal, M. (1971). *J. Immunol.* **106**, 969–974.
98. Butel, J. S., Tevethia, S. S., and Melnick, J. L. (1972). *Advan. Cancer Res.* **15**, 1–55.
99. Canaani, E., and Duesberg, P. (1972). *J. Virol.* **10**, 23–31.
100. Cassingena, R., and Tournier, P. (1968). *C. R. Acad. Sci. Paris* **267**, 2251–2254.
101. Cassingena, R., Tournier, P., May, E., Estrade, S., and Bourali, M.-F. (1969). *C. R. Acad. Sci. Paris* **268**, 2834–2837.
102. Charney, J., and Moore, D. H. (1971). *Nature (London)* **229**, 627–628.
103. Chopra, H. C., and Dutcher, R. M. (1970). *In* "Comparative Leukemia Research 1969" (R. M. Dutcher, ed.), pp. 584–592. Karger, Basel.
104. Chopra, H. C., and Mason, M. M. (1970). *Cancer Res.* **30**, 2081–2086.
105. Ciuffo, G. (1907). *Giorn. Ital. Mal. Vener.* **48**, 12–17.
106. Coffin, J. M. (1972). *J. Virol.* **10**, 153–156.
107. Coffin, J. M., and Temin, H. M. (1971). *J. Virol.* **7**, 625–634.
108. Coffin, J. M., and Temin, H. M. (1972). *J. Virol.* **9**, 766–775.
109. Coggin, J. H., Larson, V. M., and Hilleman, M. R. (1967). *Proc. Soc. Exp. Biol. Med.* **124**, 1295–1302.
110. Crawford, L. V. (1964). *J. Mol. Biol.* **8**, 489–495.
111. Crawford, L. V. (1965). *J. Mol. Biol.* **13**, 362–372.
112. Crawford, L. V. (1969). *Advan. Virus Res.* **14**, 89–148.
113. Crawford, L. V., and Black, P. H. (1964). *Virology* **24**, 388–392.
114. Crawford, L. V., and Crawford, E. M. (1963). *Virology* **21**, 258–263.
115. Creech, G. T. (1929). *J. Agr. Res.* **39**, 723–737.
116. Culp, L. A., and Black, P. H. (1972). *J. Virol.* **9**, 611–620.
117. Cuzin, F., Vogt, M., Dieckmann, M., and Berg, P. (1970). *J. Mol. Biol.* **47**, 317–333.
118. Cuzin, F., Blangy, D., and Rouget, P. (1971). *C. R. Acad. Sci. Paris* **273**, 2650–2653.
119. Dalton, A. J., de Harven, E., Dmochowski, L., Feldman, D., Haguenau, F., Harris, W. W., Howatson, A. F., Moore, D., Pitelka, D., Smith, K., Uzman, B., and Zeigel, R. (1966). *J. Nat. Cancer Inst.* **37**, 395–397.
120. Davis, B. D., Dulbecco, R., Eisen, H. N., Ginsberg, H. S., and Wood, W. B., Jr. (1967). *In* "Microbiology," pp. 1413–1444. Harper, New York.
121. Deal, D. R., Gerber, P., and Chisari, F. V. (1971). *J. Nat. Cancer Inst.* **47**, 771–780.
122. Defendi, V. (1963). *Proc. Soc. Exp. Biol. Med.* **113**, 12–16.
123. Diechman, G. I. (1969). *Advan. Cancer Res.* **12**, 101–136.
124. Deinhardt, F., Wolfe, L. G., Theilen, G. H., and Snyder, S. P. (1970). *Science* **167**, 881.
125. De Monbreun, W. A., and Goodpasture, E. W. (1932). *Amer. J. Pathol.* **8**, 43–55.
126. De-Thé, G., and O'Connor, T. E. (1966). *Virology* **28**, 713–728.
127. De Thé, G., Ambrosini, J. C., Ho, H. C., and Kwan, H. C. (1969). *Nature (London)* **221**, 770–771.
128. Diehl, V., Henle, G., Henle, W., and Kohn, G. (1968). *J. Virol.* **2**, 663–669.
129. Di Mayorca, G. A., Eddy, B. E., Stewart, S. E., Hunter, W. S., Friend, C., and Bendich, A. (1959). *Proc. Nat. Acad. Sci. U.S.* **45**, 1805–1808.
130. Dmochowski, L. (1960). *Cancer Res.* **20**, 977–1015.
131. Dougherty, R. M., and Di Stefano, H. S. (1965). *Virology* **27**, 351–359.

132. Dougherty, R. M., Di Stefano, H. S., and Roth, F. K. (1967). *Proc. Nat. Acad. Sci. U.S.* **58**, 808–817.
133. Dougherty, R. M., Marucci, A. A., and Distefano, H. S. (1972). *J. Gen. Virol.* **15**, 149–162.
134. Dreesman, G. D., Suriano, J. R., Swartz, S. K., and McCombs, R. M. (1972). *Virology* **50**, 528–534.
135. Dubbs, D. R., Kit, S., de Torres, R. A., and Anken, M. (1967). *J. Virol.* **1**, 968–979.
136. Duesberg, P. H. (1968). *Proc. Nat. Acad. Sci. U.S.* **60**, 1511–1518.
137. Duesberg, P. H. (1970). *Current Topics Microbiol. Immunol.* **51**, 79–104.
138. Duesberg, P. H., and Canaani, E. (1970). *Virology* **42**, 783–788.
139. Duesberg, P. H., and Cardiff, R. D. (1968). *Virology* **36**, 696–700.
140. Duesberg, P. H., and Vogt, P. K. (1970). *Proc. Nat. Acad. Sci. U.S.* **67**, 1673–1680.
141. Duesberg, P. H., Martin, G. S., and Vogt, P. K. (1970). *Virology* **41**, 631–646.
142. Duesberg, P., Helm, K. V. D., and Canaani, E. (1971). *Proc. Nat. Acad. Sci. U.S.* **68**, 747–751.
143. Duesberg, P., Helm, K. V. D., and Canaani, E. (1971). *Proc. Nat. Acad. Sci. U.S.* **68**, 2505–2509.
144. Duesberg, P. H., Vogt, P. K., and Canaani, E. (1971). *In* "The Biology of Oncogenic Viruses" (L. G. Silvestri, ed.), pp. 154–166. North-Holland Publ., Amsterdam.
145. Duff, R., and Rapp, F. (1970). *J. Virol.* **5**, 568–577.
146. Duff, R., and Rapp, F. (1970). *J. Immunol.* **105**, 521–523.
147. Duff, R., and Rapp, F. (1971). *Nature New Biol.* **233**, 48–50.
148. Duff, R., and Rapp, F. (1971). *J. Virol.* **8**, 469–477.
149. Duff, R., and Rapp, F. (1973). *Proc. Amer. Ass. Cancer Res.* 147–159.
150. Dulbecco, R. (1969). *Ann. Int. Med.* **70**, 1019–1030.
151. Dulbecco, R. (1969). *Science* **166**, 962–968.
152. Dulbecco, R., and Eckhart, W. (1970). *Proc. Nat. Acad. Sci. U.S.* **67**, 1775–1781.
153. Dulbecco, R., and Vogt, M. (1963). *Proc. Nat. Acad. Sci. Paris* **50**, 236–243.
154. Eagle, H., Foley, G. E., Koprowski, H., Lazarus, H., Levine, E. M., and Adams, R. A. (1970). *J. Exp. Med.* **131**, 863–879.
155. Eckhart, W., Dulbecco, R., and Burger, M. M. (1971). *Proc. Nat. Acad. Sci. U.S.* **68**, 283–286.
156. Eddy, B. E. (1964). *Progr. Exp. Tumor Res.* **4**, 1–26.
157. Eddy, B. E. (1972). *Progr. Exp. Tumor Res.* **16**, 454–496.
158. Eddy, B. E., Stewart, S. E., Young, R., and Mider, G. B. (1958). *J. Nat. Cancer Inst.* **20**, 747–756.
159. Eddy, B. E., Stewart, S. E., Stanton, M. F., and Marcotte, J. M. (1959). *J. Nat. Cancer Inst.* **22**, 161–171.
160. Eddy, B. E., Borman, G. S., Grubbs, G. E., and Young, R. D. (1962). *Virology* **17**, 65–75.
161. Eilber, F. R., and Morton, D. L. (1970). *Nature (London)* **225**, 1137–1138.
162. Ellerman, V., and Bang, O. (1908). *Zentralbl. Bakteriol. Parasitenk.* **46**, 595–609.
163. Enders, J. F. (1965). *In* "The Harvey Lectures," Series 59, pp. 113–154. Academic Press, New York.
164. Epstein, M. A. (1970). *Advan. Cancer Res.* **13**, 383–411.
165. Epstein, M. A. (1971). *Lancet* **1**, 1344–1347.
166. Epstein, M. A. (1972). *In* "Oncogenesis and Herpesviruses" (P. M. Biggs, G. De-Thé, and L. N. Payne, eds.), pp. 261–268. Int. Agency for Res. on Cancer, Lyon.
167. Epstein, M. A., Achong, B. G., and Barr, Y. M. (1964). *Lancet* **1**, 702–703.
168. Erikson, R. L. (1969). *Virology* **37**, 124–131.
169. Erikson, E., and Erikson, R. L. (1970). *J. Mol. Biol.* **52**, 387–390.
170. Erikson, E., and Erikson, R. L. (1971). *J. Virol.* **8**, 254–256.
170a. Estes, M. K. Personal communication.
171. Estes, M. K., Huang, E.-S., and Pagano, J. S. (1971). *J. Virol.* **7**, 635–641.
172. Evans, A. S. (1971). *J. Infect. Dis.* **124**, 330–337.

173. Evans, A. S., Niederman, J. C., and McCollum, R. W. (1968). *New England J. Med.* **279**, 1121–1127.
174. Evans, A. S., Rothfield, N. F., and Niederman, J. C. (1971). *Lancet* **1**, 167–168.
175. Fenner, F. (1968). "The Biology of Animal Viruses." Academic Press, New York.
176. Fields, B. N., and Joklik, W. K. (1969). *Virology* **37**, 335–342.
177. Finkel, M. P., Biskis, B. O., and Jinkins, P. B. (1966). *Science* **151**, 698–701.
178. Fischer, H., and Sauer, G. (1972). *J. Virol.* **9**, 1–9.
179. Fischinger, P. J., and O'Connor, T. E. (1968). *J. Nat. Cancer Inst.* **40**, 1199–1212.
180. Fischinger, P. J., and O'Connor, T. E. (1969). *Science* **165**, 714–716.
181. Fischinger, P. J., Nomura, S., Peebles, P. T., Haapala, D. K., and Bassin, R. H. (1972). *Science* **176**, 1033–1035.
182. Fischinger, P. J., Schäfer, W., and Seifert, E. (1972). *Virology* **47**, 229–235.
183. Fleissner, E. (1971). *J. Virol.* **8**, 778–785.
184. Frearson, P. M., and Crawford, L. V. (1972). *J. Gen. Virol.* **14**, 141–155.
185. Friend, C. (1957). *J. Exp. Med.* **105**, 307–318.
186. Friis, R. R., Toyoshima, K., and Vogt, P. K. (1971). *Virology* **43**, 375–389.
187. Gallo, R. C., Yang, S. S., and Ting, R. C. (1970). *Nature (London)* **228**, 927–929.
188. Gantt, R. R., Stromberg, K. J., and De Oca, F. M. (1971). *Nature (London)* **234**, 35–37.
189. Garapin, A.-C., Fanshier, L., Leong, J.-A., Jackson, J., Levinson, W., and Bishop, J. M. (1971). *J. Virol.* **7**, 227–232.
190. Garapin, A. C., Leong, J., Fanshier, L., Levinson, W. E., and Bishop, J. M. (1971). *Biochem. Biophys. Res. Commun.* **42**, 919–925.
191. Gardner, M. B., Rongey, R. W., Arnstein, P., Estes, J. D., Sarma, P., Huebner, R. J., and Rickard, C. G. (1970). *Nature (London)* **226**, 807–809.
192. Gardner, S. D., Field, A. M., Coleman, D. V., and Hulme, B. (1971). *Lancet* 1253–1257.
193. Gazdar, A. F., Phillips, L. A., Sarma, P. S., Peebles, P. T., and Chopra, H. C. (1971). *Nature New Biol.* **234**, 69–72.
194. Gazdar, A. F., Chopra, H. C., and Sarma, P. S. (1972). *Int. J. Cancer* **9**, 219–233.
195. Gazdar, A. F., Sarma, P. S., and Bassin, R. H. (1972). *Int. J. Cancer* **9**, 234–241.
196. Geering, G., Old, L. J., and Boyse, E. A. (1966). *J. Exp. Med.* **124**, 753–772.
197. Geering, G., Aoki, T., and Old, L. J. (1970). *Nature (London)* **226**, 265–266.
198. Gelb, L. D., Aaronson, S. A., and Martin, M. A. (1971). *Science* **172**, 1353–1355.
199. Gelb, L. D., Kohne, D. E., and Martin, M. A. (1971). *J. Mol. Biol.* **57**, 129–145.
200. Gerber, P. (1964). *Science* **145**, 833.
201. Gerber, P. (1966). *Virology* **28**, 501–509.
202. Gerber, P., and Kirschstein, R. L. (1962). *Virology* **18**, 582–588.
203. Gerber, P., and Monroe, J. H. (1968). *J. Nat. Cancer Inst.* **40**, 855–866.
204. Gerber, P., Whang-Peng, J., and Monroe, J. H. (1969). *Proc. Nat. Acad. Sci. U.S.* **63**, 740–747.
205. Gerwin, B. I., Todaro, J. J., Zeve, V., Scolnick, E. M., and Aaronson, S. A. (1970). *Nature (London)* **228**, 435–438.
206. Gilden, R. V., and Oroszlan, S. (1972). *Proc. Nat. Acad. Sci. U.S.* **69**, 1021–1025.
207. Gilden, R. V., Kern, J., Lee, Y. K., Rapp, F., Melnick, J. L., Riggs, J. L., Lennette, E. H., Zbar, B., Rapp, H. J., Turner, H. C. and Huebner, R. J. (1970). *Amer. J. Epidemiol.* **91**, 500–509.
208. Gilden, R. V., Lee, Y. K., Oroszlan, S., Walker, J. L., and Huebner, R. J. (1970). *Virology* **41**, 187–190.
209. Gilden, R. V., Oroszlan, S., and Huebner, R. J. (1971). *Virology* **43**, 722–724.
210. Gilden, R. V., Oroszlan, S., and Huebner, R. J. (1971). *Nature New Biol.* **231**, 107–108.
211. Gilden, R. V., Parks, W. P., Huebner, R. J., and Todaro, G. J. (1971). *Nature (London)* **233**, 102–103.
212. Gillespie, D., Marshall, S., and Gallo, R. C. (1972). *Nature New Biol.* **236**, 227–231.
213. Ginsberg, H. S. (1969). *In* "The Biochemistry of Viruses" (H. B. Levy, ed.), pp. 329–359. Dekker, New York.

214. Girardi, A. J. (1965). *Proc. Nat. Acad. Sci. U.S.* **54**, 445–451.
215. Girardi, A. J., and Defendi, V. (1970). *Virology* **42**, 688–698.
216. Girardi, A. J., Sweet, B. H., Slotnick, V. B., and Hilleman, M. R. (1962). *Proc. Soc. Exp. Biol. Med.* ·**109**, 649–660.
217. Goffe, A. P., Hale, J., and Gardner, P. S. (1961). *Lancet* **1**, 612.
218. Gold, P. (1971). *Ann. Rev. Med.* **22**, 85–94.
219. Goldé, A. (1970). *Virology* **40**, 1022–1029.
220. Gold, P., and Freedman, S. O. (1965). *J. Exp. Med.* **121**, 439–462.
221. Goodman, N. C., and Spiegelman, S. (1971). *Proc. Nat. Acad. Sci. U.S.* **68**, 2203–2206.
222. Grady, L., Axelrod, D., and Trilling, D. (1970). *Proc. Nat. Acad. Sci. U.S.* **67**, 1886–1893.
223. Graf, T., Bauer, H., Gelderblom, H., and Bolognesi, D. P. (1971). *Virology* **43**, 427–441.
224. Graffi, A., Schramm, T., Bender, E., Graffi, I., Horn, K. H., and Bierwolf, D. (1968). *Brit. J. Cancer* **22**, 577–581.
225. Graham, B. J., Ludwig, H., Bronson, D. L., Benyesh-Melnick, M., and Biswal, N. (1972). *Biochim. Biophys. Acta* **259**, 13–23.
226. Granoff, A. (1972). *In* "Oncogenesis and Herpesviruses" (P. M. Biggs, G. De Thé, and L. N. Payne, eds.), pp. 171–182. Int. Agency for Res. on Cancer, Lyon.
227. Green, M. (1970). *Ann. Rev. Biochem.* **39**, 701–756.
228. Green, M., and Cartas, M. (1972). *Proc. Nat. Acad. Sci. U.S.* **69**, 791–794.
229. Green, M., Piña, M., Kimes, R., Wensink, P. C., MacHattie, L. A., and Thomas, C. A. Jr. (1967). *Proc. Nat. Acad. Sci. U.S.* **57**, 1302–1309.
230. Green, M., Rokutanda, H., and Rokutanda, M. (1971). *Nature New Biol.* **230**, 229–232.
231. Gregoriades, A., and Old, L. J. (1969). *Virology* **37**, 189–202.
232. Gross, L. (1951). *Proc. Soc. Exp. Biol. Med.* **76**, 27–32.
233. Gross, L. (1953). *Proc. Soc. Exp. Biol. Med.* **83**, 414–421.
234. Gross, L. (1970). "Oncogenic Viruses." Pergamon, Oxford.
235. Gutterman, J. U., Mavligit, G., McCredie, K. B., Bodey, G. P., Sr., Freireich, E. J., and Hersh, E. M. (1972). *Science* **177**, 1114–1115.
236. Habel, K. (1961). *Proc. Soc. Exp. Biol. Med.* **106**, 722–725.
237. Habel, K. (1969). *Advan. Immunol.* **10**, 229–250.
238. Habel, K., and Eddy, B. E. (1963). *Proc. Soc. Exp. Biol. Med.* **113**, 1–4.
239. Hampar, B., Kelloff, G. J., Martos, L. M., Oroszlan, S., Gilden, R. V., and Walker, J. L. (1970). *Nature (London)* **228**, 857–859.
240. Hanafusa, H. (1969). *Proc. Nat. Acad. Sci. U.S.* **63**, 318–325.
241. Hanafusa, H. (1970). *Current Topics Microbiol. Immunol.* **51**, 114–123.
242. Hanafusa, H., and Hanafusa, T. (1966). *Proc. Nat. Acad. Sci. U.S.* **55**, 532–538.
243. Hanafusa, H., and Hanafusa, T. (1971). *Virology* **43**, 313–316.
244. Hanafusa, H., Hanafusa, T., and Rubin, H. (1964). *Proc. Nat. Acad. Sci. U.S.* **51**, 41–48.
245. Hanafusa, T., Hanafusa, H., and Miyamoto, T. (1970). *Proc. Nat. Acad. Sci. U.S.* **67**, 1797–1803.
246. Hanafusa, H., Miyamoto, T., and Hanafusa, T. (1970). *Proc. Nat. Acad. Sci. U.S.* **66**, 314–321.
247. Hanafusa, H., Hanafusa, T., and Miyamoto, T. (1971). *In* "The Biology of Oncogenic Viruses" (Silvestri, L. G., ed.), pp. 170–175. North-Holland Publ., Amsterdam.
248. Hanafusa, T., Hanafusa, H., Miyamoto, T., and Fleissner, E. (1972). *Virology* **47**, 475–482.
249. Hare, J. D. (1967). *Virology* **31**, 625–632.
250. Harris, H., and Watkins, J. F. (1965). *Nature (London)* **205**, 640–646.
251. Hartley, J. W., and Rowe, W. P. (1966). *Proc. Nat. Acad. Sci. U.S.* **55**, 780–786.
252. Hartley, J. S., Rowe, W. P., Capps, W. I., and Huebner, R. J. (1965). *Proc. Nat. Acad. Sci. U.S.* **53**, 931–938.
253. Hartley, J. W., Rowe, W. P., Capps, W. I., and Huebner, R. J. (1969). *J. Virol.* **3**, 126–132.
254. Hartley, J. W., Rowe, W. P., and Huebner, R. J. (1970). *J. Virol.* **5**, 221–225.

255. Harvey, J. J. (1964). *Nature* (*London*) **204**, 1104–1105.
256. Hatanaka, M., and Hanafusa, H. (1970). *Virology* **41**, 647–652.
257. Hatanaka, M., Huebner, R. J., and Gilden, R. V. (1969). *J. Nat. Cancer Inst.* **43**, 1091–1096.
258. Haughton, G., and Nash, D. R. (1969). *Progr. Med. Virol.* **11**, 248–306.
259. Häyry, P., and Defendi, V. (1968). *Virology* **36**, 317–321.
260. Häyry, P., and Defendi, V. (1970). *Virology* **41**, 22–29.
261. Hehlmann, R., Kufe, D., and Spiegelman, S. (1972). *Proc. Nat. Acad. Sci. U.S.* **69**, 435–439.
262. Hehlmann, R., Kufe, D., and Spiegelman, S. (1972). *Proc. Nat. Acad. Sci. U.S.* **69**, 1727–1731.
263. Hellström, K. E., and Hellström, I. (1969). *Advan. Cancer Res.* **12**, 167–223.
264. Hellström, K. E., and Hellström, I. (1970). *Ann. Rev. Microbiol.* **24**, 373–398.
265. Hellström, I. E., Hellström, K. E., Pierce, G. E., and Bill, A. H. (1968). *Proc. Nat. Acad. Sci. U.S.* **60**, 1231–1238.
266. Hellström, I., Hellström, K. E., Bill, A. H., Pierce, G. E., and Yang, J. P. S. (1970). *Int. J. Cancer* **6**, 172–188.
267. Hellström, K. E., Hellström, I., Sjögren, H. O., and Warner, G. A. (1971). *Int. J. Cancer* **7**, 1–16.
268. Helinski, D. R., and Clewell, D. B. (1971). *Ann. Rev. Biochem.* **40**, 899–942.
269. Henle, G., and Henle, W. (1966). *J. Bacteriol.* **91**, 1248–1256.
270. Henle, W., Diehl, V., Kohn, G., Zur Hausen, H., and Henle, G. (1967). *Science* **157**, 1064–1065.
271. Henle, G., Henle, W., and Diehl, V. (1968). *Proc. Nat. Acad. Sci. U.S.* **59**, 94–101.
272. Henle, G., Henle, W., Clifford, P., Diehl, V., Kafuko, G. W., Kirya, B. G. , Klein, G., Morrow, R. H., Munube, G. M. R., Pike, M. C., Tukei, P. M., and Ziegler, J. L. (1969). *J. Nat. Cancer Inst.* **43**, 1147–1157.
273. Henle, W., Henle, G., Ho, H. C., Burtin, P., Cachin, Y., Clifford, P., de Schryver, A., de Thé, G., Diehl, V., and Klein, G. (1970). *J. Nat. Cancer Inst.* **44**, 225–231.
274. Hill, M., and Hillova, J. (1972). *Nature New Biol.* **237**, 35–39.
275. Hill, M., and Hillova, J. (1972). *Virology* **49**, 309–313.
276. Hilleman, M. R., and Werner, J. H. (1954). *Proc. Soc. Exp. Biol. Med.* **85**, 183–188.
277. Hillova, J., Goubin, G., and Hill, M. (1972). *C. R. Acad. Sci. Paris* **274**, 1970–1973.
278. Hinze, H. C. (1971). *Infect. Immun.* **3**, 350–354.
279. Hinze, H. C. (1971). *Int. J. Cancer* **8**, 514–522.
280. Hirshaut, Y., Glade, P., Vieira, L. O. B. D., Ainbender, E., Dvorak, B., and Siltzbach, L. E. (1970). *N. Engl. J. Med.* **283**, 502–505.
281. Hirst, G. K. (1962). *Cold Spring Harbor Symp. Quant. Biol.* **27**, 303–309.
282. Hirt, B. (1967). *J. Mol. Biol.* **26**, 365–369.
283. Hsiung, G. D., and Gaylord, W. H., Jr. (1961). *J. Exp. Med.* **114**, 975–985.
284. Ho, H. C. (1968). *Un. Int. Contre le Cancer Monogr.* **10**, 58–63.
285. Huang, E.-S., Estes, M. K., and Pagano, J. S. (1972). *J. Virol.* **9**, 923–929.
286. Huebner, R. J. (1967). *Proc. Nat. Acad. Sci. U.S.* **58**, 835–842.
287. Huebner, R. J., and Todaro, G. J. (1969). *Proc. Nat. Acad. Sci. U.S.* **64**, 1087–1094.
288. Huebner, R. J., Rowe, W. P., Turner, H. C., and Lane, W. T. (1963). *Proc. Nat. Acad. Sci. U.S.* **50**, 379–389.
289. Huebner, R. J., Armstrong, D., Okuyan, M., Sarma, P. S., and Turner, H. C. (1964). *Proc. Nat. Acad. Sci. U.S.* **51**, 742–750.
290. Huebner, R. J., Hartley, J. W., Rowe, W. P., Lane, W. T., and Capps, W. I. (1966). *Proc. Nat. Acad. Sci. U.S.* **56**, 1164–1169.
291. Huebner, R. J., Kelloff, G. J., Sarma, P. S., Lane, W. T., Turner, H. C., Gilden, R. V., Oroszlan, S., Meier, H., Myers, D. D., and Peters, R. L. (1970). *Proc. Nat. Acad. Sci. U.S.* **67**, 366–376.
292. Huebner, R. J., Sarma, P. S., Kelloff, G. J., Gilden, R. V., Meier, H., Myers, D. D., and Peters, R. L. (1971). *Ann. N.Y. Acad. Sci.* **181**, 246–271.

293. Hung, P. P., Robinson, H. L., and Robinson, W. S. (1971). *Virology* **43**, 251–266.
294. Hurwitz, J., and Leis, J. P. (1972). *J. Virol.* **9**, 116–129.
295. Igel, H. J., and Black, P. H. (1967). *J. Exp. Med.* **125**, 647–656.
296. Inbar, M., Rabinowitz, Z., and Sachs, L. (1969). *Int. J. Cancer* **4**, 690–696.
297. Ioachim, H. L., and Berwick, L. (1970). *In* "Comparative Leukemia Research 1969" (R. M. Dutcher, ed.), pp. 566–573. Karger, Basel.
298. Ito, Y., and Evans, C. A. (1961). *J. Exp. Med.* **114**, 485–500.
299. Jarrett, W. F. H., Martin, W. B., Crighton, G. W., Dalton, R. G., and Stewart, M. F. (1964). *Nature (London)* **202**, 566–567.
300. Jensen, F. C., and Koprowski, H. (1969). *Virology* **37**, 687–690.
301. Jensen, E. M., Zelljadt, I., Chopra, H. C., and Mason, M. M. (1970). *Cancer Res.* **30**, 2388–2393.
302. Johansson, B., Klein, G., Henle, W., and Henle, G. (1970). *Int. J. Cancer* **6**, 450–462.
303. Johnson, M., and Mora, P. T. (1967). *Virology* **31**, 230–237.
304. Joklik, W. K. (1966). *Bacteriol. Rev.* **30**, 33–66.
305. Joklik, W. K., and Merigan, T. C. (1966). *Proc. Nat. Acad. Sci. U.S.* **56**, 558–565.
306. Kacian, D. L., Watson, K. F., Burny, A., and Spiegelman, S. (1971). *Biochim. Biophys. Acta* **246**, 365–383.
307. Kakefuda, T., and Bader, J. P. (1969). *J. Virol.* **4**, 460–474.
308. Kaplan, H. S. (1967). *Cancer* Res. **27**, 1325–1340.
309. Kaplan, J. C., Wilbert, S. M., and Black, P. H. (1972). *J. Virol.* **9**, 800–803.
310. Kawai, S., and Hanafusa, H. (1971). *Virology* **46**, 470–479.
311. Kawai, S., and Hanafusa, H. (1972). *Virology* **48**, 126–135.
312. Kawai, S., and Hanafusa, H. (1972). *Virology* **49**, 37–44.
313. Kawai, S., Metroka, C. E., and Hanafusa, H. (1972). *Virology* **49**, 302–304.
314. Kawakami, T. G., Huff, S. D., Buckley, P. M., Dungworth, D. L., Snyder, S. P., and Gilden, R. V. (1972). *Nature New Biol.* **235**, 170–171.
315. Kawamura, M., King, D. J., and Anderson, D. P. (1969). *Avian Dis.* **13**, 853–863.
316. Kelloff, G., and Vogt, P. K. (1966). *Virology* **29**, 377–384.
317. Kelloff, G., Huebner, R. J., Chang, N. H., Lee, Y. K., and Gilden, R. V. (1970). *J. Gen. Virol.* **9**, 19–26.
318. Kelloff, G., Huebner, R. J., Lee, Y. K., Toni, R., and Gilden, R. (1970). *Proc. Nat. Acad. Sci. U.S.* **65**, 310–317.
319. Kelloff, G., Huebner, R. J., Oroszlan, S., Toni, R., and Gilden, R. V. (1970). *J. Gen. Virol.* **9**, 27–33.
320. Kelloff, G. J., Huebner, R. J., and Gilden, R. V. (1971). *J. Gen. Virol.* **13**, 289–294.
321. Kelloff, G. J., Hatanaka, M., and Gilden, R. V. (1972). *Virology* **48**, 266–269.
322. Kelly, T. J., Jr., and Rose, J. A. (1971). *Proc. Nat. Acad. Sci. U.S.* **68**, 1037–1041.
323. Khera, K. S., Ashkenazi, A., Rapp, F., and Melnick, J. L. (1963). *J. Immunol.* **91**, 604–613.
324. Khoury, G., and Martin, M. A. (1972). *Nature New Biol.* **238**, 4–6.
325. Khoury, G., Byrne, J. C., and Martin, M. A. (1972). *Proc. Nat. Acad. Sci. U.S.* **69**, 1925–1928.
326. Kidwell, W. R., Saral, R., Martin, R. G., and Ozer, H. L. (1972). *J. Virol.* **10**, 410–416.
327. Kieff, E. D., Bachenheimer, S. L., and Roizman, B. (1971). *J. Virol.* **8**, 125–132.
328. Kieff, E., Hoyer, B., Bachenheimer, S., and Roizman, B. (1972). *J. Virol.* **9**, 738–745.
329. Kirschstein, R. C., and Gerber, P. (1962). *Nature (London)* **195**, 299–300.
330. Kirsten, W. H., and Mayer, L. A. (1967). *J. Nat. Cancer Inst.* **39**, 311–335.
331. Kit, S., and Brown, M. (1969). *J. Virol.* **4**, 226–230.
332. Kit, S., Kurimura, T., Salvi, M. L., and Dubbs, D. R. (1968). *Proc. Nat. Acad. Sci. U.S.* **60**, 1239–1246.
333. Kit, S., Kurimura, T., Brown, M., and Dubbs, D. R. (1970). *J. Virol.* **6**, 69–77.
334. Kit, S., Dubbs, D. R., and Somers, K. (1971). *In Ciba Foundation Symp. Strategy Viral Genome* (G. E. W. Wolstenholme and M. O'Connor, eds.), pp. 229–265. Churchill, London.

335. Klein, G. (1966). *Ann. Rev. Microbiol.* **20**, 223–252.
336. Klein, G. (1969). *Fed. Proc.* **28**, 1739–1753.
337. Klein, G. (1971). *Israel J. Med. Sci.* **7**, 111–131.
338. Klein, G. (1971). *Advan. Immunol.* **14**, 187–250.
339. Klein, G. (1972). *Proc. Nat. Acad. Sci. U.S.* **69**, 1056–1064.
340. Kleinschmidt, A. K., Kass, S. J., Williams, R. C., and Knight, C. A. (1965). *J. Mol. Biol.* **13**, 749–756.
341. Klement, V., Hartley, J. W., Rowe, W. P., and Huebner, R. J. (1969). *J. Nat. Cancer Inst.* **43**, 925–934.
342. Klement, V., Rowe, W. P., Hartley, J. W., and Pugh, W. E. (1969). *Proc. Nat. Acad. Sci. U.S.* **63**, 753–758.
343. Klement, V., Nicolson, M. O., Gilden, R. V., Orozlan, S., Sarma, P. S., Rongey, R. W., and Gardner, M. B. (1972). *Nature New Biol.* **238**, 234–237.
344. Koch, M. A., and Sabin, A. B. (1963). *Proc. Soc. Exp. Biol. Med.* **113**, 4–12.
345. Koch, M. A., Becht, H., and Anderer, F. A. (1971). *Virology* **43**, 235–242.
346. Koprowski, H., Jensen, F. C., and Steplewski, Z. (1967). *Proc. Nat. Acad. Sci. U.S.* **58**, 127–133.
347. Kufe, D., Hehlmann, R., and Spiegelman, S. (1972). *Science* **175**, 182–185.
348. Lai, M. M. C., and Duesberg, P. H. (1972). *Nature (London)* **235**, 383–386.
349. Latarjet, R., Cramer, R., and Montagnier, L. (1967). *Virology* **33**, 104–111.
350. Lausch, R. N., Tevethia, S. S., and Rapp, F. (1968). *J. Immunol.* **101**, 645–649.
351. Lee, L. F., Kieff, E. D., Bachenheimer, S. L., Roizman, B., Spear, P. G., Burmester, B. R., and Nazerian, K. (1971). *J. Virol.* **7**, 289–294.
352. Leis, J. P., and Hurwitz, J. (1972). *J. Virol.* **9**, 130–142.
353. Leong, J.-A., Garapin, A.-C., Jackson, N., Fanshier, L., Levinson, W., and Bishop, J. M. (1972). *J. Virol.* **9**, 891–902.
354. Leventhal, B. G., Halterman, R. H., Rosenberg, E. B., and Herberman, R. B. (1972). *Cancer Res.* **32**, 1820–1825.
355. Levin, M. J., Black, P. H., Coghill, S. L., Dixon, C. B., and Henry, P. H. (1969). *J. Virol.* **4**, 704–711.
356. Levine, A. J., and Teresky, A. K. (1970). *J. Virol.* **5**, 451–457.
357. Levine, A. S., Oxman, M. N., Henry, P. H., Levin, M. J., Diamandopoulos, G. T., and Enders, J. F. (1970). *J. Virol.* **6**, 199–207.
358. Levinson, W., Bishop, J. M., Quintrell, N., and Jackson, J. (1970). *Nature (London)* **227**, 1023–1025.
359. Levinson, W. E., Varmus, H. E., Garapin, A.-C., and Bishop, J. M. (1972). *Science* **175**, 76–78.
360. Levy, H. B. (1969). "The Biochemistry of Viruses." Dekker, New York.
361. Lewis, A. M. Jr., and Rowe, W. P. (1971). *J. Virol.* **7**, 189–197.
362. Lewis, A. M. Jr., Levin, M. J., Wiese, W. H., Crumpacker, C. S., and Henry, P. H. (1969). *Proc. Nat. Acad. Sci. U.S.* **63**, 1128–1135.
363. Lindberg, U., and Darnell, J. E. (1970). *Proc. Nat. Acad. Sci. U.S.* **65**, 1089–1096.
364. Lindstrom, D. M., and Dulbecco, R. (1972). *Proc. Nat. Acad. Sci. U.S.* **69**, 1517–1520.
365. Livingston, D. M., Scolnick, E. M., Parks, W. P., and Todaro, G. J. (1972). *Proc. Nat. Acad. Sci. U.S.* **69**, 393–397.
366. Lo Gerfo, P., Herter, F. P., and Bennett, S. J. (1972). *Int. J. Cancer* **9**, 344–348.
367. Lowy, D. R., Rowe, W. P., Teich, N., and Hartley, J. W. (1971). *Science* **174**, 155–156.
368. Lucké, B. (1934). *Amer. J. Cancer* **20**, 352–379.
369. Ludwig, H. O., Biswal, N., and Benyesh-Melnick, M. (1972). *Virology* **49**, 95–101.
370. Luftig, R. B., and Kilham, S. S. (1971). *Virology* **46**, 277–297.
371. Lyons, M. J., and Moore, D. H. (1965). *J. Nat. Cancer Inst.* **35**, 549–566.
372. Macpherson, I. A. (1970). *Advan. Cancer Res.* **13**, 169–215.
373. Macpherson, I. A. (1971). *Proc. Roy. Soc. London B* **177**, 41–48.
374. Maizel, J. V. Jr., White, D. O., and Scharff, M. D. (1968). *Virology* **36**, 126–136.

375. Manly, K. F., Smoler, D. F., Bromfeld, E., and Baltimore, D. (1971). *J. Virol.* **7,** 106–111.
376. Maramorosch, K., and Kurstak, E. (1971). "Comparative Virology." Academic Press, New York.
377. Marcus, P. I., and Salb, J. M. (1966). *Virology* **30,** 502–516.
378. Margalith, M., Margalith, E., Nasialski, T., and Goldblum, N. (1970). *J. Virol.* **5,** 305–308.
379. Margalith, M., Margolith, E., and Spira, G. (1972). *Arch. Ges. Virusforsch.* **36,** 398–400.
380. Marin, G., and Macpherson, I. (1969). *J. Virol.* **3,** 146–149.
381. Markham, R. V., Jr., Sutherland, J. C., Cimino, E. F., Drake, W. P., and Mardiney, M. R., Jr. (1972). *Rev. Eur. Etudes Clin. Biol.* **17,** 11–17.
382. Martin, G. S. (1970). *Nature (London)* **227,** 1021–1023.
383. Martin, M. A., and Axelrod, D. (1969). *Proc. Nat. Acad. Sci. U.S.* **64,** 1203–1210.
384. Martin, G. S., and Duesberg, P. H. (1972). *Virology* **47,** 494–497.
385. May, J. T., Somers, K. D., and Kit, S. (1972). *J. Gen. Virol.* **16,** 223–226.
386. Mayor, H. D., Stinebaugh, S. E., Jamison, R. M., Jordan, L. E., and Melnick, J. L. (1962). *Exp. Mol. Pathol.* **1,** 397–416.
387. McAllister, R. M. (1973). *Progr. Med. Virol.* **16,** (in press).
388. McAllister, R. M., Nelson-Rees, W. A., Johnson, E. Y., Rongey, R. W., and Gardner, M. B. (1971). *J. Nat. Cancer Inst.* **47,** 603–611.
389. McAllister, R. M., Gilden, R. V., and Green, M. (1972). *Lancet* **i,** 831–833.
390. McAllister, R. M., Nicolson, M., Gardner, M. B., Rongey, R. W., Rasheed, S., Sarma, P. S., Huebner, R. J., Hatanaka, M., Oroszlan, S., Gilden, R. V., Kabigting, A., and Vernon, L. (1972). *Nature New Biol.* **235,** 3–6.
391. McCain, B., Biswal, N., and Benyesh-Melnick, M. (1973). *J. Gen. Virol.* **18,** 69–74.
392. McDonald, R., Wolfe, L. G., and Deinhardt, F. (1972). *Int. J. Cancer* **9,** 57–65.
393. Melendez, L. V., Daniel, M. D., Hunt, R. D., and Garcia, F. G. (1968). *Lab. Anim. Care* **18,** 374–381.
394. Melendez, L. V., Hunt, R. D., Daniel, M. D., Fraser, C. E. O., Barahona, H. H., Garcia, F. G., and King, N. W. (1972). *In* "Oncogenesis and Herpesviruses" (P. M. Biggs, G. De-Thé, and L. N. Payne, eds.), pp. 451–461. Int. Agency for Res. on Cancer, Lyon.
395. Melnick, J. L. (1962). *Science* **135,** 1128–1130.
396. Metzgar, R. S., and Oleinick, S. R. (1968). *Cancer Res.* **28,** 1366–1371.
397. Michel, M. R., Hirt, B., and Weil, R. (1967). *Proc. Nat. Acad. Sci. U.S.* **58,** 1381–1388.
398. Miller, J. M., Miller, L. D., Olson, C., and Gillette, K. G. (1969). *J. Nat. Cancer Inst.* **43,** 1297–1305.
399. Mizell, M. (1969). *In* "Recent Results in Cancer Research," pp. 1–25. Springer-Verlag, New York.
400. Mizutani, S., and Temin, H. M. (1971). *J. Virol.* **8,** 409–416.
401. Mölling, K., Bolognesi, D. P., Bauer, H., Büsen, W., Plassmann, H. W., and Hausen, P. (1971). *Nature New Biol.* **234,** 240–243.
402. Moloney, J. B. (1960). *J. Nat. Cancer Inst.* **24,** 933–951.
403. Moloney, J. B. (1966). *Nat. Cancer Inst. Monogr.* **22,** 139–142.
404. Montagnier, L., and Vigier, P. (1972). *C. R. Acad. Sci. Paris* **224,** 1977–1980.
405. Montagnier, L., Goldé, A., and Vigier, P. (1969). *J. Gen. Virol.* **4,** 449–452.
406. Moore, G. E., Gerner, R. E., and Franklin, H. A. (1967). *J. Amer. Med. Ass.* **199,** 519–524.
407. Moore, D. H., Charney, J., Kramarsky, B., Lasfargues, E. Y., Sarkar, N. H., Brennan, M. J., Burrows, J. H., Sirsat, S. M., Paymaster, J. C., and Vaidya, A. B. (1971). *Nature (London)* **229,** 611–614.
408. Moroni, C. (1972). *Virology* **47,** 1–7.
409. Morton, D. L., Malmgren, R. A., Holmes, E. C., and Ketcham, A. S. (1968). *Surgery* **64,** 233–240.

410. Morton, D. L., Malmgren, R. A., Hall, W. T., and Schidlovsky, G. (1969). *Surgery* **66**, 152–161.
411. Müller, M., and Grossmann, H. (1972). *Nature New Biol.* **237**, 116–117.
412. Nahmias, A. J., Josey, W. E., Naib, Z. M., Luce, C. F., and Duffey, A. (1970). *Amer. J. Epidemiol.* **91**, 539–546
413. Nahmias, A. J., Dowdle, W. R., Naib, J. M., Josey, W. E., McLone, D., and Domescik, G. (1969). *Brit. J. Vener. Dis.* **45**, 294–298.
414. Nahmias, A. J., Josey, W. E., Naib, Z. M., Luce, C. F., and Guest, B. A. (1970). *Amer. J. Epidemiol.* **91**, 547–552.
415. Nazerian, K. (1972). *In* "Oncogenesis and Herpesvirus" (P. M. Biggs, G. De-Thé, and L. N. Payne, eds.), pp. 59–73. Int. Agency for Res. on Cancer, Lyon.
416. Newell, G. R., Harris, W. W., Bowman, K. O., Boone, C. W., and Anderson, N. G. (1968). *New England J. Med.* **278**, 1185–1191.
417. Nicolson, M. O., and McAllister, R. M. (1972). *Virology* **48**, 14–21.
418. Niederman, J. C., McCollum, R. W., Henle, G. *et al.* (1968). *J. Amer. Med. Ass.* **203**, 205–209.
419. Niederman, J. C., Evans, A. S., Subrahmanyan, L., and McCollum, R. W. (1970). *New England J. Med.* **282**, 361–365.
420. Nomura, S., Fischinger, P. J., Mattern, C. F. T., Peebles, P. T., Bassin, R. H., and Friedman, G. P. (1972). *Virology* **50**, 51–64.
421. Nonoyama, M., and Pagano, J. S. (1971). *Nature New Biol.* **233**, 103–106.
422. Norrby, E. (1971). *In* "Comparative Virology" (K. Maramorosch and E. Kurstak, eds.), pp. 105–134. Academic Press, New York.
423. Nowinski, R. C., and Sarkar, N. H. (1972). *J. Nat. Cancer Inst.* **48**, 1169–1176.
424. Nowinski, R. C., Old, L. J., Sarkar, N. H., and Moore, D. H. (1970). *Virology* **42**, 1152–1157.
425. Nowinski, R. C., Edynak, E., and Sarkar, N. H. (1971). *Proc. Nat. Acad. Sci. U.S.* **68**, 1608–1612.
426. Nowinski, R. C., Sarkar, N. H., Old, L. J., Moore, D. H., Scheer, D. I., and Hilgers, J. (1971). *Virology* **46**, 21–38.
427. Nowinski, R. C., Fleissner, E., Sarkar, N. H., and Aoki, T. (1972). *J. Virol.* **9**, 359–366.
428. Oda, K., and Dulbecco, R. (1968). *Proc. Nat. Acad. Sci. U.S.* **60**, 525–532.
429. Old, L. J., and Boyse, E. A. (1964). *Ann. Rev. Med.* **15**, 167–186.
430. Old, L. J., Boyse, E. A., and Stockert, E. (1965). *Cancer Res.* **25**, 813–819.
431. Old, L. J., Boyse, E. A., Geering, G., and Oettgen, H. F. (1968). *Cancer Res.* **28**, 1288–1299.
432. Oldstone, M. B. A., Aoki, T., and Dixon, F. J. (1972). *Proc. Nat. Acad. Sci. U.S.* **69**, 134–138.
433. Order, S. E., Porter, M., and Hellman, S. (1971). *N. Engl. J. Med.* **285**, 471–474.
434. Oroszlan, S., Fisher, C. L., Stanley, T. B., and Gilden, R. V. (1970). *J. Gen. Virol.* **8**, 1–10.
435. Oroszlan, S., Foreman, C., Kelloff, G., and Gilden, R. V. (1971). *Virology* **43**, 665–674.
436. Oroszlan, S., Huebner, R. J., and Gilden, R. V. (1971). *Proc. Nat. Acad. Sci. U.S.* **68**, 901–904.
437. Oroszlan, S., Bova, D., White, M. H. M., Toni, R., Foreman, C., and Gilden, R. V. (1972). *Proc. Nat. Acad. Sci. U.S.* **69**, 1211–1215.
438. Oxman, M. N., Baron, S., Black, P. H., Takemoto, K. K., Habel, K., and Rowe, W. P. (1967). *Virology* **32**, 122–127.
439. Padgett, B. L., Walker, D. L., ZuRhein, G. M., Eckroade, R. J., and Dessel, B. H. (1971). *Lancet* 1257–1260.
440. Pagano, J. S. (1970). *Progr. Med. Virol.* **12**, 1–48.
441. Papageorgiou, P. S., Sorokin, C., Kouzoutzakoglou, K., and Glade, P. R. (1971). *Nature (London)* **231**, 47–49.
442. Parkman, R., Levy, J. A., and Ting, R. C. (1970). *Science* **168**, 387–389.

443. Parks, W. P., and Todaro, G. J. (1972). *Virology* **47**, 673–683.
444. Parks, W. P., and Scolnick, E. M. (1972). *Proc. Nat. Acad. Sci. U.S.* **69**, 1766–1770.
445. Parks, W. P., Todaro, G. J., Scolnick, E. M., and Aaronson, S. A. (1971). *Nature (London)* **229**, 258–260.
446. Parks, W. P., Scolnick, H. M., Ross, J., Todaro, G. J., and Aaronson, S. A. (1972). *J. Virol.* **9**, 110–115.
447. Pasternak, G. (1969). *Advan. Cancer Res.* **12**, 1–99.
448. Payne, L. N., and Chubb, R. C. (1968). *J. Gen. Virol.* **3**, 379–391.
449. Payne, F. E., Solomon, J. J., and Purchase, H. G. (1966). *Proc. Nat. Acad. Sci. U.S.* **55**, 341–349.
450. Payne, L. N., Crittenden, L. B., and Okazaki, W. (1968). *J. Nat. Cancer Inst.* **40**, 907–916.
451. Payne, L. N., Pani, P. K., and Weiss, R. A. (1971). *J. Gen. Virol.* **13**, 455–462.
452. Peebles, P. T., Haapala, D. K., and Gazdar, A. F. (1972). *J. Virol.* **9**, 488–493.
453. Pereira, M. S., Blake, J. M., and Macrae, A. D. (1969). *Brit. Med. J.* **4**, 526–527.
454. Perk, K., Viola, M. V., Smith, K. L., Wivel, N. A., and Moloney, J. B. (1969). *Cancer Res.* **29**, 1089–1102.
455. Phillips, C. F., Benyesh-Melnick, M., Seidel, E. H., and Fernbach, D. J. (1965). *Brit. Med. J.* **i**, 286–288.
456. Pincus, T., Hartley, J. W., and Rowe, W. P. (1971). *J. Exp. Med.* **133**, 1219–1233.
457. Pincus, T., Rowe, W. P., and Lilly, F. (1971). *J. Exp. Med.* **133**, 1234–1241.
458. Pollack, R. E., Green, H., and Todaro, G. J. (1968). *Proc. Nat. Acad. Sci. U.S.* **60**, 126–133.
459. Pontén, J. (1971). *Virol. Monogr. 8.* Springer-Verlag, New York.
460. Pope, J. H., and Rowe, W. P. (1964). *J. Exp. Med.* **120**, 121–128.
461. Pope, J. H., Horne, M. K., and Scott, W. (1968). *Int. J. Cancer* **3**, 857–866.
462. Porter, D. D., Wimberly, I., and Benyesh-Melnick, M. (1969). *J. Amer. Med. Ass.* **208**, 1675–1679.
463. Prince, A. M., and Adams, W. R. (1966). *J. Nat. Cancer Inst.* **37**, 153–166.
464. Priori, E. S., Dmochowski, L., Myers, B., and Wilbur, J. R. (1971). *Nature New Biol.* **232**, 61–62.
465. Purchase, H. G., Witter, R. L., Okazaki, W., and Burmester, B. R. (1971). *In* "Perspectives in Virology" (M. Pollard, ed.), pp. 91–110. Academic Press, New York.
466. Qasba, P. K., and Aposhian, H. V. (1971). *Proc. Nat. Acad. Sci. U.S.* **68**, 2345–2349.
467. Quigley, J. P., Rifkin, D. B., and Reich, E. (1971). *Virology* **46**, 106–116.
468. Rabinowitz, Z., and Sachs, L. (1968). *Nature (London)* **220**, 1203–1206.
469. Rabinowitz, Z., and Sachs, L. (1969). *Virology* **38**, 336–342.
470. Rabinowitz, Z., and Sachs, L. (1969). *Virology* **38**, 343–346.
471. Rabinowitz, Z., and Sachs, L. (1970). *Virology* **40**, 193–198.
472. Rabinowitz, Z., and Sachs, L. (1970). *Nature (London)* **225**, 136–139.
473. Randerath, K., Rosenthal, L. J., and Zamecnik, P. C. (1971). *Proc. Nat. Acad. Sci. U.S.* **68**, 3233–3237.
474. Rapp, F. (1967). *Methods Cancer Res.* **1**, 451–544.
475. Rapp, F. (1969). *Ann. Rev. Microbiol.* **23**, 293–316.
476. Rapp, F., and Melnick, J. L. (1966). *Progr. Med. Virol.* **8**, 349–399.
477. Rapp, F., Butel, J. S., and Melnick, J. L. (1964). *Proc. Soc. Exp. Biol. Med.* **116**, 1131–1135.
478. Rapp, F., Kitahara, T., Butel, J. S., and Melnick, J. L. (1964). *Proc. Nat. Acad. Sci. U.S.* **52**, 1138–1142.
479. Rapp, F., Butel, J. S., Feldman, L. A., Kitahara, T., and Melnick, J. L. (1965). *J. Exp. Med.* **121**, 935–944.
480. Rapp, F., Butel, J. S., Tevethia, S. S., Katz, M., and Melnick, J. L. (1966). *J. Immunol.* **97**, 833–839.
481. Rapp, F., Melnick, J. L., and Levy, B. (1967). *Amer. J. Pathol.* **50**, 849–859.
482. Rapp, F., Pauluzzi, S., and Butel, J. S. (1969). *J. Virol.* **4**, 626–631.

483. Rauscher, F. J., Jr. (1962). *J. Nat. Cancer Inst.* **29**, 515–543.
484. Rauscher, F. J., Jr. (1970). *Proc. Nat. Cancer Conf.* **6**, 93–106.
485. Rawls, W. E. (1973). *In* "The Herpesviruses" (A. S. Kaplan, ed.). Academic Press, New York (in press).
486. Rawls, W. E., Tompkins, W. A. F., Figueroa, M. E., and Melnick, J. L. (1968). *Science* **161**, 1255–1256.
487. Rawls, W. E., Gardner, H. L., Flanders, R. W., Lowry, S. P., Kaufman, R. H., and Melnick, J. L. (1971). *Amer. J. Obstet. Gynecol.* **110**, 682–689.
488. Reich, P. R., Black, P. H., and Weissman, S. M. (1966). *Proc. Nat. Acad. Sci. U.S.* **56**, 78–85.
489. Renger, H. C. (1972). *Nature New Biol.* **240**, 19–21.
490. Renger, H. C., and Basilico, C. (1972). *Proc. Nat. Acad. Sci. U.S.* **69**, 109–114.
491. Rich, M. A., and Siegler, R. (1967). *Ann. Rev. Microbiol.* **21**, 529–572.
492. Richardson, L. S., and Butel, J. S. (1971). *Int. J. Cancer* **7**, 75–85.
493. Rickard, C. G., Post, J. E., Noronha, F., and Barr, L. M. (1969). *J. Nat. Cancer Inst.* **42**, 987–1014.
494. Říman, J., and Beaudreau, G. S. (1970). *Nature (London)* **228**, 427–430.
495. Robinson, H. L. (1967). *Proc. Nat. Acad. Sci. U.S.* **57**, 1655–1662.
496. Robinson, W. S., and Duesberg, P. H. (1968). *In* "Molecular Basis of Virology" (H. Fraenkel-Conrat, ed.), pp. 306–331. Van Nostrand Reinhold, Princeton, New Jersey.
497. Robinson, W. S., and Robinson, H. L. (1971). *Virology* **44**, 457–462.
498. Roblin, R., Härle, E., and Dulbecco, R. (1971). *Virology* **45**, 555–566.
499. Roizman, B. (1969). *In* "The Biochemistry of Viruses" (H. B. Levy, ed.), pp. 415–482. Dekker, New York.
500. Roizman, B., and Spear, P. G. (1971). *In* "Comparative Virology" (K. Maramorosch and E. Kurstak, eds.), pp. 135–168. Academic Press, New York.
501. Rokutanda, M., Rokutanda, H., Green, M., Fujinaga, K., Ray, R. K., and Gurgo, C. (1970). *Nature (London)* **227**, 1026–1028.
502. Rosenthal, P. N., Robinson, H. L., Robinson, W. S., Hanafusa, T., and Hanafusa, H. (1971). *Proc. Nat. Acad. Sci. U.S.* **68**, 2336–2340.
503. Ross, J., Scolnick, E. M., Todaro, G. J., and Aaronson, S. A. (1971). *Nature New Biol.* **231**, 163–167.
504. Ross, J., Tronick, S. R., and Scolnick, E. M. (1972). *Virology* **49**, 230–235.
505. Roth, F. K., Meyers, P., and Dougherty, R. M. (1971). *Virology* **45**, 265–274.
506. Rothschild, H., and Black, P. H. (1970). *Virology* **42**, 251–256.
507. Rous, P. (1911). *J. Exp. Med.* **13**, 397–411.
508. Rowe, W. P. (1971). *Virology* **46**, 369–374.
509. Rowe, W. P. (1972). *J. Exp. Med.* **136**, 1272–1285.
510. Rowe, W. P., and Hartley, J. W. (1972). *J. Exp. Med.* **136**, 1286–1301.
511. Rowe, W. P., Huebner, R. J., Gilmore, L. K., Parrott, R. H., and Ward, T. G. (1953). *Proc. Soc. Exp. Biol. Med.* **84**, 570–573.
512. Rowe, W. P., Pugh, W. E., and Hartley, J. W. (1970). *Virology* **42**, 1136–1139.
513. Rowe, W. P., Hartley, J. W., Lander, M. R., Pugh, W. E., and Teich, N. (1971). *Virology* **46**, 866–876.
514. Rowe, W. P., Hartley, J. W., and Bremner, T. (1972). *Science* **178**, 860–862.
515. Rowe, W. P., Lowy, D. R., Teich, N., and Hartley, J. W. (1972). *Proc. Nat. Acad. Sci. U.S.* **69**, 1033–1035.
516. Rowson, K. E. K., and Mahy, B. W. J. (1967). *Bacteriol. Rev.* **31**, 110–131.
517. Rubin, H. (1960). *Proc. Nat. Acad. Sci. U.S.* **46**, 1105–1119.
518. Rubin, H., Cornelius, A., and Fanshier, L. (1961). *Proc. Nat. Acad. Sci. U.S.* **47**, 1058–1060.
519. Rubin, H., Fanshier, L., Cornelius, A., and Hughes, W. F. (1962). *Virology* **17**, 143–156.
520. Sabin, A. B., and Koch, M. A. (1963). *Proc. Nat. Acad. Sci. U.S.* **49**, 304–311.
521. Sabin, A. B., and Koch, M. A. (1963). *Proc. Nat. Acad. Sci. U.S.* **50**, 407–417.
522. Sabin, A. B., and Koch, M. A. (1964). *Proc. Nat. Acad. Sci. U.S.* **52**, 1131–1138.

523. Sachs, L. (1965). *Nature* (*London*) **107**, 1272–1274.
524. Salzman, N. P. (1971). *In Vitro* **6**, 349–354.
525. Sambrook, J. (1972). *Advan. Cancer Res.* **16**, 141–180.
526. Sambrook, J., Westphal, H., Srinivasan, P. R., and Dulbecco, R. (1968). *Proc. Nat. Acad. Sci. U.S.* **60**, 1288–1295.
527. Sambrook, J., Sharp, P. A., and Keller, W. (1972). *J. Mol. Biol.* **70**, 57–71.
528. Sarkar, N. H., and Moore, D. H. (1972). *Nature* (*London*) **236**, 103–106.
529. Sarkar, N. H., Nowinski, R. C., and Moore, D. H. (1971). *J. Virol.* **8**, 564–572.
530. Sarkar, N. H., Nowinski, R. C., and Moore, D. H. (1971). *Virology* **46**, 1–20.
531. Sarma, P. S., and Log, T. (1971). *Virology* **44**, 352–358.
532. Sarma, P. S., Turner, H. C., and Huebner, R. J. (1964). *Virology* **23**, 313–321.
533. Sarma, P. S., Cheong, M. P., Hartley, J. W., and Huebner, R. J. (1967). *Virology* **33**, 180–184.
534. Sarma, P. S., Gilden, R. V., and Huebner, R. J. (1971). *Virology* **44**, 137–145.
535. Sarma, P. S., Huebner, R. J., Basker, J. F., Vernon, L., and Gilden, R. V. (1970). *Science* **168**, 1098–1100.
536. Sarma, P. S., Log, T., and Heubner, R. J. (1970). *Proc. Nat. Acad. Sci. U.S.* **65**, 81–87.
537. Sarma, P. S., Gilden, R. V., and Huebner, R. J. (1971). *Virology* **44**, 137–145.
538. Sarngadharan, M. G., Sarin, P. S., Reitz, M. S., and Gallo, R. C. (1972). *Nature New Biol.* **240**, 67–72.
539. Sauer, G. (1971). *Nature New Biol.* **231**, 135–138.
540. Sauer, G., and Kidwai, J. R. (1968). *Proc. Nat. Acad. Sci. U.S.* **61**, 1256–1263.
541. Savage, T., Roizman, B., and Heine, J. W. (1972). *J. Gen. Virol.* **17**, 31–48.
542. Schäfer, W., Lange, J., Bolognesi, D. P., De Noronha, F., Post, J. E., and Rickard, C. G. (1971). *Virology* **44**, 73–82.
543. Schäfer, W., Fischinger, P. J., Lange, J., and Pister, L. (1972). *Virology* **47**, 197–209.
544. Schäfer, W., Lange, J., Fischinger, P. J., Frank, H., Bolognesi, D. P., and Pister, L. (1972). *Virology* **47**, 210–228.
545. Schlesinger, R. W. (1969). *Advan. Virus Res.* **14**, 1–61.
546. Schlom, J., and Spiegelman, S. (1971). *Science* **174**, 840–843.
547. Schlom, J., Harter, D. H., Burny, A., and Spiegelman, S. (1971). *Proc. Nat. Acad. Sci. U.S.* **68**, 182–186.
548. Schlom, J., Spiegelman, S., and Moore, D. H. (1972). *Science* **175**, 542–544.
549. Scolnick, E. M., Parks, W. P., and Todaro, G. J. (1972). *Science* **177**, 1119–1121.
550. Scolnick, E. M., Parks, W. P., Todaro, G. J., and Aaronson, S. A. (1972). *Nature New Biol.* **235**, 35–40.
551. Scolnick, E. M., Stephenson, J. R., and Aaronson, S. A. (1972). *J. Virol.* **10**, 653–657.
552. Shope, R. E. (1933). *J. Exp. Med.* **58**, 607–624.
553. Sjögren, H. O. (1965). *Progr. Exp. Tumor Res.* **6**, 289–322.
554. Sjögren, H. O., Hellström, J., and Klein, G. (1961). *Exp. Cell Res.* **23**, 204–208.
555. Sjögren, H. O., Hellström, I., Bansal, S. C., Warner, G. A., and Hellström, K. E. (1972). *Int. J. Cancer* **9**, 274–283.
556. Smith, R. T., and Bausher, J. C. (1972). *Ann. Rev. Med.* **23**, 39–56.
557. Smith, K. O., Benyesh-Melnick, M., and Fernbach, D. J. (1964). *J. Nat. Cancer Inst.* **33**, 557–570.
558. Smith, R. W., Morganroth, J., and Mora, P. T. (1970). *Nature* (*London*) **227**, 141–145.
559. Smoler, D., Molineux, I., and Baltimore, D. (1971). *J. Biol. Chem.* **246**, 7697–7700.
560. Snyder, S. P., and Theilen, G. H. (1969). *Nature* (*London*) **221**, 1074–1075.
561. Sohier, R., Chardonnet, Y., and Prunieras, M. (1965). *Progr. Med. Virol.* **7**, 253–325.
562. Somers, K., and Kit, S. (1971). *Virology* **46**, 774–785.
563. Spear, P. G., and Roizman, B. (1972). *J. Virol.* **9**, 143–159.
564. Spiegelman, S. (1973). Personal communication.
565. Spiegelman, S., Burny, A., Das, M. R., Keydar, J., Schlom, J., Travnicek, M., and Watson, K. (1970). *Nature* (*London*) **227**, 563–567.

566. Spiegelman, S., Burny, A., Das, M. R., Keydar, J., Schlom, J., Travnicek, M., and Watson, K. (1970). *Nature (London)* **227**, 1029–1031.
567. Spiegleman, S., Burny, A., Das, M. R., Keydar, J., Scholm, J., Trávníček, M., and Watson, K. (1970). *Nature (London)* **228**, 430–432.
568. Stenback, W. A., Van Hoosier, G. L. Jr., and Trentin, J. J. (1968). *J. Virol.* **2**, 1115–1121.
569. Stephenson, J. R., and Aaronson, S. A. (1972). *J. Exp. Med.* **136**, 175–184.
570. Stewart, S. E., Eddy, B. E., Gochenour, A. M., Borgese, N. G., and Grubbs, G. E. (1957). *Virology* **3**, 380–400.
571. Stewart, S. E., Kasnic, G., Jr., Draycott, C., and Ben, T. (1972). *Science* **175**, 198–199.
572. Stewart, S. E., Kasnic, G., Jr., Draycott, C., Feller, W., Golden, A., Mitchell, E., and Ben, T. (1972). *J. Nat. Cancer Inst.* **48**, 273–277.
573. Stock, N. D., and Ferrer, J. F. (1972). *J. Nat. Cancer Inst.* **48**, 985–996.
574. Stone, L. B., Scolnick, E., Takemoto, K. K., and Aaronson, S. A. (1971). *Nature (London)* **229**, 257–258.
575. Stone, L. B., Takemoto, K. K., and Martin, M. A. (1971). *J. Virol.* **8**, 573–578.
576. Strand, M., and August, J. T. (1971). *Nature New Biol.* **233**, 137–140.
577. Stromberg, K. (1972). *J. Virol.* **9**, 684–697.
578. Svobodá, J., and Hložánek, I. (1970). *Advan. Cancer Res.* **13**, 217–269.
579. Svoboda, J., Machala, O., Donner, L., and Sovová, V. (1971). *Int. J. Cancer* **8**, 391–400.
580. Sweet, B. H., and Hilleman, M. R. (1960). *Proc. Soc. Exp. Biol. Med.* **105**, 420–427.
581. Swetly, P., Barbanti Brodano, G., Knowles, B., and Koprowski, H. (1969). *J. Virol.* **4**, 348–355.
582. Takemoto, K. K., and Habel, K. (1966). *Virology* **30**, 20–28.
583. Takemoto, K. K., and Stone, L. B. (1971). *J. Virol.* **7**, 770–775.
584. Takemoto, K. K., Todaro, G. J., and Habel, K. (1968). *Virology* **35**, 1–8.
585. Takemoto, K. K., Mattern, C. F. T., and Murakami, W. T. (1971). In "Comparative Virology" (K. Maramorosch and E. Kurstak, eds.), pp. 81–104. Academic Press, New York.
586. Taylor, B. A., Meier, H., and Myers, D. D. (1971). *Proc. Nat. Acad. Sci. U.S.* **68**, 3190–3194.
587. Temin, H. M. (1964). *Virology* **23**, 486–494.
588. Temin, H. M. (1971). *Ann. Rev. Microbiol.* **25**, 609–648.
589. Temin, H. M. (1971). *J. Nat. Cancer Inst.* **46**, III–VII.
590. Temin, H. M. (1972). *Proc. Nat. Acad. Sci. U.S.* **69**, 1016–1020.
591. Temin, H. M., and Baltimore, D. (1972). *Advan. Virus Res.* **17**, 129–186.
592. Temin, H. M., and Mizutani, S. (1970). *Nature (London)* **226**, 1211–1213.
593. Temin, H. M., and Rubin, H. (1958). *Virology* **6**, 669–688.
594. Tevethia, S. S., and Rapp, F. (1966). *Proc. Soc. Exp. Biol. Med.* **123**, 612–615.
595. Tevethia, S. S., Katz, M., and Rapp, F. (1965). *Proc. Soc. Exp. Biol. Med.* **119**, 896–901.
596. Tevethia, S. S., Diamandopoulos, G. Th., Rapp, F., and Enders, J. F. (1968). *J. Immunol.* **101**, 1192–1198.
597. Tevethia, S. S., Crouch, N. A., Melnick, J. L., and Rapp, F. (1970). *Int. J. Cancer* **5**, 176–184.
598. Tevethia, S. S., McMillan, V. L., Kaplan, P. M., and Bushong, S. C. (1971). *J. Immunol.* **106**, 1295–1300.
599. Theilen, G. H., Gould, D., Fowler, M., and Dungworth, D. L. (1971). *J. Nat. Cancer Inst.* **47**, 881–889.
600. Ting, R. C. (1968). *J. Virol.* **2**, 865–868.
601. Todaro, G. J., and Baron, S. (1965). *Proc. Nat. Acad. Sci. U.S.* **54**, 752–756.
602. Todaro, G. J., and Green, H. (1965). *Science* **147**, 513–514.
603. Todaro, G. J., and Green, H. (1966). *Virology* **28**, 756–759.
604. Todaro, G. J., and Green, H. (1966). *Proc. Nat. Acad. Sci. U.S.* **55**, 302–308.
605. Todaro, G. J., and Green, H. (1967). *J. Virol.* **1**, 115–119.
606. Todaro, G. J., and Huebner, R. J. (1972). *Proc. Nat. Acad. Sci. U.S.* **69**, 1009–1015.

607. Todaro, G. J., and Takemoto, K. K. (1969). *Proc. Nat. Acad. Sci. U.S.* **62**, 1031–1037.
608. Todaro, G. J., Habel, K., and Green, H. (1965). *Virology* **27**, 179–185.
609. Todaro, G. J., Zeve, V., and Aaronson, S. A. (1971). *In Vitro* **6**, 355–361.
610. Tournier, P., Cassingena, R., Wicker, R., Coppey, J., and Suarez, H. (1967). *Int. J. Cancer* **2**, 117–132.
611. Toyoshima, K., Friis, R. R., and Vogt, P. K. (1970). *Virology* **42**, 163–170.
612. Travnicek, M. (1969). *Biochim. Biophys. Acta* **182**, 427–439.
613. Travnicek, M., and Riman, J. (1970). *Biochim. Biophys. Acta* **199**, 283–285.
614. Trentin, J. J., Yabe, Y., and Taylor, G. (1962). *Science* **137**, 835–841.
615. Trilling, D. M., and Axelrod, D. (1970). *Science* **168**, 268–271.
616. Trkula, D., Kit, S., Kurimura, T., and Nakajima, K. (1971). *J. Gen. Virol.* **10**, 221–229.
617. Tsuchida, N., Robin, M. S., and Green, M. (1972). *Science* **176**, 1418–1420.
618. Tsuei, D., Fujinaga, K., and Green, M. (1972). *Proc. Nat. Acad. Sci. U.S.* **69**, 427–430.
619. Ubertini, T. R. (1972). *Infect. Immun.* **5**, 400–405.
620. Van Griensven, L., Emanoil-Ravicovitch, R., and Boiron, M. (1970). *C. R. Acad. Sci. Paris* **270**, 1723–1726.
621. Varmus, H. E., Levinson, W. E., and Bishop, J. M. (1971). *Nature New Biol.* **233**, 19–21.
622. Varmus, H. E., Bishop, J. M., Nowinski, R. C., and Sarkar, N. H. (1972). *Nature New Biol.* **238**, 189–191.
623. Varmus, H. E., Weiss, R. A., Friis, R. R., Levinson, W., and Bishop, J. M. (1972). *Proc. Nat. Acad. Sci. U.S.* **69**, 20–24.
624. Verma, I. M., Meuth, N. L., Bromfeld, E., Manly, K. F., and Baltimore, D. (1971). *Nature New Biol.* **233**, 131–134.
625. Vigier, P. (1970). *Progr. Med. Virol.* **12**, 240.
626. Vigier, P. (1972). *Int. J. Cancer* **9**, 150–161.
627. Vinograd, J., Lebowitz, J., Radloff, R., Watson, R., and Laipis, P. (1965). *Proc. Nat. Acad. Sci. U.S.* **53**, 1104–1111.
628. Vogt, P. K. (1965). *Advan. Virus Res.* **11**, 293–385.
629. Vogt, P. K. (1967). *Proc. Nat. Acad. Sci. U.S.* **58**, 801–808.
630. Vogt, M. (1970). *J. Mol. Biol.* **47**, 307–316.
631. Vogt, P. K. (1970). *In* "Comparative Leukemia Research 1969" (R. M. Dutcher, ed.), pp. 153–167. Karger, Basel.
632. Vogt, P. K. (1971). *Virology* **46**, 939–946.
633. Vogt, P. K. (1971). *Virology* **46**, 947–952.
634. Vogt, P. K. (1971). *In* "Viruses Affecting Man and Animals" (M. Sanders and M. Schaeffer, eds.), pp. 175–190. Green, St. Louis, Missouri.
635. Vogt, P. K., and Friis, R. R. (1971). *Virology* **43**, 223–234.
636. Wall, R., and Darnell, J. E. (1971). *Nature New Biol.* **232**, 73–76.
637. Walter, G., Roblin, R., and Dulbecco, R. (1972). *Proc. Nat. Acad. Sci. U.S.* **69**, 921–924.
638. Watkins, J. F., and Dulbecco, R. (1967). *Proc. Nat. Acad. Sci. U.S.* **58**, 1396–1403.
639. Watson, K. F., and Beaudreau, G. S. (1969). *Biochem. Biophys. Res. Commun.* **37**, 925–932.
640. Weil, R. (1963). *Proc. Nat. Acad. Sci. U.S.* **49**, 480–487.
641. Weil, R., and Vinograd, J. (1963). *Proc. Nat. Acad. Sci. U.S.* **50**, 730–738.
642. Weiner, L. P., Herndon, R. M., Narayan, O., Johnson, R. T., Shah, K., Rubinstein, L. J., Prejiosi, T. J., and Conley, F. K. (1972). *New England J. Med.* **286**, 385–390.
643. Weiss, R. (1967). *Virology* **32**, 719–723.
644. Weiss, R. A. (1969). *J. Gen. Virol.* **5**, 511–528.
645. Weiss, R. A., and Payne, L. N. (1971). *Virology* **45**, 508–515.
646. Weiss, R. A., Friis, R. R., Katz, E., and Vogt, P. K. (1971). *Virology* **46**, 920–938.
647. Westphal, H., and Dulbecco, R. (1968). *Proc. Nat. Acad. Sci. U.S.* **59**, 1158–1165.
648. Winocour, E. (1967). *Virology* **31**, 15–28.
649. Winocour, E. (1968). *Virology* **34**, 571–582.

650. Witter, R. L., Nazerian, K., Purchase, H. G., and Burgoyne, G. H. (1970). *Amer. J. Vet. Res.* **31**, 525–538.
651. Wolfe, L. G., Deinhardt, F., Theilen, G. H., Rabin, H., Kawakami, T., and Bustad, L. K. (1971). *J. Nat. Cancer Inst.* **47**, 1115–1120.
652. Wright, P. W., and Law, L. W. (1971). *Proc. Nat. Acad. Sci. U.S.* **68**, 973–976.
653. Yoshida, K., Smith, K. L., and Pinkel, D. (1966). *Proc. Soc. Exp. Biol. Med.* **121**, 72–81.
654. Zeigel, R. F., and Clark, H. F. (1969). *J. Nat. Cancer Inst.* **43**, 1097–1102.
655. Zilber, L. A. (1965). *Progr. Exp. Tumor Res.* **7**, 1–48.
656. Zur Hausen, H., and Schulte-Holthausen, H. (1970). *Nature (London)* **227**, 245–248.
657. Zur Hausen, H., Schulte-Holthausen, H., Klein, G., Henle, W., Henle, G., Clifford, P., and Santesson, L. (1970). *Nature (London)* **228**, 1056–1058.
658. Zur Hausen, H., Diehl, V., Wolf, H., Schulte-Holthausen, H., and Schneider, U. (1972). *Nature New Biol.* **237**, 189–190.

CHAPTER XII

Molecular Correlation Concept

GEORGE WEBER

I. Introduction

The goal of this chapter is to outline the approaches of the molecular correlation concept of neoplasia and to present the recent advances and implications achieved with application of this concept.

A. Conceptual Background

In our investigations of the biochemistry of cancer cells we anticipated the presence of a meaningful pattern that correlates with the degrees of malignancy. In a first attempt to describe the biochemistry of a hepatoma in terms of a meaningful enzymic and metabolic imbalance it was noted: "A careful comparison of the metabolism, histology, and biological behavior may bring a new understanding of the role of biochemical alterations in the pathological behavior of various liver tumors" (42). The hepatic tumor used for detailed studies was the very rapidly growing, very malignant, Novikoff hepatoma. The Novikoff tumor appeared to represent the end point of neoplastic transformation where all molecular symptoms and signs of neoplasia are expressed in the fullest degree (30). It was anticipated that a deeper understanding of the metabolism of tumors might be reached if other types of hepatomas with different degrees of malignant transformation were available. Because various liver tumors differ in their histological structure, cellular population, biological behavior, and growth rate, it was expected that the biochemical alterations which underlie morphological and biological differences would be present in varying qualitative or quantitative extents. Such a concept agrees well with clinical experience of many gradations of the same disease, from subclinical through mild or severe manifestations to the rarely encountered, full-blown case in which all symptoms and signs are present to their maximum development.

The operation of ordered and correlated expressions of morphological, biological, and metabolic behavior in neoplastic cells is apparently linked with the expression of their malignancy and growth rate (30). To test the validity of this concept and the existence of such an ordered and linked pattern at the molecular level, a prerequisite was the availability of a spectrum of neoplasms of the same cell type where the molecular imbalance could be examined in a graded and quantitative manner (33). When the spectrum of hepatomas of different growth rates became available (15, 16) the prerequisite was fulfilled for a biological system where the progression of neoplastic transformation could be conveniently investigated (32, 43, 45). The analysis of gene expression in the hepatoma spectrum was approached with the molecular correlation concept.

B. General Theory of the Molecular Correlation Concept

The molecular correlation concept was developed as a conceptual and experimental method for studying gene expression at the molecular level. This concept is based on the assumption that the various cellular functions can be analyzed, correlated, and understood in terms of events at the molecular level. The approaches of the general theory were outlined elsewhere (39, 39a) and here only the most salient features are referred to.

It was recognized that in analyzing the pattern of gene expression there are at least 5 aspects that should be identified in order to elucidate the relationship between cellular functions and molecular events. (1) It is necessary to carefully define the function (e.g., gluconeogenesis, muscular contraction, cellular respiration, etc.), its scope (biological and homeostatic role), and the different degrees of its expression. This identifies the overall events in gene expression for which the covariants at the molecular level are to be determined. An advance in understanding the control of gene expression should come from identifying for each function the covariants as (2) quantitative or (3) qualitative discriminants and establishing the extent of their covariance with the degrees in the expression of the various physiological functions. (4) As a result of such studies, one should be able to identify an integrated pattern in gene expression that characterizes specifically the function in question and the degrees of its expression. (5) Finally, it is essential to ascertain the selective biological advantage that the cellular function and its graded amplification and regulation provide for the biological system.

Whereas the general theory refers to the molecular events linked with various normal cellular functions, the special theory refers to the application of the molecular correlation concept to a special case: neoplasia.

C. Special Theory: The Molecular Correlation Concept of Neoplasia

The special theory seeks to elucidate the pattern of control of gene expression in normal and neoplastic growth. This is important, since a genetic basis for

TABLE 12.1

THE MOLECULAR CORRELATION CONCEPT OF NEOPLASIA: THE SPECIAL THEORY SHOULD
IDENTIFY THE PATTERN IN THE FOLLOWING ASPECTS OF GENE EXPRESSION[a]

1. Degrees in biological behavior of cancer cells	The extent of expression of neoplastic transformation: replicative function, growth rate
2. Key quantitative discriminants	Activities of key enzymes, antagonistic enzymes, and metabolic pathways
3. Key qualitative discriminants	Quantitative changes of several orders of magnitude; alterations opposite in direction to those of control tissues of similar growth rates; shift in isozyme pattern
4. Integrated pattern of discriminants	Diagnostic pattern of metabolic imbalance that specifically discriminates cancer cells from normal control tissues of similar growth rates (e.g., regenerating, differentiating or fetal tissues)
5. The selective biological advantage	That the imbalance in control of gene expression for replication and for metabolic pattern confers to cancer cells

[a] From (39).

malignancy must be assumed as pointed out (3): "The genetic transmission of the cancer trait from mother to daughter cells is one of the cardinal features of the neoplastic process." The molecular correlation concept analyzes the link between the progressive degrees of malignant transformation and the degrees of expression of metabolic imbalance in cancer cells (39a).

In order to elucidate the link between the degrees of neoplastic transformation and metabolic imbalance, the molecular correlation concept of neoplasia should lead to the identification of a pattern in the various aspects of gene expression indicated in Table 12.1.

D. Neoplastic Transformation: Degrees of Its Expression

There is a need for delineation of the different degrees of malignant transformation. Malignancy here will be defined as "the ability of tumor cells to grow progressively and kill their host" (9). The different degrees in the expression of the replicative potential (the integral of cell renewal rate and the extent of growth fraction in the cell population) are manifestations of the biological malignancy of the cancer cells. Malignancy in a tumor spectrum can be quantified by measuring the growth rate of the neoplasms. Thus, the different degrees in the expression of the neoplastic transformation can be characterized by measurement of tumor growth rate (30, 32, 37). As will be discussed, growth rate can be determined by several independent methods which provide an assurance of quantitation of malignancy. Thus, the covariants at the molecular level, the molecular correlates of malignancy, can be correlated with malignancy or growth rate. The covariants can characterize neoplastic growth rate quantitatively and qualitatively.

E. Key Quantitative Discriminants

It has been recognized by application of the molecular correlation concept that the activities of key enzymes of opposing and competing metabolic pathways and the ratios of the pathways and of the key antagonistic enzymes can be used to provide quantitative correlates and measures of malignancy (7, 49, 51).

F. Key Qualitative Discriminants

The reprogramming of gene expression in cancer cells also entails qualitative alterations. As an operational definition we consider qualitative alterations the following changes in gene expression: (a) a quantitative biochemical change in the neoplasms that deviates by several orders of magnitude from the levels observed in control, normal cells; (b) an alteration opposite in direction to those in control tissues of similar growth rates (for instance, hexokinase activity was markedly increased in the rapidly growing hepatomas, but it was decreased in the rapidly growing differentiating and fetal liver); and (c) isozyme shift. By critical examination of the behavior of isozymes of key enzymes in carbohydrate metabolism (27, 33, 34) a pattern was recognized which entailed a decrease in the amount of the high K_m nutritionally and hormonally responsive isozymes, whereas the low K_m isozymes increased in parallel with tumor growth rate (33, 34, 38). An example of this isozyme shift is the decrease in the amount of the liver type glucokinase and pyruvate kinase isozymes and an increase in the hexokinase and muscle type pyruvate kinase.

G. Integrated Pattern of Discriminants

With sufficient insight into the metabolic imbalance it should be possible to identify an integrated array of discriminants that provides an ordered and specific diagnostic pattern which successfully distinguishes cancer cells from resting normal cells and from rapidly growing control cells (39).

H. The Selective Biological Advantage

The essential role of alterations in gene expression and their significance in neoplasia should be evaluated for recognizing the selective advantages that the metabolic imbalance confers to the tumor cells (38, 39). This should lead to an understanding of the meaningful nature of the reprogramming of gene expression that occurs in a malignancy linked pattern in the neoplasms. In turn this should lead to the pinpointing of potential enzymic targets for selective chemotherapy against neoplastic cells.

I. Spectrum of Tumors of Different Malignancy

To test the approaches of the molecular correlation concept and the existence of a malignancy linked pattern at the molecular level, a prerequisite was the availability of a spectrum of neoplasms of the same cell type in which the molecular events of cancer could be studied in a graded and quantitative manner, (30, 33, 34). When the spectrum of liver tumors of different growth rates became available the prerequisites were fulfilled for a biological system where the progression of neoplastic transformation could be meaningfully studied (30, 32).

Origin and Properties of the Hepatoma Spectrum. The spectrum of hepatomas of different growth rates was produced by chemical carcinogenesis (15, 16). The hepatomas were maintained through serial transplantation in inbred strains of rats. All tumors were of the same cell type, thus providing a series of neoplasms of the liver parenchymal cells. The hepatomas exhibited different rates of growth; however, the individual tumor lines showed considerable biological stability which permitted the repeatability of the studies in many laboratories.* In this laboratory, we employed the spectrum of hepatomas as a model system where the spheres of gene action, the indicators of the reprogramming of gene expression, and the degrees of metabolic imbalance can be correlated with the different stages in the expression of the neoplastic transformation (30, 32, 38, 39). An overview of the progressive neoplastic departure from the biological behavior and the enzymic and metabolic balance of the normal resting liver as it is reflected in the different degrees of altered gene expression in different lines of transplantable liver tumors is given in Table 12.2.

In recent years a spectrum of kidney tumors was developed with different growth rates (17) and comparisons have been made with tumors of other cell origins, which provided a spectrum of neoplasms of different growth rates (13, 57). Thus, it was possible to test the general applicability of the molecular correlation concept of neoplasia.

J. Identification and Selection for Analysis of Opposing Key Enzymes and Metabolic Pathways

With the molecular correlation concept it was recognized that for an understanding of the regulation of the biochemical pattern and its correlation with the biological behavior of the neoplasms, it is necessary to concentrate the investigation on key enzymes and overall metabolic pathways. With the advance in understanding of regulation of intermediary metabolism, it has been feasible to pinpoint those metabolic areas where the prediction of covariants that correlate with biological behavior became possible. Thus, it was recognized that

---

* Since most of the transplantation and distribution of the tumors was carried out in collaborative work by Dr. Harold P. Morris of Howard University, this minimized variations in tumor lines from laboratory to laboratory that might have occurred otherwise.

TABLE 12.2

SPECTRUM OF HEPATOMAS OF DIFFERENT MALIGNANCY: MODEL SYSTEM FOR ELUCIDATION
OF MOLECULAR BASIS OF NEOPLASTIC TRANSFORMATION[a]

Spheres of gene action	Indicators of reprogramming of gene expression	Degrees in expression of neoplastic transformation (Extent of change from normal)		
		Slight	Intermediate	Extensive
Biological behavior	Growth rate	Low	Medium	Rapid
Morphology	Differentiation	Near normal	Medium	Poor
Genetic apparatus	Chromosome number	Normal	Increased	High
	Chromosome karyo-type	Normal	Altered	Deranged
Energy generation	Respiration	Normal	Moderately low	Low
	Glycolysis	Low	Normal or increased	High
Replication and functions	Imbalance in opposing pathways of synthesis and degradation	Moderate	Advanced	Pronounced
Isozyme pattern	Isozyme shift	Moderate	Advanced	Pronounced

[a] From (39).

meaningful correlations can be discovered by studying the following covariants: (a) activities of key enzymes that oppose each other in synthetic and degradative pathways; (b) ratios of antagonistic or competing key enzymes; (c) overall activities of synthetic and degradative metabolic pathways; (d) ratios of opposing or competing synthetic and degradative pathways; and (e) shift in the isozyme pattern of key enzymes (39a). It was also useful to pinpoint the conceptual and technical errors that would lead to failure in detecting biochemical correlations with metabolic functions or malignant transformations (37).

K. Measurement of Degrees of Malignancy: Tumor Growth Rate as a Key Determinant

The malignancy of the transplanted hepatoma line can be measured by determining the growth rate of the neoplasm. Growth rate is an important indicator of gene expression with which other indicators of gene expression manifested in the biochemical phenotype can be correlated.

1. METHODS OF MEASURING GROWTH RATE

Tumor growth rate can be measured by three independent techniques which provide the ranking of the hepatomas in order of their growth rate (Table 12.3). Since growth rate can be quantitated with precision and confidence, it is an

TABLE 12.3
MEASURING METHODS FOR RANKING TUMORS OF THE
HEPATOMA SPECTRUM BY GROWTH RATE[a]

Type of method	Description
Biological	Tumor size and volume
	Tumor weight
	Average time between transplantations
	Time required to kill host
Cytological	Mitotic counts, mitotic index
Biochemical	Study of thymidine (Tdr) metabolism
In vivo	Injection of Tdr: extraction and counting of DNA
In vitro	Incubation of tissue slices with Tdr: determining the ratio of incorporation into DNA and degradation to CO_2; using Tdr in autoradiography

[a] Growth rate is measurable with precision with one or several of the above methods which all give similar ranking.

operational advantage to relate the biochemical events to growth rate. It has been suggested that the biochemical alterations should be related with the state of differentiation or dedifferentiation of the tumors. However, as pointed out elsewhere there is no conceptual or methodological advantage in this; rather there are a number of disadvantages in the attempt to use the state of differentiation as a measure (37). Histological grading is not easily available to biochemists nor is it as precise a quantification as the different methods of measuring growth rates provide. It is reassuring that both growth rate and histological grading yield essentially the same ranking order for the various tumor lines in the spectrum.

2. THE BIOLOGICAL AND CLINICAL SIGNIFICANCE OF TUMOR GROWTH RATE

Growth rate is an expression of the degree of malignant transformation. This alone would mark it as a center of attention. Moreover, consideration of growth rate enters into the diagnosis and prognosis of clinical neoplasia. It also plays a role in the design and evaluation of various therapeutic measures. As pointed out recently the susceptibility of human tumors to chemotherapy relates to their growth rates (8, 59).

The selection of growth rate as an important parameter to which other expressions of neoplasia are related does not mean that one should overlook other significant aspects of malignancy such as the tendency to invade, to spread, and to set up metastatic lesions until the death of the organism occurs (43). However, growth rate can be quantitated.

In the selection of growth rate as an indicator of the different degrees of neoplastic transformation, it is advantageous in conducting a critical enquiry to choose a process which can be measured with precision by three independent techniques: biological, cytological, and biochemical methods (37).

L. The Three Classes of the Molecular Correlation Concept

The systematic investigation carried out in my laboratories demonstrated that the metabolic parameters in the tumors can be classified into three groups according to their relation to the degrees of neoplastic transformation as measured by the growth rates in the hepatoma spectrum (39a).

Class 1: Malignancy linked alterations. Parameters that correlate positively or negatively with growth rate are included in this group. These malignancy linked changes in gene expression can be used to characterize and to measure the progressive expression of malignancy in the tumor spectrum.

Class 2: Ubiquitous changes. Parameters that are increased in all, or decreased in all, tumors with possibly one or two exceptions are included in this group. These are ubiquitous changes where malignancy is expressed in a discontinuous fashion in the alterations of gene expression which occur in all or nearly all neoplasms in the spectrum.

Class 3: Coincidental alterations. Parameters that exhibit no correlation with tumor growth rate are included in this group. In the case of enzymes, they usually are the ones that are present in great excess and are involved in the catalysis of reversible reactions. These parameters may represent coincidental and nonessential lesions as compared to those in classes 1 and 2 which should be the essential ones closely linked with the core of neoplastic transformation. The classification of the molecular signs in relation to growth rate has been analyzed in detail (32, 43).

For a description of the biological behavior of the spectrum, its histology and growth rate, the methods of transplantation (15), karyotype (19), and the detailed analysis of the biochemical pattern, the reader is referred to several reviews and to the original papers (30–32, 37–39a, 52b).

M. Selection of Appropriate Control Tissues

1. THE NORMAL LIVER

The proper controls include normal rats of the same age, weight, strain, and sex, without tumors, as the source of appropriate control tissues. For the hepatoma spectrum, the control tissue is the liver of the normal adult rat. Suitable numbers of such control rats should be sacrificed at the same time as the tumor-bearing rats.

The liver of the tumor-bearing rat, i.e., the host liver, is not an appropriate control because it may reflect the effect of the stress of carrying the tumor and various other artifacts arising from the tumor-host relationship (30, 43, 44). Even though the host liver may have a useful role when dietary or hormonal

regulation is studied, there is still a need for the additional use of normal rats
with the tumor-bearing animals.

2. The Use of Fetal and Newborn Rat Liver as Controls

The employment of fetal liver is fraught with problems. The fetal liver is
really a hemopoietic organ in the rat and only a small portion can be identified
as liver cells (30, 40). Moreover, the ratio of hemopoietic to normal cells changes
during gestation. Unless this is taken into consideration, results obtained in
fetal liver and expressed on a gram wet weight basis are well-nigh impossible
to evaluate. Therefore, the fetal liver is not an appropriate control tissue and
results must be used with caution. After birth the hemopoietic foci rapidly
disappear and by day 5 or 6 the overwhelming majority of the cells are liver
cells. The 5-day liver of the newborn rat and the various subsequent stages
of development can be used as a system of differentiating liver and if the results
are expressed per cell they can be evaluated meaningfully (49).

3. Regenerating Liver as a Control

The regenerating liver is probably the best and the most relevant control
tissue available. The regenerating liver should be produced in the inbred
strains where the tumors are carried and in this fashion rapidly growing hepatic
tissue is available in the adult rat. Another advantage is that the growth rate
of the regenerating liver is similar to that of the most rapidly growing liver
tumors (12).

N. Expression and Evaluation of Biochemical Results

For a number of very cogent reasons all techniques in killing the animals
and preparing the tissues for the assays should be precisely standardized (30).
Special care is taken to remove necrotic, hemorrhagic, and nontumorous materials and only viable hepatoma tissue is used. A sample is preserved for
histological staining and another sample is analyzed for thymidine ratios. These
procedures are useful in the grading of the tumors.

For the expression of the biochemical results and of the enzyme assays see
references (30, 43). The conclusions from the various considerations for the
appropriateness of the different bases of expression are the following: The
biochemical parameters can be expressed per gram wet weight of tissue, per
dry weight, per protein or nitrogen content, per DNA or per average cell.
Under most circumstances the meaningful basis of expression is per average
cell. The method for counting cells is a simple one (41) which is both quick
and precise. The cellularity of the normal liver in fetal, newborn, differentiating,
and adult rat liver was reported elsewhere (49).

In examining the correlation of biochemical parameters with growth rate various simple plots and calculation of Spearman's rank correlation coefficients can
be used and examples of these are given in our work (37, 49).

II. Carbohydrate Metabolism: Pattern of Imbalance

A. Enzyme Activities: Correlation with Growth Rate

Previous work demonstrated that in the hepatoma spectrum in parallel with increasing tumor growth rate the activity of the key gluconeogenic enzymes decreased, whereas those of the key glycolytic enzymes increased (Fig. 12.1). These results are good representations of the antagonistic behavior of opposing

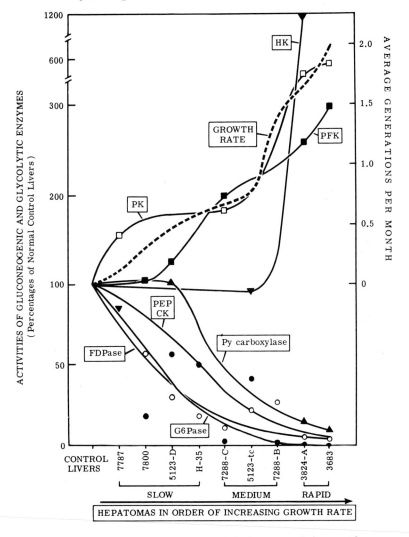

Fig. 12.1. Correlation of key enzymes of carbohydrate metabolism with tumor growth rate. The key glycolytic enzymes exhibit a positive, and the key gluconeogenic enzymes show a negative, correlation with the growth rate of hepatomas. The growth rate is indicated by the interrupted line (from 43).

key enzymes that may be used as discriminants in characterizing the progressive degrees of neoplastic transformation. These data support the molecular correlation concept (32, 43).

B. Ratios of Enzyme Activities: Correlation with Growth Rate

In more recent studies in order to investigate how closely the imbalance of the antagonistic key enzymes is linked with growth rate, the ratios of the activities of the opposing key enzymes were calculated and correlated with hepatoma growth rate. Figure 12.2 shows that the ratios of the activities of the glycolytic/gluconeogenic enzymes (hexokinase/glucose-6-phosphatase; phosphofructokinase/fructose-1,6-diphosphatase) correlate closely with hepatoma growth rate over a wide range (49).

C. Opposing Metabolic Pathways: Correlation with Growth Rate

The opposing pathways of glycolysis and gluconeogenesis also relate to growth rate (14, 30). It was first recognized in my laboratories that aerobic glycolysis increased in parallel with tumor growth rate (24, 30, 46) and that gluconeogenesis decreased in parallel with the rise in hepatoma growth rate (24, 30, 46). Thus, the metabolic imbalance correlates with the degrees of malignant transformation.

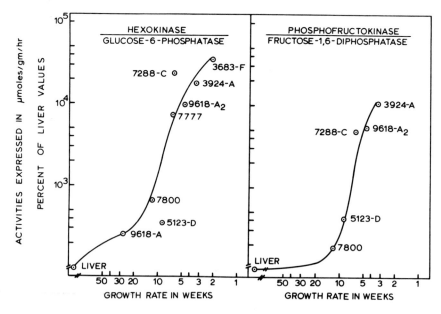

Fig. 12.2. Correlation of the ratios of opposing key glycolytic/key gluconeogenic enzymes with growth rate of hepatomas (from 49).

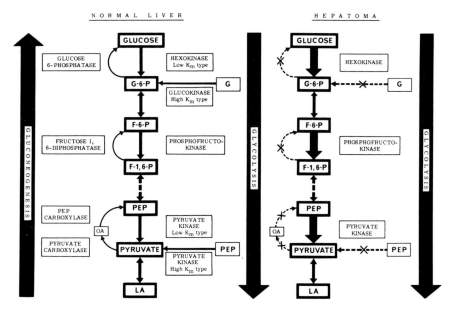

Fig. 12.3. Three of the main changes in carbohydrate metabolism are illustrated: decrease in activities of key gluconeogenic enzymes, increase in activities of key glycolytic enzymes, and the shift in isozyme pattern (from 35).

D. Isozyme Shift: Correlation with Growth Rate

The reprogramming of gene expression in the hepatoma spectrum is also revealed in the isozyme shift. In the hepatoma the emergence of such qualitative discriminants was recognized in the critical examination of the isozyme pattern of key enzymes in carbohydrate metabolism (33, 34, 39). In analyzing the relative amount of the low and high K_m isozymes of glycolysis the operation of a pattern was recognized (Fig. 12.3). This pattern entailed a decrease in the amounts of the high K_m, nutritionally and hormonally responsive isozymes such as the liver type glucokinase and pyruvate kinase. In contrast, the low K_m isozymes such as the hexokinase and muscle type pyruvate kinase increased in parallel with tumor growth rate (27, 34). A similar shift in the isozyme pattern was also recognized for the isozymes of cAMP phosphodiesterase (4, 38).

E. The Three Classes of Metabolic Alterations in Carbohydrate Metabolism

When the relation of the metabolic imbalance to the degrees of neoplastic transformation was examined, it was observed that many of the alterations now outlined and those reported earlier correlate with growth rate and thus belong to class 1 (31). A more complete listing of the parameters in carbohydrate metabolism that correlate with growth rate is given in Table 12.10 (p. 518). As pointed out in an earlier analysis there are a number of parameters in carbohydrate metabolism that may be grouped into classes 2 and 3 (43). For example, the following parameters belong in class 2. There was an increase in glucose-6-phosphate dehydrogenase activity in all the hepatomas. In contrast, in all the liver tumors there was a decrease in glycogen content, in fructose uptake, in the activity of phosphoglucomutase, and in the activity of the pathways of fructose to CO_2. The transformation of glucose to fatty acids was decreased in all hepatomas (31).

In class 3 are the parameters that do not relate to growth rate: the activities of phosphohexoseisomerase, lactate dehydrogenase, phosphoglycerate kinase, and 3-phosphoglyceraldehyde dehydrogenase. The activities of 6-phosphogluconate dehydrogenase or the malate enzyme or the activation of phosphoglucomutase show no relationship to growth rate (47).

F. Selective Advantages That the Metabolic Imbalance Confers to Cancer Cells

An analysis of the biological role of the altered gene expression in carbohydrate metabolism indicates that it confers a selective advantage to the cancer cells (30, 39, 50). This conclusion is based on the fact that the imbalance in the ratios of glycolytic/gluconeogenic enzymes results in a biochemical pattern that is favorable to glycolysis and eliminates gluconeogenic recycling. In consequence, the available glucose precursor can be channelled into glycolysis and indeed the glycolytic rate did increase in parallel with the growth rate of the hepatomas. The increase in the activity of glucose-6-phosphate dehydrogenase should provide an increased amount of the ribose and NADPH for biosynthesis in nucleic acid metabolism. The pattern of isozyme shift occurs in such a fashion that the high K_m isozymes that were subject to nutritional, hormonal, and feedback controls decreased and were gradually replaced by the low K_m isozymes that were not subject to nutritional and hormonal regulation and were much less subject to allosteric regulation by physiological signals coming from other cells of the organism. In consequence, the isozyme shift leads to a decreased responsiveness to physiological control (Fig. 12.4). This provides a partial explanation, at the molecular level, for the tendency of the cancer cells to be less responsive to regulation (33, 34, 39).

Thus, the reprogramming of gene expression confers selective advantages to cancer cells in that it insures the predominance of glycolysis, eliminates the functioning of the opposing pathway, gluconeogenesis, increases the potential for the production of ribose and NADPH and results through the isozyme shift in the cancer cells in a decreased susceptibility to regulatory signals that arise from other cells of the organism (Table 12.4).

III. DNA Metabolism: Pattern of Imbalance

It was pointed out earlier that the sum of collected evidence suggested that there was a progressive increase in the biosynthesis and a gradual decrease in the degradation of nucleic acids. Both of these processes were correlated

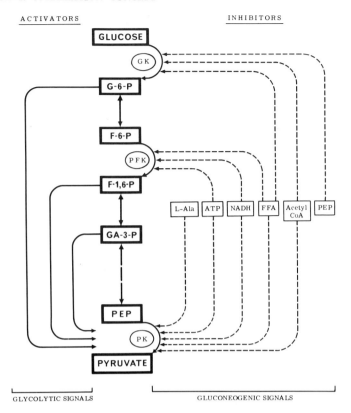

Fig. 12.4. Array of regulating molecules that modulate the enzymes of gluconeogenesis and glycolysis in liver (from 34). With the loss of glucokinase and liver-type pyruvate kinase the sensitivity to control by phosphoenolpyruvate and L-alanine is lost and the sensitivity to inhibition by ATP is decreased by an order of magnitude. The sensitivity to inhibition by acetyl-CoA is also markedly diminished.

with the increase in tumor growth rate (32, 43). The results chiefly documented the gradual rise in the biosynthesis of DNA. Recently it has been demonstrated that the reprogramming of gene expression also profoundly affected the balance of UMP and pyrimidine metabolism (7, 21, 49).

A. DNA Level: Increased with Rise in Growth Rate

A great deal of evidence accumulated that the pathways of DNA synthesis were increased and concurrently the opposing pathways of catabolism were decreased in parallel with the rise in tumor growth rate. From this, one may expect a rise in the DNA content that may correlate with the hepatoma growth rate.

It was demonstrated that the DNA per cell was in normal range in the slow growing hepatomas, but it was increased to 177% in the intermediate growth rate hepatoma 7288C, and to about 250% in the rapidly growing tumors 3924A and 3683 (12). Because of these alterations in the DNA content which roughly

TABLE 12.4

CARBOHYDRATE METABOLISM: PHENOTYPIC EVIDENCE FOR REPROGRAMMING
OF GENE EXPRESSION IN NEOPLASIA[a]

1. Synthetic enzymes:	Key gluconeogenic enzymes[b]	Decreased
2. Catabolic enzymes:	Key glycolytic enzymes[c]	Increased
3. Metabolic imbalance:	Ratios of key glycolytic/key gluconeo-genic enzymes	Increased
4. Isozyme shift:	High K_m isozymes[d]	Decreased
	Low K_m isozymes[e]	Increased
5. Relation to malignancy:	Alterations are covariant with growth rate	Malignancy-linked imbalance
6. Biological role:	Imbalance in glycolytic/gluconeogenic enzymes leads to increase in glycolysis Isozyme shift leads to decreased responsiveness to physiological controls	Confers selective advantages to cancer cells

[a] From (39a).

[b] Glucose-6-phosphatase, fructose 1,6-diphosphatase, phosphoenolpyruvate carboxykinase, pyruvate carboxylase.

[c] Hexokinase, phosphofructokinase, pyruvate kinase.

[d] Glucokinase, liver type pyruvate kinase.

[e] Hexokinase, muscle type pyruvate kinase.

correspond to alterations in chromosome number in these tumors (19), the DNA level is not recommended as a basis for expression of the biochemical results. The DNA content in the regenerating liver was in the normal range (12).

B. DNA Biosynthesis: Overall Pathway Increased with Rise in Tumor Growth Rate

In vivo studies employing injection of labeled thymidine showed that the incorporation of thymidine into DNA increased in parallel with tumor growth rate (12).

C. Enzymes of DNA Synthesis and Degradation

An examination of the enzymes involved in DNA synthesis indicated that most of these enzymes exhibited a correlation to varying extents with the growth rate of the hepatomas (Fig. 12.5).

Since growth rate and replication are intimately linked with the operation and control of pyrimidine and DNA metabolism, systematic investigations were recently carried out to discover the pattern and the relationship of these metabolic functions to the degrees of neoplastic transformation in the hepatoma spectrum. Much of these results can now be integrated into a meaningful metabolic pattern.

The activities of the synthetic and catabolic enzymes of pyrimidine and DNA metabolism are compared in Table 12.5. To make the results comparable, all enzyme activities were recalculated and expressed on the same basis (49).

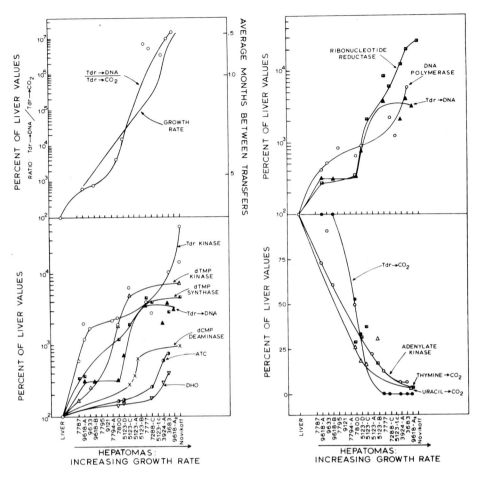

Fig. 12.5. Correlation of enzymes of pyrimidine and DNA metabolism with hepatoma growth rate (from 49).

A pattern was recognized in that the enzymes that exhibited the lowest activity in the normal resting liver of the adult rat were the ones that increased to the greatest extent in the most rapidly growing hepatomas: ribonucleotide reductase (6) and DNA polymerase (20). In turn, the synthetic enzymes that had the highest activity in the liver exhibited the smallest extent of rise in the rapidly growing neoplasms: aspartate transcarbamylase, dihydroorotase (25, 26), and nucleoside diphosphate kinase (37).

The enzymes involved in the catabolism of the pyrimidines, dihydrouracil dehydrogenase, thymidine phosphorylase, etc., (49) had in general much higher activities than the rate-limiting enzymes of the synthetic pathways, such as the ribonucleotide reductase in the *de novo* pathway and the DNA polymerase in the final common path of the *de novo* and salvage pathways.

Any comparison of absolute activities of "opposing" enzymes of synthesis and catabolism must be done with great caution since compartmentation, endogenous substrate levels, transport of precursors, the concentration of metabolites and

TABLE 12.5

DNA Metabolism: Comparison of Activities of Enzymes Involved in Synthetic and Degradative Pathways[a]

	Livers		Hepatomas (rapidly growing)	
Enzymes	Normal fed[b]	Regen. 24 hr[c]	Novikoff[c]	3683F[c]
Anabolic				
Ribonucleotide reductase	3		25,300	20,800
DNA polymerase	56	540		5,810
dTMP synthase	180	1,140	4,510	2,860
dTMP kinase	420	1,620	7,100	
TdR kinase	2,400	680	14,000	10,200
Uridine kinase	6,200	210		
dCMP deaminase	12,000	350	900	750
OMP pyrophosphorylase	20,000	380		
OMP decarboxylase	71,000			
CP synthase	94,000	96		
Aspartate transcarbamylase	123,000	127	480	796
Dihydroorotase	246,000	108		418
Nucleosidediphosphate kinase	1,200,000			200
Catabolic				
Dihydrouracil dehydrogenase	26,000	78		9
β-Ureidopropionase	144,000	58		
Dihydrouracil hydrase	276,000	66		
TdR phosphorylase	234,000	106		31

[a] Modified from Weber et al. (49). In order to achieve a comparison, all data were recalculated in $\mu\mu$moles of substrate metabolized/mg protein/hour. In calculations the values of 0.2 gm protein/gm wet weight of tissue for homogenates and 0.08 gm protein/gm wet weight for supernatant fluids were used.

[b] Values expressed as $\mu\mu$m/mg protein/hour.

[c] Values expressed as % liver.

cofactors, pH, and various modulating molecules might strongly influence the *in vivo* situation. Nevertheless, the working hypothesis is supported by data in Table 12.5 which suggested that in the hepatoma spectrum one could predict an increase in the key synthetic enzyme activities and a decrease in the key catabolic activities that should parallel hepatoma growth rate (37, 49).

D. Metabolic Imbalance: Correlation with Growth Rate

The integrated pattern of the metabolic imbalance that occurs for pyrimidine and DNA metabolizing enzymes in the hepatoma spectrum is illustrated in Fig. 12.7. The data given in Tables 12.5 and 12.6 and Figs. 12.5, 12.6, and 12.7 indicate the phenotypic evidence for reprogramming of gene expression in nucleic acid metabolism. The key enzymes of UMP, TTP, and DNA synthesis increased, and the rate limiting enzymes of UMP and TdR catabolism decreased in parallel with tumor growth rate. As a result, an imbalance emerged between the synthetic

TABLE 12.6

TdR METABOLISM: CORRELATION OF IMBALANCE OF SYNTHETIC AND CATABOLIC DEGRADATIVE PATHWAYS WITH HEPATOMA GROWTH RATE[a]

Tissue	Growth rate (av. months between transfers)	No. of observations	Thymidine to DNA		Thymidine to CO_2		$\dfrac{\text{Thymidine to DNA}}{\text{Thymidine to } CO_2}$	
			DPM/gm/hour	%	DPM/gm/hour	%		%
Control (normal liver)		44	11,330 ± 250	100	1,065,000 ± 17,000	100	0.0100 ± 0.0003	100
Hepatomas								
Slow								
66	13.0	6	12,300 ± 100	109	827,000 ± 90,000	78	0.0148 ± 0.0010	148
47-C	8.0	8	16,000 ± 1300	143	593,000 ± 40,000	56	0.0300 ± 0.0028	300
7787	7.0	4	51,000 ± 1000	450	987,000 ± 53,000	93	0.0510 ± 0.0030	510
9618-A	5.8	10	33,000 ± 5000	291	555,000 ± 50,000	52	0.0590 ± 0.0030	590
9618-B	4.5	7	33,000 ± 2000	292	387,000 ± 30,000	36	0.0810 ± 0.0040	810
8999		5	44,000 ± 3000	388	275,000 ± 28,000	26	0.165 ± 0.002	1650
9633	3.3	4	73,000 ± 12,000	660	436,000 ± 25,000	41	0.170 ± 0.020	1700
Medium								
7800	3.0	8	77,300 ± 4000	683	127,000 ± 13,000	12	0.666 ± 0.013	6660
5123-D	2.5	5	80,000 ± 22,700	706	68,700 ± 7340	6.5	1.350 ± 0.390	13,500
Rapid								
3924-A	1.0	10	230,000 ± 7000	2030	1000 ± 90	0.094	240 ± 21	2,400,000
7288-C	0.8	16	268,000 ± 9340	2370	534 ± 67	0.050	562 ± 61	5,620,000
7777	0.8	6	378,000 ± 13,400	3340	600 ± 110	0.056	630 ± 100	6,300,000
3683-F	0.5	12	465,000 ± 31,000	4100	500 ± 60	0.047	946 ± 27	9,460,000
9618-A2	0.4	7	444,000 ± 69,000	3920	400 ± 47	0.038	1100 ± 120	11,000,000

[a] From (51).

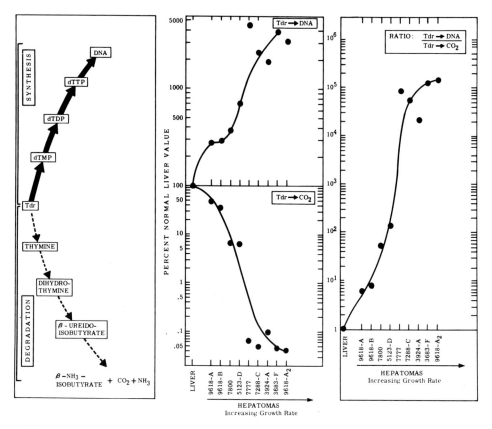

Fig. 12.6. Correlation of the behavior of the opposing pathways of thymidine metabolism with hepatoma growth rate (from 36).

and catabolic enzymes and between the overall pathways of synthesis and degradation.

This metabolic imbalance was especially reflected in the close correlation between the ratios of the incorporation of TdR to DNA/degradation of TdR to CO_2 and the hepatoma growth rate (49). These thymidine ratios showed the best correlation with tumor growth rate among all the biochemical factors examined to date and the ratios can be used to biochemically measure the growth rate in the hepatoma spectrum (36, 49). The enzyme that showed the greatest extent of increase and correlated the best with hepatoma growth rate was the ribonucleotide reductase as demonstrated by Elford *et al.* (6).

Since a number of enzymic and metabolic alterations in nucleic acid metabolism were covariant with the growth rate in the hepatoma spectrum, these parameters represent malignancy linked phenotypic expressions of neoplasia.

E. Purine Metabolism

There is relatively little known about the precise pattern of purine metabolism in the hepatoma spectrum. This important metabolic area warrants extensive further investigation.

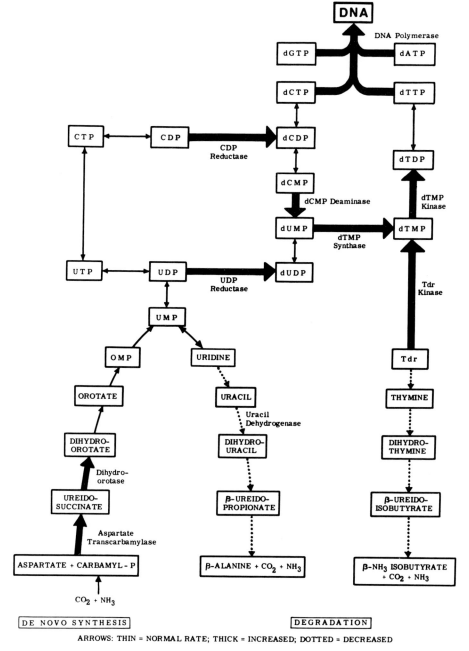

Fig. 12.7. Pattern of metabolic imbalance in pyrimidine and DNA metabolism (from 49).

F. Purine Biosynthesis: Increased with Rise in Growth Rate

A good correlation was observed between the extent of formate incorporation *in vivo* and the growth rate of hepatomas (48, 53). The incorporation of labeled formate and adenine into RNA also correlated well with the growth rate of hepatomas. In contrast, the incorporation of these precursors into RNA was increased in all the tumors examined. Thus, these latter parameters belong to class 2.

G. Purine Catabolism: Decreased with Rise in Tumor Growth Rate

Two enzymes involved in catabolism, xanthine oxidase (58) and uricase (18), in the slow growing hepatoma 5123 had 50 to 85% of the total activities of normal liver. The activities decreased to traces or appeared to be absent in the rapidly growing hepatomas (5, 18, 58).

On the basis of the present evidence, the increase in purine synthesis is, in part, unopposed by the decreased activities of the purine catabolizing enzymes.

H. RNA Metabolism

The total RNA content of liver tumors was not correlated with growth rate (18, 48). When this was first analyzed (43) it was noted, "It may be worth mentioning that the relative proportions of different molecular species of RNA and the turnover rates should be more characteristic and relevant to the problems of neoplasia and these may prove to be different in the different tumors." It is relevant to point out that tRNA methylase was highly increased in the Novikoff tumor and it was unaltered in the regenerating liver (2, 29; see Chapter VI). The hepatoma spectrum (2, 23) shows that the activity of tRNA methylase increases in parallel with the rise in hepatoma growth rate (Fig. 12.8).

I. Selective Biological Advantages

The imbalance in the ratio of synthetic/catabolic enzymes of pyrimidine, purine, and DNA metabolism leads to a biochemical pattern that highly favors synthetic utilization of precursors and effectively eliminates recycling by the marked decrease and abolition of the key catabolic enzymes (39, 43). In consequence, the available precursors can be utilized primarily for purine, pyrimidine, and DNA biosynthesis. The observations obtained by studying the ratios of rate of thymidine synthesis versus catabolic disposition are in good agreement with this prediction. Thus, in purine, pyrimidine, and DNA metabolism the reprogramming of gene expression confers selective advantages on the cancer cells by insuring the predominance of synthesis and by eliminating the operation of the opposing degradative pathways (Table 12.7).

IV. Ornithine Metabolism: Pattern of Imbalance

Since ornithine occupies a central position in several metabolic pathways, it may be assumed that this metabolite might reflect a biochemical imbalance that is linked with growth rate (51, 52, 54). Since ornithine is not contained

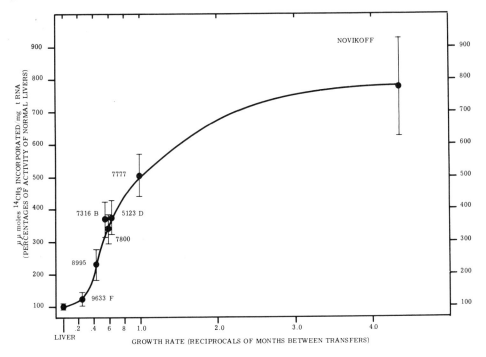

Fig. 12.8. Correlation of tRNA methylase activity with hepatoma growth rate. The means and standard errors were calculated from the original data (from 2, 23) and plotted as percentages of the values of normal liver from appropriate control rats.

TABLE 12.7

DNA METABOLISM: PHENOTYPIC EVIDENCE FOR REPROGRAMMING OF
GENE EXPRESSION IN LIVER NEOPLASIA[a]

1. Synthetic enzymes:	Key enzymes of UMP,[a] TTP,[b] and DNA[c] synthesis	Increased
2. Degradative enzymes:	Key enzymes of UMP and TdR catabolism[d]	Decreased
3. Enzymic imbalance:	Ratios of synthetic/catabolic enzymes	Increased
4. Metabolic imbalance:	Ratios of TdR to DNA/TdR to CO_2 pathways	Increased
5. Relation to malignancy:	Alterations are covariant with growth rate	Malignancy-linked imbalance
6. Biological role:	Imbalance in anabolic/catabolic enzymes of UMP metabolism leads to increased de novo DNA synthesis Imbalance in anabolic/catabolic enzymes of TdR metabolism leads to increased salvage pathway to DNA synthesis	Confers selective advantages to cancer cells

[a] Aspartate carbamyltransferase, dihydroorotase.
[b] Ribonucleotide reductase, dCMP deaminase, dTMP synthase, TdR kinase, dTMP kinase.
[c] DNA polymerase.
[d] Dihydrouracil dehydrogenase, dihydrothymine dehydrogenase.

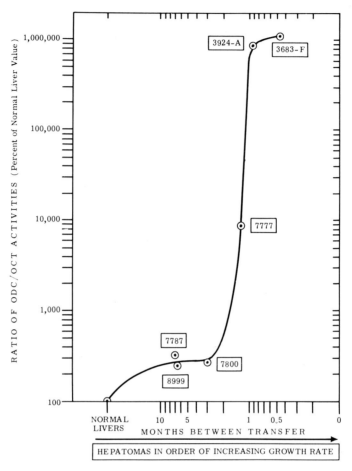

Fig. 12.9. Correlation of the ratios of ornithine decarboxylase/ornithine carbamyltransferase activities with hepatoma growth rate (from 51).

in proteins it functions elsewhere (55), i.e., it is: (a) involved in urea synthesis by ornithine carbamyltransferase activity; (b) metabolized by ornithine decarboxylase channelling it into polyamine formation; or (c) metabolized by ornithine transaminase. Ornithine is involved in the urea cycle and is involved in polyamine biosynthesis. Since the urea cycle competes with purine and pyrimidine biosynthesis for two important precursors (aspartate, carbamyl phosphate), it seemed that the operation of such a competitive situation might provide a target area for a metabolic imbalance in the hepatoma spectrum where correlations with growth rate might well be predicted (51, 52, 54). Another fact that prompted interest in ornithine metabolism is that ornithine is the only known precursor for polyamine biosynthesis and the role of polyamines in cell replication in neoplasia is as yet undefined. A systematic study carried out on the hepatoma spectrum (52, 54, 56) resulted in the discovery of an imbalance in ornithine metabolism that is linked with tumor growth rate (39a).

A. Ornithine Carbamyltransferase: Decreased with Rise in Growth Rate

Studies on the behavior of ornithine carbamyltransferase demonstrated that this enzyme activity decreased in parallel with the increase in hepatoma growth rate (52). In contrast, the activity of ornithine decarboxylase increased in most of the hepatomas and there was also an indication of an increase in the levels of certain polyamines.

B. Ornithine Decarboxylase and Polyamines: Increased

The activity of ornithine decarboxylase and the concentration of putrescine increased roughly in parallel with hepatoma growth rate. The ratio of the enzyme that channels ornithine into the urea cycle and the one that routes ornithine into polyamine synthesis, i.e., ornithine decarboxylase/ornithine carbamyltransferase (Fig. 12.9), increased in parallel with hepatoma growth rate (51, 52).

C. Ornithine Transaminase: Decreased

Preliminary studies suggest that the ornithine transaminase activity decreases in parallel with hepatoma growth rate exhibiting low activities in the rapidly growing neoplasms (28a).

D. Selective Biological Advantages of Imbalance in Ornithine Metabolism

The biological significance of the imbalance in ornithine metabolism can be perceived from the results discussed and the data illustrated in Fig. 12.10. Of the metabolic pathways of ornithine, only ornithine decarboxylase activity is retained and increased in rapidly growing liver tumors. Since there is a decrease in ornithine carbamyltransferase activity, there should be a decline in the utilization of aspartate and carbamyl phosphate for urea synthesis and, consequently, there precursors might be preferentially spared for the synthesis of DNA and RNA.

The first two enzymes of orotate synthesis (aspartate transcarbamylase, dihydroorotase) increased in parallel with hepatoma growth rate, indicating that these precursors might indeed be preferentially utilized for nucleic acid biosynthesis (25, 26).

In consequence, the metabolic imbalance manifested in the ratios of ornithine decarboxylase/ornithine carbamyltransferase might confer a selective biological advantage on the cancer cell as this imbalance becomes progressively more pronounced in parallel with the increase in tumor growth rate. Thus, for this area as well, the phenotypic evidence indicates a reprogramming of gene expression that is linked with tumor growth rate and confers a biological advantage on the neoplastic cells (51, 52).

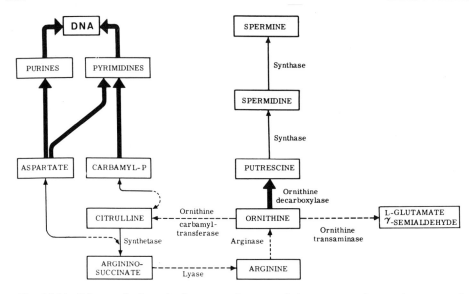

Fig. 12.10. Selective biological advantages that an imbalance in ornithine utilization might confer on neoplastic cells (from 38).

V. cAMP Metabolism: Pattern of Imbalance

Extensive studies have been carried out on numerous aspects of cAMP metabolism; however, application of the molecular correlation concept to cAMP metabolism in the hepatoma spectrum has been carried out only recently (38, 39a).

A. Application of the Molecular Correlation Concept to cAMP Metabolism

In order to apply the approaches of the molecular correlation concept, cAMP metabolism was examined from the following points of view: (a) behavior of the synthetic pathway (adenylate cyclase activity); (b) behavior of the degradative pathway (cAMP phosphodiesterase activity); (c) level of cAMP; and (d) isozyme shift.

If the reprogramming of gene expression is also manifested in the cAMP system and if the pattern resembles that observed for carbohydrate, pyrimidine, purine, DNA, and ornithine metabolism, the solution of the following problems should be undertaken (38).

(1) An imbalance in cAMP metabolism could emerge as a consequence of an alteration in the ratio of the activities of the synthetic enzyme (adenylate cyclase) and the catabolic enzyme (cAMP phosphodiesterase) that control the steady-state level of cAMP. (2) An isozyme shift might be revealed by examining the responsiveness to regulation and the kinetic behavior of the synthetic and catabolic enzymes. (3) The biological significance of an anticipated imbalance might be reflected in assays of the cAMP concentrations in normal and neoplastic tissues. (4) A linking of the anticipated imbalance in cAMP metabolism with

malignancy should be detected in the model system of the spectrum of hepatomas where alterations in gene expression can be studied in a graded and quantitative approach. The results of these investigations are integrated in Table 12.8.

B. Evidence for Reprogramming of Gene Expression in cAMP Metabolism

A comparison of the absolute activities of adenylate cyclase and phosphodiesterase in the liver suggested that at optimum substrate concentrations (which for both enzymes may not occur in the cell) the activities of these two opposing enzymes would be very unequal. The activity of phosphodiesterase would be several orders of magnitude higher than that of the synthetic enzyme, adenylate cyclase. On the other hand, the cyclase activity can be markedly increased by glucagon or epinephrine stimulation. Nevertheless, one might anticipate that the neoplastic alterations would involve a decrease in the activity of the synthetic enzyme, cyclase, and an increase in the activity of the catabolic enzyme, phosphodiesterase. Since the relevant metabolic actions of cAMP are supposed to take place in the cell membrane, these predictions would primarily pertain to the activity of these enzymes and of the cAMP level in the cell membrane of normal and tumor cells (38, 39a, 52a).

C. Adenylate Cyclase and cAMP Phosphodiesterase Activities in Hepatomas

1. ADENYLATE CYCLASE ACTIVITY IN HEPATOMAS

Adenylate cyclase activity was unaltered in the total homogenate in the various hepatomas of different growth rates and in the regenerating liver (1). However, this synthetic enzyme activity was decreased in the cell membrane of the rapidly growing hepatomas (22, 28, 52a).

2. cAMP PHOSPHODIESTERASE ACTIVITY IN HEPATOMAS

The activity of the catabolic enzyme, phosphodiesterase, when it was measured in the supernatant fluid, was decreased in the hepatomas, but it was unchanged in the regenerating liver (4). However, when the phosphodiesterase activity was measured in the cell membrane of rapidly growing hepatomas, it was observed that this enzyme activity was markedly increased (22, 28, 52a).

D. Regulation and Isozyme Shift in Enzymes Involved in cAMP Metabolism

1. ADENYLATE CYCLASE: STUDY OF STIMULATION OF ENZYME ACTIVITY

In a spectrum of hepatomas of different growth rates it was shown that the homogenate adenylate cyclase activity was markedly stimulated by sodium fluoride to the same extent as it was in normal or in regenerating liver. In contrast, studies with glucagon demonstrated a different pattern. Glucagon stimulation caused a statistically significant rise in adenylate cyclase activities in all normal and regenerating liver tissues. The hormone increased liver activities by 2- to 3-fold. A similar rise was observed in the slow growing hepatomas; however, there was only a minor elevation in the medium growth rate hepatoma studied and in the rapidly growing tumors there was no response to glucagon stimulation.

These results indicate that there was a decline in the responsiveness to glucagon stimulation in the adenylate cyclase system in parallel with the increase in hepatoma growth rate (1, 38). The results are compatible with the suggestion that there is an isozyme shift in the hepatomas and that there is a growth-rate linked decrease in the liver type glucagon-sensitive adenylate cyclase isozyme.

2. cAMP Phosphodiesterase: Isozyme Shift

Kinetic studies on the behavior of the supernatant fluid phosphodiesterase activity carried out at 1 mM cAMP (high K_m enzyme) and at 1 μM cAMP (low K_m enzyme) suggested that two phosphodiesterases were present in normal liver and in slow and rapidly growing hepatomas, one with a low apparent $K_m = 2$ to 3 μM and another with an apparent $K_m = 100$ to 500 μM. The high K_m phosphodiesterase activity was decreased in both slowly and rapidly growing hepatomas. In contrast, the low K_m phosphodiesterase activity in the slow and rapidly growing hepatomas increased to 185 and 265%, respectively. This alteration in the isozyme pattern of cAMP phosphodiesterase is specific to the neoplastic process, inasmuch as no similar isozyme shift was observed in the rapidly growing differentiating or regenerating liver (4).

The behavior of the cAMP phosphodiesterase isozymes is in line with the pattern of isozyme shift for the high and low K_m glucokinase-hexokinase and the hepatic muscle type pyruvate kinase systems. Thus, the observation for the phosphodiesterase isozyme shift supports the predictions of the molecular correlation concept that the neoplastic transformation entails a progressive emergence of a reprogramming of gene expression that appears to be linked with tumor growth rate (38).

E. Selective Biological Advantages

The evidence for the reprogramming of gene expression in neoplasia as manifested in the cAMP system (Table 12.8) is suggestive that the pattern of imbalance is basically similar to that found for carbohydrate, purine, pyrimidine, DNA, and ornithine metabolism. Thus, the enzyme involved in the synthesis of cAMP, although unaltered in the total homogenate, was decreased in the cell membrane of the rapidly growing hepatoma. In contrast, the activity of the catabolic enzyme, phosphodiesterase, which was decreased in the supernatant fluid, was increased in the cell membrane.

A decrease in the susceptibility to regulatory influence and the emergence of an isozyme shift were recognized in the decrease in glucagon sensitivity for the cyclase and in the increased low K_m phosphodiesterase activity in the

TABLE 12.8

cAMP METABOLISM: PHENOTYPIC EVIDENCE FOR REPROGRAMMING OF
GENE EXPRESSION IN LIVER NEOPLASIA[a]

1. cAMP level:	Overall concentration, subcellular compartmentation, turnover	Not certain
2. Synthetic enzyme:	Adenylate cyclase	
	Total cell activity	Unchanged
	Sensitivity to NaF stimulation	Unchanged
	Sensitivity to glucagon stimulation	Decreased with increase in growth rate
	Activity in membrane	Decreased
3. Catabolic enzyme:	cAMP phosphodiesterase	
	Total soluble activity	Decreased
	Activity in membrane	Increased
4. Isozyme shift:	Glucagon responsive cyclase	Decrease in hormone sensitivity
	Phosphodiesterase	
	High K_m isozyme	Decreased
	Low K_m isozyme	Increased
5. Enzymic imbalance:	Hormone responsive cyclase	Decreased
	Low K_m phosphodiesterase	Increased
	Activity in membrane	
	Adenylate cylase	Decreased
	Phosphodiesterase	Increased
	Phosphodiesterase/cyclase ratio	Increased
6. Biological role:	Imbalance in membrane phosphodiesterase/cyclase ratio / Isozyme shifts for phosphodiesterase and cyclase	Might confer selective advantages

[a] From (38).

rapidly growing hepatomas. It appears that the imbalance in the cAMP system relates to the malignancy of the hepatomas.

It has been postulated, with the evidence chiefly pertaining to tissue culture studies with normal and neoplastic fibroblasts, that the level of cAMP was low in the transformed cells and high in the normal, slow growing fibroblasts. However, preliminary studies in this laboratory, and in other centers, indicated that the total cAMP content was not altered in the hepatomas of different growth rates (38). No information is available on the cAMP concentration in the cell membrane or on cAMP turnover in various subcellular organelles.

In view of these uncertainties, the present results can only be taken as an indication that the alterations in the cAMP system are generally similar to those in other areas of imbalance in intermediary metabolism as found by application of the molecular correlation concept of neoplasia (39a, 52a).

VI. Specificity of Metabolic Phenotype to Malignancy

In view of the various claims in the literature suggesting that the neoplastic condition is a disease of differentiation or a reestablishment of the fetal condition,

TABLE 12.9

DISCRIMINATING POWER OF BIOCHEMICAL PATTERN: KEY DIFFERENCES
BETWEEN RAPIDLY GROWING NEOPLASTIC, FETAL, NEWBORN,
AND REGENERATING LIVER

Markers of gene expression	Livers[a]			
	Neoplastic (rapidly growing)	Newborn (6-day-old)	Fetal (17-day-old)	Regenerating (24 hr)
Glucose-6-phosphatase	<1	350[b]	12[b]	100[b]
Fructose-1,6-diphosphatase	<1	175[b]	7.1[b]	100[b]
Phosphoenolpyruvate carboxykinase	<1	160[b]		100[b]
Pyruvate carboxylase	<1	275[b]		100[b]
Hexokinase	500	36	83[b]	100[b]
Phosphofructokinase	229	44	49[b]	100[b]
Pyruvate kinase	499	15	11[b]	100[b]
Glucose-6-phosphate dehydrogenase	751	50	26[b]	100[b]
6-Phosphogluconate dehydrogenase	48	18	26	100[b]
HK/G-6-Pase	8,800	57[b]	690[b]	100[b]
PFK/FDPase	6,463	86[b]	674[b]	100[b]
G-6-P DH/6PG DH	1,120	288[c]	100[b]	100[b]
Thymidine into DNA	3,900	1,224[c]	3,083	910[c]
Thymidine to CO₂	<0.1	68[b]	5	64[b]
TdR to DNA/TdR to CO₂	11,500,000	1,788[c]	54,550[c]	1,450[b]
DNA/cell	250	87		100
TdR phosphorylase	32		2.0[b]	126
Uridine phosphorylase	375		1.8[b]	106
Dihydrouracil dehydrogenase	<10			78
TdR kinase/dihydrouracil dehydrogenase	>1,000			<10
Ornithine carbamyltransferase	1	33[b]	6.6[b]	83[b]

[a] Modified from (39). Values are expressed as percent of normal adult liver.

[b] Qualitative discriminant.

[c] Quantitative discriminant.

it is pertinent to examine the evidence provided by metabolic examination of these conditions because the biochemical phenotype should provide support for or against such contentions (38, 39).

To investigate the specificity of the changes in gene expression for neoplasia, it is necessary to compare the tumor metabolic pattern to a series of control tissues that exhibit similar biological properties in terms of proliferation rate. For tumor tissue the rapidly growing hepatomas were selected because these highly malignant neoplasms display the full expression of the enzymic and metabolic imbalance in neoplasia. The control tissues were provided by the rapidly growing, regenerating liver in the adult rat, the near term (19-day-old) differentiating, fetal liver, and developing liver in the 6-day-old rat (39).

The key biochemical alterations and the ratios in carbohydrate, pyrimidine, DNA, and ornithine metabolism for normal, neoplastic, regenerating, fetal, and newborn liver are compared in Table 12.9. All enzyme activities were calculated in micromoles of substrate metabolized per hour per gram wet weight of tissue and expressed as micromoles of substrate metabolized per hour per cell. For a meaningful comparison, the results in this table are in percentages, taking the values of the liver of the adult rat as 100%.

Key Differences between Rapidly Growing Neoplastic, Fetal, Newborn, and Regenerating Liver

A contrast of the enzymic and metabolic phenotype in the rapidly growing hepatomas with the pattern observed in normal and fetal liver (Table 12.9) demonstrates the vastly different biochemical pattern of the cancer cells. It is also possible to clearly discriminate between the metabolic pattern of the hepatoma cells and that of the regenerating liver, especially since carbohydrate metabolism is essentially unaltered after partial hepatectomy.

The discriminating power of the biochemical pattern provides no support at the biochemical level for suggestions that neoplasia is a disease of differentiation or that it is a regression to the fetal biochemical pattern. While there might be some coincidental overlapping in the metabolic pattern, it is more relevant that a critical examination reveals numerous differences between the biochemical phenotype of the hepatoma and those of the differentiating or fetal liver in the rat. These differences are the more important because all of these liver tissues and the rapidly growing hepatomas have similar growth rates. Therefore, one may conclude that there is a definitive pattern of quantitative and qualitative discriminants that distinguishes malignant cells from normal control tissues of similar growth rates, such as the regenerating, differentiating, or fetal tissues. The evidence indicates that the overall molecular pattern of the cancer cells is ordered, it is linked with the degree of malignant transformation, and it is specific to neoplasia (39, 39a, 52a).

VII. Conclusions: Phenotypic Evidence for Reprogramming of Gene Expression in Cancer Cells

A. Molecular Correlates of Malignancy

The molecular correlation concept provides a pattern for understanding and evaluating biochemical alterations in neoplasms. Table 12.10 summarizes most of the biochemical alterations that correlate with hepatoma growth rate; these are the alterations that have been grouped into class 1. In the progressive nature of these alterations the different degrees of biological malignancy are expressed at the molecular level. For such molecular targets, chemotherapeutic approaches

TABLE 12.10   BIOCHEMICAL DISCRIMINANTS THAT CORRELATE WITH GROWTH RATE IN HEPATOMAS[a]

Carbohydrate metabolism	Nucleic acid metabolism	Protein and amino acid metabolism	Other metabolic areas
Glucose synthesis: Decreased	DNA synthesis: Increased	Protein synthesis: Increased	Polyamine synthesis: Increased
Pyruvate conversion to glucose	DNA content	Amino acid incorporation into protein (alanine, aspartate, glycine, serine, isoleucine, valine)	Ornithine decarboxylase
Glucose-6-phosphatase	Thymidine incorporation into DNA		Putrescine content
Fructose-1,6-diphosphatase	Formate into DNA		Urea cycle: Decreased
Phosphoenolpyruvate carboxy-kinase	Adenine into DNA	Activity of the postmicrosomal protein synthesizing system	Ornithine carbamyltransferase
Pyruvate carboxylase	Thymidine kinase	Ratio of total free amino acid to total protein content	Lipid metabolism: Decreased
Glucose catabolism: Increased	DNA polymerase		Lipid content
Glycolysis	Thymidylate synthetase	Decrease: S-adenosylmeth-ionine synthetase	α-Glycerophosphate dehydro-genase
Hexokinase	Deoxycytidylate deaminase	Enzymes catabolizing amino acids: Decreased	Butyrate to acetoacetate
Phosphofructokinase	DNA nucleotidyltransferases		Respiratory activity: Decreased
Pyruvate kinase	Ribonucleotide reductase	Decreased	Oxygen consumption
Glycolytic ATP production	DNA catabolism: Decreased	Tryptophan pyrrolase	Mitochondrial protein content
Pentose phosphate pathway: Increased	Thymine degradation to CO_2	Serotonin deaminase	Respiratory ATP production
C-1/C-6 oxidation of glucose	RNA synthesis: Increased	5-Hydroxytryptophan decar-boxylase	
Specific phosphorylating enzymes: Decreased	Formate into RNA	Glutamate dehydrogenase	
Fructokinase and glucokinase	Dihydroorotase	Glutamate-oxaloacetate transaminase	
Fructose metabolism: Decreased	Aspartate carbamyltransferase		
Fructose incorporation into glycogen through fructokinase	tRNA methylase		
Thiokinase	G content of rapidly sediment-ing nuclear RNA		
Aldolase	GU content of 4–7S nuclear RNA		
Responsiveness to glucocorticoid stimulation: Decreased	RNA catabolism: Decreased		
Response of gluconeogenic enzymes	Xanthine oxidase		
Glycogenic response	Uricase		
Isozyme shift	RNA metabolic response to glucocorticoid stimulation: Decreased:		
High K_m isozymes: decreased	Precursor incorporation into total tumor RNA after steroid injection		
Low K_m isozymes: increased			

[a] From (39a).

TABLE 12.11

GENERALIZATION OF THE PHENOTYPIC EVIDENCE: REPROGRAMMING OF GENE
EXPRESSION IN CANCER CELLS[a]

1. Metabolic imbalance	In activities of opposing key enzymes and metabolic pathways
2. Shift in isozyme pattern	Decrease in high K_m and increase in low K_m isozymes
3. Decreased responsiveness to regulation	Hormonal stimulation, feedback, and allosteric controls
4. Relation to biological behavior (malignancy)	Biochemical alterations are progressive and correlate with growth rate

[a] From (39a).

may be designed. Therefore, the identification and elucidation of the control mechanisms that pertain to these molecular correlates of malignancy should have clinical significance for chemotherapy.

B. Generalization of the Phenotypic Evidence: Reprogramming of Gene Expression in Cancer Cells

As a result of application of the approaches of the molecular correlation concept of neoplasia, the following generalizations may be drawn from the evaluation of the experimental results (Table 12.11).

In the spectrum of hepatomas of different malignancy a metabolic imbalance is revealed in the activities of opposing key enzymes and metabolic pathways of synthesis and catabolism in the areas of carbohydrate, purine, pyrimidine, DNA, ornithine, and cAMP metabolism. There is a shift in isozyme pattern that is manifested in a decrease in the high K_m and an increase in the low K_m isozymes in carbohydrate metabolism and in the cAMP phosphodiesterases. A decreased responsiveness to regulation was recognized in the decline in the susceptibility to hormonal stimulation, feedback, and allosteric control mechanisms. Thus, in the biochemical phenotype the reprogramming of gene expression is linked with the progressive malignant transformation as revealed in the spectrum of tumors of different growth rates.

The above outlined analysis of the results of the conceptual and experimental approaches achieved by application of the molecular correlation concept of neoplasia led to the recognition of an ordered and specific pattern of gene expression in the hepatoma spectrum (37, 39, 39a).

VIII. Applicability of the Pattern Observed in the Hepatomas to Other Neoplasms

A detailed analysis of the general applicability of the molecular correlation concept to neoplasms other than hepatomas will be provided elsewhere. It is pertinent to point out here that a number of publications provide evidence that the correlation of metabolic alterations and tumor growth rate also applies to kidney tumors (13, 57), mammary cancer (11), and other neoplasms of different growth rates (10). Therefore, the available evidence supports the view that the molecular correlation concept is valid not only for hepatomas but for the various other types of neoplasms that have been subjected to appropriate examination (37, 39a).

Acknowledgments

The research work of the author was supported by grants from the United States Public Health Service, National Cancer Institute, Grant Nos. CA-13526 and CA-05034, the Damon Runyon-Walter Winchell Cancer Fund, and Goldblatt Brothers Employees Nathan Goldblatt Cancer Research Fund.

References

1. Allen, D. O., Munshower, J., Morris, H. P., and Weber, G. (1971). *Cancer Res.* **31**, 557–560.
2. Borek, E. (1968). *Annu. Symp. Fundamental Cancer Res.*, 22nd (R. B. Hurlbert, ed.), pp. 165–190. Univ. of Texas Press, Houston, Texas.
3. Busch, H. (1962). "An Introduction to the Biochemistry of the Cancer Cell." Academic Press, New York.
4. Clark, J. F., Morris, H. P., and Weber, G. (1973). *Cancer Res.* **33**, 356–361.
5. De Lamirande, G., Allard, C., and Cantero, A. (1958). *Cancer Res.* **18**, 952–958.
6. Elford, H. L., Freese, M., Passamani, E., and Morris, H. P. (1970). *J. Biol. Chem.* **245**, 5228–5233.
7. Ferdinandus, J. A., Morris, H. P., and Weber, G. (1971). *Cancer Res.* **31**, 550–556.
8. Frei, E., III (1972). *Cancer Res.* **32**, 2593–2607.
9. Klein, G., Bregula, U., Wiener, F., and Harris, H. (1971). *J. Cell Sci.* **8**, 659–691.
10. Knox, W. E., Horowitz, M. L., and Friedell, G. H. (1969). *Cancer Res.* **29**, 669–680.
11. Knox, W. E., Linder, M., and Friedell, G. H. (1970). *Cancer Res.* **30**, 283–287.
12. Lea, M. A., Morris, H. P., and Weber, G. (1966). *Cancer Res.* **26**, 465–469.
13. Lea, M. A., Morris, H. P., and Weber, G. (1968). *Cancer Res.* **28**, 71–74.
14. Lo, C., Cristofalo, V. J., Morris, H. P., and Weinhouse, S. (1968). *Cancer Res.* **28**, 1–10.
15. Morris, H. P. (1965). *Advan. Cancer Res.* **9**, 227–302.
16. Morris, H. P., Dyer, H. M., Wagner, B. P., Miyaji, H., and Rechcigl, M., Jr. (1964). *Advan. Enzyme Regulat.* **2**, 321–333.
17. Morris, H. P., Wagner, B. P., and Meranze, D. R. (1970). *Cancer Res.* **30**, 1362–1369.
18. Novikoff, A. B. (1960). *In* "Cell Physiology of Neoplasia" (T. C. Hsu, ed.), pp. 219–268. Univ. of Texas Press, Austin, Texas.
19. Nowell, P. C., Morris, H. P., and Potter, V. R. (1967). *Cancer Res.* **27**, 1565–1579.
20. Ove, P., Jenkins, M. D., and Laszlo, J. (1970). *Cancer Res.* **30**, 535–539.
21. Queener, S. F., Morris, H. P., and Weber, G. (1971). *Cancer Res.* **31**, 1004–1009.
22. Rethy, A., Vaczi, L., Toth, F. D., and Boldogh, I. (1973). *In* "Carcinogenesis and Cyclic AMP." Miami Winter Symposia Ser., 153–177.
23. Sheid, B., Wilson, S. M., and Morris, H. P. (1971). *Cancer Res.* **31**, 774–777.
24. Sweeney, M. J., Ashmore, J., Morris, H. P., and Weber, G. (1963). *Cancer Res.* **23**, 995–1002.
25. Sweeney, M. J., Hoffman, D. H., and Poore, G. A. (1967). *Proc. Amer. Ass. Cancer Res.* **8**, 66.

26. Sweeney, M. J., Hoffman, D. H., and Poore, G. A. (1971). *Advan. Enzyme Regulat.* **9**, 51–61.
27. Taylor, C. B., Morris, H. P., and Weber, G. (1969). *Life Sci.* **8**, 635–644.
28. Tomasi, V., Rethy, A., and Trevisani, A. (1973). *In* "Carcinogenesis and Cyclic AMP." Miami Winter Symposia Ser., pp. 127–144.
28a. Tomino, I., Katunuma, N., Morris, H. P., and Weber, G. Submitted for publication.
29. Tsutsui, E., Srinivasan, P. R., and Borek, E. (1966). *Proc. Nat. Acad. Sci. U.S.* **56**, 1003–1009.
30. Weber, G. (1961). *Advan. Cancer Res.* **6**, 403–494.
31. Weber, G. (1963). *Advan. Enzyme Regulat.* **1**, 321–340.
32. Weber, G. (1966). *Gann Monogr.* **1**, 151–178.
33. Weber, G. (1968). *Naturwissenschaften* **55**, 418–429.
34. Weber, G. (1969). *Advan. Enzyme Regulat.* **7**, 15–40.
35. Weber, G. (1969). *Annu. Symp. Fundamental Cancer Res.*, 22nd (R. B. Hurlbert, ed.), pp. 527–566. Univ. of Texas Press, Houston, Texas.
36. Weber, G. (1971). *Proc. Int. Cancer Congr., 10th, 1970* **1**, 837–867. Yearbook Med. Publ., Chicago, Illinois.
37. Weber, G. (1972). *Gann Monogr. Cancer Res.* **13**, 47–77.
38. Weber, G. (1973). *In* "Carcinogenesis and Cyclic AMP." Miami Winter Symposia Ser., pp. 57–94.
39. Weber, G. (1973). *Advan. Enzyme Regulat.* **11**, 79–102.
39a. Weber, G. "Biochemical Strategy of the Cancer Cell," (in press).
40. Weber, G., and Cantero, A. (1955). *Cancer Res.* **15**, 679–684.
41. Weber, G., and Cantero, A. (1957). *Endocrinology* **61**, 701–712.
42. Weber, G., and Cantero, A. (1959). *Cancer Res.* **19**, 763–768.
43. Weber, G., and Lea, M. A. (1967). *In* "Methods in Cancer Research" (H. Busch, ed.), Vol. 2, pp. 523–578. Academic Press, New York.
44. Weber, G., and Morris, H. P. (1963). *Cancer Res.* **23**, 987–994.
45. Weber, G., Banerjee, G., and Morris, H. P. (1961). *Cancer Res.* **21**, 933–937.
46. Weber, G., Morris, H. P., Love, W. C., and Ashmore, J. (1961). *Cancer Res.* **21**, 1406–1411.
47. Weber, G., Henry, M., Wagle, S. R., and Wagle, D. S. (1964). *Advan. Enzyme Regulat.* **2**, 335–346.
48. Weber, G., Singhal, R. L., and Srivastava, S. K. (1965). *Advan. Enzyme Regulat.* **3**, 369–387.
49. Weber, G., Queener, S. F., and Ferdinandus, J. A. (1971). *Advan. Enzyme Regulat.* **9**, 63–95.
50. Weber, G., Stubbs, M., and Morris, H. P. (1971). *Cancer Res.* **31**, 2177–2183.
51. Weber, G., Ferdinandus, J. A., Queener, S. F., Dunaway, G. A., Jr., and Trahan L. J-P (1972). *Advan. Enzyme Regulat.* **10**, 39–62.
52. Weber, G., Queener, S. F., and Morris, H. P. (1972). *Cancer Res.* **32**, 1933–1940.
52a. Weber, G., Trevisani, A., Heinrich, C. P., and Ferdinandus, J. A. (1974). *Advan. Enzyme Regulat.*, in press.
52b. Weinhouse, S. (1972). *Cancer Res.* **32**, 2007–2016.
53. Wheeler, G. P., Alexander, J. A., and Morris, H. P. (1964). *Advan. Enzyme Regulat.* **2**, 347–369.
54. Williams-Ashman, H. G., Coppoc, G. L., and Weber, G. (1972). *Cancer Res.* **32**, 1924–1932.
55. Williams-Ashman, H. G., Janne, J., Coppoc, G. L., Geroch, M. E., and Schenone, A. (1972). *Advan. Enzyme Regulat.* **10**, 225–245.
56. Williams-Ashman, H. G., Coppoc, G. L., Schenone, A., and Weber, G. (1973). *In* "Polyamines and Cancer." pp. 181–197. Raven Press, New York.
57. Williamson, D. H., Krebs, H. A., Stubbs, M., Page, M. A., Morris, H. P., and Weber, G. (1970). *Cancer Res.* **30**, 2049–2054.
58. Wu, C., and Bauer, J. M. (1962). *Cancer Res.* **22**, 1239–1245.
59. Zubrod, C. G. (1972). *Proc. Nat. Acad. Sci. U.S.* **69**, 1042–1047.

CHAPTER XIII

Phenotypic Variability as a Manifestation of Translational Control

HENRY C. PITOT, THOMAS K. SHIRES,
GEOFFREY MOYER, and CARLETON T. GARRETT

I. Introduction

The pathologist bases the anatomical diagnosis of cancer on histological criteria, some of which are based on the morphology of the tissue from which the neoplasm arose. From the very beginnings of cellular pathology, the diversity and morphological heterogeneity of neoplasms, even derived from the same tissue or cell type, has been one of the hallmarks of cancer. In contrast, the early investigations on the biochemistry of cancer (14, 53) demonstrated by rates of glycolysis that there is a tendency of cancer cells towards a single biochemical phenotype. The resolution of these two opposing view points, one of the pathologist and the other of the biochemist, is one of the major problems in oncology.

II. Phenotypic Heterogeneity in Hepatomas

While Greenstein and others espoused the concept of convergency of the biochemical phenotype of all neoplasms, they recognized exceptions to this proposed generalization. In fact, from Greenstein's experiments (14) one can see variation in enzyme levels in several hepatomas (Fig. 13.1). It is apparent that the overall phenotype of the several lesions presented here is quite divergent.

In the early 1960's, the biochemical phenotypes of several highly differentiated hepatocellular carcinomas were analyzed (33, 36, 39). Since that time studies in a number of laboratories have demonstrated that none of the biochemical phenotypes of hepatocellular carcinomas is the same. Some 40 or more neoplasms have been investigated to varying extents and in all instances as more enzyme activities are assayed it is apparent that phenotypically each neoplasm is unique and is different from the liver, the parent tissue. The data from a number of Morris hepatomas is seen in Fig. 13.2 (40). Not only do the levels of the four enzymes studied vary among neoplasms, but their regulation by dietary protein also varies. While examination of a single enzyme activity demonstrates that some neoplasms have equivalent enzyme amounts among each other or even with liver, if one examines the activities and the regulation by dietary protein of all four enzymes, the pattern of each neoplasm is unique unto itself (12, 30).

In other studies with mouse hepatomas (8, 43) similar findings have been described. The enzymic profile or biochemical phenotype of both spontaneous and transplanted mouse hepatomas were unique to the particular lesion. On continued transplantation transplantable neoplasms retain their own unique phenotype, a phenomenon also found in hepatocellular carcinomas of the rat.

III. Phenotypic Variability in Other Neoplasms

While the majority of the biochemical studies carried out in experimental oncology have been with hepatomas, within the last decade the biochemical characterization of a number of neoplasms of other tissues has been studied. In a series of primary and transplanted mammary carcinomas of the rat (15–17), like those of the hepatocellular carcinoma series, each neoplasm is biochemically

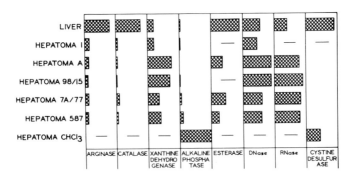

Fig. 13.1. Enzyme levels in liver and hepatomas of the mouse. The hatched bars represent relative activity of each enzyme as specified below for each of the 6 hepatomas and liver. Data excerpted from Greenstein (14).

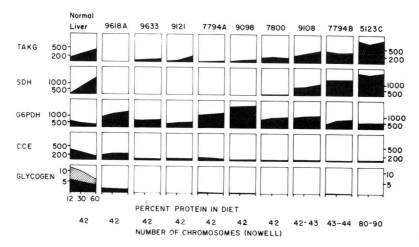

Fig. 13.2. Activities of four enzymes and glycogen content of liver and nine Morris hepatomas with chromosome numbers shown below. Each box shows by means of the blacked-in area the level of each of the 4 enzymes and the glycogen content of animals on a 12, 30, and 60% casein diet fed for at least 1 week. Abbreviations are as follows: TAKG; tyrosine aminotransferase, SDH; serine dehydratase, G6PDH; glucose-6-phosphate dehydrogenase, CCE; citrate cleavage enzyme. This chart is reproduced from the work of Potter *et al.* (40).

unique with respect to its set of quantitative enzyme levels and in the environmental mechanisms regulating the level of enzymes in these neoplasms.

A better example of the biochemical heterogeneity in one class of neoplasms is exemplified in the myelomas (Chapter XIV). For many years the protein produced by this neoplasm in any one patient differed from that of other patients with similar neoplasms (31). In a large series of mouse myelomas, the protein produced by each neoplasm is unique to that tumor (38–40). In view of the extreme diversity of the potential structures of antibody molecules, diversity of myeloma globulins was presumably due to the excessive production of a single antibody species in each neoplasm. In this instance the biochemical heterogeneity afforded by this set of neoplasms is exemplified by the diversity seen in one protein species secreted by the tumor.

There is also variation in ^{131}I uptake in a series of experimental thyroid tumors (54). While this is only a single biochemical parameter, taken with the histological variation seen in the series, it is apparent that these tumors exhibit the same phenomena of phenotypic variability found in mammary and myeloma neoplasms.

IV. Phenotypic Variability in Preneoplasia

While the examples cited earlier show that in carefully studied situations phenotypic variability is the rule rather than the exception for most classes of neoplasms, relatively little work has been done in the phenotypic characterization of the so-called "preneoplastic lesion." The original experiments of Berenblum (3) indicated that carcinogenesis occurs in at least two steps, initiation followed by promotion; thus a cell type must exist having the inherent potential of neoplasia but not necessarily exhibiting neoplasia. This has given rise to the idea of the preneoplastic lesion. In man, a number of examples of such lesions include leucoplakia, certain skin lesions, and cervical dysplasia (11). Experimentally the two best studied examples of preneoplastic lesions are the regenerating hepatic nodule and the hyperplastic mammary nodule. In the case of the former, a recent investigation (2) indicated that serum protein synthesized by regenerating liver nodules produced by feeding 2-fluorenylacetamide had patterns unique to each nodule investigated. Earlier investigations by others (22) have also suggested that each regenerating nodule is not biochemically identical with another, although the investigations such as outlined with the hepatocellular carcinomas have not yet been carried out. In preliminary investigations in this laboratory the levels of five enzymes of carbohydrate and lipid metabolism have a unique quantitative pattern in each of a series of six hyperplastic mammary nodules.

These investigations suggest that the phenomenon of phenotypic variability and biochemical heterogeneity may be a characteristic which occurs shortly after or even at the time of the initial transformation of a normal to a neoplastic cell.

V. Mechanisms of Phenotypic Variability

A. Genetic

The varied phenotypes demonstrated by neoplasms may well be related to the mechanism of the transformation event, especially since there is some evidence that even the initiated cell may already exhibit this phenotypic variability.

Since the neoplastic transformation itself is a heritable event, one of the most likely mechanisms for these effects are that they are the result of direct mutations or changes in the genetic apparatus. Direct evidence that neoplasia is the result of a specific genetic alteration has not yet been forthcoming. No abnormal protein has been described as unique to one or more neoplasms, although it is quite apparent that many tumors produce proteins which their tissue of origin is not normally capable of producing (7). On the other hand, cytogenetic evidence that the total genome of many, if not most neoplasms, is different from that of the parent tissue has been well substantiated (6, 29, see Chapters I, III). Yet, there are numerous examples of perfectly diploid karyotypes seen in highly differentiated neoplasms including experimental hepatocellular carcinomas (see Fig. 13.2), human neoplasms (13, 46, 52), and other experimental situations (25). Thus, while it is true that most tumors do exhibit cytogenetic abnormalities, those closest to the initiated cell may not. In view of the fact that at least preliminary evidence suggests that the biochemical heterogeneity seen in autonomous neoplasms is also present in the preneoplastic situation or the initiated cell, it would not appear that cytogenetic abnormalities can totally explain the phenotypic aberrations.

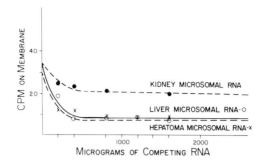

Fig. 13.3. DNA-RNA hybridization of rat liver DNA with labeled rat liver nuclear RNA and competition by microsomal RNA from kidney, liver, and hepatomas 5123. See text for references to techniques utilized.

On the other hand, experiments may be carried out to determine whether or not the genetic information coding for cytoplasmic proteins of the neoplastic cell is the same or different from the normal tissue giving rise to the neoplasm. Unfortunately, techniques to answer this question unequivocally have not yet been forthcoming. Specifically, the technique of DNA-RNA hybridization and hybridization competition in eukaryotic systems has many difficulties (4, 27). At sufficiently high RNA/DNA ratios nonspecific intramolecular interactions are minimized (44). Under these conditions the cytoplasmic RNA population in liver and the Morris hepatocellular carcinoma 5123 were not distinguishable by these techniques although cytoplasmic RNA from kidney was clearly distinguishable from liver cytoplasmic RNA (Fig. 13.3). These experiments suggest that no major differences were readily discerned between the cytoplasmic RNA population of this neoplasm and the tissue of origin, despite the extensive enzymic differences seen in this tumor as compared to liver (Fig. 13.2). This data would suggest that there may not be a great loss or gain of genetic information in the cytoplasm of this neoplasm. Both the genome and its transcription in this neoplastic tissue are remarkably similar to the tissue from which it arose, yet in many respects the phenotype of the two tissues are as different as are liver and kidney (see also Chapters V, VIII).

B. Translational Mechanisms

The arguments presented suggest that mechanisms other than defects in the genome may be important in the mechanisms of the neoplastic transformation. Examples have been reported of the specific control of genetic expression in mammalian liver at the translational level. The synthesis of tryptophan oxygenase may be doubled in the absence of RNA synthesis by administration of tryptophan to adrenalectomized animals fed on low protein diet (10). Similarly, the synthesis of serine dehydratase may be increased 3-fold upon the administration of a mixture of amino acids to animals during a period in which the synthesis of the enzyme has previously been shown to be independent of RNA synthesis

TABLE 13.1

ESTIMATED mRNA TEMPLATE LIFETIME FOR ENZYMES IN RAT TISSUES *In Vivo*

Enzyme	Liver	Hepatocellular carcinoma
Serine dehydratase	6–8 hours	H–35 = <1 hour
		5123 = >2 weeks
Ornithine aminotransferase	18–24 hours	5123 = >24 hours
Tryptophan oxygenase	>2 weeks	H–35 = <12 hours
		5123, 7316, 7800 = <30 minutes
Tyrosine aminotransferase (induced)	2–3 hours	H–35 = >6 hours
Thymidine kinase	<3 hours	H–35 = >12 hours

Enzyme	Mammary gland[a]	Mammary carcinoma (R3230AC)
Glucose-6-phosphate dehydrogenase	<2 days	>2 days
Malic enzyme	<2 days	>2 days

[a] Data adapted from the study of Hilf *et al.* (15).

(20). Furthermore, in this and other laboratories (18, 24, 32) the administration of glucose effectively suppresses the synthesis of several gluconeogenic enzymes in the absence of concomitant RNA synthesis. By utilizing doses of inhibitors that suppress total RNA synthesis better than 95%, it was found that a number of enzymes have finite time periods after their synthesis is initiated during which their synthesis is entirely translational and independent of further transcription. These time periods have been termed the template lifetime for an enzyme; the lifetime for each enzyme so far investigated is different.

In several hepatocellular carcinomas, the template lifetimes for each enzyme were not only different in the neoplasms, but also different from the values in liver (Table 13.1). There is variation in template lifetimes in the hepatomas studied in comparison with normal liver. Accordingly, the phenotypic variability (Fig. 13.2) may reflect the variability in template lifetimes of the enzymes. If a template is very unstable and is translated for only short periods of time, the enzyme synthesized from the template would be at low levels in the cytoplasm (tryptophan oxygenase in the Morris 7800 hepatoma). On the other hand, if the template lifetime for an enzyme is very extended, such as that for serine dehydratase in the 5123 hepatoma, a considerable amount of enzyme would be found in the neoplasm. Thus, the present data suggest that phenotypic variability depends on template lifetime variability, and a major question becomes that of the nature of the stable template.

VI. Mechanisms of Template Stability—The Membron

It has been proposed that the stable template is a structure consisting of a combination of a functioning polysome with an intracellular membrane (33–37). This functioning regulatable translating unit has been termed the "membron" in analogy to the operon, a functioning regulatable unit of the genome. A number of experiments directed towards establishing or refuting the existence and structure of the membron have been carried out in this laboratory and some supportive evidence has been forthcoming from other laboratories.

1. After prelabeling of nascent chains from bound and free polysomes *in vivo* (19), the subsequent release of these chains by *in vitro* incubation with puromycin demonstrated that only polysomes bound to the endoplasmic reticulum were capable of releasing labeled chains with the immunological specificity of the soluble intracellular enzyme, serine dehydratase, whose template stability had been previously demonstrated (Table 13.1).

2. Immunologically reactive serine dehydratase has been found that is bound to polysomes associated with the endoplasmic reticulum.

3. As has been previously described in this laboratory and subsequently in a number of laboratories, polysomes readily bind *in vitro* to membranes of the rough endoplasmic reticulum from which ribosomes have previously been removed (9, 21, 41, 45, 47, 48). They do not bind, or bind relatively poorly, to membranes of the smooth endoplasmic reticulum at low temperatures (49). Conditions utilized for polysome binding *in vitro* produce negligible binding of individual ribosomal subunits.

4. Previous binding of poly GC to membranes of the rough endoplasmic reticulum from which polysomes have been removed inhibits subsequent polysome binding.

5. Brief treatment of membranes with trypsin, but not with neuramidinase, lipase, or ribonuclease, prevents binding of polysomes to membranes of the endoplasmic reticulum from which ribosomes have been removed. Furthermore, freezing and thawing of the membrane markedly inhibits its binding ability.

6. To demonstrate the differences between "functional" binding of polysomes and "nonfunctional" binding, experiments were carried out to determine whether or not reconstituted rough membranes possess the capability of transmembrane injection of polypeptide chains as seen in native preparations from secretory organs such as the liver (42). Reconstituted rough membranes or native rough membranes were added in equal amounts in a complete amino acid incorporating system (Table 13.2) and incubated. After seven minutes puromycin was added and the incubation was continued for 13 more minutes (experiments A and B). The reaction was stopped with cold buffer and the mixture centrifuged. All the precipitable activity in the supernatant was considered extravesicular and not associated with the vesicles of the endoplasmic reticulum. The membrane pellet consisting of ribosomes bound to the vesicles of the endoplasmic reticulum were then resuspended, treated with deoxycholate (DOC) and sedimented again at high speed. This procedure separated detergent(DOC)-released material and a ribosomal pellet. Total precipitable radioactive macromolecules and the distribution of radioactivity after puromycin were generally similar for both the native and reconstituted rough membranes. Activity in the detergent-soluble fraction (after puromycin) represented about one-fourth of the total radioactivity and about one-half of the released nonribosomal activity for both membrane preparations. Replacement of the detergent step with sonication of

TABLE 13.2

PUROMYCIN EFFECT ON THE DISTRIBUTION OF POLYPEPTIDE RADIOACTIVITY AMONG
COMPONENTS OF NATIVE ROUGH MICROSOMAL AND RECONSTITUTED ROUGH
MEMBRANES AND RELATED SYSTEMS[a]

	Percent [³H]leucine DPM			
	Extra-vesicular supernatant	Ribosomes	Deoxycho-late-released	Total precipi-table DPM
A. Native rough microsomes				
No puromycin	25.3	67.6	5.1	1950
Puromycin	23.8	-52.9	23.3	1900
B. Reconstituted rough microsomes				
No puromycin	11.1	80.1	8.8	1900
Puromycin	25.6	49.9	24.5	1850
C. Polysomes mixed with RNase-treated membranes at start of incubation				
No puromycin	9.5	86.5	4.0	1700
Puromycin	29.9	59.5	10.5	1000
D. Polysomes mixed with tryp-sinized rough microsomes				
No puromycin	36.4	50.4	13.2	2650
Puromycin	53.9	30.2	15.9	3550
E. Polysomes (no membranes)				
No puromycin	38.3	57.6	4.1	4500
Puromycin	69.3	25.8	4.9	4400

[a] Triplicate tubes with a complete amino acid incorporation system were incubated 10 minutes at 37°C and puromycin added to a final concentration of 1 mM. Control tubes received an equal volume of TKM. All tubes were then incubated an additional 20 minutes. Mixtures were chilled and centrifuged at 275,000 g for 1 hour. Supernatant was precipitated with 5% TCA and the pellet resuspended in TKM and treated with 0.5% deoxycholate. After centrifugation, the ribosomal pellets and supernatants containing intravesicular material were treated with 5% TCA. Acid precipitates were handled as described (19).

the membrane vesicle after puromycin release yielded approximately the same final distribution of radioactivity.

It appears that polysome-membrane complexes formed *in vitro* are very similar to rough microsomes in their transmembrane injection activity. Furthermore, these results speak for both the correct choice by polysomes of operational sites and possibly for the correct positioning of polysomes on these sites. To test whether or not it was necessary for polysomes to be bound to obtain transmembrane injection of labeled protein, polysomes were added to treated membranes at the start of the incubation utilizing a cell-free incorporating system (experiment C). Control studies with labeled polysomes showed that about 50% of the polysomes were bound to the membranes and the rest remained free. These studies demonstrate that only a portion of the labeled protein was found in the detergent-soluble fraction. Thus, association of polysome and membrane are required for this process.

At 37°C, binding of polysomes to membranes of the smooth endoplasmic reticulum occurs as well as to trypsin-treated membrane, but this binding does not produce a functional transmembrane injection of the growing chain (experiment D, DOC-released). These studies therefore demonstrate that the *in vitro* investigation of polysomes binding to membranes is a reasonable reproduction of the *in vivo* situation and the conclusions drawn from these studies concerning the structure of the membron may be applicable to an understanding of the process of translation.

Studies from this (23) and other laboratories (5) have demonstrated the relative resistance of polysomes bound to membrane to the effects of ribonuclease and similar enzymes. These experiments suggest, along with those in bacterial systems (1), that the membrane-bound polysome is much more stable and resistant to environmental factors than the free polysome, making the former an ideal candidate for the stable template role. Furthermore (51), the physiological situation where polysomes break down *in vivo* and are then reconstituted in the absence of further RNA synthesis suggests that template stability results from an association of the messenger RNA with the membrane rather than the total polysome with the membrane. Many of the details of the exact structure of the stable translating unit of the cytoplasm termed the "membron" remain to be determined. The experimental evidence to date argues that the interaction between the membrane and the polysome gives structural integrity to the stable mRNA template.

VII. Phenotypic Variability and Membrane Protein Turnover—Relation to the Stable Template

Thus far, the mechanism of phenotypic variability has been related to the alteration in template lifetime and the stable template which is the membrane-bound polysome, termed the membron. There remains the problem of the relationship of altered template stability to the structure of the membron.

Recent studies in this laboratory (28) have demonstrated that certain membrane proteins of the endoplasmic reticulum from neoplasms have different decay characteristics than the presumed homologous protein from normal tissue. Specifically Fig. 13.4 shows that turnovers are different for three such membrane proteins, separated on the basis of their molecular weight by SDS-urea-polyacrylamide gels from host liver and Morris hepatoma 7800. As is seen, the half-lives of two of the three proteins appear comparable in liver and hepatoma, while the third, protein (A), decays at a considerably slower rate. Further studies carried out in a morphologically better differentiated tumor, the Morris hepatoma 9618A, in which six homologous proteins were analyzed revealed differences in the rate of decay of most of these proteins in the neoplasm as compared to the host liver. Thus another aspect of phenotypic variability associated specifically with the intracellular membrane population appears. One would like to relate this effect to the variation in template lifetime and the biochemical heterogeneity seen in these neoplasms.

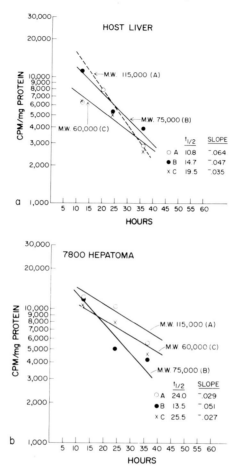

Fig. 13.4. (a) Radioactive decay rates of 3 molecular sizes of proteins separated from the endoplasmic reticulum using sodium dodecyl sulfate acrylamide gel electrophoresis. The $t_{1/2}$'s are given both in hours and as a slope in the lower right-hand corner. (b) Sodium dodecyl sulfate acrylamide gel electrophoresis separation of 3 molecular weight protein families from the endoplasmic reticulum of the Morris 7800 hepatoma. The $t_{1/2}$'s and slopes are given as for the host liver. The experimental conditions are those employed by Moyer and Pitot (28).

Since the basis of the membron concept is an association between the messenger RNA ribonucleoprotein of the functioning polysome and certain membrane structures, presumably protein, variations in protein turnover in the membrane may result in a variation in membron stability. Theoretical aspects of the membron structure have previously been described (50). In these considerations, the most likely interaction between polysome and membrane which could explain the experimental data was thought to be protein–protein interaction, probably between the protein associated with the messenger RNA itself (informosome protein) and some protein structure in the membrane itself. While the primary mechanisms for altered template stability have been postulated as resulting from an environmentally induced alteration in the 3-dimensional mosaic pattern of the intracellular membrane, it is relatively easy to understand that a combination of an altered 3-dimensional structure with a super-imposed change in protein turnover would serve further to alter the binding sites between polysome and membrane.

VIII. Conclusions

The experimental and theoretical arguments proposed in this chapter have been addressed to a description of the morphological and biochemical heterogeneity of human and experimental neoplasia as one of the major pervading characteristics of cancer in general. The finding of altered template stability in experimental hepatocellular carcinomas is one that can be utilized to explain in a mechanistic fashion the extremely varied phenotype found in these tumors and perhaps in all differentiated neoplasms. The membron concept is a theoretical model proposed to explain messenger RNA template stability in differentiated mammalian tissues. The logical corollary is that alterations in template lifetime and template stability may result from changes in the membron structure which consists of ribosomes, messenger RNA and the membrane. Most of the arguments relate to changes in membrane structure, but it is obvious that changes in the message itself or in membrane structural protein (34) may lead to some or all of the alterations that have been described. A major problem is to delineate the contributions of the genome and the environment to the neoplastic transformation.

Acknowledgment

Portions of the work reported herein was supported in part by grants from the National Cancer Institute (CA-07175) and the American Cancer Society (E-588).

References

1. Aronson, A. (1965). *J. Mol. Biol.* **13**, 92–104.
2. Becker, F. F., Klein, K. M., and Asofsky, R. (1972). *Cancer Res.* **32**, 914–920.
3. Berenblum, I. (1954). *Advan. Cancer Res.* **2**, 129–159.
4. Birnboim, H. C., Pene, J. J., and Darnell, J. E. (1967). *Proc. Nat. Acad. Sci. U.S.* **58**, 320–327.
5. Blobel, G., and Potter, V. R. (1967). *J. Mol. Biol.* **26**, 293–305.
6. Boveri, T. (1929). "The Origin of Malignant Tumors" (Transl. by M. Boveri). Williams and Wilkins, Baltimore, Maryland.
7. Bower, B. F., and Gordon, G. S. (1965). *Ann. Rev. Med.* **16**, 83–118.
8. Bresnick, E., Mayfield, E. D., Liebelt, A. G., and Liebelt, R. A. (1971). *Cancer Res.* **31**, 743–751.
9. Burka, E. R., and Schickling, L. F. (1970). *Biochemistry* **9**, 459–463.
10. Cho-Chung, Y. S., and Pitot, H. C. (1968). *Eur. J. Biochem.* **3**, 401–406.
11. Dunham, A. J. (1972). *Cancer Res.* **32**, 1359–1374.
12. Emmelot, P. (1964). *Acta Un. Int. Contra Cancer* **20**, 902–908.
13. Granberg, I. (1971). *Hereditas* **68**, 165–218.

14. Greenstein, J. P. (1954). "Biochemistry of Cancer," 2nd ed. Academic Press, New York.
15. Hilf, R., Michel, I., Silverstein, G., and Bell, C. (1965). *Cancer Res.* **25**, 1854–1868.
16. Hilf, R. (1968). *Cancer Res.* **28**, 1888–1890.
17. Hilf, R., Goldenberg, H., Greenstein, M., Meranze, D. R., and Shimkin, M. B. (1970). *Cancer Res.* **30**, 1223–1230.
18. Jervell, K. F., Christoffersen, T., and Morland, J. (1965). *Arch. Biochem. Biophys.* **111**, 15–22.
19. Jost, J.-P., Khairallah, E. A., and Pilot, H. C. (1968). *J. Biol. Chem.* **243**, 3057–3066.
20. Jost, J.-P., and Pitot, H. C. (1968). *In* "Regulatory Mechanisms for Protein Synthesis in Mammalian Cells" (A. San Pietro, M. R. Lamborg and F. T. Kenney, eds.), pp. 283–298. Academic Press, New York.
21. Khawaja, J. A., and Raino, A. (1970). *Biochem. Biophys. Res. Commun.* **41**, 152–518.
22. Kitagawa, T. (1971). *Gann* **62**, 217–224.
23. Lamar, C., Prival, M., and Pitot, H. C. (1966). *Cancer Res.* **26**, 1909–1914.
24. Lee, S. C., Tews, J. K., Morris, M. L., and Harper, A. E. (1972). *J. Nutr.* **102**, 319–330.
25. Mark, J. (1969). *Eur. J. Cancer* **5**, 307–315.
26. McIntire, K. R., and Potter, M. (1964). *J. Nat. Cancer Inst.* **33**, 631–648.
27. Melli, M., Whitfield, C., Rao, K. V., Richardson, M., and Bishop, J. O. (1971). *Nature New Biol.* **231**, 8–12.
28. Moyer, G., and Pitot, H. C. (1972). *Fed. Proc.* **31**, 611.
29. Ohno, S. (1971). *Physiol. Rev.* **51**, 496–526.
30. Ono, T. (1966). *Gann Monogr.* **1**, 189–206.
31. Osserman, E. F., and Tabatsuki, K. (1963). *Medicine* **42**, 357–384.
32. Peraino, C., and Pitot, H. C. (1964). *J. Biol. Chem.* **239**, 4308–4313.
33. Pitot, H. C. (1960). *Cancer Res.* **20**, 1262–1268.
34. Pitot, H. C. (1968). *Cancer Res.* **28**, 1880–1887.
35. Pitot, H. C. (1969). *Arch. Path.* **87**, 212–222.
36. Pitot, H. C., Peraino, C., Bottomley, R. H., and Morris, H. P. (1963). *Cancer Res.* **23**, 135–142.
37. Pitot, H. C., Sladek, N., Ragland, W., Murray, R. K., Moyer, G., Soling, H. D., and Jost, J-P. (1969). *In* "Microsomes and Drug Oxidations," pp. 59–79. Academic Press, New York.
38. Potter, M. (1962). *J. Exp. Med.* **115**, 339–356.
39. Potter, V. R., Pitot, H. C., Ono, T., and Morris, H. P. (1960). *Cancer Res.* **20**, 1255–1261.
40. Potter, V. R., Watanabe, M., Pitot, H. C., and Morris, H. P. (1969). *Cancer Res.* **29**, 55–78.
41. Ragland, W. L., Shires, T. K., and Pitot, H. C. (1971). *Biochem. J.* **121**, 271–278.
42. Redman, C. M., and Cherian, M. G. (1972). *J. Cell Biol.* **52**, 231–245.
43. Reynolds, R. D., Potter, V. R., Pitot, H. C., and Revbar, M. D. (1971). *Cancer Res.* **31**, 808–812.
44. Riggsby, W. S., and Merrian, V. (1968). *Science* **161**, 570–571.
45. Roobal, A., and Rabin, B. R. (1971). *FEBS Lett.* **14**, 165–169.
46. Sandberg, A. A., Ishihara, T., Mirva, T., and Hauschba, T. S. (1961). *Cancer Res.* **21**, 678–689.
47. Scott-Burden, T., and Hawtrey, A. O. (1971). *Hoppe-Seyler's Z. Physiol. Chem.* **352**, 575–582.
48. Shires, T. K., Narurkar, L., and Pitot, H. C. (1971). *Biochem. J.* **125**, 67–79.
49. Shires, T., Narurkar, L. M., and Pitot, H. C. (1971). *Biochem. Biophys. Res. Commun.* **45**, 1212–1218.
50. Shires, T. K., Kauffman, S. A., and Pitot, H. C. (1973). *In* "Biomembranes," Vol. 3, Dekker, New York (in press).
51. Stewart, G. A., and Farber, E. (1967). *Science* **157**, 67–69.
52. Tseung, P.-Y., and Jones, H. W. (1969). *Obstet. Gynecol.* **33**, 741–752.
53. Warburg, O. (1930). "Metabolism of Tumors." Arnold, London.
54. Wollman, S. H. (1963). *Rec. Progr. Hor. Res.* **15**, 579–618.

CHAPTER XIV

Plasmacytomas

MICHAEL POTTER

The plasmacytomas in mice* are a homolog for the malignant plasma cell tumor referred to as multiple myeloma in man. The major difference in the plasma cell tumors in the two species is the tissue site in which they appear to develop. Patients with multiple myeloma develop multiple tumors in the bone marrow cavities. It is clear though from the homogeneous nature of the immunoglobulin produced by the multiple tumors that the tumor process which involves multiple bones simultaneously originates from a single source and spreads to the different bone marrow cavities. In the mouse, plasmacytomas

---

* Abbreviations: MOPC = mineral oil plasmacytoma, MPC = Merwin plasmacytoma, McPC = MacIntire's plasmacytoma, ASC = antigen-sensitive cells. These tumors have been developed in different laboratories and assigned different experimental numbers.

can be evoked by several procedures and the tumors do not arise in bone marrow cavities but rather in the peritoneal connective tissues.

In both mouse and man, plasmacytomas synthesize and secrete homogeneous immunoglobulin. By definition antibodies are a heterogeneous group of immunoglobulin molecules that bind the same antigen. A question that has interested many has been what relation the plasmacytoma has to antibody-producing cells. For a long time the immunoglobulin molecules produced by plasmacytomas were regarded as abnormal, chiefly, because they were produced by tumor cells and hence had no relation to antibody-producing cells. More recently immunochemical study of homogeneous immunoglobulins produced by tumors has provided strong evidence that the homogeneous immunoglobulins of tumor origin resemble normal immunoglobulins. Thus plasmacytomas are related to the normal antibody-producing cell system in the organism.

I. Introduction

The physiological function of the plasma cell is the synthesis and secretion of immunoglobulin. The immunoglobulin produced by a single plasma cell, however, is almost always a single molecular type. This is a remarkable phenomenon because the vertebrate organism is endowed genetically with the capacity to produce a very great variety of immunoglobulins. The developmental process, whereby a single plasma cell becomes restricted to producing but one immunoglobulin, is the result of two mechanisms, one in which the immunoglobulin genome becomes differentiated and a second process of cellular specialization. These two events are coupled and develop in parallel.

This chapter presents current status of information on an unusual form of carcinogenesis, the development of plasmacytomas in the inbred BALB/c strain of mice. Plasmacytomas do not occur spontaneously in these mice but can be evoked in high frequency by the intraperitoneal implantation of plastic discs or injection of mineral oils. Plasmacytomas are of interest to molecular biologists because they are tumors of highly differentiated and specialized cell types. This provides a system for examining the critical differences between normal and neoplastic plasma cells. It is hypothesized that from an analysis of the development and performance of various functions of the cell, e.g., its special biosynthetic processes, its mode of proliferation, its cell surface receptors that orient the cell in the multicellular system, and its metabolism, that the defects that determine neoplastic behavior will be identified. The neoplastic change may be established by a transformation of a fully developed cell or it may occur during a developmental or maturational process when various controls in the cell are changing.

The plasmacytomas will be discussed from these two aspects: (1) the determinative events that take place in the somatic genome that result in restricted immunoglobulin production and (2) the development of the specialized cell.

II. Differentiation of the Immunoglobulin Genome

Immunoglobulin synthesis is a multistep process which can be divided into four basic processes: (1) activation and stabilization of the specialized immunoglobulin genome; (2) transcription of L and H chain messenger RNA; (3) synthesis and assembly on light and heavy polysomes of 4-chain monomers; and (4) attachment of carbohydrate side chains, intracellular transit, and secretion across the cell membrane (Fig. 14.1). IgA and IgM polymer formation occurs extracellularly after release of monomers from the membrane, or possibly as a final step on the membrane itself.

While all of the immunoglobulin biosynthetic pathway is potentially relevant to a discussion of the molecular biology of plasmacytomas, emphasis here will be given to the differentiation process and its stability. First, the differentiation process provides the basis for understanding the development of normal plasma cells; secondly, the most common disorders in immunoglobulin synthesis in

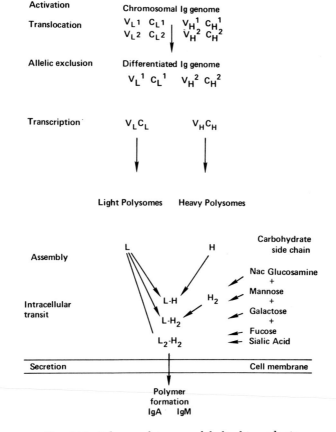

Fig. 14.1. Scheme of immunoglobulin biosynthesis.

plasmacytomas appear to involve the stability of the "differentiated" immuno-globulin genome. No doubt there are many abnormal forms of immunoglobulin biosynthesis in plasmacytomas that have been described and which will be found on further study, but the fact remains that many plasmacytomas are capable of synthesizing and secreting normal immunoglobulin molecules and this makes it unlikely that the immunoglobulin-producing apparatus is directly involved in the neoplastic process (9, 83, 96, 114).

A. The Immunoglobulin Molecule: Genetic Control

The molecular unit of secreted immunoglobulins is a four polypeptide chain structure. Each unit has a molecular weight of approximately 150,000 and is composed of two identical light (L) polypeptide chains (each of about 24,000 molecular weight) and two identical heavy (H) polypeptide chains (each of about 53,000 MW). The basic structural characteristics of immunoglobulin mole-cules, including important landmarks, are shown schematically in Fig. 14.2.

The genetic control of immunoglobulin L (light) and H (heavy) chain struc-tures has proved to be unusual. Although both of these types are single chains linked throughout by covalent peptide bonds, each type L and H is controlled not by one but by two structural genes.

The evidence that led to the development of the two gene-one polypeptide chain theory for immunoglobulins came from comparative amino acid sequence studies of immunoglobulin chains derived from myeloma proteins from man and the inbred BALB/c mouse (26, 27, 35).

The structural comparisons of L and H chains indicated each chain type was divisible into two segments. L Chains within a species vary in length from 213 to 218 amino acids and are divided into two polypeptide segments: a V_L (variable, light chain) polypeptide segment, which varies in length from amino terminal residue 1 to residue 106 to 111, and the C_L (constant, light chain) polypeptide segment of constant length consisting of the carboxyl terminal 107 amino acids. Heavy chains are divided into the V_H (variable, heavy chain) polypeptide of about 110 amino acids again beginning at the amino terminus and ending about one-fourth of the length of the chain and C_H (constant, heavy chain) which begins at about the 110th amino acid and extends to the carboxyl terminus (containing about 330 or more residues).

The reason why the amino terminal segments of L and H chains are called "variable" is that IgL or H chains isolated from a single species all possess the same species-specific sequence in the carboxyl terminal segment (constant segment), but individual chains differ from each other in the amino terminal seg-ment. The first suspicion that an unusual form of genetic control was operating developed when it became apparent that there were marked differences among the species in the C-region sequences for homologous structures. This made unlikely the existence of a large series of light or heavy chain genes each with a part controlling a different V polypeptide and another controlling the same species specific C polypeptide. Such a system would require a means for repeat-

IMMUNOGLOBULIN MOLECULE

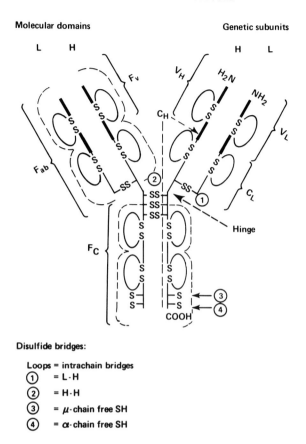

Fig. 14.2. The model of the immunoglobulin molecule shows the hypothetical molecular domains on the left with proteolytic fragments indicated by brackets, and molecular domains (31, 50, 76a, 79a) indicated by dotted lines on the left. Three proteolytic fragments are indicated Fab (fragment containing the antigen binding site), Fc (crystallizable fragment), and a recently isolated fragment Fv (50) which contains V_L and V_H polypeptides. Domains are segments of polypeptide chains that appear as globular regions in X-ray crystallographic analysis (76a, 79a).

The disulfide bridges and free disulfides are indicated. Each of the domains contains one intrachain disulfide bridge, which is schematically shown as a loop. While the schematic molecule depicts an L–H disulfide, some IgA molecules in the mouse lack this type of bridge and in these molecules the L chains are joined to each other by a disulfide bridge and is labelled according to the domain of origin (2).

The angle at the hinge region varies with different classes of molecules, in IgG the Fab fragments are nearly 180° apart while in IgA the angle is closer to 90°. The restricted extension of the Fab fragments in mouse IgA may explain why IgA monomers in the mouse cannot precipitate or agglutinate while IgG monomers are able to carry out these cross-linking functions.

The genetically determined structural segments are shown on the right: V_L (variable light chain), C_L (constant light chain), V_H (variable light chain), and C_H constant heavy chain. The V segments are at the aminoterminal ends of both chains.

ing many times on the chromosome a DNA with a characteristic sequence and, further, some method for maintaining these sequences the same and free of mutations.

The more facile explanation was by postulating (26) that there were two types of genes one for V and one for C. The genomes of vertebrates have many V genes and relatively few C genes. Genetic proof of the separate structural gene control of the V and C polypeptides has not been completely proved, but all of the evidence, to date, strongly supports the two-gene polypeptide chain interpretation. In the transition from a stem cell to an ASC cell four structural genes are activated among a very much larger available source; the result is the formation of a highly specialized immunoglobulin product. First, a unique antigen-binding specificity is established by the V_L and V_H genes and second, other physiological functions are established by the variability of C_H gene, which includes complement-binding capability, polymer formation, tissue binding and transplacental migration secretion across epithelial cells. It remains to be demonstrated whether there is special C_H function that permits immunoglobulin molecules to be incorporated into cell membranes.

B. Varieties of Immunoglobulin Genes

Different classes of C_L, C_H, V_L, and V_H structural genes are found in a single species and for a single genome. Analysis of the immunoglobulin genes of the mouse (Table 14.1) showed there are only three C_L genes and six C_H genes. By contrast there are an unestimated but larger number of V_L and V_H genes. An important characteristic of immunoglobulin genes are the "rules of association." Specific sets of V polypeptides associate with one or more C polypeptides and

TABLE 14.1

IMMUNOGLOBULIN STRUCTURAL GENES IN THE MOUSE

	Lambda				Kappa		Heavy chain						
	$C_{\lambda1}$	$V_{\lambda1}$	$C_{\lambda2}{}^a$	$V_{\lambda2}{}^a$	C_κ	V_κ	C_μ	$C_{\gamma3}$	C_α	C_γ	C_η	C_ϕ	V_H
Number of related genes per haploid set	1	b	1	1	1	35[c]	1	1	1	1	1	1	Many[c]

[a] MOPC 315 protein L chain is the only protein in this class so far isolated (98).

[b] Of 11 $V_{\lambda1}$ sequences sequenced 8 are identical, the others differ at only three positions (119).

[c] Total number is not yet known. Based on partial amino acid sequences over 35 V_κ varieties have been isolated (46, 47). Many more are suspected. Only limited data is available on V_H sequences, many genes based on sequence differences are suspected. The C_α, C_γ, C_η, and C_ϕ genes are very tightly linked in the mouse in the IgC_H locus (42, 86). Other commonly used names for C_H genes are $C_\gamma = C_{\gamma2a}$; $C_\eta = C_{\gamma2b}$, and $C_\phi = C_{\gamma1}$ (see ref. 83).

these are not interchangeable. The three association groups in the mouse are V_κ with C_κ; V_λ with C_λ, and V_H with all six of the C_H genes. The C_H and V_H association is based thus far on limited data, but the same association has been found in man where more data is available (45, 53).

It is not yet established how the immunoglobulin genes are arranged on the chromosome. The evidence clearly favors the existence of three complex loci, one each for kappa, lambda, and the heavy chains; within each are C and V genes. Genetic studies in the mouse using allotypic and idiotypic serological markers have given some data on the structure of the IgC_H V_H complex locus. Several of the IgC_H genes are tightly linked onto one chromosomal region (42, 86). Further, differences in immune responses have been demonstrated in congenic stocks of mice that differ from the parental strain in IgC_H genes (14, 76). These observations provide genetic evidence for linkage of V_H and C_H genes.

The antigen-binding sites are determined by V_L and V_H polypeptides (50). It is not known whether all of the possible antigen-binding sites can be generated by germ line V_L and V_H genes. The variety of immunoglobulins is so great that a germ line mechanism may not be plausible (18, 56). It has been proposed that another process occurs in somatic cells and acts on V_L and V_H genes to create further variations. A number of different mechanisms for somatic variation have been proposed but none is yet established. The supporting evidence for somatic variations are the minimal sequence differences that have been observed in $V_{\lambda 1}$ (119) and within subclasses of V_κ (64, 66, 83). Chains differing in only 1 to 3 positions have been isolated from different BALB/c plasmacytomas. It is argued that a somatic rather than a germ line basis for minimal differences is more plausible.

C. Activation

The first step in immunoglobulin synthesis is the activation of the four immunoglobulin structural genes which occurs as stem cells differentiate into ASC-B lymphocytes (Fig. 14.3). Factors regulating this developmental step are not known. It is generally assumed that some automated process exists that develops varieties of ASC in the absence of antigen. Most workers today do not think antigen "instructs" stem cells to differentiate specific cell types.

While the biochemical basis for activation remains to be elucidated, key steps in differentiation can be reconstructed from structural characteristics of immunoglobulins produced by single cells.

1. ALLELIC EXCLUSION

A plasmacytoma or a single normal plasma cell synthesizes immunoglobulin from one or the other of the available alleles, but not from both simultaneously. This phenomenon called "allelic exclusion" was originally observed in myeloma proteins derived from individuals that were heterozygous for immunoglobulin

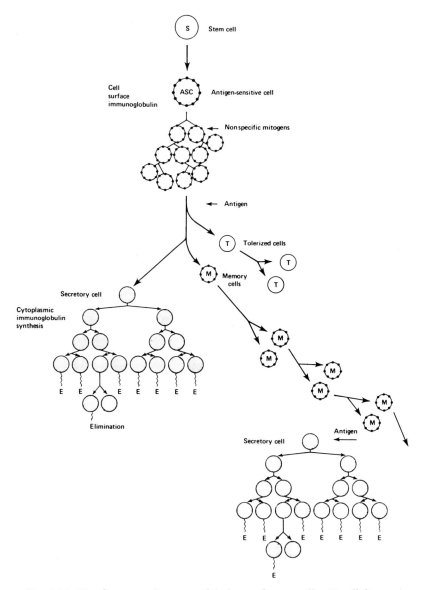

Fig. 14.3. Development of immunoglobulin-producing cells (B-cell lineage).

structural genes (39, 117). In each case, only one of the two possible genetic markers was expressed in the myeloma protein and hence in the cell.

The phenomenon of allelic exclusion reveals that activation involves only one chromosome. Since activation of an immunoglobulin locus, e.g., kappa, lambda, or heavy chain, also involves both a V and a C gene, it might be asked whether the V and C genes must be linked on one chromosome, or whether they can be derived from different chromosomes.

This problem has been studied in the rabbit where antigenic markers for both V_H and C_H genes are available. Nearly 99% of all immunoglobulins are made from genes from the same chromosome (61). Using special techniques, however, it was found that about 1% of heavy chains can be produced from V and C genes from different chromosomes. These results suggest the feasibility of activation of V and C genes in the trans position, but some caution must be exercised in that the same result might occur from a prior somatic recombination. The more favorable activation process occurs on V and C genes in the cis arrangement.

Additional evidence that suggests C and V genes must be physically close to each other in the activation process is the fact that specific sets of V genes associate with exclusively specific C genes.

2. TRANSLOCATION

To explain the origin of covalently linked polypeptide chains containing both C and V elements, the translocation of 2 DNA segments has been hypothesized (27). In the translocation hypothesis the continuous chromosomal DNA is nicked at the beginning and end of the C gene and at the end of the V gene. The two DNA segments are joined. This could involve the formation of an extra chromosomal DNA segment. Alternatively, the process could occur in situ on the chromosome and thus involve only two DNA nicks. Such a linkage, however, might be very unstable and broken during mitosis and DNA synthesis. The stability of the differentiated 2-gene complex could be maintained by an extra-chromosomal DNA template. There is a precedent for this mechanism in amphibian oocyte peripheral nucleolus formation where during oogenesis thousands of copies of nucleolar genes are delaminated from the chromosome in the form ringlike structures (69). There has been, however, no direct demonstration in plasma cells of nonchromosomal template DNA. An alternative to the covalent DNA template concept is that the activated genes on the chromosomes are used in the initial step in synthesis and the joining is accomplished at the RNA level.

One approach to this problem is to isolate messenger RNA for light or heavy chains and determine if the length corresponds to the polypeptide chain length. While the plasmacytoma cell seems to be an ideal system for isolating a single species of messenger RNA, this has not yet been accomplished. This is due in part to the presence of other messenger RNA's in plasmacytomas, as only 10% to 30% of the total intracellular protein synthesized in a plasmacytoma is immunoglobulin (83). An RNA fraction has been isolated (103) that was highly enriched with light chain mRNA from microsomes. The microsomal fractions were extracted with 1% SDS and purified by sucrose density gradient centrifugation. The 9 S and 13 S fractions obtained were pooled and used as mRNA in a cell free synthesis rabbit reticulocyte system. Of the total protein synthesized, only 20 to 27% was light chain. More recently polysomes were isolated from the MOPC 41 plasmacytoma by sucrose gradient centrifugation, and RNA extracted from this fraction was placed on an oligo T (d-thymidine) cellulose column that anneals RNA rich in adenylic acid sequences (108). Ninety-eight percent of the RNA from MOPC 41 applied to the column was not bound. The 2% that was bound was eluted from the column in two small peaks. One was very active in directing synthesis of light chain. This RNA was not homogeneous, however, and contained several different components that were capable of directing light chain synthesis, including one that was 13 S and another that was 19 S. The light chain messenger is apparently monocistronic (covalent) and approximately 200 nucleotides longer than required for the synthesis of light chain. This extra RNA is extraneous and not involved in controlling light chain synthesis. The finding indicates the mRNA for the L chain, at least, is a single covalent strand and further suggests the origin of the covalent mRNA is a covalent DNA sequence.

3. Intraclonal Switch Mechanism for IgC_H Genes

There is evidence from several sources that cells differentiated to produce immunoglobulin can vary the type of IgC_H gene. Using fluorescent antibody techniques, lymphocytes in immunized rabbits have been identified that have IgM on the cell surface and IgG in the cytoplasm. These cells were obtained from rabbits that were heterozygous for IgC_L IgV_H genes, and in the study fluorescent antisera specific for allotypic markers were used (77). In the double producing cells it was possible to demonstrate by double staining procedures that the same IgC_L and IgV_H genes were in both immunoglobulins. This is strong evidence against the possibility that the cell surface immunoglobulin was passively absorbed. In studies of anti-idiotypic antibodies in rabbits it has further been noted that rabbits can produce IgM and IgG antibodies with the same highly specific idiotype (75).

The most direct evidence for the intraclonal switch phenomenon has been obtained from studies on a human immunoglobulin-producing lymphoma in which two homogeneous proteins were found in the serum, one an IgM protein and the other IgG (32). Partial amino acid sequence studies extending for 38 residues from the amino terminus of the V_κ part of the light chain and 34 residues from V_H parts of the γ and μ chains were identical in both cases. In addition, peptide maps of the isolated chains' light chains were the same. Idiotypic antisera prepared to the IgM and IgG proteins reacted with both proteins (34).

Immunofluorescent studies of the tumor cells from this patient revealed the presence of two cell populations, one making the IgG and the other the IgM. Both cell populations were stained with the antiidiotypic antiserum (57). It is thought an IgM cell differentiates continuously to IgG producing cell derivatives.

Hypothetically, in the intraclonal switch mechanism, an immunoglobulin-producing cell differentiates two different programs of synthesis based upon the type of IgC_H gene. Conceivably, the ASC-B lymphocyte could produce simultaneously two classes of immunoglobulin with the same F_V, an IgM and an IgG form. As the cell matures, only the capacity to make the IgM or IgG form persists.

D. Abnormalities in Immunoglobulin Synthesis

The major forms of abnormal synthesis in plasmacytomas are (1) cells that synthesize and secrete only light chains (Bence Jones protein-producing cells) and (2) the cells that no longer synthesize and secrete any immunoglobulin (nonproducers). These phenomena have been associated with both multiple myeloma in man and the mouse plasmacytomas, and are apparently common forms of defectiveness inherent to these highly differentiated tumors. L chain-secreting variants have been observed to occur frequently *in vivo* during plasmacytoma development (85)

L chain-secreting variants have also been induced *in vivo* by transplanting plasmacytomas into immunized hosts (60). BALB/c mice, immunized to the MOPC 315 myeloma protein, can resist grafts of 10^3 to 10^4 cells. Most of the mice completely destroyed the tumor, but in others the tumor was only partially eliminated and ultimately killed the host. Transplant lines initiated from such mice were often composed of only L chain-secreting variants. Adaptation of plasmacytomas to *in vitro* conditions is frequently associated with appearance of L chain-secreting variants.

Quantitative *in vitro* assays have been developed detecting defectiveness of immunoglobulin production. For example, the MPC-11 tissue culture adapted plasmacytoma has a cloning efficiency of 90 to 100% when plated on in agar on top of a feeder layer of primary, secondary, or tertiary mouse embryo cells. After three days of incubation, cultures are overlayed with another layer of soft agar containing anti-immunoglobulin serum. Sera specific for heavy and light chains were used; colonies secreting immunoglobulin with antigenic determinants recognized by the antiserum are found to be overlayed by immune precipitate (Fig. 14.4), while those no longer making immunoglobulin recognized by the antiserum were not overlayed with precipitate (13, 96, 97).

When MPC 11 cells were plated and tested for their ability to make heavy chains, 29 of 4993 colonies examined failed to make heavy chains. These colonies were isolated and grown into mass culture and tested for immunoglobulin synthesis and it was found that all were able to form light chains, but were completely unable to make heavy chains intracellularly. A reversion to heavy chain synthesis was never observed in over 23,000 colonies examined. Further, when light chain-only producers were plated and tested for their ability to make light chains some L chain clones gave rise to nonproducing cells (other lines were stable and did not give rise to nonproducers).

The rate of development of these defective forms was found to be roughly similar in several tumors tested. The striking characteristic of defectiveness is its high rate of development and lack of back mutations.

While the rate of these defects could be increased by mutagens, their spon-

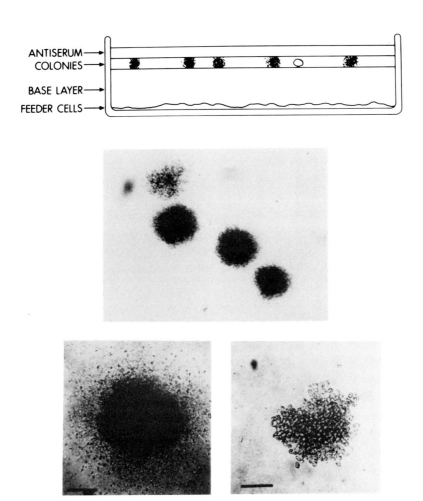

ANTISERUM→
COLONIES→
BASE LAYER→
FEEDER CELLS→

Fig. 14.4. Agar cloning method of Coffino and Scharff. See text for explanation.

taneous origin suggests that a process affecting the stability of activated genes is continuously operative in neoplastic plasma cells. Functions that are not essential for viability can be deleted to the advantage of the cell providing more energy for growth. If the defects in immunoglobulin synthesis are representative of a general internal process that affects other genes as well, these observations are important to the concept of phenotypic repression in cancer cells (Chapter I).

E. Immunoglobulins Produced by Neoplastic Plasma Cells: The Question of Abnormality

Most studies to date have dealt with immunoglobulins secreted by plasma cells and little, if anything, has been reported about the molecular structure of membrane associated immunoglobulin. The 4-chain monomer and polymer immunoglobulins secreted by most plasmacytomas (myeloma proteins) are normal in structure, i.e., they have the characteristic chain structure and a molecular weight similar to normal immunoglobulin. The older literature frequently refers to myeloma proteins as abnormal proteins. The evidence cited for abnormality was the excessive concentration, the electrophoretic homogeneity and, most important, the fact that patients whose sera contained a myeloma protein usually were deficient in protective antibodies and were prone to infections.

These phenomena can now be explained as due to excessive growth of cells within a differentiated clone of Ig-producing cells and the production of homogeneous immunoglobulin. The acceptance of this concept leads to a new question, i.e., if the immunoglobulin produced by a plasma cell tumor is structurally normal it should be able to bind antigens.

The screening of mouse myeloma proteins for antigen-binding activity has been productive of a considerably high yield of antigen-binding proteins approaching 5% in many of the series tested (81–83, 89). Mouse proteins have been found that bind a variety of different ligands. The chemical study of the interaction of these homogenous immunoglobulins with their respective ligands has revealed that proteins can precipitate, agglutinate, fix complement and bind free hapten in equilibrium dialysis states (see 83 for references). These molecules interact with ligand as would be predicted for a single molecular species of immunoglobulin in antibody (antibody by definition is a heterogeous group of normal immunoglobulins that bind the same antigen).

Recently, evidence has been presented that demonstrates the close structural similarities of normal immunoglobulins and myeloma proteins, using antigenic markers specific for individual species of F_V called idiotypes. Essentially, it is possible to produce antibodies either in the same inbred strain (syngeneic immunization) in genetically different animals of the same species (allogeneically), or in members of other species (xenogeneic immunization) that are specific for a determinant on the F_V fragment. Because there are so many different immunoglobulins these antigenic markers are highly specific and when they are assigned to antigen-binding proteins the double use of idiotype and antigen-binding activity becomes an extremely useful marker system. A characteristic of some idiotypic determinants is their proximity and relation to antigen-binding sites. This is demonstrable by examining the antigenicity of the myeloma protein in the presence and absence of its specific ligand (15, 102). Many idiotypic determinant sites are blocked when the ligand is bound in the site, thus demonstrating that the idiotypic determinant is in a region contiguous to the antigen-binding (15, 102) site. Since anti-idiotypic antibody can be prepared allogeneically to virtually every myeloma protein, it became possible to search for idiotypic similarities between myeloma proteins of independent origin. Attempts to find similarities were made by screening hundreds of proteins with 25 highly specific sera without finding convincing evidence for idiotypic similarity among randomly chosen myeloma proteins. However, when idiotypic antibodies were prepared to myeloma proteins with the same antigen-binding activity as was done for the group of eight available phosphorylcholine-binding proteins, five of the eight had an identical idiotype, the S63-T15 idiotype (87). Each of these proteins was derived from a plasmacytoma that arose in a different mouse.[*] Thus, 5 plasmacytomas of independent origin can produce the same unique type of immunoglobulin, but further detailed sequence studies will be necessary for final proof.

Antibodies have been prepared to the S63-T15 idiotype and normal antibodies to phosphorylcholine have been tested to see if any have this idiotype (20). Mice were immunized with the R36 strain of pneumococcus which lacks a capsular polysaccharide and has apparently a considerable amount of the pneumococcus C polysaccharide on its surface. The cell population that responded to this antigen was tested for its ability to produce plaques in agar plates containing sheep red blood cells (SRBC) coupled with phosphorylcholine. The initial response was almost entirely inhibited by the antiidiotypic antibody, prepared to the S63-T15 idiotype indicating the normal immunoglobulin releasing cells were producing immunoglobulins with the same F_V as was found on the myeloma proteins. A related result has been obtained in the $\alpha 1 \rightarrow 3$ dextran response in mice (14) when anti-idiotypic antisera was prepared to the J558 myeloma protein that binds dextrans containing $\alpha 1 \rightarrow 3$ oligosaccharides. The normal antibodies elicited to $\alpha 1 \rightarrow 3$ dextran had idiotypic specificities related to those on the J558 myeloma protein.

The ultimate means for structurally comparing myeloma proteins and individual molecular species in antibody will be by comparing the structures of antigen-binding sites. The antigen-binding site has been studied indirectly through the use of affinity labeling reagents, and by the specificity of homogenous immunoglobulins for structurally related ligands. All of these methods are indirect and a direct visualization of the site will depend on a crystallographic study of the antigen-binding site. Recently, there has been some success in this area. The MOPC 315 pepsin Fab fragment has been crystallized and the crystals bind dinitrophenyl-containing ligands (51). Unfortunately, these crystals were long needles and were not useful for high resolution X-ray crystallography. However, crystals of the pepsin Fab fragment from the McPC 603 myeloma protein that binds phosphorylcholine ligands have been obtained (95). These crystals have diffraction spots out to 2.8 Å, sufficient for constructing high resolution electron density maps and ultimately a model of an antigen-binding immunoglobulin. Attempts are in progress to crystallize other antigen-binding myeloma proteins. Among the first 15 proteins tried only one gives a useful crystal. However, the great value of the mouse system is reproducibility. By merely screening myeloma proteins for binding activity, an unlimited supply of active proteins can be obtained.

The X-ray crystallographic data will reveal the topology of the combining site. The phosphorylcholine binding site on the McPC 603 has been located on a 4.5 Å electron density map (Fig. 14.5) (76a). The comparative study of several crystals will show whether this site always occurs in the same region

---

[*] Two of the five tumors were induced in Dr. Melvin Cohn's laboratory in La Jolla and three in our laboratory at the N.I.H. Partial amino acid sequence peptide map studies of two of the proteins has not, as yet, revealed any structural differences. (L. Hood, S. Rudikoff, W. Konigsberg, M. Potter, work in progress.)

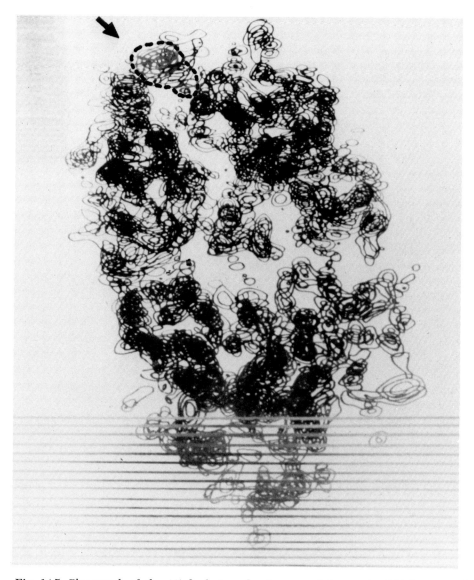

Fig. 14.5. Photograph of the 4.5 Å electron density map of the pepsin Fab′ fragment of McPC603 myeloma protein. This protein binds specifically phosphorylcholine (81, 87) and precipitates antigens that contain phosphorylcholine groups (82, 87). The Fab′ fragment can be crystallized in 42% solutions of ammonium sulfate (95), and the crystals are suitable for high resolution X-ray crystallographic analysis out to 3 Å. Shown here is an electron density map at low resolution. Four distinct globular regions corresponding to the four domains V_κ, C_κ, V_H, and C_{H1} can be discerned. The large space beginning just under the dotted area in the upper left of the map and traversing towards the center lies between the V_κ and the V_H. The division between C_κ and C_{H1} is not clearly visible in this photograph. However the space between the V and C regions is clearly visible from the center to the right side of the photograph.

The crystal in the photograph was prepared in the presence of a specific heavy metal derivative of phosphorylcholine: 2-(5′-acetoxy-mercuri-2′-thienyl)ethylphosphorylcholine (AMTEPC) (76a). The AMTEPC compound was located by Fourier difference techniques (see area enclosed in heavy dotted line). The regions between the V_κ and the V_H at one end of the molecule are believed to represent the specific combining site of the homogeneous antibodylike McPC603 myeloma protein.

of the molecule or whether it may be formed randomly on different parts of the F_V region. With this information it should be possible then to make the comparison between normal homogeneous antibody which can be obtained under special experimental conditions and myeloma proteins.

1. FUNCTIONALLY ABNORMAL PROTEINS

The findings in mice, based upon the relatively high frequency of antigen-binding proteins, substantiate the hypothesis that plasmacytomas produce normally structured immunoglobulins, but this is still only a small percentage and a nagging question still is can many of the proteins be abnormal and, if so, in what way? It may be argued that some myeloma proteins lack combining sites for any antigen. Reasons for this inertness can be hypothesized. First according to the clonal selection theory V_L and V_H genes are independently activated. Each cell expresses only one of each, and hence only one V_L, V_H pair. Some V_L, V_H combinations may be essentially degenerate, i.e., have combining sites for antigens the mouse will never encounter. If the cells producing these useless immunoglobulins can be converted to neoplasms then their homogeneous immunoglobulin products would appear to be functionally inert.

2. STRUCTURALLY ABNORMAL PROTEINS

In the mouse plasmacytoma system, two forms of abnormal proteins have been identified. The more common are the incomplete proteins, the Bence Jones proteins that are composed of only light chains. These forms are due to a disorder in immunoglobulin synthesis rather than an abnormality in structural genes (cf. above).

The one structurally abnormal protein found in mice is the 2-chain IgA myeloma protein. Thus far, six examples have been observed. All of the proteins were discovered first in the urine of mice bearing the tumors; like free light chains they induce renal tubular casts (myeloma kidney). The proteins also appear in the serum. The 2-chain IgA proteins have a molecular weight of about 70,000 and contain a complete light chain and an incomplete alpha heavy chain. The molecular weights of two of these chains have been determined (72, 99) and found to be 40,000 (MOPC47A) and 46,000 (AdjPC6C). It is thus possible there are several abnormal forms. The evidence currently suggests the defective alpha chains lack a carboxyl terminal segment of the Cα amino acid sequence. This includes the part of the chain that contains the free sulfhydryl employed in linking polymers of IgA. Further, none of the inter-heavy chain bridges form. The molecular basis for these abnormalities have not yet been established.

F. Summary

Some important concepts to emerge from these studies include the following.
1. The unusual nature of the two gene: one polypeptide chain mechanism for immunoglobulin light and heavy chains requires a special means of gene differ-

entiation. Relevant phenomena now known about this process are the association of specific C and V genes, allelic exclusion, hypothetical mechanisms of translocation, and the feasibility of an intraclonal switching of IgC_H genes. The basis of antibody diversity is thought to result largely from inherited V_L and V_H structural genes. However, the immune potential is so great it has long been argued that modifications of structural genes are necessary to produce all the varieties of immunoglobulins that the vertebrate organism is capable of making. These modifications could hypothetically develop in antigen-sensitive cells or memory cells and possibly are responsible for the "minimal" amino acid sequence differences that have been found in certain classes of V_L genes. There is no evidence yet that any mechanism of variation related to the specificity of antibody can develop in plasma cells or plasmacytoma cells. However, this possibility has not been completely ruled out by quantitative study of the critical V-region amino acids in immunoglobulins derived from a plasmacytoma. The crystallization of antigen-binding myeloma proteins from the mouse and the localization of the active site will provide a basis for examining this problem in more detail.

2. In many plasmacytomas immunoglobulin synthesis results in the production of 4-chain monomer immunoglobulins, just as would be expected in normal plasma cells. Immunoglobulin synthesis per se probably has little, if anything, to do with the neoplastic state in these tumors.

3. An antigen-binding activity has been found for about 5% of myeloma proteins in the mouse, suggesting that in these cases the plasmacytoma cells were derived from antigen-selected cells. Recent evidence, using idiotypic antisera, has revealed idiotypic similarities between naturally induced antibodies to $\alpha 1 \rightarrow 3$ dextrans, and phosphorylcholine and myeloma proteins with respective antigen-binding activities.

4. A common abnormality in immunoglobulin synthesis, found in many plasmacytomas, is the loss of the ability to produce heavy chains resulting in cell types that produce only light chains, or a more extreme disorder in which all immunoglobulin synthesis ceases. These abnormalities are interpreted as being due to a failure to maintain genes in an activated state.

5. A few structurally abnormal forms of immunoglobulin made in plasmacytomas have been described, i.e., the rare 2-chain IgA molecules. Most monomeric and polymeric immunoglobulins have a normal structure.

6. A possible origin of plasmacytoma from cells that have not been selected by antigen has not been ruled out.

III. Plasma Cell Development and Maturation

A. Differentiation of Antigen-Sensitive Cells (ASC)

The process of cell differentiation in plasma cells results in the development of cells that are restricted to producing immunoglobulin with only a single type antigen-binding specificity. Since each vertebrate organism is genetically endowed with the capability of producing thousands of different molecular types of immunoglobulin, the specialization of the single plasma cell is an extraordinary form of differentiation.

Each newly differentiated immunoglobulin-producing cell can potentially be "one of a kind" at the time of its origin and represent the beginning of an immunoglobulin-producing clone. An immunoglobulin-producing clone (the B-cell lineage) consists of all the cells derived from the initial differentiation and includes antigen-sensitive B lymphocytes, memory cells, immunoglobulin secreting cells (plasma cells and lymphoplasmacytes), and cells that are paralyzed (tolerized cells).

The first stage in the immunoglobulin-producing series is a cell that synthesizes and incorporates homogeneous immunoglobulin into the cell membrane. It is not known from existing data whether membrane immunoglobulin is similar to one of the classes of immunoglobulin secreted by plasma cells.

Three B-cell developmental pathways have been delineated: (1) development to a secretory cell (plasma cell) which is usually associated with a rapid burst of cellular proliferation culminating in maturation, loss of DNA synthesis, and senescence (64, 74); (2) development to a memory cell that remains morphologically lymphoid in character and divides slowly and continuously for extensive periods (10, 19, 62); or (3) development to a paralyzed cell which, like the memory cell, can also persist but does not secrete immunoglobulin. Under appropriate and specific conditions memory and paralyzed cells can become actively secreting cell types (24, 70).

B. B-Cell Receptors; Fluid Mosaic Model of Membrane Structure

Protein receptors are normally distributed all over the cell surface. Until recently very little was known about their relation to the cell membrane structure. The fluid mosaic model of the cell membrane (32, 101) has brought together into a single theory a new dynamic concept on the organization of the cell membrane. This model challenged the long held trilaminar model of the membrane in which the central phospholipid bilayer extended continuously between outer and inner layers of protein. The arrangement in the trilaminar model may not be thermodynamically stable, chiefly because the hydrophobic and hydrophilic interactions of phospholipids, proteins, and aqueous environment are not maximized (101). In the mosaic model of membrane structure proteins are embedded in a fluid lipid matrix. An essential property of membrane proteins is that they have available for interaction both polar and nonpolar residues. The nonpolar portions of the molecules would interact with the fatty acid hydrophobic component of the phospholipid layer, while the polar regions would extend outward and inward.

Two types of membrane associated proteins are the "peripheral" proteins that are relatively easily dissociated from the membrane by chelating agents and high salt concentrations and integral proteins which comprise about 70% of membrane-associated protein, and which is tightly associated with the phospholipid of the membrane. Integral proteins are dissociated with difficulty; this requires more drastic conditions, including use of detergents, and even then the proteins are often not clearly separated from the membrane. According to some of the criteria (101), immunoglobulin, phytomitogen, and H_2 receptors on B lymphocytes are integral proteins.

The amphipathic nature of immunoglobulins is assumed since globular proteins are thought to have both polar and nonpolar groups on their surfaces. However, it is not known whether membrane immunoglobulin can be distinguished from circulating immunoglobulin by the class of heavy chain. Possibly, some classes of immunoglobulins have available more nonpolar groups than others, thereby making them more suitable for integration into membranes.

The major predictions of the fluid mosaic model are (1) there is no "long range" order in the distribution of protein in the membrane; (2) short range order is feasible; and (3) under physiological conditions the lipids of functional cell membranes are in a fluid rather than crystalline state (101).

Evidence that protein molecules in membranes are mobile has been demonstrated in several experiments. After fusion of human and mouse cells, the distribution of human and murine cell surface markers was followed (33). Within 40 minutes of fusion the human and mouse membrane proteins were intermingled throughout the surface of the new heterokaryon (33). Since this was not sufficient time for new synthesis, the phenomenon was attributed to redistribution of preformed cell surface protein. Studies of antigens on lymphocytes (11) on the phenomenon of antigenic modulation have repeatedly demonstrated that cell surface proteins on lymphocytes are mobile (25, 52, 110, 115). With the use of fluorescence microscopy and radioautography the movement of cell surface proteins (receptors) has been traced. These movements require the interaction of a reactive substance with the membrane bound receptor which will be called here a reactor. Protein receptors normally distributed all over the cell surface can be aggregated by interaction with reactor. Aggregates, depending upon the interaction, can coalesce at one pole of the cell (called the uropod) where they are visualized by fluorescence microscopy as a cap. The aggregated complex is usually then internalized into the cytoplasm of the cell (115). Cap formation and internalization (or endocytosis) are temperature dependent. For example, reactor and receptor can interact at 4°C, but cap formation and internalization requires the cells be brought to 37°C (115). Essentially, then, the interaction of receptor with reactor clears the cell surface of receptor.

Clearance is followed by regeneration of receptor by new synthesis. The further development, proliferation, and maturation of B cells is generally thought to be regulated by the interaction of cell surface receptors and various reactive factors. The significant receptor is the specific differentiated immunoglobulin produced by that cell.

Many reactors used in experimental systems such as antibody prepared to cell surface proteins probably do not occur naturally and hence do not yet have biological significance. However, others are clearly important biologically and can be found in the *milieu interne* of the organism. For the cells in the B lineage the most important of all reactors is antigen. Antigen reacts with the cell surface immunoglobulin and this reaction is thought to control the further development of the cell. The appropriate concentration of antigen triggers the development of the B lymphocyte to an immunoglobulin-secreting plasma cell and concommittently the cell undergoes a rapid burst of mitotic activity. The pathway by which this process is regulated is not known. However, the existing evidence indicates that the clearance of immunoglobulin from the cell surface is followed by a more intense production of immunoglobulin (25). Thus, the clearance process sets in motion active synthesis that involves immunoglobulin-producing genes. The presence of excessive antigen can paralyze cells so that all of the cell surface immunoglobulin is bound and clearance does not follow (25). Such cells are paralyzed or tolerized by antigen.

In addition, receptors for aggregated immunoglobulin (11, 12, 28) and for phytomitogens, such as concanavalin A and phytohemagglutinin stimulate mitosis (5, 36). A relatively specific mitogen for B lymphocytes is lipopolysaccharide or endotoxin (6). While the receptor for lipopolysaccharide has not been characterized, it is known to be independent of specific immunoglobulin receptor (6). The C3 (and possibly the Fc) receptors for aggregated immunoglobulin have been suggested to play a role in attracting B cells to the lymphoid follicles (28). Extensive comparisons of receptors on B cells and plasmacytomas have not yet been made. Most but not all plasmacytomas lack the Fc receptor; an exceptional plasmacytoma, HPC6, does however carry this receptor (17). It is not known how antigen is involved with the regulation of mitotic activity. Conceivably, at some stages of development, there is a pathway that can be stimulated by the interaction cell surface immunoglobulin and antigen. Plasmacytomas in all probability can proliferate in the absence of antigen and, thus, are dissociated from this control, but how this comes about is not known.

For molecular biology the fluid mosaic theory dispells the old concept of a fixed ordered membrane structure, and in its place depicts the cell surface as a highly reactive organelle. The short-range order, i.e., potential interaction of membrane proteins with each other to establish biological function provides new possibilities for the molecular biologist to explain cellular physiology and regulation (32). Also significant is the dynamic aspect of regenerating cell surface protein which places continued demands on the cell to maintain the integrity of its outer surface. The beginning application of these principles to the B cell differentation has been briefly outlined.

C. Origin of Plasmacytomas

While plasmacytomas are composed of immunoglobulin-secreting cells, i.e., mature cell types in the B-cell lineage, it is not at all clear where the critical changes leading to neoplasia first develop, and what relationship these changes have to specific cells in the B-cell lineage. For example, the genetic changes could begin in ASC-B lymphocytes but are not expressed until the cells mature to a further stage. Alternatively, genetic changes leading to the neoplastic state may depend upon the specific developmental state of the genome that prevails when a cell has matured to the secretory cell stage.

1. POSSIBLE ROLE OF ANTIGEN

Several lines of evidence suggest that some plasmacytomas are derived from antigen-selected cells; this could implicate ASC, memory cells, tolerized cells, and secreting cells. First, the high proportion of mineral oil-induced plasmacytomas that produce immunoglobulins of the IgA class (66%) (83) is evidence in favor of previous antigenic selection. Immunocytes producing IgA immunoglobulins are not usually found in abundance in lymphoreticular tissues such as the spleen and lymph nodes, but instead are concentrated in the lamina propria of the gut and respiratory tracts where they constitute around 80% of the entire plasma cell population (16, 22). Interestingly, the lamina propria of the gut is a tissue that normally has a high plasma cell population. The concentration of plasma cells in the lamina propria is believed to be related to the fact that IgA immunoglobulin molecules following liberation from the plasma cell can be taken up and secreted across epithelial cells into the lumen of the gut, respiratory, urinary, mammary and salivary tracts (112, 113).

The IgA system of cells, then, is strategically located at tissue sites where the organism is constantly challenged by exogenous antigen. The IgA immunoglobulins secreted across epithelia presumably aid in impeding the entry of microbes and viruses into the organism (122).

The development of the IgA system of cells in the lamina propria is not yet completely understood but available evidence suggests that antigens entering the organism across the mucosal lining stimulate the formation of the lamina propria system of cells and, further, can specifically trigger an IgA immune response (37). Two lines of evidence support this hypothesis. First, germfree mice which lack a microbial flora have a paucity of immunoglobulin producing cells in the lamina propria of their gastrointestinal tracts (21). Second, it has been possible to immunize mice by the oral administration of a protein antigen and show that the predominant, almost exclusive cellular response, is an IgA response in the lamina propria of the gut (41, 73). To demonstrate this fact, germ free mice had to be used chiefly because protein antigens are normally digested normal bacterial flora. In other experiments it has been demonstrated that antigens administered orally to germfree mice stimulate the formation of IgA-producing cells that appear in the spleen and mesenteric lymph nodes.

Recent studies have shown that IgA-producing lamina propria cells have a half-life of 4.7 days (62a), indicating a rapid turnover of this population, and are another example of the dynamic nature of immunocyte development.

Anatomically plasmacytomas do not arise in a tissue that is in direct continuity with the lamina propria and to explain the peritoneal location of the plasmacytomas it is necessary to postulate that IgA-committed cells migrate or circulate and then become diverted into the peritoneal site. Evidence for the circulation of IgA-committed cells has been obtained in several studies (22, 37).

Other findings suggesting a direct relationship of plasmacytomas to antigen-selected cells is the drastically reduced incidence of plasmacytomas in mineral oil-treated, germfree mice (63). Germfree mice lack a normal microbial flora and hence a major source of antigenic stimulation. Further, evidence that plasmacytomas are related to antigen-selected immunocytes is the consistent finding of antigen-binding myeloma proteins in mice. As might be anticipated most of these proteins are IgA in class (Table 14.2). In a number of screening tests that have been reported, the incidence of antigen-binding proteins has been in the range of 1 to 5%, depending on the particular series and the number of antigens screened (83).

TABLE 14.2
Mouse Myeloma Proteins with Antigen-Binding Activity

Antigen[a]	Specificity	Myeloma proteins		
		IgM	IgA	IgG
?	Nitrophenyl		MOPC 315 (λ2) MOPC 460 (κ) XRPC 25 (κ)	
Lactobacillus Ag[b]	Phosphorylcholine		S63 (κ)	ALPC 43 (G3)
Pneumococcus C ps			S107 (κ)	MOV 26 (G3)
Trichoderma ps.[b]			TEPC 15 (κ)	
Aspergillus sp, ps[b]			HOPC 8 (κ)	
Ascaris			MOPC 299 (κ)	
			MCPC 603 (κ)	
			MOPC 167 (κ)	
			MOPC 511 (κ)	
Wheat extract[b]	B1 $\rightarrow$ 6 D-Galactan		J539 (κ)	
Hardwood bedding[b]			TEPC 191 (κ)	
Arabinogalactan			SAPC 10 (κ)	
Gum ghatti			JPC 1 (κ)	
			XRPC 24 (κ)	
Wheat extract	Pronase sensitive		TEPC 521	
Leuconostoc meserentoides dextran	α1 $\rightarrow$ 3 dextran	MOPC 104 E (λ1)	J558 (λ1)	
B. subtilis levan[b]	Fructosan			J606 (G3) κ
B. circulans levan[b]				UPC 10 (G)
Inulin				
Proteus mirabilis	α-Methyl D-glactoside		MOPC 384	
	α-Methyl D-mannoside		McPC 870	
Salm weslaco lps	N-Acetyl D-mannosamine		MOPC 406 (κ)	
Salmonella and *Pasteurella* HE Ag	Trypsin-sensitive		MOPC 467	

[a] Ag = Antigen; Ps = polysaccharide; sp = species; lps = lipopolysaccharide; HE = heat extract.

[b] Antigen isolated from microbial flora, dietary constituent, or environment of the BALB/c mouse.

A group of antigens for which antigen-binding myeloma proteins have been repeatedly found are $\alpha 1 \to 3$ dextrans $B1 \to 6$ D-galactans, fructosans, phosphorylcholine, and nitrophenyl (Table 14.2). For each of these antigens, multiple proteins have been isolated (83, 89) suggesting that these particular antigens are prevalent in the environment of the mouse and that the plasmacytoma population reflects, in some way, the normal immunocyte population. Antigens here have been described according to the antigenic determinant that is recognized by the myeloma protein. Different natural products from plant, microbial, and animal sources may contain these determinants and be possible natural immunogens in the mouse. Natural sources for many of these antigens have been identified in the mouse (77, 81).

2. In Which Cell Does the Neoplastic Change Occur?

It is not known which cell in the B cell differentiation developmental pathway (Fig. 14.3) is the target for the neoplastic transformation. The long latent period between the first injection of oil and the development of many plasmacytomas suggests that the transformation is not sudden but rather evolves through several steps. If so, the rapidly proliferating Ig-secreting plasma cells associated with the active phases of the secondary responses are unlikely candidates because these cells quickly lose the capacity to synthesize DNA and presumably are eliminated by cell death (62, 74). The more likely candidates are long lived memory cells that divide more slowly, or which hypothetically can be perpetuated by antigen, or even ASC-B lymphocytes. Long-lived lymphocytes are well known from many studies, but in addition, long-lived plasma cells have been found in lymph nodes as long as 6 months after antigen exposure (68a).

Memory cells, for example, that have been repeatedly stimulated by antigen could accumulate the types of genetic damage, outlined above, in a nonspecific way. Such cells might be relatively more prone to giving rise to neoplastic clones. This would account for the repeated appearance of myeloma proteins with the same binding activity. Since ASC-B cells are lymphocytes, it might be expected that neoplasms derived from such cells would be lymphomatous in character, i.e., have a predilection for selectively growing in lymphoreticular tissues. Since plasmacytomas rarely grow in this way, at least in the primary host, or in the early transplant generation hosts, it seems unlikely that ASC-B cells are directly transformed into plasmacytomas. Lymphomatous immunoglobulin-producing tumors in mice have been described and these differ from plasmacytomas in their growth behavior. Essentially, they behave as lymphomas by originating and growing in lymph nodes, spleen, and Peyer's patches (30, 83). Thus, it appears the neoplastic property in plasmacytoma development depends upon maturation to a plasma cell.

D. Role of Mineral Oil

Plasmacytomas can be induced in the inbred BALB/c strain of mice with two contrasting types of materials, solid plastic discs and mineral oils. The most effective solid plastic materials are large plastic discs usually with rough edges, or Millipore diffusion chambers (plastic rings onto which are cemented Millipore membranes) (67). In addition, rough edged Lucite borings are equally effective (67). The plastic materials induce plasmacytomas and fibrosarcomas. Because of the ease of introducing mineral oils into the peritoneum the mineral oil method of induction has been the most widely studied.

BALB/c mice (usually females) are given three intraperitoneal (0.5 ml) injections of mineral oil at two month intervals beginning when the mice are one to three months of age (84). The intraperitoneal injection of oil or pristane causes the formation of an oil granuloma on the surface of the peritoneum. Within weeks after the third injection some mice begin developing a hemorraghic ascites, which is caused by plasmacytoma growing on the peritoneal surfaces. In others, tumors continue to develop over the next year and half or longer (Fig. 14.6). A good yield of plasmacytomas is about 60 to 70%.

With the exception of metastases to the superior mediastinal lymph nodes, the plasmacytoma remains confined to the peritoneum (88). Thus far, only two inbred strains have been shown to be susceptible BALB/c and NZB (67, 80, 116). A few tumors can be induced in F_1 hybrids of BALB/c and other strains (80). The strict dependence of plasmacytoma induction on the specific inbred strains clearly implicates a powerful genetic influence on susceptibility.

Mineral oil is probably not a direct carcinogen, that is, it does not contain a chemical component which resembles any known chemical carcinogen. There have been two studies made on mineral oils to determine if they contain polycyclic unsaturated hydrocarbons but none have been found (58, 92). Pure alkanes, possible components of mineral oil, such as 2,6,10,14-tetramethylpentadecane, 7-N-hexyloctadecane, and phytane have been shown to be highly effective in inducing plasmacytomas (3, 4, 83). Also, pristane induces tumors more rapidly than oil (Fig. 14.6). Pristane is more irritating than oils containing mixed compounds. Most of the alkanes injected are probably not metabolized, but some limited degree of oxidation can occur which may result in the formation of fatty acids. Oil injected intraperitoneally usually remains in situ, either as free oil or a part of the granulomatous response.

The general assumption made from all of these facts is that mineral oil or pristane does not interact directly with plasma cells. Rather, it is hypothesized the primary effect of mineral oil or plastic is to induce a change in the tissue environment and the physiology of the peritoneum.

Mineral oil treatment alters the peritoneal environment in such a way that plasmacytoma cells can proliferate when normally they could not. Paradoxically, ascites tumor cells of primary plasmacytomas do not grow well and establish transplant lines when transplanted to the normal peritoneal cavity (90). By contrast, when small numbers of primary (10^2 to 10^5) ascites cells are transplanted, mice that have been pretreated with mineral oil nearly 100% of all tumors can be established in transplant. In a series of fifteen different primary tumors studied, all were established in primed mice, but only three in nonprimed mice. Further, some of the tumors maintained this apparent dependence for

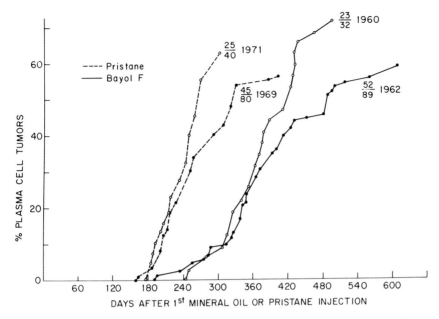

Fig. 14.6. Development of plasma cell tumors following 3 bimonthly intraperitoneal injections of mineral oil.

several generations. The tumors grew at different rates in the conditioned mice, but most produced ascites within several weeks of transplantation.

The growth of primary plasmacytomas in primed mice suggests that in the primary host mineral oil creates a favorable environment for growth and permits tumors to proliferate. These same cells may lack the ability to grow in other sites or in the normal peritoneum. This difference could be due to several different types of causes: (1) the abnormal peritoneal environment supplies a factor essential for growth, a factor much like the colony stimulating factor for granulocytes (68); (2) the mineral oil or some product resulting from it blocks the ability of normal cell eliminating processes (immunological surveillance), or (3) the oil acts as an adjuvant and stimulates the production of an immune response to clones which, in turn, generates antibody which has enhancing properties.

A systematic study of all of these factors has not been completed, however it is clear that plasmacytoma cells have several varieties of cell-associated antigens including the cell membrane-associated Ig itself (38). Under certain circumstances the BALB/c mouse, for example, can make anti-idiotype antibodies to its own myeloma proteins (60, 102). Further, mice making these antibodies are able to resist challenge of living tumor cells. The immunoglobulin idiotypes of plasma cells then are potentially tumor-specific antigens. Other antigens have, as previously mentioned, been found on plasmacytoma cells, i.e., the PC1 allo-antigen and the xVEA antigens (2, 4, 111). Other tumor-specific antigens, not yet identified structurally, have also been found (81, 93).

In the early stages of development most plasmacytoma cells (i.e., primary plasmacytoma cells) have many potential antigens and these cells can be eliminated by an immunological surveillance mechanism, e.g., macrophages or cytotoxic T cells that recognize and destroys these cells. If the surveillance mechanism is blocked, however, the plasmacytoma cells can proliferate. To experimentally explore this possibility, mice were immunized to the AdjPC5 plasmacytomas (91). This has been transplanted for many generations, but nonetheless has a transplantation antigen. Further, the AdjPC5 plasmacytoma is extremely sensitive to the alkylating agent, aniline mustard. Mice with large tumors were treated with this compound and 80% of them after regressing the tumor were immune to reinoculation of 10^5 tumor cells subcutaneously or 10^3 to 10^4 tumor cells intraperitoneally (91, 120, 121).

Mice immunized to the AdjPC5 plasmacytoma were then given pristane intraperitoneally and one to four weeks later were challenged with AdjPC5 cells (91). In contrast to immune nonpristane-treated mice which were resistant to intraperitoneal challenge the primed mice were susceptible. This result indicates that in the face of a strong tumor cell immunity mineral oil or pristane can directly or indirectly block the tumor destroying process locally.

The possibility that blocking immune functions is a factor in plasmacytoma development is supported by the finding that antithymocyte serum given during the first four months of treatment with mineral oil can enhance plasmacytoma development (65).

E. Possible Role of Viruses in Plasmacytoma Development

RNA-containing viruses which produce C particles have been shown to induce various types of immunohematopoietic neoplasms in several different species of vertebrates. The avian leukosis (ALV) and murine leukemia viruses (MuLV) have been extensively studied. In each system a group of C-type RNA viruses have been found. Within a system, the viruses all share a common group specific antigen (gs antigen) that is located in an internal protein of the virion. Viruses within the group can differ from each other in virion envelope antigens. In the mouse common envelop variants are shared by several viruses. Different viruses induce, or are associated with, different neoplastic types: the Friend virus induces a form of erythroleukemia in mice, while the Gross Passage A and RadLV induce thymic lymphocytic neoplasms. C-type RNA viruses, in the MuLV system, have been associated with other immunohematopoietic neoplasms. For example, C-type RNA viruses have been associated with reticulum cell neoplasms in mice. These reticulum cell neoplasms occur spontaneously in old mice of different strains sometimes quite frequently (29). They are the principle neoplasms that occur spontaneously in 80% of SJL/J mice at about one year of age (71, 100) and are the predominant neoplasms in allogeneic disease (7, 8). C-type RNA viruses have also been associated with plasmacytomas in mice (Table 14.3). This association raises a number of questions concerning the role of C-type RNA viruses of the MuLV complex in the development of immunohematopoietic

TABLE 14.3
VIRUSES ASSOCIATED WITH MURINE PLASMACYTOMAS AND BALB/c MICE[a]

Viruses	Internal virion antigen	Envelope antigen	Cell surface antigen	Source	Ref.
C-type					
MuLV (gross related)	gs	G (Gross)	GCSA Gix.	TC lines TX lines 1° Tumors	48, 106 118
MuMA (myeloma associated)	gs	xVEA(PC.1)	PC.1	TC lines Transplants 1° Tumors Norm. P.C.	2b, 2c, 40, 111
MuLV (N tropic)	gs	Not determined	—	BALB/c (3–24 mos)	1, 78, 79
(B tropic)	gs	Not determined	—	BALB/c (7–24 mos)	1, 78, 79
Intracisternal A particle	Intracisternal A particle structural protein	—	—	1° tumors TC and TX lines Normal TD Cells	54

[a] P.C. = plasmacytoma; TC = tissue culture; TD = thoracic duct; TX = transplant lines; gs = group specific.

neoplasms. The frequent finding of C-type viruses with a specific immunohematopoietic neoplasm suggests a possible role of the virus in the neoplastic development. However, in many of these associations infectious virus that reproduces the disease has not been isolated. This fact does not necessarily mean the virus has not had an inductive role, but does make the association of virus and neoplasm indirect. A further complication is that murine leukemia viruses are virtually ubiquitous in mice being found in normal mice of almost all stains.

Three viral agents have been found in mouse plasmacytomas: (1) the agent believed to be a virus that produces the intracisternal A particles (2) a C-type RNA virus that is related to the Gross agent, and (3) a C-type RNA virus that does not carry Gross related antigens but has xVEA envelope antigen.

Every BALB/c plasmacytoma that has been examined by electron microscopy has been shown to contain intracisternal A particles often these are in great abundance (23, 54). The intracisternal A particle is associated with a small amount of RNA, a characteristic protein which differs electrophoretically and serologically from other viral antigens and an unusual DNA polymerase enzyme (123). These findings suggest the particles are produced by viruses. However, no one has succeeded in transmitting the intracisternal A particles and no biological activity has been demonstrated for them.

MuLV C-type RNA virus related to the Gross type virus have been found in plasmacytomas in several studies (2, 49, 106, 118). Identification of the MuLV (Gross) was made chiefly by finding two cell surface antigens GCSA (Gross cell surface antigen) and Gix (99, 106). The GCSA antigen is detected on the surface of cells, using a cytotoxic assay system. Antiserum prepared in C57B6/6 mice by immunization with AKR leukemic cells is reacted with C57BL/6 leukemic cells from a tumor induced by Gross passage—A virus. This serum is cytotoxic for C57BL/6 leukemic cells. The presence of GCSA on test cells is determined by absorption. The GCSA antigen is thought to be invariably associated with MuLV (Gross) infection (106). The majority of myelomas examined were GCSA positive for this antigen (106).

The Gix antigen is another cell surface antigen that is also found during MuLV (Gross) production. For example, it is expressed on normal strain 129 thymocytes. Although Gix is not expressed on normal BALB/c cells, most plasmacytomas have this antigen.

An extremely interesting MuLV-C-RNA virus, not Gross virus-related, has recently been identified in plasmacytomas (2). This was found in an unexpected way. Previously an antiserum had been produced in DBA/2 mice by immunization with MOPC70A plasmacytoma cells which recognized an antigen called PC.1. This was present on all BALB/c plasmacytomas studied but absent from lymphocytic neoplasms. Further, the antigen showed a characteristic strain distribution being present on normal cells in BALB/c, C3H/He, A, AKR, SJL/J, NZB, MA, and CE, etc. but absent in C57BL/6, DBA/2, C3H/Bi, and others (111). It was considered to be an alloantigen based strain distribution and a differentiation antigen based on its association with plasma cells (and some other tissues). An attempt was made to localize the source of this antigen by immunoelectron microscopy. In this technique a specific hybrid antibody is artificially prepared that has specificity for both PC.1 and an electron-dense particle such as Southern Bean virus or ferritin (2). The target cell is exposed to the reagent and electronphotomicrographs are made. The antiserum can also be specifically absorbed. It was discovered by this sensitive technique that antiPC.1 antisera (2) contained three different types of specificities: (a) for GCSA, (b) for PC.1 and (c) for the virions of a C-type particle that budded from the surface of plasmacytoma cells. These particles were not Gross virus, for MuLV (Gross) particles were unable to absorb out the activity. It was concluded the predominant activity of the antiserum was directed to another type of MuLV virus.

The possible etiological significance of the particle comes from cytotoxic assays studies with mouse plasmacytoma cells where it was observed that normal BALB/c serum and complement were cytotoxic for plasmacytoma cells (40). This was due to the presence of a naturally occurring antibody in mouse serum including BALB/c which had the same specificity as allogeneically prepared antiPC.1 sera. This natural antiserum also labeled the virions of the C-type particles lacking the Gross envelope antigen.

The strain distribution of the natural antibody was unusual and was found in both PC.1+ and PC.1- strains. All of the evidence suggests that mice carry C-type RNA virus that is present on transplantable plasmacytomas and also on normal plasma cells, as antiPC.1 antiserum was cytotoxic for some normal plasma cells producing antibody to sheep red blood cells (SRBC) (111).

In the studies described above the C-type RNA viruses have been found in long-term transplants. C-type virus production increases in normal BALB/c mice with age (78, 79) or can be activated *in vitro* in BALB/c cells by bromo- or iododeoxyuridine (59, 104, 105). Mixed lymphocyte reactions and graft versus host reactions can also activate C-type viruses (44, 45). C-type virus production in long-term transplants may have no pathogenetic significance in plasmacytoma development. Recently though 3 types of C-type viruses have been found in primary plasmacytomas (1a), particles with (1) Gross type envelope antigen, (2) xVEA antigen, and (3) neither envelope antigen. This suggests several viruses were activated during the development of the plasmacytoma.

Direct evidence that viruses can play a role in plasmacytoma development has been recently obtained with the Abelson virus (MLV-A). This virus (2a), originally isolated from a BALB/c mouse that had been continuously treated from birth with prednisolone and infected with Moloney virus at one month of age, rapidly induces lymphosarcomas in newborn and adult mice, in as short a period as 21 days. MLV-A complex contains infective Moloney leukemia virus, a defective virus MLV-A and LDV (lactic dehydrogenase virus) (90a). When MLV-A complex is injected intraperitoneally into mice that have been given a single injection of 0.5 ml pristane 36 to 57 days previously, about 25% develop plasmacytomas within 21 to 80 days (long before plasmacytomas appear following pristane alone) and another 60% develop nonthymic lymphosarcomas during the same period. As with oil-only evoked plasmacytomas, 60 to 65% of MLV-A associated plasmacytomas produce IgA type myeloma proteins (90a). The rapid action of MLV-A complex indicates viruses can initiate plasmacytoma development, thus raising the possibility that activation of endogenous viruses in appropriate cells may be the critical initiating event in mice given only mineral oil.

The association of C-type viruses with plasmacytomas suggests a basis for explaining the unusual genetic susceptibility of BALB/c mice to plasmacytoma formation. A number of genes have identified and mapped in inbred strains of mice which regulate C-type virus production (1, 49, 94, 104, 105, 107, 109). BALB/c mice may carry (as an integrated viral gene) a special C-type virus, or have a unique type of genetic locus that regulates virus production in the key target cell.

F. Summary

Membrane receptors associated with B lymphocyte plasma cell development form a set of characteristics that are linked to the regulation of cell division and maturation. In the fluid mosaic model of membrane structure clearance of cell receptors by aggregation and internalization is followed in some cases by vigorous new synthesis. This establishes a chain of events beginning on the cell surface to biosynthesis controlled ultimately in the nucleus. This process illustrates the dynamic aspect of cell membrane protein synthesis. A relatively high number of myeloma proteins in the mouse bind natural antigens which are continuously present in the environment, e.g., antigens containing phosphorylcholine, dextrans, levans, and galactans. Possibly some property of these antigens cause clones to proliferate over a long period and thus increases the opportunity for neoplastic change.

In the mineral oil induction model of plasmacytomas formation mineral oil probably is not the proximate inducing agent (carcinogen). The function of mineral oil or plastic is probably to produce an abnormal tissue environment in the peritoneal cavity, where plasmacytoma development selectively occurs. One effect of the intraperitoneal injection of mineral oil that occurs relatively rapidly, i.e., within weeks is to block an established tumor immunity (local immunosuppression). Since plasmacytomas carry tumor specific antigens (specific immunoglobulin and other antigens) the local oil-related immunosuppression could play an important role in plasmacytoma development.

Plasmacytoma formation in mice has a genetic basis, for these tumors can only be induced in a few strains (BALB/c, NZB). Genes regulating the production of C-RNA viruses (in the MuLV system) may be factors. Several C-RNA viruses in the MuLV system have been associated with plasmacytomas and BALB/c mice. Activation of these viruses in key cells in the B-cell lineage might initiate neoplastic change.

References

1. Aaronson, S. A., and Stephenson, J. R. (1973). *Proc. Nat. Acad. Sci. U.S.* **70**, 2055–2058.
2. Abel, C. A., and Grey, H. M. (1968). *Biochemistry* **7**, 2682–2688.
2a. Abelson, H. T., and Rabstein, L. S. (1970). *Cancer Res.* **30**, 2213–2222.
2b. Aoki, T., Potter, M., and Sturm, M. M. (1973). *J. Nat. Cancer Inst.* In press.
2c. Aoki, T., and Takahashi, T. (1972). *J. Exp. Med.* **135**, 433–457.
3. Anderson, P. N. (1970). *Proc. Amer. Ass. Cancer Res.* **11**, 3.
4. Anderson, P. N., and Potter, M .(1969). *Nature (London)* **222**, 994–995.
5. Anderson, J., Edelman, G. M., Möller, G., and Sjöberg, O. (1972). *Eur. J. Immun.* **2**, 233–235.
6. Andersson, J., Möller, G., and Sjöberg, O. (1972). *Cell. Immun.* **4**, 381–393.
7. Armstrong, M. Y. K., Gleichmann, E., Gleichmann, H., Beldotti, L., Andre-Schwartz, and Schwartz, R. (1970). *J. Exp. Med.* **132-4**, 417–439.
8. Armstrong, M. Y. K., Schwartz, R. S., and Beldotti, L. (1967). *Transplantation* **6**, 1380–1392.
9. Askonas, B. A., Williamson, A. R., and Awdeh, Z. L. (1969). *Gamma Globulin Struct. Biosynthe. London Acad. Fed. Eur. Biol. Soc. Symp.* **15**, 105–116.
10. Askonas, B. A., Williamson, A. R., and Wright, B. E. G. (1970). *Proc. Nat. Acad. Sci. U.S.* **67**, 1398–1403.
11. Basten A., Miller, J. F. A. P., Sprent, J., and Pye, J. (1972). *J. Exp. Med.* **135**, 610–626.
12. Basten, A., Warner, N. L., and Mandel, T. (1972). *J. Med.* **135**, 627–642.
13. Baumal, R., Coffino, P., Bargellesi, A., Buxbaum, J., Laskov, R., and Scharff, M. D. (1971). *Ann. N.Y. Acad. Sci.* **190**, 235–249.
14. Blomberg, B., Geckler, W. R., and Weigert, M. G. (1972). *Science* **177**, 178–180.
15. Brient, B. W., and Nisonoff, A. (1970). *J. Exp. Med.* **132**, 951–962.
16. Cebra, J. J. (1969). *Bacteriol. Rev.* **33**, 159–171.
17. Cline, M. J., Sprent, J., Warner, N. L., and Harris, A. W. (1972). *J. Immun.* **108**, 1126–1128.
18. Cohn, M. (1971). *Cell. Immunol.* **1**, 468–475.
19. Cooper, G. N., and Turner, K. (1969). *J. Reticuloendothelial Soc.* **6**, 419–434.

20. Cosenza, H., and Kohler, H. (1972). *Science* **176**, 1027–1029.
21. Crabbé, P. A., Nash, D. R., Bazin, H., Eyssen, H., and Heremans, J. F. (1970). *Lab. Investigat.* **22**, 448–457.
22. Craig, S. W., and Cebra, J. J. (1971). *J. Exp. Med.* **134**, 188–200.
23. Dalton, A. J., Potter, M., and Merwin, R. M. (1961). *J. Nat. Cancer Inst.* **26**, 1221–1267.
24. Diener, E., and Feldmann, M. (1972). *Transplant. Rev.* **8**, 76–103.
25. Diener, E., and Paetkau, V. H. (1972). *Proc. Nat. Acad. Sci. U.S.* **69**, 2364–2368.
26. Dreyer, W. J., and Bennett, C. J. (1965). *Proc. Nat. Acad. Sci. U.S.* **54**, 864–868.
27. Dreyer, W. J., Gray, W. R., and Hood, L. (1967). *Cold Spring Harbor Symp. Quant. Biol.* **32**, 353–367.
28. Dukor, P., Bianco, C., and Nussenzweig, V. (1970). *Proc. Nat. Acad. Sci. U.S.* **67**, 991–997.
29. Dunn, T. B., and Dunn, T. B., and Deringer, M. K. (1968). *J. Nat. Cancer Inst.* **40**, 771–821.
30. Ebbesen, P., Rask-Nielsen, R., and McIntire, K. R. (1968). *J. Nat. Cancer Inst.* **41**, 473–493.
31. Edelman, G. M. (1971). *Ann. N.Y. Acad. Sci.* **190**, 5–25.
32. Fox, C. F. (1972). *Sci. Amer.* **226**, 31–38.
33. Frye, C. D., and Eddidin, M. (1970). *J. Cell Sci.* **7**, 319–335.
34. Fudenberg, H. H., Wang, A. C., Pink, J. R. L., and Levin, A. S. (1971). *Ann. N.Y. Acad. Sci.* **190**, 501–506.
35. Gray, W. R., Dreyer, W. J., and Hood, L. (1967). *Science* **155**, 465–467.
36. Greaves, M. F., and Bauminger S. (1972). *Nature New Biol.* **235**, 67–70.
37. Halstead, T. E., and Hall, J. G. (1972). *Transplantation* **14**, 339–346.
38. Hannestad, K., Kao, M. S., and Eisen, H. N. (1972). *Proc. Nat. Acad. Sci. U.S.* **69**, 2295–2299.
39. Harboe, M., Osterland, C. K., Mannik, M., and Kunkel, H. G. (1962). *J. Exp. Med.* **116**, 719–738.
40. Herberman, R. B., and Aoki, T. (1972). *J. Exp. Med.* **136**, 94–111.
41. Heremans, J. F., and Bazin, H. (1971). *Ann. N.Y. Acad. Sci.* **190**, 268–274.
42. Herzenberg, L. A., McDevitt, H. O., and Herzenberg, L. A. (1968). *Ann. Rev. Genet.* **2**, 209–244.
43. Hirsch, M. S., Black, P. H., Tracy, G. S., Leibowitz, S., and Schwartz, R. S. (1970). *Proc. Nat. Acad. Sci. U.S.* **67**, 1914–1917.
44. Hirsch, M. S., Phillips, S. M., Solnik, C., Black, P. H., Schwartz, R. S., and Carpenter, C. B. (1972). *Proc. Nat. Acad. Sci. U.S.* **69**, 1069–1072.
45. Hood, L., and Ein, D. (1968). *Nature (London)* **220**, 764–767.
46. Hood, L., McKean, D. J., Farnsworth, V., and Potter, M. (1973). *Biochemistry* **12**, 741–749.
47. Hood, L., McKean, D., and Potter, M. (1970). *Science* **170**, 1207–1209.
48. Hyman, R., Ralph, P., and Sarkar, S. (1972). *J. Nat. Cancer Inst.* **48**, 173–184.
49. Ikeda, H., Stockert, E., Rowe, W. P., Boyse, E. A., Lilly, F., Sato, H., Jacobs, S., and Old, L. J. (1973). *J. Exp. Med.* **137**, 1103–1107.
50. Inbar, D., Hochman, J., and Givol, D. (1971). *Proc. Nat. Acad. Sci. U.S.* **69**, 2659–2662.
51. Inbar, D., Rotman, M., and Givol, D. (1971). *J. Biol. Chem.* **246**, 6272–6275.
52. Karnovsky, M. J., Unanue, E. R., and Levinthal, M. (1972). *J. Exp. Med.* **136**, 907–930.
53. Kohler, H., Shimizu, A., Paul, C., Moore, V., and Putnam, F. W. (1970). *Nature (London)* **227**, 1318–1320.
54. Kuff, E. L., Luefers, K. K., Ozer, H. L., and Wivel, N. A. (1972). *Proc. Nat. Acad. Sci. U.S.* **69**, 218–222.
55. Landucci-Tosi, S., and Tosi, R. M. (1973). *Immunochemistry* **10**, 65–71.
56. Lederberg, J. (1959). *Science* **129**, 1649–1653.
57. Levin, A. S., Fudenberg, H. H., Hopper, J. E., Wilson, S. K., and Nisonoff, A. (1971). *Proc. Nat. Acad. Sci. U.S.* **68**, 169–171.

58. Lijinsky, W., Somaki, I., Mason, G., Ramahi, H. Y., and Safari, T. (1963). *Anal. Chem.* **35**, 952–956.
59. Lowy, D. R., Rowe, W. P., Teich, N., and Hartley, J. W. (1971). *Science* **174**, 155–156.
60. Lynch, R. G., Graff, R. J., Sirisinha, S., Simms, E. S., and Eisen, H. N. (1972). *Proc. Nat. Acad. Sci. U.S.* **69**, 1540–1544.
61. Mage, R. (1971). "Progress in Immunology," (B. Amos, ed.), pp. 47–59. Academic Press, New York.
62. Makela, O., and Nossal, G. J. V. (1962). *J. Exp. Med.* **115**, 231.
62a. Mattioli, C. A., and Tomasi, T. B., Jr. (1973). *J. Exp. Med.* **138**, 452–460.
63. McIntire, K. R., and Princler, G. L. (1969). *Immunology* **17**, 481–487.
64. McKean, D. J., Potter, M., and Hood, L. (1973). *Biochemistry* **12**, 749–759.
65. Mandel, M. A., and Decosse, J. J. (1972). *J. Immunol.* **109**, 360–365.
66. McKean, D. J., Potter, M., and Hood, L. (1973). *Biochemistry* **12**, 760–771.
67. Merwin, R. M., and Redmon, L. W. (1963). *J. Nat. Cancer Inst.* **31**, 998–1017.
68. Metcalf, D., Chan, S. H., Stanley, E. R., Moore, M. A. S., Gunz, F. W., and Vincent, P. C. (1972). In "The Nature of Leukemia," *Proc. Int. Cancer Conf. Syndey, Australia,* pp. 173–186.
68a. Miller, J. J., III. (1963). *J. Immun.* **92**, 673–681.
69. Miller, O. L., Jr. (1966). *Nat. Cancer Inst. Monogr.* **23**, 53–66.
70. Möller, E., and Sjöberg, O. (1972). *Transplant Rev.* **8**, 26–49.
71. Murphy, E. D. (1963). *Proc. Amer. Ass. Cancer Res.* **4**, 46.
72. Mushinski, J. F. (1971). *J. Immunol.* **106**, 41–50.
73. Nash, D. R., Crabbe, P. A., Bazin, H., Eyssen, E., and Heremans, J. F. (1970). *Experientia* **25**, 1094–1096.
74. Nossal, J. G. V., and Makela, O. (1962). *J. Exp. Med.* **115**, 209–230.
75. Oudin, J., and Michel, M. (1969). *J. Exp. Med.* **130**, 619–642.
76. Pawlak, L. L., Mushinski, E. B., Nisonoff, A., and Potter, M. (1973). *J. Exp. Med.* **137**, 22–31.
76a. Padlan, E. A., Segal, D. M., Spante, T. F., Davies, D. R., Rudikoff, S., and Potter, M. (1973). *Nature (London).* In press.
77. Pernis, B., Forni, L., and Amanti, L. (1971). *Ann. N.Y. Acad. Sci.* **190**, 420–429.
78. Peters, R. L., Hartley, J. W., Spahn, G. J., Rabstein, L. S., Whitmire, C. E., Turner, H. C., and Huebner, R. J. (1972). *Int. J. Cancer* **10**, 283–289.
79. Peters, R. L., Rabstein, L. S., Spahn, G. J., Madison, R. M., and Huebner, R. J. (1972). *Int. J. Cancer* **10**, 273–282.
79a. Poljak, R. J., Amzel, L. M., Avey, H. P., Becker, L. N., and Nisonoff, A. (1973). *Nature New Biol.* **235**, 137–138.
80. Potter, M. (1967). *Methods Cancer Res.* **11**, 105–157.
81. Potter, M. (1970). *Fed. Proc.* **29**, 85–91.
82. Potter, M. (1971). *Ann. N.Y. Acad. Sci.* **190**, 306–321.
83. Potter, M. (1972). *Physiol. Rev.* **52**, 631–719.
84. Potter, M., and Boyce, C. R. (1962). *Nature (London)* **193**, 1086–1087.
85. Potter, M., and Kuff, E. L. (1964). *J. Mol. Biol.* **9**, 537–544.
86. Potter, M., and Lieberman, R. (1967). *Cold Spring Harbor Symp. Quant. Biol.* **32**, 187–202.
87. Potter, M., and Lieberman, R. (1970). *J. Exp. Med.* **132**, 737–751.
88. Potter, M., and MacCardle, R. C. (1964). *J. Nat. Cancer Inst.* **33**, 497–515.
89. Potter, M., Mushinski, E. B., Rudikoff, S., and Appella, E. (1972). *Int. Convocation Immunol., 3rd Buffalo* (in press).
90. Potter, M., Pumphrey, J. G., and Walters, J. L. (1972). *J. Nat. Cancer Inst.* **49**, 305–308.
90a. Potter, M., Sklar, M., and Rowe, W. P. (1973). *Science.* In press.
91. Potter, M., and Walters, J. L. (1973). *J. Nat. Cancer Inst.* In press.
92. Rask-Nielsen, R., and Ebbesen, P. (1965). *J. Nat. Cancer Inst.* **35**, 83–94.

93. Röllinghoff, M., Rouse, B. T., and Warner, N. L. (1973). *J. Nat. Cancer Inst.* **50**, 159–172.
94. Rowe, W. P., Hartley, J. W., and Bremmer, T. (1972). *Science* **178**, 860–862.
95. Rudikoff, S., Potter, M., Segal, D., Padlan, E., and Davies, D. L. (1972). *Proc. Nat. Acad. Sci. U.S.* **69**, 3689–3692.
96. Scharff, M. D., Bargellesi, A., Baumal, R., Buxbaum, J., Coffino, P., and Laskov, R. (1970). *J. Cell Physiol.* **76**, 331–348.
97. Scharff, M. D., and Laskov, R. (1970). *Prog. Allergy* **14**, 37–80.
98. Schulenberg, E. P., Simms, E. S., Lynch, R. G., Bradshaw, R. A., and Eisen, H. N. (1971). *Proc. Nat. Acad. Sci. U.S.* **68**, 2623–2626.
99. Seki, T., Appella, E., and Itano, H. A. (1968). *Proc. Nat. Acad. Sci. U.S.* **61**, 1071–1078.
100. Siegler, R., and Rich, M. A. (1968). *J. Nat. Cancer Inst.* **41**, 125–143.
101. Singer, S. J., and Nicoloson, G. L. (1972). *Science* **175**, 720–731.
102. Sirisinha, S., and Eisen, H. N. (1970). *Proc. Nat. Acad. Sci. U.S.* **68**, 3130–3135.
103. Stavenezer, J., and Huang, R. C. C. (1971). *Nature New Biol.* **230**, 172–176.
104. Stephenson, J. R., and Aaronson, S. A. (1972). *Proc. Nat. Acad. Sci. U.S.* **69**, 2798–2801.
105. Stephenson, J. R., and Aaronson, S. A. (1972). *J. Exp. Med.* **136**, 175–184.
106. Stockert, E., Gid, L. J., and Boyse, E. A. (1971). *J. Exp. Med.* **133**, 1334–1355.
107. Stockert, E., Sato, H. T., Itakura, K., Boyse, E. A., and Old, L. J. (1972). *Science* **178**, 862.
108. Swan, D., Aviv, H., and Leder, P. (1972). *Proc. Nat. Acad. Sci. U.S.* **69**, 1967–1971.
109. Taylor, B. A., and Meier, D. (1971). *Proc. Nat. Acad. Sci. U.S.* **68**, 3190–3194.
110. Taylor, R. B., Duffus, P. H., Raff, M. C., and dePetris, S. (1971). *Nature New Biol.* **233**, 225–229.
111. Takahashi, T., Old, L. J., and Boyse, E. A. (1970). *J. Exp. Med.* **131**, 1325–1341.
112. Tomasi, T. B. (1970). *Ann. Rev. Med.* **21**, 281–298.
113. Tomasi, T. B., and Bienenstock, J. (1968). *Advan. Immun.* **9**, 2–96.
114. Uho, J. W. (1970). *Cell. Immun.* **1**, 228–244.
115. Unanue, E. R., Perkins, W. D., and Karnovsky, M. I. (1972). *J. Exp. Med.* **136**, 885–906.
116. Warner, N. L. (1971). *J. Immun.* **107**, 937.
117. Warner, N. L., Herzenberg, L. A., and Goldstein, G. (1966). *J. Exp. Med.* **123**, 707–721.
118. Watson, J., Ralph, P., and Sarkar, S. (1970). *Proc. Nat. Acad. Sci. U.S.* **66**, 344–351.
119. Weigert, M., Cesari, M., Yonkovich, S. J., and Cohn, M. (1970). *Nature (London)* **228**, 1045–1047.
120. Whisson, M. E., and Connors, T. A. (1965). *Nature (London)* **205**, 406.
121. Whisson, M. E., and Connors, T. A. (1965). *Nature (London)* **206**, 689–691.
122. Williams, R. C., and Gibbons, R. J. (1972). *Science* **177**, 697–699.
123. Wilson, S. H., and Kuff, E. L. (1972). *Proc. Nat. Acad. Sci. U.S.* **69**, 1531–1536.

Epilogue

HARRIS BUSCH

What's past is prologue

—*Shakespeare, The Tempest II*

At a critical point in World War II, Winston Churchill announced that the war had reached the "end of the beginning." For cancer research no man has the ability to speak as an authority to advise what point will represent such a very special time. What can be said is that in the last decade there has been a truly remarkable proliferation of information regarding the machinery of the cell that is involved in translation of information from the genetic apparatus into protein synthesis. Because of the obvious importance of this subject to cancer it is not surprising that a major development in the field has been the extension of such fundamental information to the fields of carcinogenesis, determination of the cell phenotype, and other special fields of cancer research.

One of the key questions that is always being asked is how much more information will be required until some rational basis or cancer therapy of prevention can be evolved. From the point of view of the molecular biologists, the question hinges largely on the availability of information regarding fundamental mechanisms of cell regulation. Since proteins or other molecular species that may be involved in this process are probably present in cells in very limited amounts, i.e., femtogram (10^{-15} gm) quantities, it is clear that our analytical methods must be considerably extended beyond their present level for us to specifically define those molecules involved in gene control.

It remains to be seen whether the high rate of progress in evolution of such information will continue in the next decade. If it does, progress can be made from the kinds of methods shown in Fig. 8.12 (p. 334) which shows proteins present in tenths and even hundreths of picograms (10^{-12} gm) in the cell nucleus to one or two logs greater resolution. Thus, it would seem that the difficult matter of evaluation of gene control would not be beyond our grasp within a relatively short period of time.

The very high level of optimism among oncologists at the present time emerges from the concept that with such information it would not be very long until chemical solutions would evolve for the cancer problem. The key problem is the penetration into the nucleus of molecular fragments with high binding efficiency for gene sites and their special interaction with the genes involved in neoplastic growth. It is clear now that even relatively small molecules can penetrate the nucleus with high efficiency and in sufficient concentration to alter or control nuclear function. At present, it would seem optimal to supply cancer cells with controlling molecules such as peptides with sufficient information to have their own binding characteristics with special sites on DNA. If gene control proteins can be identified that limit cell growth or nontumor cells, it would clearly be advantageous to utilize the information on amino acid sequence of such molecules as a basis of production of chemotherapy agents.

Regardless of the approaches. that can be made on the basis of information that will continue to develop from molecular biological studies it seems clear that such studies need to be continued to at least define the problem for the future of chemotherapy. All of the currently available anticancer agents are limited in their usefulness by their high degree of toxicity, and only when there is adequate differentiating information available can specific targets be selected for definitive anticancer activity rather than generalized antigrowth activity. The fact that useful cancer chemotherapy has been evolved in spite of the great problems that exist is a tribute to the skill, perseverance, and intelligence of the dedicated individuals who have worked in this field. All will agree that the future of chemotherapy hinges largely upon the evolution of information on better targets. If nothing more, molecular biological approaches should provide these targets within the next decade.

Author Index

Numbers in parentheses are reference numbers and indicate that an author's work is referred to although his name is not cited in the text. Numbers in italics show the page on which the complete reference is listed.

A

Aaronson, S. A., 164 (1), 172 (398), *174,
183,* 200 (10), 211 (289), 219 (289),
237, 409 (550), 412 (3, 4), 413 (205,
550), 414 (445), 415 (6, 446, 503, 550),
427 (551), 432 (2, 3), 433 (5, 550),
435 (198), 436 (7, 569), 441 (1, 2, 3, 5,
6, 7), 451 (1), 463 (609), *468, 469, 473,
480, 481, 482, 483, 484,* 561 (1), 563
(1, 104, 105), *564, 567*
Abe, M., 30 (1), *35*
Abel, C. A., 539 (2), 559 (2), 561 (2),
562 (2), *564*
Abelev, G. I., 33 (2), *35,* 435 (8), *469*
Abell, C. W., 340 (1), *345*
Abelson, H. T., 563 (2A), *564*
Abelson, J. N., 253 (1), *271*
Abercrombie, M., 9 (3), *35*
Abraham, A. D., 207 (1), *229*
Abrams, R., 284 (100), *307*
Abrass, I. B., 190 (270), 201 (270), *236,*
364 (72), *374*
Achey, P. M., 162 (29), *174*
Achong, B. G., 441 (167), 467 (167), *472*
Adam, E., 467 (9, 10), *469*
Adams, G. H. M., 321 (2), *345*
Adams, H., 345 (249), *352*
Adams, J. M., 188 (2, 3), 191 (2, 3),
194 (2, 3), 198 (2, 3), *229*
Adams, R. A., 462 (154), *472*
Adams, R. L. P., 151 (2, 67), *174, 175*
Adams, W. R., (463), *480*
Adelman, R. C., 331 (83A), *348*
Adesnik, M., 200 (4), 201 (80), 203 (4),
229, 231
Adler, J., 287 (3), *304*
Adler, K., 329 (3), *345*
Afkham, J., 384 (28), *398*
Agarwal, M. K., 370 (1), *372*
Agrawal, K. C., 286 (75), *306*
Ainbender, E., 468 (280), *475*
Aizawa, C., 212 (18), *230*
Akao, M., 342 (4), *346*

Akino, T., 199 ((106), 204 (5), 216 (5),
229, 232
Alanen-Irjala, K., 361 (43), *373*
Alberga, A., 329 (5), 330 (5), 339 (5), *346*
Albert, A. E., 330 (6), *346*
Alberts, B. M., 114 (3), *174,* 194 (6),
215 (6), *229,* 332 (7), *346*
Alexander, H. E., 29 (175), 30 (149, 175),
39
Alexander, H. G., 47 (67), *76*
Alexander, J. A., 507 (53), *521*
Alfrey, V. G., 134 (4, 211, 284), *174, 179,
181,* 195 (208), 198 (301), 217 (208),
235, 237, 321 (94, 142, 213, 280, 280A),
322 (142, 237), 324 (10, 95, 157, 213),
325 (8, 9, 12, 94, 275), 328 (14), 329
(10–12), 331 (274), 333 (274), 334
(274), 337 (274), 338 (237, 274), 339
(158), 340 (13, 87, 158), 342 (274),
344 (280), *346, 348, 349, 350, 351, 352,
353,* 362 (2), *362, 372, 374*
Ali, J., 199 (335), *238*
Allard, C., 489 (5), 508 (5), *520*
Allen, D. O., 489 (1), 514 (1), *520*
Allen, D. W., 416 (11), 441 (11, 12), 463
(12), *469*
Allen, R. A., 70 (3), *75*
Alloway, J. L., 29 (4, 5), *35*
Aloni, Y., 441 (14), 454 (14), *469*
Al-Saadi, A., 86 (1), *105*
Altmann, H. W., 69 (1), 74 (1), *75*
Amaldi, F., 13 (7), *35,* 201 (13), 220 (7, 13),
221 (13), 222 (13), *230,* 264 (64),
265, 272, 273
Amano, M., 199 (106), 204 (5), 216 (5),
229, 232
Amanti, L., 544 (77), 557 (77), *566*
Ambrose, E. J., 9 (3), *35*
Ambrosini, J. C., 467 (127), *471*
Ames, B. N., 159 (5, 6), *174*
Ametani, T., 69 (187), 70 (187), *79*
Amodio, F. J., 332 (7), *346*
Amzel, L. M., 539 (79A), *566*
Anderer, F. A., 447 (345), *477*

571

C

Courington, D. P., 150 (40), *175*

Court Brown, W. M., 88 (46), *106*

Coutsogeorgopoulos, C., 120 (252), 121 (252)

Cowdry, E. V., 42 (36), 48 (35, 36), *75*

Cowling, G. J., 219 (73), *231*

Cox D., 341 (18A), *346*

Coyle, M. B., 168 (429), 169 (115, 430), *176, 184*

Cozarelli, N. R., 116 (116), *176*

Cozzone, A., 190 (74), *231*

Crabbé, P. A., 555 (21, 73), *565, 566*

Craddock, V. M., 153 (117, 272), *176, 180*

Craig, S. W., 555 (22), *565*

Cramer, F., 256 (142), *275*

Cramer, R., 451 (349), *477*

Crane, F. L., (32), *346*

Crane-Robinson, C., 131 (55), 133 (55), *175*, 318 (43), *347*

Crathorn, A. R., 168 (118, 381, 382, 383), 169 (382), *176, 183*

Crawford, E. M., 439 (114), *471*

Crawford, L. V., 412 (110), 439 (114), 444 (112, 113), 445 (111, 112), 447 (184), *471, 473*

Creaser, E. H., 211 (75), *231*

Creasey, W. A., 286 (91), 291 (27), 295 (50), *305, 306, 307*

Creech, G. T., 461, (115), *471*

Crepy, O., *350*

Crick, F. H. C., 32 (165, 166), 33 (165, 166), *39*, 108 (472), 109 (473), 111 (473, 474), 114, 139 (119), 141, *176, 185*, 356 (16), *373*

Crighton, G. W., 408 (299), 423 (299), *476*

Crippa, M., 63 (37), *75*, 330 (64), *347*

Cristofalo, V. J., 498 (14), *520*

Crittenden, L. B., 405 (450), *480*

Croninger, A. B., 18 (171), *39*

Crooke, S. T., 32 (32), 33 (32), *36*, 64 (120a), 77, 206 (58), 217 (200), 218 (54), 219 (54, 76), 220 (58), *231, 234*, 245 (24), 246 (24), 249 (24), 260 (24), *272*

Crosswhite, L. H., 95 (36), 96 (35), 99 (10), *105, 106*

Crothers, D. M., 61 (99), *77*

Crouch, N. A., 457 (597), *483*

Crumpacker, C. S., 456 (362), *477*

Cruz, O., 288 (55), *306*

Cuatrecasas, P., 330 (65, 66), *347*

Culp, L. A., 461 (116), *371*

Culvenor, C. C. J., 385 (20), *398* (117), *471*

Cuzin, F., 118 (212), *179*, 447 (118), 462,

D

Daams, J. H., 395 (9), *398,* 423 (49, 50), 434 (49), *470*

Dahlberg, J. E., 194 (26, 27), 196 (77), 198 (26, 27), 220 (77), *230, 231,* 250 (34a), 271 (34a), *272*

Dahmus, M. E., 130 (41), *175,* 319 (38), 329 (38, 39), 331 (38), 337 (38), *346*

Dalton, A. J., 3 (41), *36,* 404 (119), 409 (119), 410 (119), *471,* 561 (23), *565*

Dalton, R. G., 408 (299), 423 (299), *476*

Daly, J. W., 390 (57), *399*

Daly, M. M., 340 (13), *346*

Dan, K., 34 (107), *38*

Dancis, J., 302 (1), *304*

Daneholt, B., 28 (43), *36,* 190 (78), 191 (78), 196 (78), *231,* 243 (40), *273*

Daniel, M. D., 442 (393, 394), 450 (393), *478*

Dao, T. L., 378 (21), *398*

D'Ari, L., 224 (265), *236*

Darnell, J. E., Jr., 198 (243), 199 (279), 200 (4, 30, 79, 156a, 308, 349), 201 (80, 81, 252, 279, 348a), 203 (4, 308), 206 (242), 209 (79), 210 (242, 243), 217 (349), 221 (279), *229, 230, 233, 235, 236, 237, 238,* 246 (116), 263 (81), 265 (81), *274, 275,* 454 (636), *477, 484,* 527 (4), *533*

Das, M. R., 413 (565, 566), 414 (566, 567), *482, 483*

Daskal, I., 52 (87), 64 (87), 77, 211 (55), 212 (55), 213 (55), 220 (55), *231,* 329 (46), *347*

Datta, B., 151 (119a), *177*

Datta, R. K., 151 (119a), *177*

Daune, M., 157 (152), *177*

Dave, C. J., 50 (38), *76*

Davern, C. I., 117 (186), 151 (186), *178*

David, M., 73 (39), *76*

Davidson, E. H., 191 (82), 193 (45), 194 (45), 210 (45), *230, 231,* 271 (13), *272*

Davidson, J. N., 120 (411, 412), *184*

Davidson, N., 135 (213, 339), *179, 182*

Davies, D. L., 539 (76a), 548 (76a, 95), 549 (76a, 95), *567*

Davies, J., 371 (17), *373*

Davis, B. D., 404 (120), 439 (120), 443 (120), *471*

Davis, B. K., 190 (84), *231*

Davis, H. J., 441, 467, *469*

Davis, J. M. G., 50 (40), *76*

Davis, J. R., 35 (30), *36,* 329 (48), *347*

Davis, R. H., 333 (67), *347*

Sneider, T. W. *(contd.)*
184
Snyder, L., 206 (307), *237*
Snyder, S. P., 408 (124, 560), 409 (314), 423 (124, 560), *471, 476, 482*
Soave, C., 135 (112), *176*
Sobel, H. J., 67 (175), 74 (175), *79*
Sober, H. A., 331 (153), 332 (153), *349*
Soeiro, R., 55 (201), 64 (200), 79, 200 (308, 349), 203 (308), 217 (349), 222 (363), *237, 238*
Söll, D., 256 (160), *276*, 356 (58), 359, *374*
Sofer, W. H., 329 (277), *353*
Soffer, R. L., 362 (95), 363 (57, 93, 94), *374, 375*
Sohby, C. M., 370 (74), *374*
Sohier, R., 439 (561), *482*
Sokal, J. E., 99 (10), *105*
Soling, H. D., 528 (37), *534*
Solnik, C., 563 (44), *565*
Soloff, B. L., 72 (23), *75*
Solomon, J. J., 419 (449), 423 (449), *480*
Somaki, I., 558 (58), *566*
Somers, C. E., 19 (68), *37*
Somers, K. D., 425 (385), 433 (385, 562), 460 (334), *476, 478, 482*
Sonneborn, T. M., 199 (309), *237*
Sonnenberg, B. P., 328 (252a), *352*
Soriano, R. Z., 50 (105), 51 (105), *77*
Sorm, F., 282 (97), 283 (96), *307*
Sorof, S., 328 (19), 330 (19, 20), 340 (19, 20, 253, 254), *346, 352*
Sorokin, C., 468 (441), *479*
Southern, E. M., 135 (419), *184*
Sovová, V., 429 (579), *483*
Spadoni, M. A., 190 (87), 199 (87), *231*
Spahn, G. J., 561 (78, 79), 563 (78, 79), *566*
Spahr, P.-F., 188 (3), 191 (3), 194 (3, 157), 198 (3, 157), *229, 233*
Spante, T. F., 539 (76A), 548 (76A), 549 (76A), *566*
Spatz, M., 385 (121), *401*
Spear, P. G., 446 (351), 447 (500, 563), 448 (500), *477, 481, 482*
Spelsberg, T. C., 134 (193), *178*, 191 (310), 194 (310), *237*, 317 (284), 329 (258), 331 (258), 334 (61, 257), 335 (61, 257), 336 (255, 256), 338 (186, 257, 262), *347, 350, 352, 353*
Spelsberg, W. T., 338 (185A), *350*
Spencer, J. H., 151 (420), *184*, 211 (75), *231*
Speyer, J. F., 394 (122), *401*
Spiegelman, S., 195 (134, 135, 160), 198 (114), 199 (134, 135, 160, 311), 208 (114), 211 (284), 212 (17a, b, c, 120a,

137a, 159a, 283a, 311a, b), *230, 232, 233, 236, 237*, 250 (62, 77), *273, 274*, 413 (565, 566), 414 (221, 547, 566, 567), 415 (306), 425 (19), 441 (18), 464 (18, 20, 261, 262, 347, 546, 548, 564), 465 (44), *469, 474, 475, 476, 477, 482, 483*
Spielvogel, R. L., 151 (458), *185*
Spira, G., 459 (379), *478*
Spirin, A. S., 199 (312–314), 217 (312–314), *237*
Spiro, D., 127 (485), *185*
Spizizen, J., 30 (148), *39*
Spohn, W., 224 (304a, b), *237*, 243 (149), 249 (149), *275*
Sporn, M. B., 152 (123), *177, 184*, 201 (206), *235*, 340 (73), *347*
Sprent, J., 553 (11), 554 (11, 17), *564*
Sprunt, K., 30 (149), *39*
Srinivasan, D., 369 (96), *375*
Srinivasan, P. R., 151 (44, 422), 152 (44), 158 (189), *175, 178, 184*, 201 (315), *237*, 453 (526), *482*, 369 (4, 96), *373, 375, 521*
Srivastava, S. K., 507 (48), 508 (29, 48), *521*
Staehelin, M., 243 (56), 251 (56), 257 (56), *273*, 367 (97), *375*
Staehelin, T., 201 (100), 220 (100), *232*
Stahl, F. W., 32 (110), *38*, 109 (314), 110 (314), *181*
Stanislawski-Berencwajg, M., 395 (123), *401*
Stanley, E. R., 559 (68), *566*
Stanley, T. B., 418 (434), 419 (434), *479*
Stanley, W. M., Jr., 199 (274), *236*, 359 (12), *373*
Stanton, M. F., 40 (159), *472*
Stanton, R. H., 149 (341), *182*
Starbuck, W. C., 218 (60), *231*, 311 (182), 313 (183, 271, 295), 316 (182), 317 (183), 318 (183, 295), 321 (182), 325 (182), 329 (47, 50), 338 (183), *347, 350, 353*
Starr, J. L., 219 (362), *238*
Stavenezer, J., 543 (103), *567*
Steck, T. L., 410 (24), 412 (24), *469*
Stedman, E., 31 (105), *38*, 310 (259), 311 (259), *352*
Steele, W. J., 55 (77), 57 (77, 176), 65 (161a, 173a), 76, 78, 79, 189 (316), 196 (316, 317), 198 (316, 317), 208 (316, 317), 216 (316), 228 (317), *237*, 247 (109), *274*, 317 (51), 329 (51), 330 (260, 261), 339 (260), 345 (249), *347, 352*
Steggles, A. W., 191 (310), 194 (310), *237*,

Subject Index

A